Walter, Hamilton and Israel's
Principles of Pathology for Dental Students

For Churchill Livingstone

Publisher: Simon Fathers
Editorial Co-ordination: Editorial Resources Unit
Copy Editor: Alison Whitehouse
Indexer: Nina Boyd
Production Controller: Neil Dickson
Design: Design Resources Unit
Sales Promotion Executive: Duncan Jones

Walter, Hamilton and Israel's Principles of Pathology for Dental Students

J. B. Walter TD MD MRCP FRCPath
Departments of Pathology and Medicine, University of Toronto;
Department of Pathology, General Division of the Toronto Hospital;
Department of Medicine (Dermatology),
St. Michael's Hospital, Toronto, Canada

Margaret C. Grundy FDSRCS(Eng) DDS(Birm)
Formerly Department of Children's Dentistry and
Orthodontics, University of Birmingham, UK

FIFTH EDITION

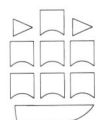

CHURCHILL LIVINGSTONE
EDINBURGH LONDON MADRID MELBOURNE NEW YORK AND TOKYO 1993

CHURCHILL LIVINGSTONE
Medical Division of Longman Group UK Limited

Distributed in the United States of America by Churchill
Livingstone Inc., 650 Avenue of the Americas, New York,
N.Y. 10011, and by associated companies, branches and
representatives throughout the world.

First edition 1967
Second edition 1971
Third edition 1974
Fourth edition 1981
Fifth edition 1992

ISBN 0 443 04124 5

British Library Cataloguing in Publication Data
A catalogue record for this book is available from the British
Library.

Library of Congress Cataloging in Publication Data

Walter, J. B. (John Brian)
    Principles of pathology for dental students/J. B. Walter and
Margaret C. Grundy. --5th ed.
        p. cm.
    Includes index.
    ISBN 0-443-04124-5
    1. Pathology. 2. Dental students. I. Grundy, Margaret C.
II. Title.
    [DNLM: 1. Pathology. QZ 4 W232p]
RB111.W16 1992
616.07'0246176--dc20
DNLM/DLC   91–34011
for Library of Congress   CIP

Produced by Longman Singapore Publishers (Pte) Ltd
Printed in Singapore

Preface

The student embarking on a career in dentistry must achieve, within a period of five years, sufficient skill to recognize, diagnose correctly and treat the diseases occurring in the oral cavity. In addition to becoming adept in many complicated practical procedures, the student must also have acquired much theoretical knowledge. This knowledge should be based on sound general principles, and Part 1 of this book is intended to cover the principles of general pathology in a manner suited to the particular needs of the dentist.

The dental surgeon treats not only diseases of the oral cavity but also people—each patient is an individual with problems that may not be confined to the mouth, but which may modify the treatment or necessitate taking special precautions. The treatment of a patient with heart disease is one example, and more recently problems have arisen related to prevention of the spread of the human immunodeficiency and hepatitis viruses. Although the dentist need not be medically qualified, the practitioner should be sufficiently well informed to appreciate the patient's general condition, so as to allow an effective co-operation with medical colleagues.

Part 2 of this book is designed to cover the basic principles of pathology pertaining to some of the special systems. Of necessity, this coverage is brief, but is intended to be adequate, so that when time and opportunity arise, the dentist will be able to consult specialized texts without the feeling of venturing into unknown lands. When the student encounters pathology for the first time, many new words and concepts are met; these we have endeavoured to define when they are first introduced, so that learning may proceed by a series of graded steps. We have appended a list of general references to each chapter in the hope of fostering enquiry in our students. Further reading and a critical approach to published material must continue during the whole of one's professional life.

Eleven years have elapsed since the fourth edition was published and many advances have been made. Electron microscopy is routinely used in the examination of many tissues, particularly tumours. Immunofluorescent and immunoperoxidase techniques have added a wealth of information relating to tumour types, particularly the lymphomata, and have contributed to our understanding of the immune response. Gene cloning and the use of DNA probes have added their quota to the general advances in our understanding of the chemical bases of disease, particularly as related to inherited disease, immunology and carcinogenesis. The study of oncogenes, their products and growth factors is at last drawing together the phenomena of healing and tumour formation. Each of the organ systems has been reviewed and some important topics either covered more adequately or introduced for the first time. These include the lipoproteins and their relationship to atherosclerosis, the acute phase response, interstitial pneumonia, the acute respiratory distress syndrome, the pathogenesis of pulmonary emphysema, tubulointerstitial disease of the kidneys, acute tubular necrosis, recently recognized infections including *Legionella pneumonia*, Lyme disease and acquired immunological deficiency, important mechanisms involved in diarrhoea, brain herniations and finally the dysplastic naevus syndrome. In summary, many changes have been made and we hope the book will serve its functions the better for them. An important change is the introduction of colour photographs—in all over 100 are included.

The previous editions were written in collaboration with Dr Martin Israel and we regret his departure. The effects of his pen will still be apparent in this edition, but his other publications and interest in counselling have left him bereft of time. With the modification of authorship, we have taken the opportunity to change Dr Hamilton to Dr Grundy, the married name by which she has been known for many years.

Toronto
Poole, 1992

J.B.W.
M.C.G.

Acknowledgements

We wish to thank The W B Saunders Company of Philadelphia for allowing us to use illustrations from Walter J B 1992 *An Introduction to the Principles of Disease*, 3rd ed. Likewise we are indebted to Lea and Febiger of Philadelphia for generously allowing us illustrations from their book Walter J B 1989 *Pathology of Human Disease*. We wish also to thank Wolfe Medical Publications Ltd for allowing us to use illustrations from Rock W P, Grundy M C and Shaw L 1988 *Diagnostic Picture Tests in Paediatric Dentistry*. The source of the material taken from these books is acknowledged under each caption. Likewise colleagues who have provided material are also acknowledged in a similar manner. Where material is used that has been published previously in journals or other books the source is similarly acknowledged.

Many figures in this book have previously been published in the sixth edition of Walter J B and Israel M S *General Pathology*, Churchill Livingstone, Edinburgh. These are not individually acknowledged. However, some of the gross specimens taken from this source are from the Wellcome Museum of Pathology, and we are grateful to the President and the Council of the Royal College of Surgeons of England for permission to publish them. In accordance with their wishes each is acknowledged at the end of each caption, and their catalogue number is indicated. A number of specimens illustrated are from the Boyd Museum of the University of Toronto, and we thank Dr M D Silver, Professor and Chairman of the Department of Pathology for permission to use these.

It is a pleasure to express our gratitude for artwork to Margot Mackay, University of Toronto, Faculty of Medicine, Department of Surgery, Division of Biomedical Communications, Toronto and to the Department of Clinical Illustrations, Birmingham Dental School. As in previous editions of this book, our thanks are due to Mrs Sonja Duda, librarian of the Banting Institute, Toronto, for valuable help in obtaining references.

J.B.W.
M.C.G.

Contents

PART 1

General pathology

1. Introduction

In the practice of medicine it is soon apparent that the majority of patients who seek help do so because of some abnormality which is causing them distress. Such *symptoms* can be dispelled by simple remedies—quite often by time and reassurance. Much of medicine is an art which its practitioners, whether doctors, dentists, nurses, or physiotherapists must learn. Nevertheless, there have always been individuals who were not content simply to observe disease and the effects of empirical time-honoured remedies upon it. They have attempted to describe and record the abnormalities in their patients in an objective manner; by introducing measurements they initiated the science which is called pathology.

Disease itself is as difficult to define as is the normal, from which it is a departure. As generally used, the term disease is employed to describe a state in which there is a sufficient departure from the normal for signs or symptoms to be produced. The variations from the normal are called *lesions*, and although generally structural in nature, the term may also be used to describe functional abnormalities, for example *biochemical lesions* (p. 40). The cause of the disease is called its *aetiology* and the development of the lesions its *pathogenesis*. Although aetiology and pathogenesis are generally described as separate entities, in practice it is often difficult to distinguish between them. Indeed, the aetiology of one era may become part of the pathogenesis of the next. An example will suffice. A patient takes a large dose of strychnine, develops convulsions, and dies. Clearly the aetiology of the disease is administration of strychnine. However, a closer consideration may reveal that the drug was self-administered during a phase of depression. The suicidal administration of strychnine would then be part of the pathogenesis of the fatal disease depression.

Although this instance may appear to be an exaggeration of the difficulty in delineating the cause of a disease, many other examples will be encountered. The great advances in bacteriology which started at the end of the nineteenth century fostered the concept that each disease had a single cause. To state that a boil is always caused by the *Staphylococcus aureus* is true, but nevertheless this is an incomplete statement. It is known that patients with diabetes mellitus are prone to develop recurrent boils. Which is the cause of the boils, the staphylococcus or the diabetes? Present doctrine would still favour the organism, but the diabetes would be labelled a major predisposing factor. Multiple causes are probably much more common than we think. The doctrine of one cause for one disease has certainly failed to be a profitable concept in the search for the aetiology of many common diseases such as cancer, arteriosclerosis, emphysema, chronic bronchitis, and dental caries.

An attempt to avoid the difficulty in defining disease has been the introduction of the term *syndrome*. This is a condition in which there occurs a defined collection of lesions, signs, or symptoms which are not necessarily always caused by the same agent. Thus Mikulicz's syndrome is defined as bilateral painless enlargement of the lacrimal and salivary glands from whatever cause. It may be found in leukaemia, but frequently the cause is unknown and it is then said to be *idiopathic*. Clearly the diseases in which the cause is not known are difficult to distinguish from syndromes. Indeed, the two terms are frequently used quite indiscriminately and interchangeably.

Pathology is the study of disease. It describes the cause, course and termination of disease. In almost all diseases the lesions are morphological or chemical, and their study is closely linked to the techniques available. Modern methods of chemical analysis have enormously added to our appreciation of the metabolic aspects of medicine. *Radiography and other imaging techniques* have enabled the physician to see images of the internal organs of living patients in much the same way that their ancestors acquired knowledge at the traditional necropsy. Thus *computed tomography* (CT) scan or CAT scan (computerized axial tomography) reveals a two-dimensional 'slice' through the patient and is of great value in detecting lesions that would remain undetected by conventional radiography. The CT scan involves exposing the patient to ionizing radiation and in order to avoid this other techniques have been developed. *Magnetic resonance imaging* is a recent innovation that involves placing the patient in a powerful magnetic field so that the hydrogen molecules of the body line up and emit a small electric current that can be analysed and displayed on the monitor. *Ultra-sound imaging* is another non-invasive technique, and has the advantage of being relatively inexpensive. It works on a principle also used in sonar and radar. The method is safe and used routinely to investigate the fetus in utero.

Pathology still relies heavily on microscopy of tissue sections. The traditional paraffin wax method and staining by haematoxylin and eosin are the mainstay of routine histopathology. Special staining is used to identify particular components. Thus the periodic acid staining (PAS) identifies glycoproteins and is useful to demonstrate basement membranes and fungi (Fig. 1.1). More recently monoclonal antibodies have been prepared against numerous tissue components. If labelled with a flurochrome such as fluorescin, the site of attachment of the antibody to the antigen in the tissue can be seen by examining the section under ultraviolet light (see Figs. 37.18 & 37.19). Alternatively the antigen may be tagged with horseradish peroxidase and subsequently visualized by addition of a suitable substrate for the enzyme. Slides prepared by this *immunoperoxidase technique* are examined by ordinary light microscopy (Fig. 1.2).

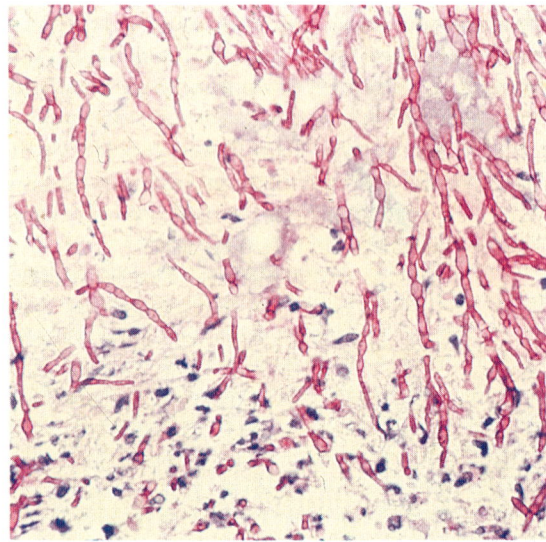

Fig. 1.1 *Candida* organisms in the base of an oral ulcer. The section has been stained by the periodic acid–Schiff (PAS) method and shows the organisms stained red. Occasional budding yeasts are present but the majority of the fungi are in the form of elongated pseudohyphae.

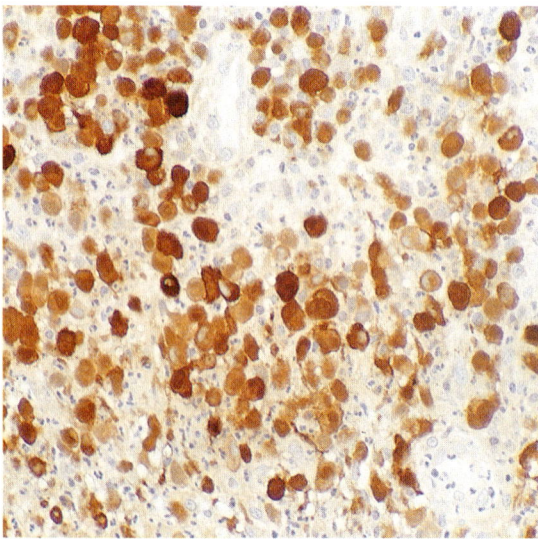

Fig. 1.2 Immunoperoxidase method. This section of skin in histiocytosis X has been stained to show the presence of S 100 protein. The large cells stained brown are malignant Langerhans' cells.

The frozen section technique, involving cutting sections embedded in ice, has been used for many years to obtain a rapid diagnosis of material removed at surgery. Thus a suspicious tumour can be identified and the correct procedure undertaken while the patient is still under the anaesthetic. The technique is also employed for some immunoperoxidase stains and for enzyme identification.

Electron microscopy with its tremendous magnification is now used routinely for showing cell details, and is particularly useful for tumour identification. It is also invaluable for virus identification and in research.

Flow cytometry is a new technique for examining cells that can be obtained in suspension —for instance blood cells and some tumour cells. The cells are marked by suitable probes and the suspension analysed automatically. The method is useful for the identification of the clonality of leukaemic and tumour cells.

GENERAL READING

Doane D W, Anderson N 1987 Electron microscopy in diagnostic virology. Cambridge University Press, Cambridge

Falini B, Taylor C R 1983 New developments in immunoperoxidase techniques and their application. Archives of Pathology and Laboratory Medicine 107:105

Mesa-Tejada R, Pascal R A, Fenoglio C M 1977 Immunoperoxidase: a sensitive immunohistological technique as a 'special stain' in the diagnostic pathology laboratory. Human Pathology 8:313

Weakley B S 1981 A beginner's handbook in biological transmission electron microscopy, 2nd edn. Churchill Livingstone, Edinburgh

2. Normal structure

The body is composed of innumerable cells which are bound together by a variable amount of intercellular material. Each cell is enclosed by an outer limiting membrane, the *cell* or *plasma membrane*, and contains a nucleus which is bounded by the *nuclear membrane.*

Development from the fertilized ovum is accomplished by two processes:

1 *Division*, whereby more cells are produced and

2 *Maturation*, or *differentiation*, whereby cells develop specific structures which enable them to perform specialized functions, e.g. contraction in the case of muscle fibres. Some highly specialized cells, e.g. neurons, lose their ability to divide as they become differentiated, but others do not, e.g. liver cells. What is lost during the process of maturation is the ability to differentiate along other lines. While the fertilized ovum is *totipotent*, i.e. capable of producing all the tissues of the body, its cellular progeny are not all alike and do not have this ability. Both cytoplasmic and nuclear factors are probably involved in differentiation, but the nature of this process, which may be regarded as a type of ageing, is not understood.

Early evidence of differentiation within the mass of cells composing the developing embryo is the formation of three distinct germ-layers. An outer layer of cells forms the *ectoderm*, while a tube develops within the mass and the cells lining it form the *endoderm*. This tube forms the basis of the future alimentary canal and the organs that bud from it—lungs, liver, pancreas, and others. The *mesoderm* consists of cells lying between the ectoderm and the endoderm. The primitive cells of each germ-layer can differentiate along two separate lines to form either epithelium or connective tissue. These are described later (see p. 22). It is evident that the cells of the body show a considerable diversity of structure and function, yet each is in fact remarkably independent. Each receives a supply of oxygen and foodstuff from the blood stream with which it must produce its own structural components and secretion, and from which it must release the energy required for mechanical, chemical, or electrical work. It is therefore not surprising that all cells are built upon a similar basic plan.

The number of chemical reactions known to occur inside the cell is so great that it would be difficult to understand how these could proceed in a structure as simple as the cell appears to be under the light microscope. The electron microscope has changed all this—from a barren wilderness, the internal structure of the cell is now seen to resemble a large industrial city with its factories, warehouses, streets, power-stations, etc. (Fig. 2.1).

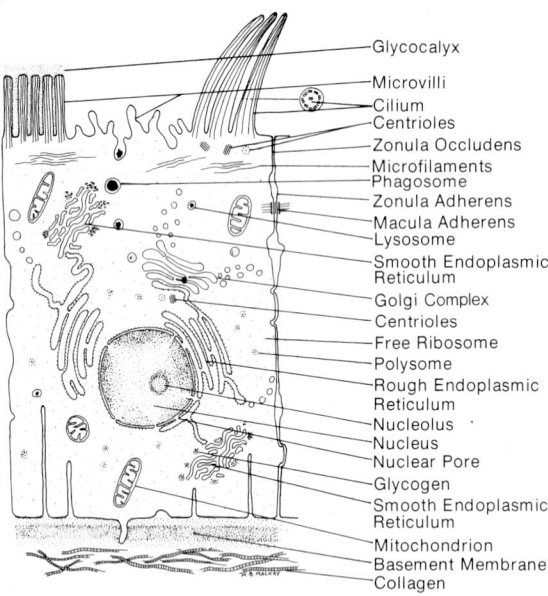

- Glycocalyx
- Microvilli
- Cilium
- Centrioles
- Zonula Occludens
- Microfilaments
- Phagosome
- Zonula Adherens
- Macula Adherens
- Lysosome
- Smooth Endoplasmic Reticulum
- Golgi Complex
- Centrioles
- Free Ribosome
- Polysome
- Rough Endoplasmic Reticulum
- Nucleolus
- Nucleus
- Nuclear Pore
- Glycogen
- Smooth Endoplasmic Reticulum
- Mitochondrion
- Basement Membrane
- Collagen

Fig. 2.1 Diagrammatic representation of a hypothetical typical epithelial cell. The free surface of the cell has projecting microvilli, which on the left are arranged regularly to form a brush border. In the centre the villi are irregular, and micropinocytotic-vacuole formation is depicted. On the right cilia are shown. The cell adjoins its neighbours with some interdigitation of their plasma membranes; one junctional complex is shown. The nucleus contains one nucleolus, and is surrounded by a double-layered membrane. Between the nucleus and the free border is the cell centre, or centrosome, and adjacent to this is one Golgi complex. There are two centrioles lying at right angles to each other. The base of the cell rests on a basement membrane, and adjacent to this collagen fibres are shown. The plasma membrane, like the other membranes of the cell, has a trilaminar structure. Ribosomes are scattered free in the cell cytoplasm, and are also attached to the rough endoplasmic reticulum and the outer nuclear envelope. (Drawn by Margot Mackay, University of Toronto.)

THE CELLS

Each cell possesses an outer limiting membrane (the cell or plasma membrane) and within its protoplasm there is another limiting membrane which encloses the nuclear material. Most cells possess a single nucleus which is centrally placed; the basal nuclei of some columnar epithelial cells and the eccentric nuclei of plasma cells are obvious exceptions to this role. Cells with more than one nucleus are called *giant*, or *multinucleate cells*. The osteoclast is an example of such a cell normally found in the body. Giant cells that are formed under pathological conditions are described later.

THE CELL MEMBRANE

The cell membrane is an extremely important structure, since it forms the interface between the cell cytoplasm and the interstitial tissue fluids, or in the lower forms of life, the exterior. Its functions may be listed as movement, cell recognition, adhesion, control of cell growth, and transfer function.

Cell movement

Examination of living cells reveals that the plasma membrane is not a rigid structure, but is in constant motion. This motility is particularly well developed in certain cells and permits them to move bodily through the tissues. The white blood cells—polymorphonuclear leucocytes, lymphocytes, and monocytes—behave in this way. The undulating surface of the macrophage is particularly characteristic. Folds of the membrane have been observed to entrap a droplet of fluid by a process known as *pinocytosis*.

Apart from locomotion, the surface movement of monocytes and polymorphonuclear leucocytes produces another effect. By pushing out projections, or *pseudopodia*, around particles, they are able to surround and finally engulf them. This process of ingestion is called *phagocytosis*.

Cell recognition

The membranes of the cell, including the plasma membrane, are associated with the antigens by which the body is able to recognize its own cells and tolerate them. Cells from another individual are regarded as aliens, and are attacked by the immune response which they provoke.

Receptor function. Many agents act on cells at specific points, or *cell receptors*. Thus influenza viruses attach themselves to specific receptors on the red-cell envelope (p. 191). Likewise drugs and hormones act on their own receptors. The presence of these specific receptors on particular cells is indeed the explanation of how hormones act only on their target cells and not on other cells. The mechanism of action of many non-steroid hormones is of great interest. The attachment of the hormone to its receptor activates the enzyme adenylate cyclase, which is situated in the cell membrane. This enzymatic activation causes ATP, which is present in abundance on the inner side of the cell membrane, to be converted into adenosine 3',5'-cyclic phosphate—a nucleotide known more widely as *cyclic AMP* or simply cAMP. This important compound has many actions. Thus, in a liver cell acted upon by adrenaline, the formation of cAMP leads to the activation of a phosphorylase that converts glycogen to glucose: this is then released from the cell. In other instances cAMP acts on the nucleus and stimulates the expression of some particular genetic information (Fig. 2.2). In this way cAMP acts as a *second messenger* for the action of glucagon, thyrotrophic hormone, ACTH, and other hormones. Some cell membrane receptors are coupled to systems other than one involving cyclic AMP; their activation may involve regulation of Ca^{2+} flux. With steroid hormone the specific cell receptors are in the cytoplasm.

Cell adhesiveness

The cell membrane is concerned with adhesiveness, which is a factor that induces cells of like constitution to stick together. If the cells of an embryo are separated from each other and are then allowed to come together again, they aggregate to form organs and tissues. This affinity which cells have for their own kind must be an important mechanism in the development and maintenance of the architecture of multicellular animals. But not all cells behave in this manner. The cells of the blood do not exhibit adhesiveness, nor to some extent do cancer cells, for they are able to infiltrate freely into the surrounding tissues.

Cell growth

The mitotic activity in epidermis is greatly increased in an area of skin adjacent to a wound. The increased production of cells continues until epidermal cells from one side of the wound meet those migrating from the other side. Contact of like cells with like then inhibits cell division; the phenomenon is called *contact inhibition* (p. 98). It appears to be a function of the cell membrane. Malignant transformation, infection of a cell by a virus, and treatment with proteolytic enzymes all appear to alter the cell membrane and release cells from this inhibition.

Transfer function

All substances which enter or leave the cell protoplasm must cross the cell membrane, and the properties of this membrane are responsible for the peculiar chemical composition of the cytoplasm.

Chemicals soluble in organic solvents enter cells much more readily than do those which are water soluble. The absorption of some substances is related to enzymatic activity occurring at or near the cell surface. How chemicals cross the membrane and the factors which regulate their passage can be understood only in relationship to

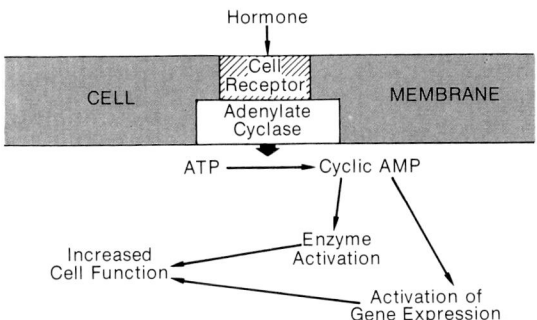

Fig. 2.2 The second-messenger concept. Many hormones act first by becoming attached to specific receptor sites on the membranes of target cells. Thus, adrenal cells have receptors that 'recognize' adrenocorticotrophin. The enzyme adenylate cyclase is activated in the cell membrane and passes into the cytoplasm where it catalyses the formation of cyclic AMP, which acts as a second messenger. It may therefore be regarded as a type of chemical switch that turns on the cell to perform specific functions.

the structure of the membrane itself, for as in other realms of pathology, structure and function are interdependent.

Membrane structure in relation to function

Electron microscopy has shown an intact membrane some 7.5 nm* in width which, in suitably prepared material, can at high magnification be resolved into two electron-dense laminae with an intervening clear space. This trilaminar structure, as first described by Robertson, is known as a *unit membrane,* and it appears to have no pores such as have been postulated to explain the observed permeability of the cell membrane.

Substances are transported across the cell membrane either by bulk transfer or by diffusion. *Bulk transfer* involves the processes of phagocytosis, pinocytosis (previously described) and micropinocytosis. In *micropinocytosis* small invaginations of the cell membrane (Fig. 2.1), the *caveolae intracellulares,* become nipped off to form vesicles; in this way small quantities of fluid or particulate matter may be imbibed by a process that resembles pinocytosis but on a small scale. Indeed, the processes of phagocytosis, pinocytosis and micropinocytosis are commonly grouped together as *endocytosis,* in contrast to *exocytosis,* in which the contents of membrane-bound vacuoles (e.g. secretions) are liberated at the cell surface by fusion of the cell membrane with the vacuolar membrane. The contents of the endocytotic vacuoles are still membrane bound and not in the cytoplasmic ground substance proper. The fusion of an endocytotic vacuole with a primary lysosome containing lytic enzymes results in the formation of a *secondary lysosome, phagosome,* or *heterophagosome,* and by the digestion of its contents may result in their being released by diffusion into the substance of the cell.

The formation of micropinocytotic vesicles on one side of a cell and their discharge from another surface by exocytosis, is one postulated mechanism whereby substances may cross a cellular barrier, e.g. blood-vessel endothelium. The process is known as *cytopempsis.*

*1 mm = 1000 μm. 1 μm = 1000 nm. The Ångström unit (Å) is a tenth of 1 nm, and is no longer used in measurement.

The *passive diffusion* of small ions across the cell membrane and the sodium pump are described on page 12.

In active transport there is the passage of chemicals across the cell membrane against a physico-chemical gradient, and the mechanism requires the expenditure of energy (Fig. 2.3). Amino-acid transport is a good example, and is of great importance in the intestine and the renal tubules. Thus there is a failure to reabsorb cystine, lysine, ornithine, and arginine in the kidney in the classical type of *cystinuria.*

The current concept of the cell membrane is that it is composed of two layers of structurally asymmetrical lipid molecules with their hydrophilic polar heads turned outwards (Fig. 2.4). Globular proteins form an integral part of the membrane and are bonded by hydrophobic inter-

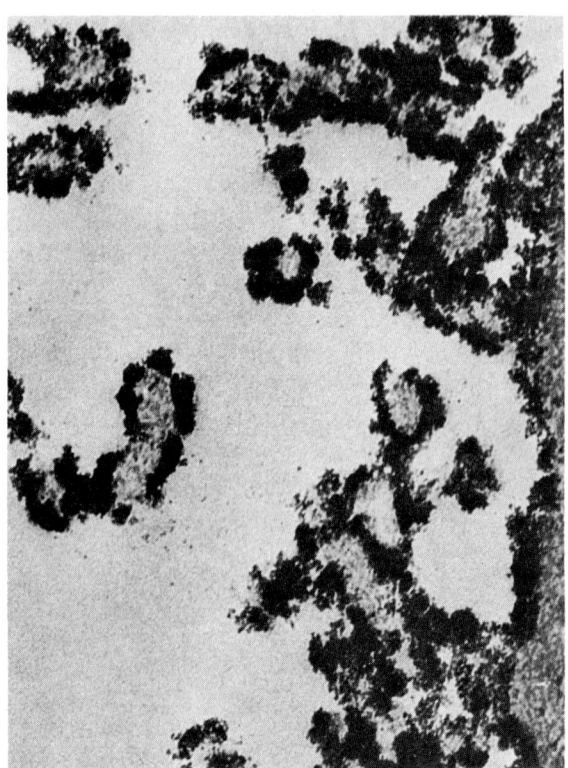

Fig. 2.3 Detail of the plasma membrane of a HeLa cell with much surface activity in the form of profuse filamentous microvilli. After staining for enzymes splitting adenosine triphosphate, dense reaction-product had been deposited with close precision at the cell membrane, indicating that the enzymes are localised there, presumably for the supply of energy requirements. × 55 000. (Electron micrograph by courtesy of Professor M A Epstein and Dr S J Holt.)

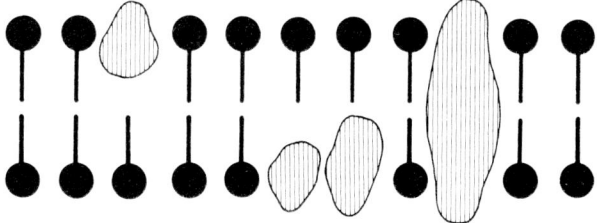

Fig. 2.4 Diagrammatic representation of the plasma membrane. The membrane is shown as a double layer of phospholipid molecules with their hydrophilic (water-loving) ends pointing outwards and their hydrophobic (water-hating) ends facing inwards. Globular proteins are partially or completely embedded in the lipid. This concept of a fluid lipid bilayer with embedded protein was described by Singer and Nicolson (*Science*, 1972, *175*:720) It is believed that the carbohydrate side-chains of the protein molecules form the glycocalyx, which is illustrated in Fig. 2.5.(Drawn by Margot Mackay, University of Toronto.)

action with lipid. These proteins are thus floating in a sea of lipid, thereby forming a fluid mosaic. The proteins can move laterally, and while some are exposed only on one side of the membrane, others traverse it completely.

The proteins of the cell membrane are heterogeneous—some act as antigens, while others are specific receptors for hormones, lectins, viruses, etc. Others have transport or enzymatic functions (Fig. 2.3).The cell receptors are probably linked to the microtubules and microfilaments of the underlying cytoplasm. The microtubules connecting one receptor with the next could be regarded as forming a cytoskeleton anchoring respective receptors. The microfilaments, on the other hand, could act as contractile elements, so that the receptors could move within the cell membrane. That such movement can occur is well known, for the attachment of an antibody to its specific receptor in the cell membrane can result in movement of the complexes to form groups, or caps, which subsequently enter the cell by endocytosis. In this way receptors can be removed from the cell surface and the corresponding antigen can enter the cell.

In summary, the structure of the plasma membrane is very complex and contains lipid and protein. It can consume energy and change its shape in response to stimuli. Its protein molecules are heterogeneous, some being responsible for the receptor sites, others for antigenicity, enzyme activity, etc.

RELATIONSHIP OF CELLS TO EACH OTHER

Epithelial cells are generally closely applied to each other, but even then there is an electron-lucent area of 15–20 nm between their adjacent cell membranes. This is probably due to a covering of mucopolysaccharide. The free surface of epithelial cells is also covered by an additional coat, the *glycocalyx*, which on high resolution electron microscopy can be seen to be filamentous (Fig. 2.5).

Cell junctions

Adjacent cells exhibit specialized junctional areas that subserve two functions:

1. They enable cells to adhere to their neighbours, and can be adapted to form a seal to prevent substances passing between them. This is particularly important in the intestinal epithelium (Fig. 2.5) and in the endothelial lining of blood vessels.

2. They form areas of close contact through which cells can *communicate* with each other. Most cells do not live in isolation; they cooperate, and coordinate their activities with those of their neighbours. How this is brought about is poorly understood, but the phenomena of peristalsis, contact inhibition (p. 98), and tissue induction may well be regulated by mechanisms that involve cell junctions.

One might speculate that these structures are also important in the organized processes of embryogenesis, repair, and regeneration, as well as in the disorganized proliferation of neoplasia.

THE CYTOPLASM

Chemical composition

The cytoplasm is that part of the protoplasm not included in the nucleus, and is composed largely of water. There is also about 8% of protein. The contents differ from the extracellular fluid in several important respects. There is a high concentration of potassium, magnesium, and phosphate which contrasts with the sodium, chloride, and bicarbonate found in the extracellular fluids. The osmotic pressure within the cells (exerted principally by protein, potassium, magnesium, and phosphate) is equal to that of the extra-

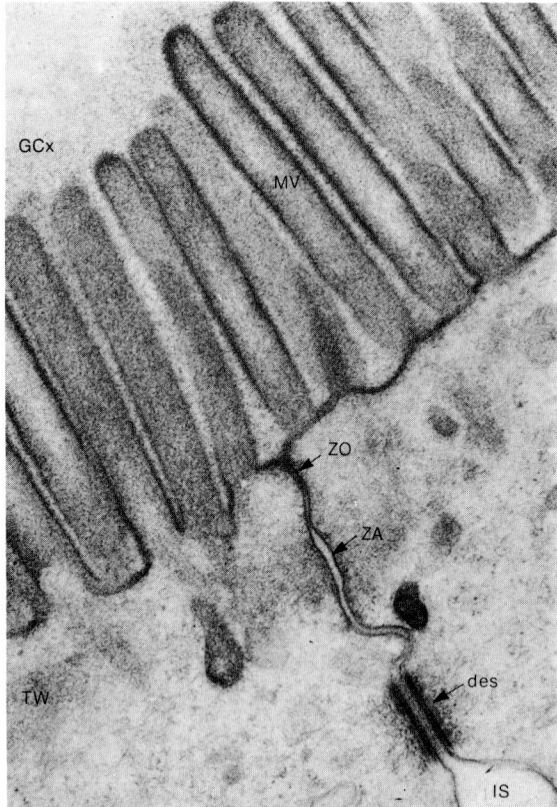

Fig. 2.5 Details of the luminal surface of an absorptive cell of the human small intestine. The apical cell membrane is thrown into regular microvilli (MV). There is a fuzzy covering, which is termed a *glycocalyx* (GCx). One junctional complex is shown. It consists of three parts: (1) The tight junction, or *zonula occludens* (ZO), which is an area where the plasma membranes of the two adjacent cells appear to fuse. 'Zonule' means an encircled band or girdle; the zone forms an effective seal between adjacent cells. It is an area where one cell can communicate with adjacent ones. (2) The *zonula adherens* (ZA), which is an area where the cell membranes are closely applied to each other but are not fused. Filaments of the terminal web are concentrated at this area. (3) The desmosomes or maculae adherentes (des), which are complex structures and are button-shaped. Numerous microfilaments converge on the desmosomes. Where junctional complexes are not present there is often a space between adjacent cells (IS = intercellular space). (× 112 000). (Photograph by courtesy of Dr Y C Bedard, Mount Sinai Hospital, Toronto.)

cellular fluid (exerted by sodium, chloride, and bicarbonate).

Water and chloride diffuse readily across the cell membrane, but potassium and sodium do so comparatively slowly, potassium diffusing about one hundred times faster than sodium. Others, phosphate and protein, do not diffuse at all. The net negative charge of protein and phosphate within the cell is balanced by potassium. In a passive diffusion system the result would be a greater concentration of ions within the cell than outside it, and the cell would swell. However, there is a mechanism in the cell membrane which actively excludes sodium. This is the '*sodium pump*', which requires ATP for its operation. The ultimate source of energy is mitochondrial cell respiration; it follows that damage to these organelles is characterized by cell swelling. In severe illnesses, such as heart failure and hepatic failure, there is an increase in the cell-membrane permeability. Potassium leaves the cells and sodium enters them. This has been called the '*sick-cell syndrome*', and is evident biochemically as hyponatraemia.

Formed structures

Electron microscopy has revealed that the structure of the cytoplasm is very complex indeed. It is subdivided into many compartments by membranes which closely resemble the plasma membrane in structure. The most extensive subdivision is effected by the *endoplasmic reticulum*, but the cytoplasm also contains many membrane-bound structures, or *organelles*—mitochondria, lysosomes, etc.

Endoplasmic reticulum

The endoplasmic reticulum is divided into rough and smooth, depending on whether there are attached ribosomes.

Rough endoplasmic reticulum. This consists of a series of membranes which are formed into an intercommunicating series of tubes, vesicles, and cisterns (Figs 2.1 and 2.6). It is in these spaces that the secretion of some glands first appears. Situated on the outer surface of the endoplasmic reticulum there are granules, about 15 nm in diameter, which are rich in *ribonucleic acid (RNA)*. These are *ribosomes,* and they give the endoplasmic reticulum a rough appearance. Similar granules lie free in the cytoplasm and are not attached to the endoplasmic reticulum. The ribosomes play a very important part in cellular metabolism because it is in relation to them that *protein synthesis* occurs (p. 18). When the ribosomes are lying free the protein is for the cell's own internal requirements. Protein for export is synthetized in relation to the endoplasmic reticulum. Sometimes ribosomes are grouped together to form polysomes (Fig. 2.6).

The endoplasmic reticulum and its associated ribosomal granules cannot be distinguished in the 'paraffin' sections used in routine pathology. The RNA content, however, is distinguished by its red staining with pyronin and its blue staining (*basophilia*) with haematoxylin—the latter, being a basic substance, combines with acids, e.g. the nucleic acids. It follows that the cytoplasm of cells actively engaged in protein synthesis appears blue or mauve in haematoxylin and eosin stained (H. & E.) sections. Plasma cells are an excellent example of this, for immunoglobulin (a glycoprotein) is formed in the rough endoplasmic reticulum. Sometimes the accumulation of glycoprotein is so excessive that the cisterns of the rough endoplasmic reticulum become greatly dilated and contain masses that are visible in light microscopy, these are called *Russell bodies*. They take the appearance of refractile, eosinophilic, PAS-positive, spherical masses, either solitary or else forming grape-like structures in the cell cytoplasm (Fig. 2.7). They are particularly frequent in chronic inflammation of the oral tissues.

Smooth endoplasmic reticulum. In some cells the endoplasmic reticulum also forms a complex lattice of tubules which has no attached ribosomes and therefore appears *smooth*. The smooth and rough elements of the endoplasmic reticulum are continuous with each other, with the outer lamina of the nuclear membrane, and perhaps also with the plasma membrane. The smooth endoplasmic reticulum has been related to the following functions:

Drug metabolism. Following the administration of barbiturates and other toxins there is an

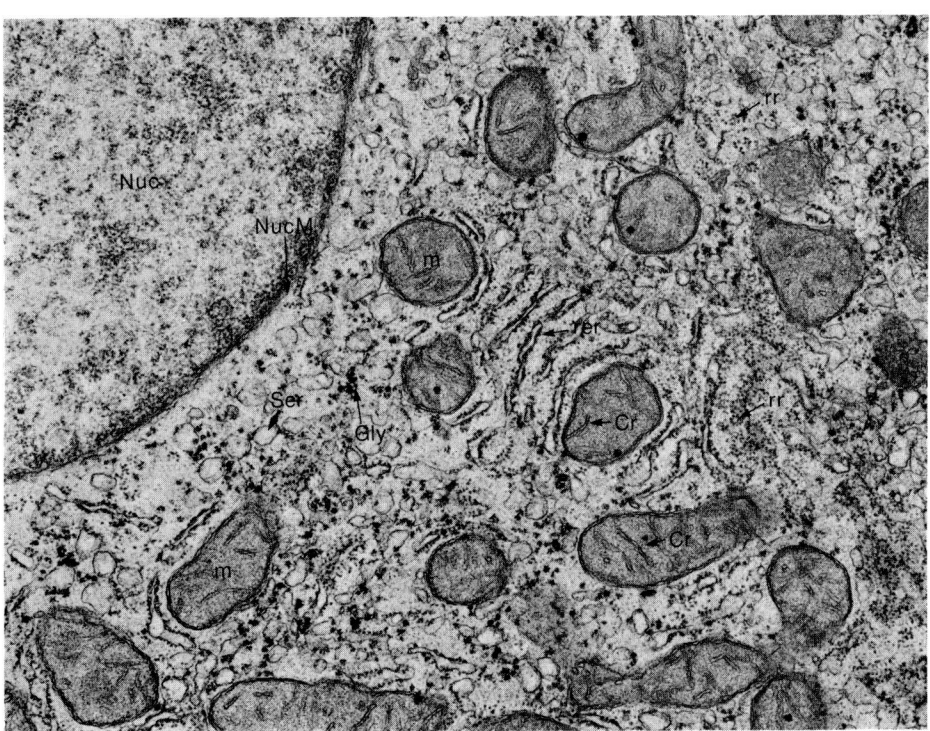

Fig. 2.6 Liver cell showing part of its nucleus (Nuc) and cytoplasmic organelles. Mitochondria (m) with their cristae (Cr) are shown along with rough endoplasmic reticulum (rer) to which are attached ribosomes (r). Smooth endoplasmic reticulum (Ser) is associated with glycogen granules (Gly). Some ribosomes appear free in the cytoplasm and are forming rosettes (rr). Note also the nuclear membrane (NucM) surrounding the nucleus (× 24 000). (Photograph by courtesy of Dr Y C Bedard, Mount Sinai Hospital, Toronto.)

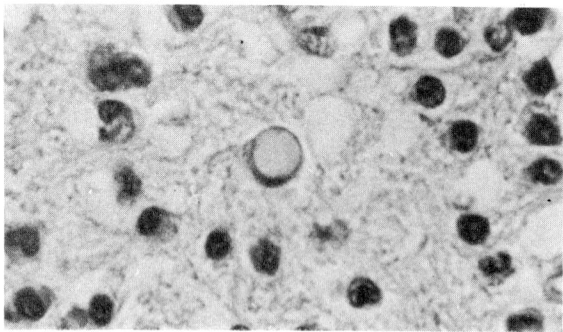

Fig. 2.7 Russell body. Chronic inflammatory granulation tissue showing one Russell body in the cytoplasm of a plasma cell. The nucleus of the cell is compressed to one side. × 600.

increase in the smooth endoplasmic reticulum of the liver cells. This appears to be an adaptive response to ensure detoxification

Steroid metabolism
Carbohydrate metabolism. In the liver glycogen synthesis occurs in close relationship to smooth endoplasmic reticulum (Fig. 2.6).

Muscle contraction. In striated muscle specialized smooth endoplasmic reticulum is important in the release and recapture of calcium ions during the contraction and relaxation of fibres.

Mitochondria

These rod-shaped bodies have a smooth outer limiting membrane and an inner electron-dense membrane which is folded into incomplete septa, or *cristae*, that subdivide the mitochondria into compartments (Fig. 2.6).

This complex structure of the mitochondria is a reflection of their function. They contain all the enzymes of the Krebs cycle and of the terminal electron transport system (cytochrome system). The *Krebs cycle* is a system whereby products of carbohydrate, fat, and protein metabolism are oxidized to produce energy (Fig. 2.8). The latter is stored in the form of the high energy bonds of adenosine triphosphate (ATP), and is utilized whenever the cell performs any kind of work. The mitochondria are the power-stations of the cell, and are among the first structures to be affected when adverse conditions prevail. Mitochondria are capable of enlargement, and

replicate by transverse division. Mitochondrial DNA may play a role in this process (see p. 17).

Golgi complex

The *Golgi complex*, or *apparatus*, consists of a series of flattened sacs and small vesicles (often arranged in curved stacks), much smaller than those of the endoplasmic reticulum. They are usually adjacent to the *centrosome*, a clear area near the centre of the cell, which contains one or more *centrioles*. The Golgi complex is best developed in glandular cells, and is usually situated close to the nucleus on the side nearest the lumen.

The main function of the Golgi complex is the modification and packaging of material synthetized in the rough endoplasmic reticulum. The material in the rough endoplasmic reticulum is pinched off in smooth covered vacuoles (*transport vesicles*) which pass to the forming face of the Golgi complex (this is generally the convex surface). The membrane of the vesicle fuses with that of the Golgi complex, and its contents pass through the stacks, being finally released from the maturing face of the Golgi complex as membrane-bound vacuoles. During its passage through the stacks the material may be condensed, sulphated (e.g. the glycoproteins of ground substance), or combined with carbohydrate. The vacuoles leaving the maturing face of the Golgi complex can be of many varieties, according to the cell type. Some are secretory vacuoles, others contain mucopolysaccharide or procollagen, others are primary lysosomes, while others pass to the cell surface and by fusing with the cell membrane, contribute material to it (Fig. 2.9).

Lysosomes

Lysosomes are rounded, membrane-bound organelles that contain lytic* enzymes active at a low pH, i.e. acid phosphatase, deoxyribonuclease, and cathepsins. The lysosomal enzymes are formed in the rough endoplasmic reticulum, and pass into the Golgi complex where they are packaged. They are released from the maturing face of the Golgi

---

*Lyse—to render soluble.

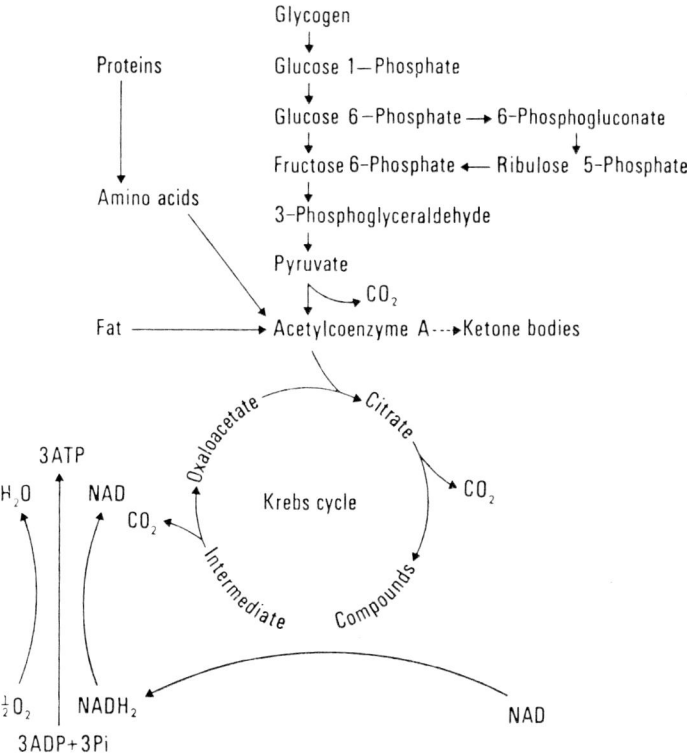

Fig. 2.8 Outline of the metabolic pathways concerned in energy production. This whole process in the oxidation of glycogen to CO_2 and water can be considered as occurring in two phases. The first, or anaerobic, phase results in the formation of pyruvate, and is known as glycolysis. The second, or aerobic, phase is the Krebs cycle. Products of carbohydrate, fat, and protein metabolism are fed into the Krebs cycle via acetylcoenzyme A. Several enzymic reactions of the Krebs cycle involve the reduction of NAD to $NADH_2$. Reoxidation of $NADH_2$ by the cytochrome system is coupled with phosphorylation of ADP to ATP, viz.

$$NADH_2 + {}^1/_2 O_2 + 3ADP + 3Pi \rightarrow NAD + H_2O + 3ATP.$$

The hexose monophosphate shunt, or pentose-phosphate pathway, leads to the formation of ribulose phosphate and is an alternative pathway in certain cells. It is an aerobic process, and in addition to its products re-entering the glycolytic sequence, sugars of 4–7 carbon atoms are formed and utilized in various synthesis processes.

Key: NAD—Nicotinamide adenine dinucleotide. $NADH_2$—Dihydronicotiamide adenine dinucleotide. Pi—Inorganic phosphate. ADP—Adenosine diphosphate. ATP—Adenosine triphosphate.

complex as *primary lysosomes*. Membrane-bound material in the form of *heterophagosomes* formed as a result of endocytosis, or as *autophagosomes* (or *cytolysomes*) containing damaged worn-out cell components, fuse with the primary lysosomes to form *secondary lysosomes*. These bodies present a variety of appearances. They contain foreign ingested material or fragments of recognizable cell components—mitochondria, endoplasmic reticulum, etc. Sometimes they contain lipid which assumes the form of a concentric lamination of myelin figures. Eventually the lysosomes contain only indigestible material, and they remain as *residual bodies* containing lipofuscin. These are the wear-and-tear pigments of light microscopy.

The stability of the lysosomal membrane can

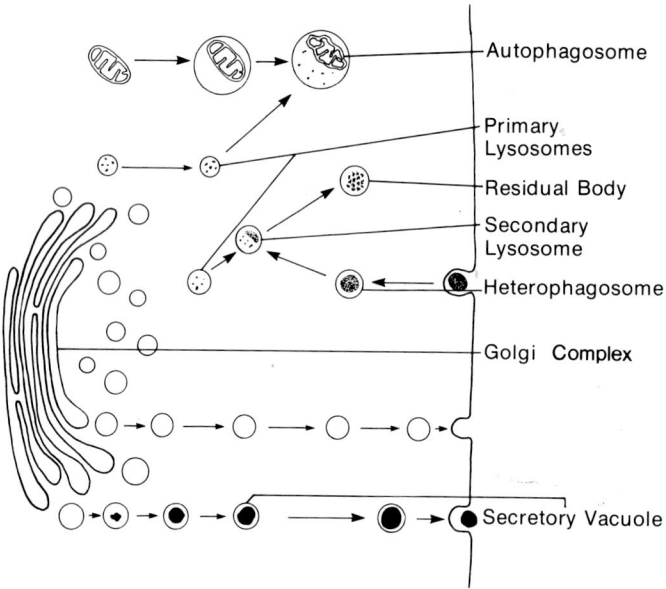

Fig. 2.9 The Golgi complex (Golgi apparatus) and its possible functions. This diagram depicts the Golgi complex as a series of flattened sacs from which numerous vacuoles arise. Some vacuoles contain secretory material that has been synthetized in the endoplasmic reticulum. Some vacuoles appear to be empty and travel to the cell surface where their membranes fuse with the cell membrane. Other vacuoles contain lytic enzymes and become primary lysosomes. These fuse with autophagosomes or heterophagosomes to form secondary lysosomes. Undigested material remains in residual bodies. (Drawn by Margot Mackay, University of Toronto. Reproduced from Walter J B (1992) An introduction to the principles of disease, 3rd edn, W B Saunders, Philadelphia with permission of the publishers.)

be increased by the action of glucocorticoids; this may be a factor in their protective action against the damaging effects produced by ultraviolet light, bacterial endotoxin, etc.

Lysosomal digestion plays a part in the removal of unwanted cells during embryonic development. Thus, after cell death the lysosomal enzymes are probably responsible for the cell's digestion and ultimate dissolution. Lysosomal enzymes also play a part as mediators of acute inflammation (p. 62), and their release from polymorphs can cause local tissue damage. This is particularly prominent in immune-complex reactions (p. 139).

Microbodies

Microbodies are membrane-bound, rounded organelles characterized by their content of oxidases, such as urate oxidase and catalase, an enzyme which acts on hydrogen peroxide and liberates oxygen. This enzyme is of some importance in the oral cavity (p. 71).

Cytoskeletal system

The cell sap or cytosol contains a number of filaments that provide the cytoplasm with some degree of rigidity but also take part in movement both within the cell, as at mitosis, and when the cell moves as a whole during locomotion. Several chemical and morphological types of filaments are known—microtubules, actin filaments, myosin filaments and intermediate filaments.

Microtubules. These are tubular structures about 25 nm in diameter. Their centres are composed of material of low electron density, and they therefore appear as hollow tubes. Microtubules are composed of protein subunits called tubulin, and can undergo rapid breakdown and reassembly. This reassembly is inhibited by the alkaloid colchicine. In some cells, e.g. diatoms, the microtubules appear to provide rigidity, acting as a cytoskeleton, and they may be responsible for the relatively fixed shape of some cells, e.g. blood platelets and podocytes. Another function of the microtubules is that of assisting the transport of material within the cell; they serve to direct secretory granules, e.g. those containing insulin, to the cell surface prior to exocytosis. Their function in relationship to cell receptors has already been described (p. 11). The filaments of the spindle at mitosis are composed of microtubules, therefore colchicine inhibits mitosis at the metaphase.

Myosin and actin filaments. Actin filaments (also called micro filaments) are small, being about 6nm in diameter. Myosin filaments (also called thick filaments) are larger, being about 15 nm in diameter. Both are involved in cell contraction and movement.

Intermediate filaments. These filaments are so named because, being about 10nm in diameter, they are intermediate in size between actin and myosin. Five major classes are recognized. Apart from their important role as part of the cyto-skeletal system in the function of the cell, they have a practical use in pathology because they can be detected in the cell by the use of specific monoclonal antibodies. In this way, the cell type of poorly differentiated tumours can be inves-tigated because the tumour cells tend to have the same intermediate filaments as the parent cell of origin. The intermediate filaments are: keratin filaments (tonofilaments) present in epithelial cells and particularly abundant in epidermis; *desmin filaments*, characteristic of muscle cells; *vimentin filaments*, present in many connective tissue cells and some epithelial cells; *neuro-filaments*, present in neurons; and *glial filaments*, present in glia and ependyma.

Centriole

The centriole is a cylindrical body about 15 nm long, which is concerned with the orien-tation of the spindle (p. 22). Each cell has two centrioles (at least) which are situated in the centrosome and divide before the onset of mitosis (Fig.2.1).

Other cytoplasmic components include glyco-gen granules, fat globules, etc. Some cells contain specialized structures, e.g. granules in eosino-phils. Furthermore, as the resolution of the elec-tron microscope is being increased, so further structures are being described. In many instances their function is not known, but there is little doubt that in due course the ultrastructure of cells will turn out to be very complex—as complex indeed as life itself.

Cytoplasmic DNA

The presence of DNA in the cytoplasm is now well established. Some is present in the mito-chondria, and appears to direct protein synthesis via specific mRNA. Many other forms of cyto-plasmic DNA are known, and have been most extensively studied in bacteria. Some can act as infectious agents (e.g. bacteriophage), or may replicate in unison with cell division and there-fore act as cytoplasmic genetic material. These agents are called *episomes,* or *plasmids,* and their presence can greatly alter the function of a cell. Thus the production of toxin by the diphtheria bacillus is related to the presence of one of these agents, as is also the development of antibiotic resistance. Their role in mammalian cells is at present speculative, but it may well be related to the inheritance of certain diseases, viral infections (for instance slow viruses), and the development of cancer.

THE NUCLEUS

Situated within the cell and enclosed by a mem-brane is the *nucleus,* an important structure because it contains, in chemical form, the coded information which is handed down from one cell to its progeny and from one generation to the next. The chemical which performs this vital function is a nucleoprotein consisting of a histone combined with *deoxyribonucleic acid (DNA).* The acidic components of the nuclear material, since they combine with basic dyes like haematoxylin, are responsible for the basophilia with H.&E. The basophilic material in the nucleus is often called *chromatin,* a name coined before the dis-covery of DNA.

Chemical structure of DNA

The DNA molecule is composed of two poly-nucleotide chains spiralled around a common axis. Each chain is composed of multiple units termed *nucleotides* (base–deoxyribose sugar–phosphate), linked together by a phosphate. The common bases are either purines (adenine and guanine) or pyrimidines (thymine and cytosine). In the DNA molecule the bases are directed towards the central axis, and are joined by hydrogen bonding between a purine and a pyrimidine. Only adenine pairs with thymine, and only guanine with cytosine (Fig. 2.10).

The DNA in the nucleus contains genetic information which is passed via RNA into the cytoplasm, where it is used in the manufacture of proteins of exact composition. The word *gene* is used to describe the hypothetical unit of heredity for any single characteristic. It is present in the nucleus as a length of DNA. The gene is broken up into segments: *exons* which are used in the formation of mRNA and *introns* which appear to act as spacers.

The order of the bases in DNA constitutes the genetic code, in which a sequence of three bases corresponds to a single amino acid. A type of RNA (messenger RNA, or mRNA) is made in the nucleus in the presence of DNA-dependent RNA polymerase. The process is termed *transcription*, and the mRNA is modelled on one of the polynucleotide chains of DNA which acts as a template. The base sequence of the RNA is complementary to that of DNA, i.e. cytosine corresponds with guanine, etc. The initial transcript is long because it contains the sequences corresponding to both exons and introns. The RNA is processed so that the information of introns is removed and only that of the exons remains in the mRNA. The mRNA passes into the cytoplasm and becomes associated with a group of ribosomes (a *polysome*). Here protein synthesis occurs. Each triplet, or codon, of the mRNA base order is responsible for one amino acid. As the ribosomes 'read' along the RNA molecule, successive amino acids are added to an ever increasing polypeptide chain. In this way a protein of exact composition is synthesized; secondary and tertiary structure are a consequence of this. The actual addition of each amino acid is effected by another type of RNA, transfer RNA or tRNA, a separate form of which exists for each amino acid. The process is complex and is described as *translation*, for the code of the DNA finally appears legible in the form of a polypeptide chain.

The discovery that certain enzymes (termed *restriction endonucleases*) can cut the DNA molecule at specific sites has been of immense importance. Thus the enzyme EcoRI isolated from *E.coli* will cut the DNA molecule as shown below:

$$\begin{array}{ccc} -\text{G A A T T C-} & & -\text{G} \quad \text{A A T T C-} \\ & \longrightarrow & + \\ -\text{C T T A A G-} & & -\text{C T T A A} \quad \text{G-} \end{array}$$

SITE
OF
CUT

The ends of the segments so produced are 'sticky', and will readily join with other DNA segments produced by the same endonuclease. Hence, using appropriate techniques, the DNA from a cell can be split into suitable lengths and inserted into the DNA of a bacterium or yeast. If the selected segment of DNA contains a particular gene, growth of the bacterium will result in the formation of numerous copies of the gene. This process is called gene cloning and has

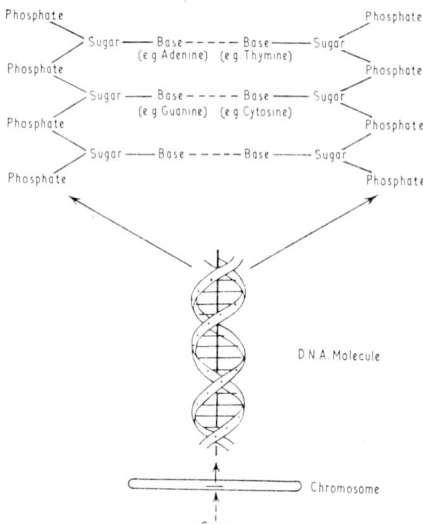

Fig. 2.10 Suggested chemical structure of DNA. The two polynucleotide chains are united by their bases, the order of which constitutes the genetic code. (After Watson J D, Crick F H C 1953 Nature (Lond) 171:737.)

numerous applications, as growth of the organism leads to production of the protein for which the gene encodes. Complex polypeptides such as growth hormone can be manufactured commercially by this technique.

In another technique, a single strand of the DNA can be tagged with radioactive material and used as a probe to detect the gene in a cell. Using this technique, the chains of the cell's DNA are first separated and the probe is applied. Its DNA will hybridize with the appropriate section of the cell's DNA.

For details of these techniques, collectively termed recombinant DNA technology, the reader is referred to specialized texts.

Control of cell growth and differentiation

Although the coordinated growth and differentiation of cells in multicellular organisms must be of great importance, relatively little is known of the mechanisms involved. The classical steroid, protein or polypeptide hormones, and vitamins play some part and act at a site distant from their formation. Other mechanisms seem to involve close cell-to-cell interaction and are effected by the production of locally acting chemicals, which include nucleotides, prostaglandins, leukotrienes and a group of peptides termed *peptide regulatory factors* (PRF). The latter appear to be particularly important. They act locally and either affect adjacent cells (paracrine effect) or the cell that secreted them (autocrine effect). They include a number of *growth factors* (e.g. epidermal growth factor, platelet-derived growth factor, haematopoietic growth factors). The *cytokines* or interleukins are similar factors that have immunoregulatory effects—*monokines* derived from monocytes and *lymphokines* from lymphocytes. *Interferons* fall into this general group. The names attached to these substances are somewhat misleading, for they were derived from their original assay systems or biological behaviour, and do not necessarily reflect their main site of origin or actions.

The regulatory peptides act on cell-surface receptors and activate various mechanisms that initiate a second message. In some cases this involves a kinase activity that phosphorylates tyrosine residues in cellular proteins. The mechanism

varies with each peptide and, indeed, some peptides appear to have receptors in the nucleus. A remarkable finding is that some of the peptides, or their receptors, are formed as a result of the activity of *cellular oncogenes* (c-*onc*). As will be described in Chapter. 21 these genes, or mutated forms of them, are important in the pathogenesis of certain, and perhaps most, malignant tumours. If cellular oncogenes are involved in the regulation of normal cell division and maturation, it would provide a starting point to our understanding of how their dysfunction could be important in the formation of cancer.

Control of gene action

It is evident that each nucleated cell of the body contains the necessary information for the manufacture of every protein of which the body is composed. That they do not do so all the time is evidence that there is some very adequate control mechanism. Thus erythroid cells manufacture haemoglobin, plasma cells immunoglobulin, etc. Nevertheless, it is not surprising that under abnormal circumstances cells produce substances which are alien to their accustomed products. This occurs in neoplasia, and an excellent example is the secretion by certain cancer cells of hormones which normally are produced only in the very specialized cells of the endocrine glands (p. 250).

Chromosomes

The DNA molecules are not lying free in the nuclear sap, but are contained in long threads called *chromosomes*. Each resting somatic cell contains a definite number of chromosomes, the *diploid*, or 2*n*, number. This corresponds to a definite amount of DNA, the 2c amount. In humans the diploid number is 46, and of these 23 are derived from each parent. Two chromosomes are related specifically to sex, and these are called the *sex chromosomes*. One is considerably larger than the other and is called a X chromosome, while the smaller one is called Y chromosome. Females have two X chromosomes whereas males have an X and a Y chromosome. The remaining 22 pairs are identical in appearance in both sexes and are called *autosomes*.

Certain exceptions to the rules are found. In normal liver with increasing age some cells are found with nuclei containing abnormal, multiple amounts of DNA, i.e. $4n$, $8n$, or $16n$ amounts. These are called *polyploid* nuclei, and are formed as the result of cells replicating their genetic material but having been blocked in the G_2 phase of the cell cycle. Polyploidy is also a feature of hypertrophied muscle, and is encountered in megaloblasts (Ch. 26). Cells may contain an amount of DNA that is not an exact multiple of the normal amount, a condition called *aneuploidy*, which is a feature of malignant cells.

During the period between cell division (interphase) the chromosomes are present in the nucleus as long drawn-out threads. These are not visible as such using the light microscope, but in some areas along the thread there is sufficient coiling for the condensation of material to render these areas recognizable as chromatin dots of the nucleus. Such chromatin (*heterochromatin*) appears as areas of deep staining, and is thought to represent regions of the chromosomes which are condensed and relatively inert metabolically. The remainder of the nucleus is lightly stained, and the dispersed chromatin material (*euchromatin*) is in an active form. It follows that the actual morphology of the nucleus varies considerably from one cell to another, and that an assessment of function can be made from nuclear structure. In active cells, e.g. neurons, the nucleus is vesicular and very little heterochromatin is present. Heterochromatin is more abundant in epithelial cells and gives the nucleus a stippled appearance. In inactive cells, e.g. small lymphocytes, late normoblasts, and spermatozoa, the heterochromatin occupies most of the nucleus which therefore appears deeply basophilic. In the mature plasma cells the heterochromatin is disposed close to the nuclear membrane in clumps to produce the cartwheel, or clock-faced, appearance so typical of this cell.

Some cells which are very large, e.g. the osteoclasts of the bone marrow, contain many nuclei and are called *multinucleate giant cells*. Some of the RNA component of the nucleus may appear as a separate structure called the *nucleolus*. This is particularly prominent in cells which are actively metabolizing—e.g. cancer cells.

The Barr body

Murray Barr first noticed the presence of a chromatin mass in the nerve cells of the female cat but not that of the male cat. In humans the *Barr body* or *sex chromatin* can easily be demonstrated as a demilune on the nuclear membrane of buccal mucosa cells (Fig. 2.11).

The Barr body is derived from a single X chromosome, and the number of Barr bodies seen in a cell is one less than the number of X chromosomes present. One X chromosome in each nucleus behaves like the autosomes. It becomes uncoiled between each cell division and therefore is not seen. If another X chromosome is present it replicates late in mitosis, remains inactive and appears as a Barr body. It follows that the normal male, having only one X chromosome, is chromatin negative while the normal female is chromatin positive, i.e. has sex chromatin.

Examination of smears for the Barr body was once an important investigation if an abnormality

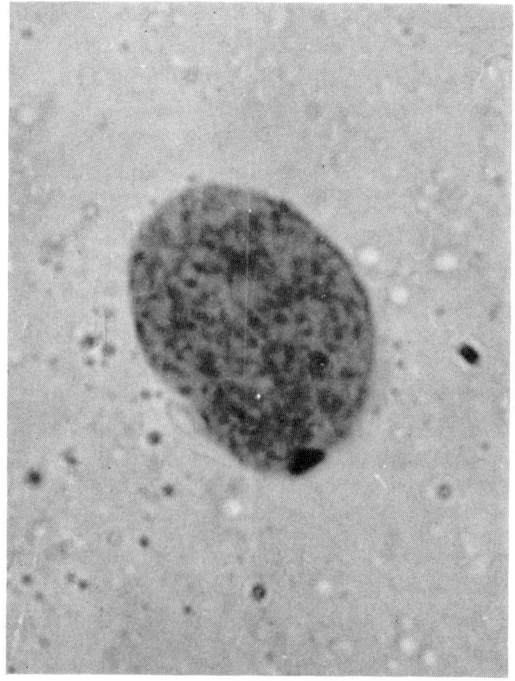

Fig. 2.11 The Barr body. Nucleus of a cell from buccal mucosal smear of a female, showing the sex chromatin mass on the nuclear membrane. Stained by acetic orecin. (Photograph by courtesy of Dr Nigel H Kemp.)

of the sex chromosomes was suspected. The method has been replaced in modern cytogenetic laboratories by complete karyotype examination.

The cell cycle. The cell cycle is reckoned to begin at the completion of one cell division (mitosis) and to end at the completion of the next division. The time taken for one cell cycle is the *generation time*.

Immediately following cell division the cell enters the first resting, or G_1 phase. The length of this phase is the most variable component of the cell cycle. Sometimes a cell may remain in this state for a long period; it is then described as having entered the G_0 phase. It may later return to the cell cycle, or else become so fully differentiated as to become incapable of further mito-sis. There are some cells, notably the neurons, which cannot undergo mitosis.

The G_1 phase is followed by a synthesis, or S, phase, during which the DNA of the nucleus replicates. There then follows a short gap, the G_2 phase, before the beginning of mitosis.

Mitosis

The mechanism whereby somatic cells divide is a complicated process in which the nuclear material is reduplicated, and then carefully divided into two equal parts, which reform the nuclei of the two daughter cells (Fig. 2.12).

During the period between mitoses (*interphase*) the chromosomes are present in the nucleus as

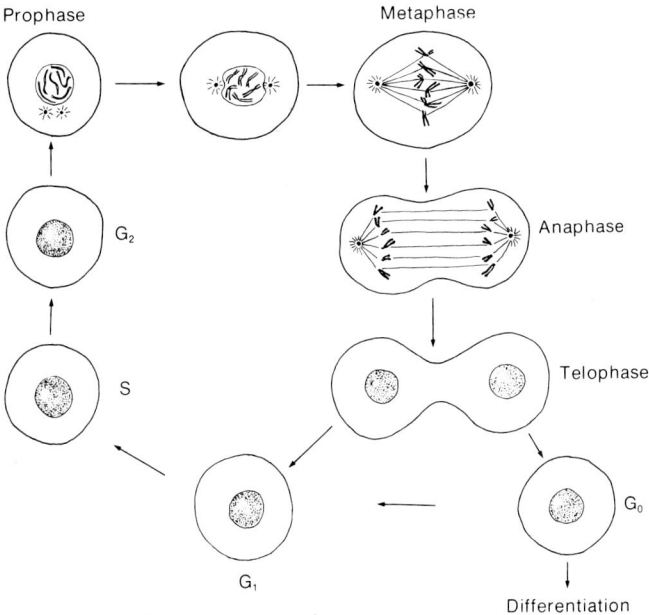

Fig. 2.12 The cell cycle. DNA reduplication occurs during the synthesis stage (S). This is followed by a short resting stage (G_2) before the cell enters mitosis. Following division the daughter cells may enter the second resting stage (G_1) before recommencing DNA synthesis. Other daughter cells can pass into a resting phase (G_0), and after a period can either re-enter the cell cycle or become differentiated and cease to be capable of mitosis. In prophase the individual chromosomes become visible—for the sake of clarity only six are shown, but the normal human cell contains 46. Each chromosome has already split into two chromatids. In metaphase the chromosomes are arranged along the equatorial plate, and the spindle is fully formed. In anaphase, the chromatids, now called chromosomes, move apart. In telophase the daughter nuclei reform, and the cytoplasm divides to produce two cells each with the amount of DNA corresponding to the normal number of chromosomes.

long drawn-out threads. These are not visible as such using the light microscope, but in areas along the thread there is sufficient coiling for the condensation of material to render these areas recognizable as the heterochromatin of the nucleus. Each chromosome is thought to contain one long DNA molecule.

Following the G_2 phase, each chromosome is seen to have divided longitudinally into two *chromatids* which are held together by a *centromere*. The chromosomes show coiling along their length; in this way they become shorter and thicker, and therefore visible. The cell has now entered into the first phase of mitosis—*prophase*. Meanwhile in the centrosome the microtubules become arranged so as to form the spindle fibres which converge on a dense body adjacent to the centrioles. The centrioles move away from each other to opposite poles of the cell, and in this way the *spindle* is formed; its microtubules are attached to the centromeres, and each centriole looks like a star, or *aster*.

Concurrently the nucleoli and nuclear membrane disappear. The cell is now in *metaphase* with the split chromosomes being arranged along a plane which bisects the cell (the 'equatorial plate').

During the next phase (*anaphase*) the centromeres divide, and each set of chromatids (now called chromosomes) is guided by the fibrils of the spindle to either pole of the cell.

The final stage (*telophase*) involves division of the cytoplasm of the cells, and the reconstitution of the nucleoli and nuclear membrane of each daughter cell.

It can be readily understood how during mitosis each chromosome reduplicates itself exactly, and each daughter cell contains an identical quota of nuclear material. It is presumed that each DNA molecule (and gene) is also reduplicated exactly. Should an error occur during mitosis such that an abnormal gene is produced, the process is called a *somatic mutation*. It is possible that cancer develops in this way.

Meiosis

In the testis and ovary the process of cell division is more complex, and is called *meiosis*. The process results in cells which contain only half the number of chromosomes (the *n*, or *haploid*, number, i.e. 23 in the human), and half the amount of DNA. These cells develop into gametes, either sperms or ova. With fertilization the diploid number of chromosomes, 46, is restored. It sometimes happens that during meiosis a pair of chromosomes fail to separate, and both are drawn into the one daughter cell. This is called *non-disjunction*. Sometimes fragments of a chromosome are lost (*deletion*), or become attached to another chromosome (*translocation*). If these abnormal gametes are fertilized, it is evident that an abnormal offspring may result. This is considered in Chapter 3.

ARRANGEMENT OF CELLS

The majority of cells in the human body do not occur separately, but are grouped together to form tissues. Traditionally, two main types of cells are distinguished—those of the epithelia and those of the connective tissues or mesenchyme.

Epithelial cells

Epithelial cells cover surfaces, e.g. the skin, or line cavities, e.g. the mouth, and in these situations they are essentially protective in function. Covering epithelium may also perform a secretory function; the respiratory epithelium, for instance, secretes mucus.

In addition to covering extensive surfaces, the secretory type of epithelial cell may be arranged to form glands. These may be simple like the mucous glands of the colon, or more elaborate, like those of the breast and salivary glands. A feature common to all epithelial cells is that they are closely contiguous to one another. This is evident on light microscopy, and even under the electron microscope these cells appear to be separated by only a thin layer of low electron density, about 15 nm in width.

Connective tissue cells

Connective tissue cells are the other type of cell present in the body. They usually separated widely from each other by *ground substance* in which are embedded fibres (usually *collagenous*).

This type of connective tissue, typified by bone, cartilage, tendon, and fibrous tissue, is primarily supportive in function. Other connective tissue cells have been endowed with specialized cytoplasm, e.g. for contraction (muscle fibres), conduction (neurons), phagocytosis (monocytes), and oxygen carriage (red cells).*

The division of the cells of the body into two groups is convenient for some purposes, as will be seen when the classification of tumours is described. Nevertheless, the division is arbitrary and in some ways unsatisfactory. Thus, the flattened cells which line the blood vessels are usually considered to be connective tissue, although they are, in fact, performing a covering function. The same may be said of the mesothelial cells lining the pleura and peritoneum, and those of the synovium.

An important group of connective tissue cells are concerned with phagocytosis but their delineation and classification have proved both difficult and controversial. The group includes cells widely called reticulum cells, but this term has been applied to several types of cell:

Histiocytic reticulum cells. These cells, also simply called 'histiocytes', are present in most tissues; they are of bone marrow origin and potentially phagocytic. They line sinuses in lymph nodes, spleen and liver (Kupffer's cells). When activated and phagocytic, histiocytic reticulum cells become macrophages.

Fibroblastic reticulum cells. The existence of these cells is controversial but they are described as forming the reticulum framework of lymph nodes and spleen.

Dendritic reticulum cells. A cell probably of bone marrow origin and found in B-cell areas of the lymphoreticular system.

Interdigitating reticulum cell. Also of bone marrow origin these cells are present in T-cell areas of the lymphoreticular system. The *Langerhans' cell* is included in this group; it is present in the epidermis and is of great importance in the immune reaction. It processes and presents antigen to lymphocytes.

---

*Some authorities prefer to restrict the connective tissues to bone, cartilage, etc., and regard the specialized elements as belonging to separate systems, e.g. haematopoietic, nervous, etc.

The term *reticuloendothelial system* (RES) was coined by Aschoff to include a group of cells that are phagocytic and capable of taking up a soluble dye such as trypan blue from the blood. The system includes mobile members (the monocytes of the blood) and fixed cells (histiocytic reticulum cells), some of which also line sinuses in lymph nodes, spleen and liver. Its cells are associated with the reticulin framework of these organs but do not produce it. Nor are the ordinary endothelial cells included. Hence the term 'reticuloendothelial' is inappropriate. At a conference held in Leiden in 1969 a group of workers proposed a new classification of cells termed the *mononuclear phagocyte system* (MPS). This includes monocytes of the blood, histiocytic reticulum cells, macrophages, and precursor cells of the bone marrow from which they are all derived. The use of this term is gaining support and it has replaced 'reticuloendothelial system' in medical literature. Yet this classification also has its drawbacks; for instance dendritic and interdigitating reticulum cells are very closely related yet are excluded because they are not phagocytic. Multinucleate cells in granulomatous inflammation are included. Another term often used is *lymphoreticular system*. It is convenient but imprecise; it includes lymphoid cells and all cells included under the terms RES and MPS.

THE INTERCELLULAR SPACE

THE GROUND SUBSTANCE

The ground substance varies in consistency from an amorphous gel forming the translucent material of hyaline cartilage to the glairy fluid found in the synovial joint cavities. It is in the molecular meshes of the ground substance that the extracellular interstitial fluid is contained. This extracellular fluid constitutes about one-third of the total body water, and lies between the blood vessels and the cells. It contains various electrolytes in a concentration similar to that of the plasma and also small uncharged solute material, such as oxygen, CO_2, glucose, and urea, which is conveyed either for cellular metabolism or for excretion. In addition the ground substance contains:

Glycoproteins

These have a protein backbone with a few attached oligosaccharide side chains covalently bonded. The group included fibronectin, laminin and some collagens (e.g. type IV). Their carbohydrate content allows them to be stained red with the PAS stain[*] and this is a useful method of demonstrating basement membrane zones.

Fibronectins. The fibronectins are a family of related glycoproteins that are manufactured by many cells types, with vascular endothelium being the principle source. They have been described as a 'molecular glue' and their presence is necessary for many cell-to-cell interactions, as well as the adhesion of fibres such as fibrin and collagen both to each other and to cells. Malignant cells have less extracellular fibronectin than their normal counterpart and this may be a factor in the invasive properties and metastasis that malignant cells exhibit.

Laminin. This glycoprotein is present in basement membrane and is involved in the attachment of epithelial cells to the collagen of the basement membrane.

Chondronectin. This has a similar role for the attachment of chondrocytes to collagen in cartilage.

Proteoglycans

Previously called mucoproteins, these consist of a protein backbone with many polysaccharide side chains which are acidic and are called *glucosaminoglycans* (previously called acid mucopolysaccharides). The proteoglycans are manufactured by fibroblasts and similar cells such as osteoblasts.

---

[*]*The periodic acid-Schiff reaction.* When periodic acid is applied to a section many carbohydrate components are oxidized to aldehydes. Aldehydes produce a red colour with Schiff's reagent (a solution of basic fuchsin decolourized by sulphurous acid). Therefore if Schiff's reagent is applied to a treated section, the parts containing carbohydrate are stained red. The PAS reaction is useful for the demonstration of glycogen, ground substance, and epithelial mucus.

They are commonly demonstrated in tissue sections by using two empirical methods —Alcian blue stain or the colloidal iron stain of Hale. Two groups of glucosaminoglycans are recognized:

Non-sulphated group. This comprises hyaluronic acid and chondroitin.

Sulphated group. This group includes chondroitin-4 sulphate, chondroitin-6 sulphate, dermatan sulphate, heparan sulphate and keratan sulphate.

The physical and presumably the chemical properties of each connective tissue depend as much on the nature of the ground substance as on the arrangement and type of its fibres. For example, keratan sulphate forms 50% of the total glucosaminoglycan content of the cornea, but is present in only small amounts in osteoid.

COLLAGEN

Collagen consists of a family of proteins which constitute about one-third of the body's protein. Its fibres form a scaffold in all tissues and is the chief component of fascia, dermis (including gingiva), cornea, dentine, and tendon, and gives these structures tensile strength. Isotope studies indicate that although much of the body's collagen is metabolically stable, some of it is rapidly synthetized and degraded; the excretion of hydroxyproline in the urine gives some indication of the amount of collagen which is being degraded. Thus the excretion is high in hyperparathyroidism. Collagen comprises almost 90% of the organic matrix of bone, and its particular composition is adapted for the deposition of the bone salts.

The collagen of connective tissue is synthetized by fibroblasts or similar cells such as are found in tendon, cornea, bone, and cartilage. An exception to this is the collagen component of basement membrane, which is formed by the adjacent epithelial or endothelial cells and differs in several respects from other collagens.

Microscopic appearance of collagen

Collagen fibres of connective tissue, such as fascia, dermis, dentine, bone, tendon, and mature scar tissue, are largely composed of type I collagen and readily stained by eosin or analine blue combined with phosphotungstic acid (Mallory's stain). They also stain red with picrofuchsin (van Gieson's stain).

Reticulin consists of fine branching fibres that form the scaffold for the parenchyma in some organs, e.g. liver, spleen and lymph node. The fibres stain poorly with eosin and are demonstrated by silver impregnation methods. Type III collagen is their major component. Electron microscopy reveals that the fibres of both collagen (Fig. 2.13) and reticulin are made up of fibrils which show a cross banding with a periodicity of about 64 nm. The fibrils are made up of collagen molecules each of which is about 280 nm long and 1.4 nm wide. The molecules are arranged with a quarter-length overlap with their lateral neighbours thereby giving the fibrils their characteristic periodicity. There is a gap of about 41 nm between the head of one molecule and the tail of the next; in osteoid tissue this serves as a nidus for calcification.

It is evident that different lateral arrangements of the molecules could form fibrils with a different periodicity, and such have been found to exist—thus, long, spaced collagen can be found at certain sites.

Chemical composition of collagen

Collagen has a characteristic X-ray diffraction pattern, and from this its structure has been surmised. The basic collagen molecule is 280 nm long and 1.4 nm wide, with a molecular weight of about 340 000 daltons. It consists of three polypeptide chains. Each of the polypeptide chains is coiled, and the three molecules are wound around a common axis like a three-stranded rope. It is thus a 'coiled coil'.

At least nine types of chain are known and various combinations of these polypeptide chains are known to combine to form five types of collagen:

Type I: $[\alpha1(I)]_2\alpha2(I)$. This type of collagen is widely distributed, and is the major component of dermis, tendon, bone, and dentine. It consists of two $\alpha1(I)$ chains and one $\alpha2(I)$ chain. Its molecular form is therefore recorded as $[\alpha1(I)]_2\alpha2(I)$.

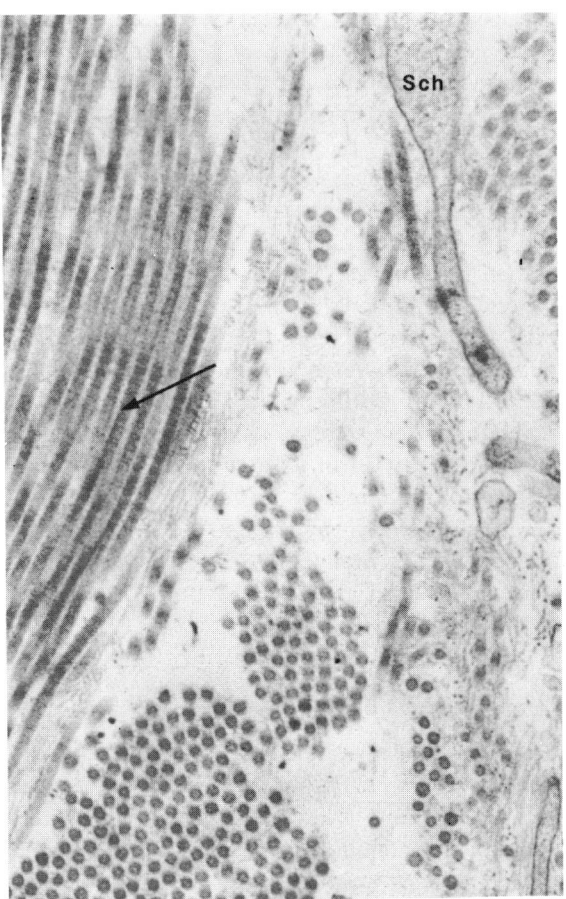

Fig. 2.13 Section of collagen fibrils in a peripheral nerve. The fibrils show the characteristic cross-banding (arrow), which is best seen where the fibrils are cut longitudinally. Part of the cytoplasm of a Schwann cell (Sch) is also shown ($\times$ 12 000). (Photograph by courtesy of Dr N B Rewcastle. From Walter J B (1992) an introduction to the principles of disease, 3rd edn, W B Saunders, Philadelphia.)

Type II: $[\alpha1(II)]_3$. This type of collagen consists of three $\alpha1(II)$ chains and is chiefly found in cartilage.

Type III: $[\alpha1(III)]_3$. This type of collagen comprises approximately 50% of the collagen of the heart valves and the major arteries.

Type IV: $[\alpha1(IV)]_3$, $[\alpha2(IV)]_3$. Collagen composed of three $\alpha1(IV)$ chains is found only in basement membranes.

Type V: $[\alpha1(V)]_2\alpha2(V)$; $[\alpha1(V)\alpha2(V)\alpha3(V)]$. This type of collagen is found in the sheaths surrounding muscle and Schwann cells, and also in basement membranes.

Each polypeptide chain consists of about 1000

amino-acid residues and has a molecular weight of about 95 000 daltons. It is coiled to form a helix in which, unlike the usual protein α-helix, there are no hydrogen bonds between adjacent amino acids on the same chain. Each helix is stabilized by hydrogen bonds with adjacent polypeptide chains. Throughout most of the chain every third amino acid is glycine, and a common sequence is glycine–proline–hydroxy-proline. Collagen is indeed characterized by its high content of glycine (33%) and proline and hydroxyproline which together constitute about 22%. Hydroxyproline is an amino acid which is not found to any great extent in other proteins, and an estimation of its amount in hydrolysates of tissue may therefore be used to measure the amount of collagen present. It is also noteworthy that collagen contains hydroxylysine, and it is to this amino acid that carbohydrate is attached (either galactose or glucogalactose).

Biosynthesis of collagen

The three polypeptide chains of collagen are formed separately under the direction of separate genes (Fig. 2.14). Each mRNA gives rise to a primary polypeptide chain (termed *preprocollagen chain* $\alpha 1(I)$ etc.). This is a helical molecule with two globular cysteine containing extensions, one at the $-NH_2$ and the other at the $-COOH$ terminal region. At the $-NH_2$ terminal extension the extension acts as a leader or signal that directs entry of the molecule into the rough endoplasmic reticulum. This signal is shortly removed and the chain that remains is termed *procollagen chain* $\alpha 1(I)$, etc. Within the endoplasmic reticulum three chains form a superhelix to form *procollagen*, but only after two essential steps— hydroxylation of prolyl and lysyl residues, and glycosylation of the hydroxylysine residues.

Hydroxylation. Hydroxylation of certain propyl and lysyl residues takes place in the presence of specific enzymes, oxygen, ferrous ions, α-ketoglutarate and ascorbic acid.

Glycosylation of hydroxylysine residues. A specific enzyme and manganese are required for this step.

Secretion of procollagen. Following the two steps described above three polypeptide chains unite to form a triple helix now called *procollagen*, which passes into the Golgi complex and is finally secreted into the extracellular space. This occurs only if all the previous steps have been carried out correctly. It follows, for example, that in vitamin C deficiency there is a lack of procollagen formation.

Formation of collagen. In the extracellular space procollagen is converted into collagen. Two enzymes are required—procollagen aminopeptidase and procollagen carboxylase. These two enzymes catalyse the removal of the polypeptide chains that form the globular extensions at the ends of the procollagen molecule. In the case of collagen types I and II, both extensions are removed and the collagen molecules align themselves with a one-quarter overlap to form immature collagen fibrils, which lack tensile strength.

Cross linkage of fibrils to form fibres. The next step is the oxidative deamination of specific lysyl or hydroxylysyl residues under the influence of the enzyme lysyl oxidase. Aldehyde groups so formed interact with adjacent chains to form a variety of cross-linkages that give the strength to the collagen. This is a relatively slow process and one can readily understand why the tensile strength of a wound steadily increases over a period of several months.

In the case of type III collagen, not all the extensions of procollagen are removed and the molecules align themselves with their neighbours to form fibrils and banded fibres. These fibres remain thin, however, and are recognized histologically as *reticulin fibres*. They are coated with much ground substance, and it is in this that silver is deposited under suitable staining. In the case of types IV and V collagen very little extracellular processing occurs and the fibrils form a meshwork, being well designed to act as a filter in a basement membrane, but lacking the banded appearance on electron microscopy.

Catabolism of collagen

Although collagen appears to be metabolically very stable, it is evident that under some circumstances it can be formed very rapidly and equally rapidly degraded and removed. The denaturation of collagen involves the actions of

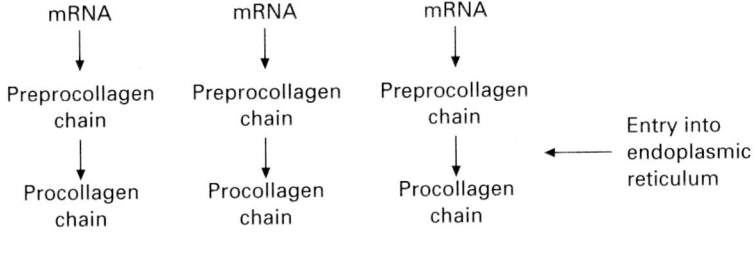

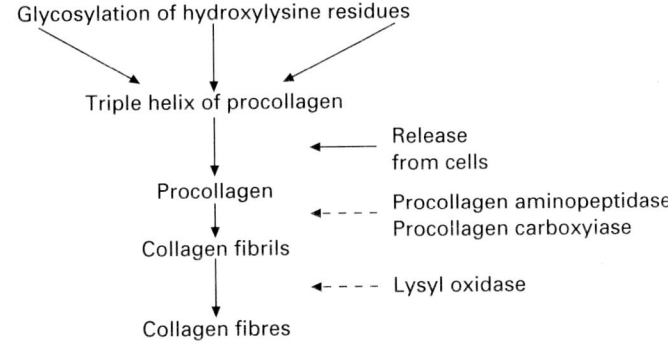

Fig. 2.14 Diagram to illustrate the biosynthesis of collagen.

proteolytic enzymes, either specific collagenases or non-specific proteases. Both play a part under some circumstances.

Non-specific proteases. Proteolytic enzymes are present in the lysosomes of neutrophils and macrophages. In inflammatory lesions these enzymes play a part in collagen degradation. Thus in suppuration the collagenous framework of a tissue is removed and an abscess formed. In other inflammatory lesions macrophages are seen to ingest collagen fibres. A good example is found in necrobiotic lesions.

Collagenases. It is now well established that specific collagenases are formed by many tissues. Thus, during post-partum involution of the uterus, and in the early stages of the regeneration of an amputated newt's arm, there is a rapid dissolution of the collagenous framework of the tissues. Likewise, in the maturation of scar tissue it is evident that collagen is removed at the same time as new collagen is laid down, so that the scar steadily becomes stronger as its tissues are remodelled. It seems likely that collagenases are important and that their function is to degrade

collagen. This action is balanced by collagen synthesis, so that under normal conditions the proper amount of collagen is present in the tissue. Increased collagen synthesis or decreased collagenase activity results in fibrosis.

Collagenase inhibitors are known to exist in plasma, but their role in collagen homeostasis is not known.

ELASTIC FIBRES

The elastic fibres of the aorta and its large branches, the ligamentum nuchae, lung, etc., appear very different from collagen on light microscopy; they stain *deep red with eosin, dark brown with orcein,* and *black with the resorcinol fuchsin stain of Weigert.* Early electron-microscopic studies have shown that elastic tissue consists of two components: one is the microfibril and the other is a homogeneous material of variable electron density. The microfibrils are obvious during the formation of elastic, but with ageing are more difficult to detect. Elastic tissue is very resistant to digestion by acids and alkalis, but is readily attacked by the enzyme elastase produced by some organisms.

Chemically elastic fibres consist of a protein, *elastin*, with polysaccharide. Elastin contains two amino acids, desmosine and isodesmosine, which are thought to be important in forming the cross-linkages which give to elastic tissue the resilience which is its characteristic physical property. With age there is an increase in the content of desmosine and isodesmosine, and this is accompanied by a loss of resilience. Calcification of elastic fibres is another feature of the ageing process; it also occurs in metastatic calcification (see p. 222).

Elastic fibres are formed by the activity of smooth muscle cells in some situations, e.g. in the aorta wall and in atheromatous plaques. In other tissues, cells which resemble fibroblasts appear to be involved. No specific 'elastoblasts' have been identified.

GENERAL READING

Cormack D H 1987 Ham's Histology, 9th edn. J B Lippincott, Philadelphia

Fawcett D W 1986 Bloom and Fawcett—A textbook of histology, 11th edn. Saunders, Philadelphia

Ghadially F N 1988 Ultrastructural pathology of the cell and matrix, 3rd edn. Butterworth, London

Hayes P C, Wolf C R, Hayes J D 1989 Blotting techniques for the study of DNA, RNA, and proteins. British Medical Journal 299:965

Lasser A 1983 The mononuclear phagocytic system. Human Pathology 14:108

Leeson C R, Leeson T S, Paparo A 1985 Textbook of histology, 5th edn. Saunders, Philadelphia

Miles J S, Wolf C R 1989 Principles of DNA cloning. British Medical Journal 299:1019

Watson J D, Tooze J 1981 The DNA story. Freeman, San Francisco

Weinberg R A 1985 The molecules of life. Scientific American 253(4):48

3. The genetic basis of disease

Traditionally much of pathology is concerned with the effects of adverse factors such as heat, trauma, and bacteria acting on a normal individual. Many diseases are regarded as being caused by particular agents—thus tuberculosis may be said to be caused by the tubercle bacillus. Such a one-sided approach to medicine is no longer tenable. If a hundred people were to be exposed to a particular dose of tubercle bacilli, only a few would develop the disease. No two people are the same, nor do they react in exactly the same way. Each individual is different, and the difference is thought to lie in the coded infor-mation (or genetic material) that is handed down to that person from his or her parents. This infor-mation is very precise, and is capable of exact analysis. Today we think of inheritance in terms of the structure of the DNA molecule and the sequence of its bases. The familial incidence of certain diseases has been noted since ancient times, but the situation was greatly clarified by Gregor Mendel, who, by observing the mode of inheritance of particular characteristics in the garden pea, noted that the characteristics be-haved as if they were determined by units which were passed unchanged from one generation to the next. To these units the name *genes* was given, and it is postulated that a pair of them is present in every somatic cell. Each gene is situated at a specific site, or *locus*, on one of a pair of chromosomes, and the genes forming a pair are called *alleles*, or *allelomorphs*. If they are alike the individual is called a *homozygote* for that particular gene, while if dissimilar the word *heterozygote* is used. The genetic makeup of an individual is called his *genotype*, and the effects which these genes produce is the *phenotype*.

MODE OF INHERITANCE

In order to explain Mendelian inheritance several assumptions have been made:

1. Genes occur in pairs
2. One gene of each pair is received from each parent
3. Genes remain unchanged through many generations
4. Some genes may be considered as dominant and some as recessive. A *dominant gene*

produces its effect both in the heterozygote and in the homozygote. *Recessive genes*, on the other hand, produce their effects only in the homozygous condition. Genes which occupy an intermediate position are described later. Sometimes a particular *locus* can be occupied by one of many possible genes. A simple example of this type is illustrated below in respect of the ABO blood groups.

Dominant genes

The pattern of inheritance of a dominant gene may be illustrated by reference to the ABO blood group. The allelic genes concerned occupy one *locus*, and may be *A*, *B*, or *O*.

A homozygous individual who has two *A* genes (genotype *AA*) has in the red cells the blood group substance A (phenotype group A). Likewise the heterozygote *AO* is also phenotypically blood group A, because the *A* gene is dominant and the *O* is recessive. The *B* gene, like *A*, is dominant, and both are described as *codominants*. The possible blood groups in this system are shown below:*

Genotype	Phenotype
AA	A
AO	A
OO	O
BB	B
BO	B
AB	AB

Thus the six genotypes produce only four recognizable blood groups. The occurrence of two or more genetically different classes of individuals with respect to a single trait is known as *polymorphism*.† The blood groups provide an excellent example, but many others are also known. Thus there are many genetically determined variants of haemoglobin and of some of the plasma proteins.

Some diseases are inherited as dominant characteristics, e.g. achondroplasia and dentinogenesis

---

* It will be appreciated that the ABO blood group is much more complex than is described in this book.
† The frequency should be greater than 1%, since very rare traits can arise by mutation and their occurrence in a population does not constitute polymorphism.

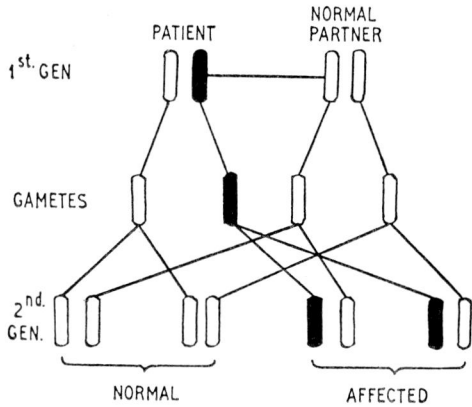

Fig. 3.1 Diagram illustrating the transmission of a disease inherited as a dominant factor. One pair of chromosomes is shown for each individual, the black chromosome being the one carrying the defective gene. It will be seen that half the children of an affected patient are themselves diseased.

imperfecta. The mode of inheritance is shown in Fig. 3.1, and it should be noted that:

1. The disease appears in every generation, or else it dies out. The occasional instance of poor penetrance (p. 32) and the occurrence of a new mutant provide exceptions to this rule. If the disease greatly reduces the breeding potential of the sufferer, it follows that most cases encountered will be sporadic and due to new mutations
2. Unaffected members do not pass on the disease (but see penetrance, p. 32)
3. The affected members are usually heterozygous, and if the breeding partner is normal, the chances of the offspring being affected are 50%.
4. Males and females are equally liable to be affected.

Recessive genes

Diseases inherited as recessive traits are frequently severe and reduce the breeding chances of the sufferer, e.g. galactosaemia (p. 33) and xeroderma pigmentosum (p. 267). The birth of an abnormal individual is often the first indication that an abnormal gene is present in the family. Figure 3.2 shows the mode of transmission, and it can be seen that both parents of the affected

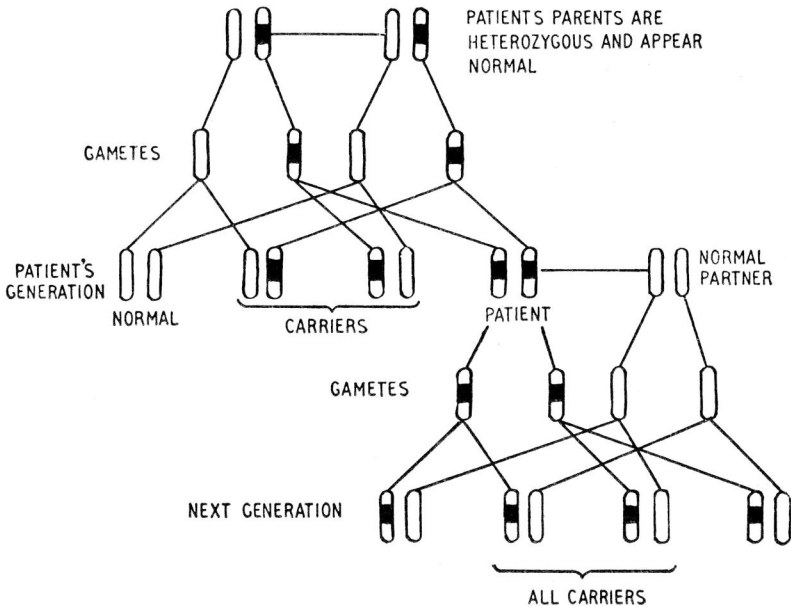

Fig. 3.2 Diagram to illustrate the transmission of a disease inherited as a recessive factor. It will be seen that the patient's parents are both unaffected heterozygotes, and that all the patient's children are likewise carriers.

individual are themselves heterozygous carriers. Most individuals are heterozygous for several harmful genes, and since some members of one family are likely to have the same recessive gene, the dangers of close interbreeding are apparent.

Sex-linked genes

A gene is said to be sex-linked when it is localized on an X or Y chromosome. Usually the gene is recessive, and is situated on the X chromosome. The bleeding diseases haemophilia and Christmas disease are inherited in this way (Fig. 3.3). Female heterozygotes are protected by the normal gene on their other X chromosome; half the carrier's sons, however, have the disease. The only Y-linked trait is hairy pinna.

Sex-linked dominant traits are recognized but are rare. Affected females convey the gene to half their sons and daughters, whereas affected males transmit it only to their daughters. Since there can be no male-to-male transmission, there is an excess of female victims. Haemolytic anaemia due to glucose 6-phosphate dehydrogenase deficiency is an example of this type of inheritance.

Gene linkage

Genes situated on the same chromosome tend to segregate together at meiosis and appear in the next generation. The closer they are together the less likely are they to separate. The genes controlling the HLA antigens are a good example and are inherited as a haplotype.

Intermediate inheritance

When the heterozygote differs from either homozygote, the inheritance is described as intermediate. A good example is sickle-cell anaemia, in which the heterozygote has the sickle-cell trait and differs both from the normal individual and the patient with sickle-cell anaemia (see p. 33).

Concept of expressivity

So far genes have been considered as behaving either as dominant or recessive. In fact the position is much more complex. A gene may produce a severe disease in one individual but only a minor deformity in another. The concept of

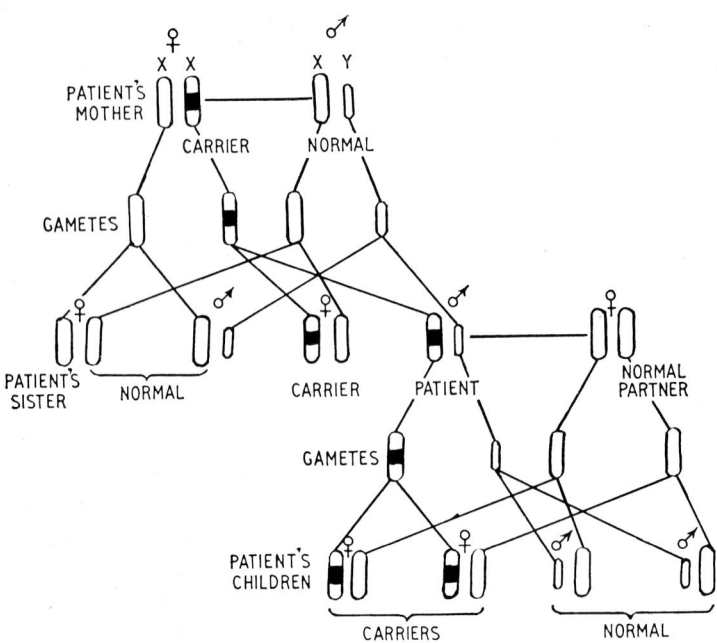

Fig. 3.3 Mode of transmission of a disease like haemophilia, which is inherited as a sex-linked recessive factor. The abnormal gene is situated on the X chromosome. and therefore produces its effect in the male but not in the female except in the rare event of her being homozygous. All the patient's daughters are carriers, but all his sons are normal.

expressivity has been introduced to explain this. If a gene which usually produces a severe effect is found to cause a minor one in a particular individual, it is said to show poor expressivity. In some instances it produces no detectable effect at all, and a dominant trait may then miss a generation. This is an example of *reduced penetrance,* a term used when some individuals with the appropriate genotype fail to express it. Another complication is the failure of a trait, in other respects behaving as a dominant, to be manifest in one sex. This is called *sex limitation.* Male pattern baldness behaves in this way, and for the gene to become manifest there must be a level of testosterone found naturally only in males.

Multifactorial or polygenic inheritance

Multifactorial inheritance, where several genes each influence one particular function, is a further complication. Diseases inherited in this way tend to be familial, but do not follow a simple Mendelian pattern. Further complications arise when environmental factors also influence the genotype.

INBORN ERRORS OF METABOLISM

If there is a point mutation, an error occurs at a particular point in the DNA of a gene, so that an abnormal protein is produced. A good example of this group of *inborn diseases of metabolism* is sickle-cell anaemia, an autosomal recessive trait found in certain individuals, usually of African stock: valine is substituted for glutamine at a specific site in one of the polypeptide chains of the globin molecule of haemoglobin. The abnormal haemoglobin is termed Hb-S. Homozygous individuals manufacture Hb-S, and its presence in their red cells renders them liable to become distorted to a sickle shape at low oxygen tension. The distorted cells block vessels and this may lead to infarction, e.g. of the spleen, bone, central nervous system and skin. The abnormal cells are more easily removed from the circulation and destroyed so that anaemia develops (*sickle-cell anaemia*).

Heterozygous individuals suffer from a mild anaemia, and are said to have the *sickle-cell trait*. Their red cells contain both normal adult haemoglobin, Hb-A, and Hb-S. It might be wondered why the sickle-cell gene, being so harmful, should not have killed off all its carriers and died out. It appears that those with the trait, although at a slight disadvantage in a temperate climate, are at a distinct advantage in the tropics, because they have greater resistance to malaria than do normal individuals. Through natural selection this apparently harmful gene has become widely distributed in tropical climates and has reached a high frequency. The haemoglobin molecule has been the object of intense study, and a large number of variants are now known. This is an example of the *genetic heterogeneity* in the population, and other instances are noted below in respect of certain enzymes.

Many other inborn errors of metabolism are known. Often the defective gene product is an enzyme and an abnormal gene gives rise to a protein with defective enzymatic activity. As examples there are at least 78 known variants of glucose 6-phosphate dehydrogenase deficiency and three of galactosaemia (described below). Enzyme-deficient red cells are considered in Chapter 26.

Galactosaemia

Babies with this defect lack an enzyme which converts galactose to glucose. The galactose, or its metabolites, derived from the lactose in milk, accumulates in the blood and interferes with the development of the brain, the eye, and the liver. Mental defect, cataracts, and cirrhosis of the liver are the results of this simple biochemical defect. The defects can be ameliorated by avoiding lactose and galactose in the diet. The ethics of condemning a child to a lifelong artificial diet might, however, be questioned.

Phenylketonuria

This disease affects between 3 and 5 persons per 100 000 of the population and is characterized by retardation of mental development. The disease is due to the absence of an enzyme that converts the amino acid phenylalanine to tyrosine. Hence, with a normal diet an affected baby develops a high blood level of phenylalanine and its keto derivatives. These are the cause of brain damage, which can be largely averted by the administration of a diet low in phenylalanine. Early diagnosis, by finding phenylalanine or its derivatives in the urine, is therefore very important. The condition is inherited as a Mendelian autosomal recessive trait; 1% of the population are heterozygotes, and can be detected by the administration of a test dose of phenylalanine, when the blood level rises. This does not occur in a normal individual. This detection of heterozygotes has a practical value. If a married couple are both carriers, their chance of producing an affected child is 25%: they can be warned of this risk. This is a good example of the kind of information offered in genetic counselling.

Pseudocholinesterase deficiency

Patients with a deficiency of this enzyme are very susceptible to suxamethonium, a drug used to produce relaxation during anaesthesia. The drug is inactivated in the normal person by the enzyme pseudocholinesterase.

α_1-Antitrypsin deficiency

α_1-Antitrypsin is a protease inhibitor, normally present in the blood, that protects the lung from damage caused by smoking and atmospheric pollution; probably the enzyme inhibits elastase released from polymorphs. Secretion of the enzyme is determined by a gene which has many known variant abnormal alleles. In those patients who have a very low plasma level of the enzyme there is a high incidence of panacinar pulmonary emphysema. For reasons that are not known the defect is also associated with neonatal hepatitis.

The lipidoses

This group, also known as the lipid-storage disease is associated with an enzyme defect that results in the accumulation of lipid material in affected cells. Gaucher's disease and Niemann–Pick disease will be described. Both are more common in Jewish children, and there are several forms of both depending on the exact genetic and enzymatic defect.

Gaucher's disease

In the common *adult form* of the disease, which has a protracted course, there is a massive accumulation of glucocerebroside due to the deficiency of the enzyme glucocerebrosidase. Glucocerebroside is probably derived from effete red and white cells in the mononuclear phagocyte system, and it is in these cells that the main accumulation of lipid is found. The swollen phagocytic cells are called Gaucher's cells and their accumulation causes massive enlargement of the spleen (causing hypersplenism) and liver. Destructive lesions may occur in the bones, especially the femur. Marrow replacement can lead to thrombocytopenia and leucopenia. In the *infantile and juvenile forms* of Gaucher's disease there is central nervous involvement with severe mental retardation and death. The glucocerebroside is derived from gangliosides which have a rapid turnover during infancy.

Niemann-Pick disease

The defect in this disease is sphingomyelinase deficiency leading to sphingomyelin accumulation in many cells types—spleen, liver, and other parenchymal tissues including the brain. Death in infancy is usual.

Lysosomal storage diseases

Lysosomal enzymes are very important in the breakdown of effete cellular components. If one of the enzymes is defective, the normal substrate accumulates in the cells, and frequently this is associated with cell damage and ultimately necrosis. There are three important groups of condition. In one type of *glycogen storage disease* there is a defective enzyme involved in the metabolism of glycogen. In the *mucopolysaccharide storage diseases* there is deficiency of the enzymes responsible for breakdown of the connective tissue components, dermatan sulphate, heparan sulphate or keratan sulphate. There are at least six syndromes, and of these Hurler's syndrome (gargoylism) is the best known. It is associated with severe skeletal deformities including a grotesque appearance of the head. The *gangliosidoses* are the third group of lysosomal diseases to be considered. The common is Tay–Sachs disease in which there is defective lysosomal hexosaminidase A. Ganglioside accumulates in the neurons of the central nervous system leading to deterioration that commences in infancy and leads to death by about the third year of life. The importance of the disease is its frequency in Ashkenazic Jews. In some groups about one person in 30 is a carrier, so that the chance of two carriers marrying and producing affected children is very high. Fortunately carriers can be detected and forewarned. Affected fetuses can be diagnosed by amniocentesis.

DISEASE ASSOCIATED WITH GENETIC CONSTITUTION

In spite of the great advances in biochemical genetics, there are many diseases in which the mechanisms involved are not understood. They appear to be more common in certain families, and are spoken of as *familial diseases,* but their occurrence and distribution cannot be predicted. High blood pressure, obesity and heart disease seem to fall into this group.

Sometimes particular characteristics are associated with certain diseases, though they themselves are not the obvious cause. The association of a particular disease with race, e.g. cancer of the breast in North American women, or with sex, e.g. goitres in women and cancer of the lung in men, is an example of this. In addition, innate immunity to infection (see p. 123) is an inherited characteristic, and so is the inherited liability to develop hypersensitivity (p. 138). The association of blood groups with disease has also been recognized; cancer of the stomach is more frequent in group A subjects, while duodenal ulceration is more common in those of group O. There is a relationship between certain histocompatibility genes and disease, e.g. HLA-B27 and ankylosing spondylitis.

DISEASES ASSOCIATED WITH GROSS CHROMOSOMAL ABNORMALITIES

As mentioned on p. 19, the human being has 46 chromosomes in each cell, of which two are sex chromosomes and the remainder autosomes. Certain individuals have been found to have more than 46 chromosomes, while others have less (Figs 3.4 and 3.5). Finally, abnormalities in the shape or form of individual chromosomes have also been noted. These abnormalities may be considered under two headings:

1. *Alteration in number of chromosomes*
2. *Alteration in structure of chromosomes.*

Although the finding of a chromosomal abnormality is regarded as uncommon, it is now apparent that those cases detected in postnatal

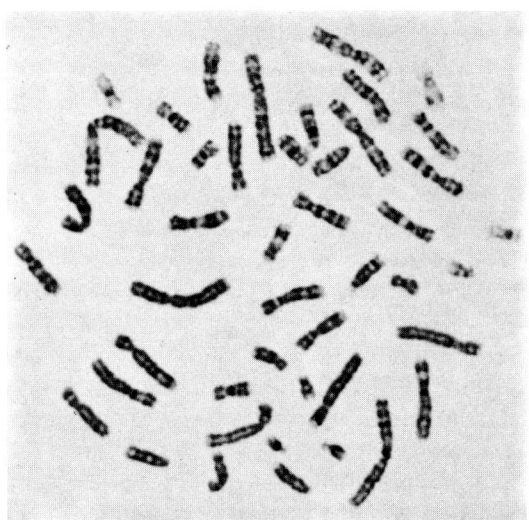

Fig. 3.4 Human chromosomes at metaphase. Lymphocytes from the blood of a normal woman were grown in culture for 72 h before colcemid (a colchicine derivative) was added. This chemical inhibits spindle formation so that mitoses are halted at metaphase. Two hours later a hypotonic solution was added to make the cells swell. The dispersed chromosomes were then stained with Giemsa after they had been pretreated with trypsin. This technique brings out the banding of the chromosomes.
    The mitosis shown contains 46 chromosomes, each of which is a divided structure joined by a centromere. The individual chromosomes can be cut out with scissors and arranged in pairs as shown in Fig. 3.5. Such an arrangement is called a karyotype. (Photography by courtesy of Dr H A Gardner, Director of Genetic Services, Oshawa General Hospital, Oshawa, Canada. From Walter J B (1992) An introduction to the principles of disease, 3rd edn, W B Saunders, Philadelphia.)

life represent only the residue of a much larger group of abnormal zygotes. About half the spontaneous abortions in the first 3 months of pregnancy have chromosomal anomalies, one of the commonest being triploidy (the cells having 69 chromosomes). About 30% of zygotes are aborted spontaneously, and gross genetic errors are clearly a major cause.

ALTERATION IN NUMBER OF CHROMOSOMES

Additional chromosomes

The commonest example is where there is one extra chromosome.

Trisomy

The presence of three chromosomes of a kind instead of two is called trisomy. An example is Down's syndrome (trisomy 21, or mongolism) in which a child is born with three of the 21 chromosome. Usually the total number of chromosomes is 47, and the karyotype is recorded as 47, XX, 21+ (or 47, XY, 21+ according to the child's sex). In occasional cases the additional 21 chromosomes is translocated to the 15 chromosome, so that the total number is 46. This *translocation mongolism* is important because the chromosomal defect is frequently present in one of the parents without producing clinical effects. In these circumstances the chromosomal defect is transmitted to many of the offspring.

The characteristic manifestations of Down's syndrome, the mongoloid facial features and the mental defect, are all too familiar, since such children are produced with an incidence of approximately 1 in every 600 live births (Fig. 3.6).

Several other syndromes are recognized in which other autosomes are trisomic, but they are rare.

The presence of additional sex chromosomes is not uncommon. Certain individuals are found to have an extra X. Some are apparent males, have the genetic constitution 47, XXY, and their cells are chromatin positive. They have small testes which fail to develop at puberty, there is little facial hair, they may have a female

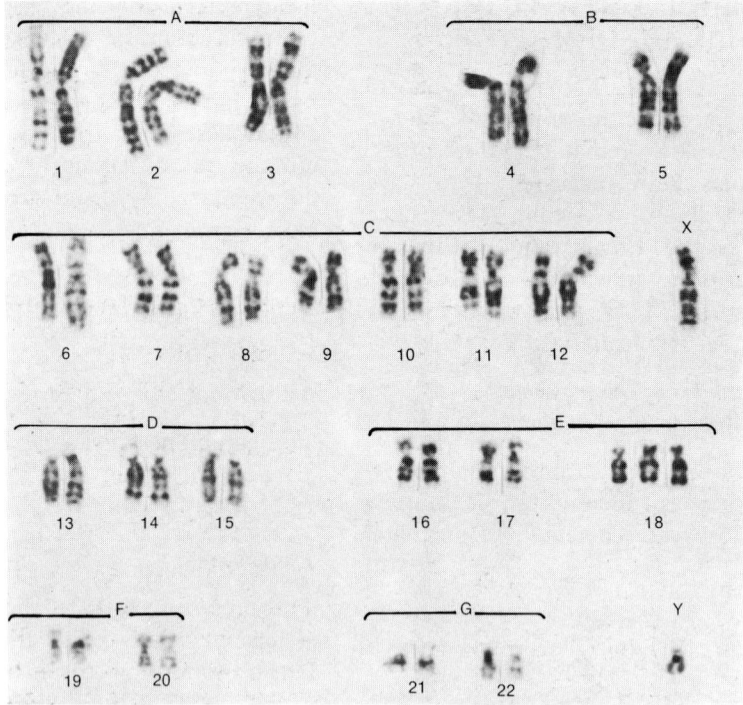

Fig. 3.5 Karyotype showing trisomy 18 from a stillborn male with cyclopia. The karyotype is that of a cell with 47 chromosomes. It is evidently from a male, since there is a Y chromosome. The anomaly must therefore be of fetal origin, since the mother had a normal 46, XX karyotype. The additional chromosome No. 18 arose by nondisjunction; its manifestations were incompatible with postuterine life. (Reproduced from Walter J B (1992) An introduction to the principles of disease, 3rd edn, W B Saunders, Philadelphia with permission of the publishers.)

type of breast development (*gynaecomastia*), and are sterile. These features become evident at puberty, and the condition is known as *Klinefelter's syndrome*. Another group of patients are the *poly-X females*, 47, XXX, who are females having an extra X.

In the 47, *XYY syndrome* there is normal male development, but some individuals are abnormally tall and exhibit a criminally aggressive temperament.

Reduction in number of chromosomes

The loss of an autosome appears to be incompatible with postuterine life. In those cases where such a state has been described, a small chromosome is involved, and it seems likely that the chromosome is in fact present but has become attached to another chromosome (i.e. it has been translocated).

The sex chromosomes appear to be less vital, and deletion of one is compatible with life. About 1 in every 3000 births produces a female with 45 chromosomes, having the normal number of autosomes but with only one X. This 45, X, or *ovarian dysgenesis syndrome*, becomes obvious at adolescence, when ovulation and menstruation fail to occur. Such individuals are short, stunted, and sterile. When accompanied by two or more of a number of somatic abnormalities, e.g. webbing of the neck, a shield-like chest with widely-spaced nipples, short fourth metacarpal bone, coarctation of the aorta, or hypoplastic nails, the eponym *Turner's syndrome* is applied. Their cells are chromatin negative, since only one X is present.

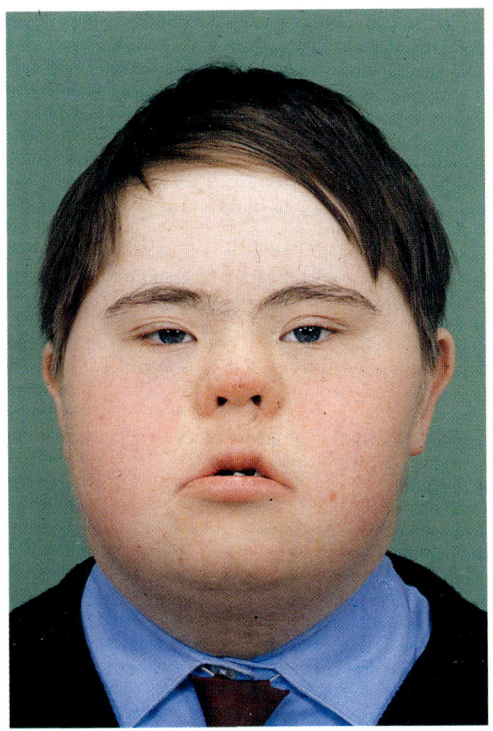

Fig. 3.6 Down's syndrome. Hypoplasia of the middle third of the face with relative mandibular prognathism. Oval slanting eyes and prominent epicanthic folds which cover the inner canthus of the eyes as in the Mongolian races. (Photograph by courtesy of the Department of Clinical Illustration, Birmingham Dental School, Birmingham, England. Previously published in Rock W P, Grundy M C, Shaw L 1988 Diagnostic picture tests in paediatric dentistry, Wolfe Medical Publications, London)

ABNORMALITIES OF CHROMOSOME STRUCTURE

Many abnormalities in the size, shape, or banding of chromosomes have been described. These will not be considered in detail. Sometimes a portion of a chromosome is deleted, and the remaining portions join together to form a *ring chromosome*. Translocation results in abnormal chromosomes (see translocation mongolism).

Although certain syndromes, many of them very uncommon, are now recognized as being accompanied by chromosomal abnormality, the actual pathogenesis is obscure. In a number of tumours the affected neoplastic cells have been found to have a constant chromosomal abnormality. The best known example of this is *chronic myeloid leukaemia*, in which the abnormal white cells and red-cell precursors, in some cases, lack one arm of chromosome 22. This small chromosome is called the *Philadelphia*, or *Ph'*, *chromosome*. Again, the significance of this finding is not understood, but the deletion is a useful diagnostic marker for this type of leukaemia.

AVOIDANCE OF GENETIC DEFECTS

Genetic counselling may serve to persuade some high-risk couples from procreation, but once conception has occurred, the only course open may be the induction of an abortion.

AMNIOCENTESIS

Screening between the 14th and 16th week involves removing 15 ml of amniotic fluid from the amniotic sac through the anterior abdominal wall. Fetal cells which have been shed into the amniotic sac are then grown. This technique is not without risk; in 1% there may be leakage of amniotic fluid. It is offered to mothers over 35 years and to those with a family history of genetic abnormality. *Down's syndrome* and other chromosomal abnormalities can be detected as can the sex of the child. *X-Linked* inherited diseases can therefore be detected, and the parents can decide whether to limit their family to girls in order to prevent the birth of a son with a serious condition. However, it must be remembered that 50% of sons will be normal. *Spina bifida* and *anacephaly* can also be detected by an assay of α-fetoprotein, a rise being due to the amount of choroid plexus exposed. More recently, DNA probes have been used to detect abnormal genes.

ULTRASOUND

This non-invasive technique can be used to detect abnormal organs and to assess fetal maturity if dates are not known or are uncertain,

FETOSOCOPY

It is possible to take blood samples from the fetus to detect *sickle-cell anaemia*, *thalassaemia* and *haemophilia*. This method is not without risk.

CHORIONIC VILLUS SAMPLING

A sample of tissue is removed from the chorion, which is genetically identical to the fetus.

The detection of abnormalities gives the parents a chance to choose termination of the pregnancy rather than produce a baby with a serious abnormality. This is not an easy choice and is based not only on the medical information but also personal, religious, social and the psychological background of the parents.

ENVIRONMENTAL FACTORS CAUSING DISEASE

Much of human pathology is concerned with those diseases which are acquired in postnatal life as a result of the action of external factors. The effects of physical and chemical agents, living organisms, and dietary deficiencies are the common causes of these *acquired diseases*. It must not be forgotten, however, that the developing fetus is also sensitive to environmental influences—in some instances much more so than is the adult. Intrauterine events may produce defects which are present at birth (*congenital*), but which are not inherited, since no genetic mechanism is involved. Some congenital lesions of acquired aetiology may copy abnormalities of genetic cause; these are therefore called *phenocopies*. For example, the condition of small brain (microcephaly) may be inherited, or may result from intrauterine irradiation, or infection with toxoplasmosis. The other causes of congenital defects—infection, ionizing radiation, drugs, etc.—are considered in greater detail in Chapter 20.

A final point deserves consideration: hereditary diseases may be congenital, e.g. achondroplasia, but they may also appear later on in life, e.g. Huntington's chorea. The time of onset of a disease gives no indication as to whether the cause is environmental or genetic.

GENERAL READING

Emery A E H 1981 Recombinant DNA technology. Lancet 2:1406

Epstein C J, et al 1983 Recent developments in the prenatal diagnosis of genetic diseases and birth defects. Annual Review of Genetics 17:49

Gardner H A 1987 The genetic basis of disease. In: Walter J B, Israel M S, General pathology. Churchill Livingstone, Edinburgh

Gartler S M, Riggs A D 1983 Mammalian X-chromosome inactivation. Annual Review of Genetics 17:155

Harnden D G, Klinger H P (eds) 1985 An international system for human cytogenetic nomenclature (1985) ISCN. Karger, Basel

Kalter H, Warkany J 1983 Congenital malformations: etiologic factors and their role in prevention. New England Journal of Medicine 308:424

Leading Article 1986 Lysosomal storage diseases. Lancet 2:898

Leading Article 1984 Molecular genetics for the clinician. Lancet 1:257

Lewin B 1985 Genes. John Wiley and Sons, New York

McKusick V A 1983 Mendelian inheritance in man, 6th edn. Johns Hopkins University Press, Baltimore

Nora J J, Fraser F C 1981 Medical genetics: principles and practice, 2nd edn. Lea & Febiger, Philadelphia

Ryder L P, Svejgaard A, Dausset J 1981 Genetics of HLA disease association. Annual Review of Genetics 15:169

Stanbury J B, Wyngaarden J B, Fredrickson D S (eds) 1983 The metabolic basis of inherited disease, 5th edn. McGraw-Hill, New York

Thompson J S, Thompson M W 1986 Genetics in medicine, 4th edn. Saunders, Philadelphia

4. Cell and tissue damage

CELL DAMAGE

Since the tissues of the body are all ultimately derived from a single cell, the fertilized ovum, it is reasonable to assume that all the complex functions of the body and all the intricacies of disease will ultimately be explicable in terms of the function and disorders of individual cells. The concept of *pathology as a cellular study* stems from the invention of the compound microscope by Van Leeuwenhoek in the seventeenth century, and blossomed in the nineteenth century with its application to disease by the German school of pathology headed by Virchow. Recent advances in technology have extended this approach. Electron microscopy, with its resolution several hundred times greater than that of the light microscope, has enabled pathology to enter a subcellular phase. The damaged cells in disease can now be described at a subcellular, or even a molecular, level. This study has been augmented by applying chemistry to the examination of cells, using the techniques of *histochemistry*. Methods are now available for the intracellular identification of complex proteins, such as enzymes and antibodies, as well as relatively simple substances such as glycogen and haemosiderin.

Chemists have, however, exerted a quite different influence on the study of disease by adopting another approach. Instead of concentrating on the individual cell or its organelles, they have turned their attention to specific chemical reactions. Thus, in respect of the metabolism of galactose, most cells can be regarded as behaving in a standard way. One important feature in the metabolism of galactose is the enzyme galactose 1-phosphate uridyl transferase, which converts galactose 1-phosphate to glucose 1-phosphate. Deficiency of this enzyme produces the disease *galactosaemia*, which can therefore be explained without recourse to a microscope or the study of individual cells. This second approach to pathology has been of immense value both in the delineation of disease processes and in the treatment of individual patients. Ultimately this broad concept of biochemical disorder must be reduced to a cellular level. In the inborn errors of metabolism, this has already happened.

CELL DEGENERATION AND ADAPTATION

Various types of cellular degeneration or adaptation may result from the cells being submitted to a wide variety of adverse circumstances which may be either internal or external events. These may be summarized:

Internal events: *genetic error*—enzyme defects.
*deprivation of essential
chemicals*—e.g. hormones,
vitamins, oxygen, etc.
*immunologically mediated
damage*
loss of blood supply.

External agents: *physical*—heat, cold, trauma,
radiation
chemical—poisons, lack of
oxygen
microbial—microbial invasion
and the effects of toxins.

The agents that have been most studied are chemicals and hypoxia, and these will be described in more detail.

Damage caused by chemicals—biochemical lesions

The first hint of the mechanism of damage caused by chemicals was provided by the observation by Rudolf Peters that pigeons subjected to a thiamine-deficient diet developed severe neurological symptoms and died. No abnormality could be detected by histological examination of the brain, and it was surmised that a *biochemical lesion* was present and responsible for the symptoms. Peters found that thiamine is necessary for cell metabolism and energy production. Nerve cells, with their high metabolic requirements, are among the first cells to be affected, and this explains the nervous manifestations of thiamine deficiency. Many diseases are known in which a genetic error leads to the formation of a defective enzyme and a block in some metabolic reaction. These are the inborn errors of metabolism alluded to in Chapter 3.

Chemicals can produce biochemical lesions in a variety of ways. The chemical may closely resemble a normal metabolite. For example, cells fed with 5-fluorouracil respond to the agent as if it were uracil, but the abnormal end-product blocks other essential processes. This deliberate sabotage of cellular metabolism has been called *lethal synthesis* by Peters, and has been used with some success in the treatment of malignant disease. Thus local applications of 5-fluorouracil destroys the abnormal cells in actinic keratosis and actinic cheilitis. Another example of lethal synthesis is

the action of chemotherapeutic agents on bacteria. Thus, sulphonamides are treated as *para*-aminobenzoic acid by some bacteria. This ultimately blocks cellular metabolism. Likewise, penicillin blocks cell-wall synthesis, thus rendering the bacteria extremely fragile and easily destroyed by osmotic effects.

Chemicals can produce biochemical lesions in more complex ways. Although not toxic themselves they may be metabolized (generally in the liver) to toxic metabolites such as free radicals. Some of these are carcinogenic, others cause cell damage. A good example of the latter is the drug acetaminophen, which in large doses can cause liver necrosis. The effects of the toxic products can be neutralized by cysteine or one of its derivatives, and this provides an effective antidote.

Hypoxic cell damage

Hypoxia causes a reduction of aerobic respiration and therefore ATP production. This has many consequences. Active cells, such as muscle, cease to contract. Anaerobic glycolysis leads to the production of lactic acid within the cells and if the area involved is large there is acidosis. The sodium pump is impaired and the cells swell. Protein synthesis is reduced and if the changes are marked the cell dies.

The mechanism of cell death in hypoxia, generally due to ischaemia, is not as simple as it may at first sight appear. Much of the cell damage in hypoxia is produced not during the initial period of ischaemia, but during the later phase when the tissue is perfused again and reoxygenated. During this phase it is suggested that damaging powerful oxidants such as the superoxide radical are formed. Experimentally it has been found that the administration of agents that convert these active agents to less damaging substances reduce the amount of tissue damage. Such a procedure could possibly reduce the damage of an acute ischaemic episode, e.g. a coronary thrombosis or spasm.

The morphology of the degenerations

Various morphological types of cellular degeneration can result from cells being subjected to a wide variety of adverse circumstances. The names attached to these degenerative or reactive processes are mainly descriptive; while some are appropriate, others are frankly misleading. Two main groups are described. Firstly, there is a group associated with an *excessive accumulation of water* in the cell: these are *cloudy swelling*, *vacuolar degeneration*, and *hydropic degeneration*. Secondly, there is *fatty change*, which in the past has been subdivided into fatty degeneration and fatty infiltration.

Changes associated with accumulation of water

Cloudy swelling. This is generally described in specialized cells, e.g. those of the heart, liver, and kidney. The affected organ is swollen. Microscopically the cells are swollen and the cytoplasm is granular. From being a common descriptive term, cloudy swelling has now largely fallen into disuse.

Vacuolar or hydropic degeneration. The cells show great swelling (ballooning) due to an accumulation of fluid. This is the most severe form of this group of degenerative changes, and, although it is reversible, the affected cells frequently rupture and die. Examples of this are to be seen in the liver cells in acute viral hepatitis and in the basal cells of the epidermis in lupus erythematosus.

Changes associated with the accumulation of fat

An accumulation of excess stainable fat is a frequent finding in parenchymal cells; it is especially common in the liver, and its causes are the same as those of cloudy swelling. A fatty liver is enlarged, and is soft in consistency. On section its cut surface bulges and appears greasy. Its colour is pale and in severe cases yellow (Fig. 4.1).

Nature of fatty change. Electron microscopy has revealed that many normal cells contain small droplets of lipid, but (with the obvious exception of adipose cells) these are not visible on light microscopy. The lipid is found within the endoplasmic reticulum; this is well shown in the intestinal epithelial cells during fat absorption. Excessive accumulation of fat are found in

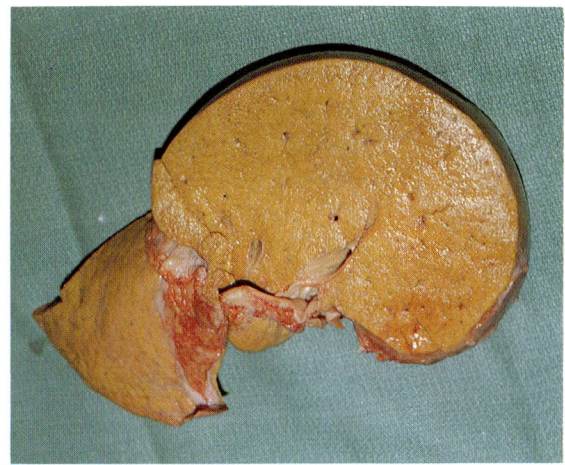

Fig. 4.1 Fatty liver. The cut surface of the liver shows the characteristic yellow colour of severe fatty change.

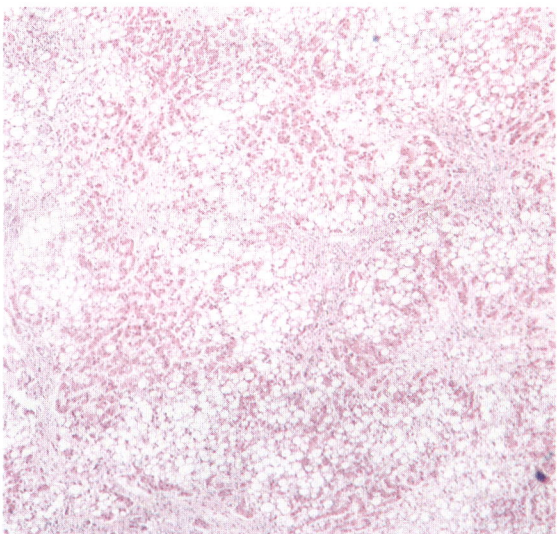

Fig. 4.2 Fatty liver. The normal lobular pattern of the liver is present but many of the hepatocytes are distended with fat globules that appear as empty spaces in the cytoplasm.

response to many adverse conditions, e.g. hypoxia and poisoning. This occurs readily in the liver, and the lipid accumulations appear in the rough endoplasmic reticulum and sacs of the Golgi complex. Such membrane-bound lipid droplets are termed *liposomes*. Later, if the adverse conditions persist, much larger, non-membrane-bound lipid droplets appear and gradually fuse together until one droplet comes to occupy much of the cytoplasm. Precisely how the liposomes evolve into these droplets is not known, but the process may be related to a defect in the synthesis of components needed to package lipid in the Golgi complex. The excess of fat that appears in damaged cells is derived from the fat depots in adipose tissue.

Depot fat is composed mostly of neutral fat, and when it is mobilized it is transported in the blood as free fatty acid bound to albumin. This is removed by the tissues and utilized for metabolic purposes. If the cells are damaged by hypoxia, poisoned, etc., their metabolic activity is impaired and the fat normally brought to them is inadequately utilized; it accumulates as droplets which are at first small, but later fuse into large globules (Fig. 4.2).

In the past the appearance of fine droplets was labelled *fatty degeneration,* while cells showing a large globule were said to show *fatty infiltration.* Clearly the pathogenesis is the same in each condition, and to avoid confusion both these terms have now been dropped, and *fatty change,* or *fatty metamorphosis,* substituted. It should not be confused with the accumulation of true fat cells in the tissues such as commonly occurs in the heart and pancreas of obese people. Similar local deposits of fat are also sometimes found accompanying chronic inflammation and following atrophy, e.g. of lymph nodes and thymus. These conditions are sometimes called fatty infiltration, but confusion is most easily avoided if the term *adiposity* is used. *Interstitial fatty infiltration* is an alternative name, but it must be clearly understood that the condition bears no relationship to the lesion depicted in Fig. 4.1 in which the excess neutral fat is in parenchymal cells.

Fatty change in the liver due to inadequate diet. The liver occupies a central position in fat metabolism. Non-esterified fatty acid derived from the adipose tissue is brought to it, metabolized, e.g. by conversion into phospholipids such as lecithin (phosphatidyl choline), and finally passed into the blood in the form of lipoproteins. If because of an inadequate diet there is a deficiency of choline, conversion cannot take place and neutral fat accumulates in the cells. This mechanism is the most probable cause of the fatty liver seen in starvation, and is particularly severe in kwashiorkor (p. 206).

Paradoxically, overfed animals may also show fatty livers; this may be due to a relative deficiency of lipotropic substances. The fatty liver of chronic alcoholism may in part be due to malnutrition, but in addition there is the factor of a direct action on the liver of large amounts of ethanol, and cirrhosis is an important complication.

Nature of the changes

It is often assumed that the cellular changes of cloudy swelling or hydropic degeneration are the same regardless of the organ affected, be it liver, kidney, or islets of Langerhans. Such is not the case. Electron microscopy has revealed a great variety of changes.

It is not easy to give a clear generalized account of the cell's response to injury, since relatively few cell-types have been investigated to any extent. Most work has been carried out on liver and kidney subjected to a variety of chemical poisons, e.g. carbon tetrachloride, ethionine, barbiturates, ethanol, etc. Some of the changes in the cell's components will be described.

Nuclear changes

A variety of nuclear changes have been described in poisoned cells. One of the earliest is clumping of the chromatin along the nuclear membrane and around the nucleolus. The nucleoli show loss of their granular component, and the fibrillar material is sometimes dispersed into separate segments. Nucleoli are therefore smaller but more numerous. The loss of granular material may indicate impaired synthesis of ribosomal material and messenger RNA. Reduced RNA synthesis is found in damaged cells, and this is reflected in the cytoplasm as reduced protein synthesis. It should be stressed that by light microscopy nuclear changes are not obvious or characteristic in cells showing degeneration.

Cytoplasmic changes

These may be considered under five headings.

Evidence of increased cell function. Cellular components may proliferate or reorganize in a manner which suggests a state of *hyperfunction* and adaptation. In response to certain poisons, e.g. phenobarbitone, the smooth endoplasmic reticulum becomes more abundant and forms complex whorls or gyrations (Fig. 4.3); this is regarded as an adaptive mechanism and indicates an attempt to increase the cell's ability to detoxify the substance.

It may also be the morphological expression of a drug-induced enzyme induction. Thus phenobarbitone causes an increase in smooth endoplasmic reticulum as well as leading to enzyme induction. The latter has the effect of increasing the metabolism of coumarin anticoagulants, a fact that must be borne in mind if the two drugs are given simultaneously. There is also increased enzymatic glucuronidation of bilirubin, an effect of therapeutic value. However, some agents, including carcinogens, cause a proliferation of smooth endoplasmic reticulum that is accompanied by decreased enzymatic activity. Likewise free ribosomes, rough endoplasmic reticulum, and the Golgi complex may proliferate; the number of lysosomes may increase, and mitochondria become more abundant, enlarge, and exhibit an increase in their internal complexity. Evidently the cell's metabolism is increased, for protein synthesis, ATP production, and catabolic activity may all be stimulated as may sometimes glycogen synthesis.

Micropinocytotic activity may increase, and this results in the appearance of numerous vacuoles in the cytoplasm.

Evidence of decreased cell function. Cellular components may become less numerous and show evidence of *hypofunction*. In damaged liver cells the rough endoplasmic reticulum shows dilatation of its sacs and loss of attached ribosomes. Polysomes are reduced in number. These changes are particularly associated with hydropic degeneration, and indicate *impaired protein synthesis*.

Mitochondrial changes are frequent. These organelles may show swelling and a loss of cristae. An increase in calcium content has also been described. Impaired function results in reduced oxidative phosphorylation, and ATP production is reduced. Since this substance forms the main immediately available source of energy for cellular

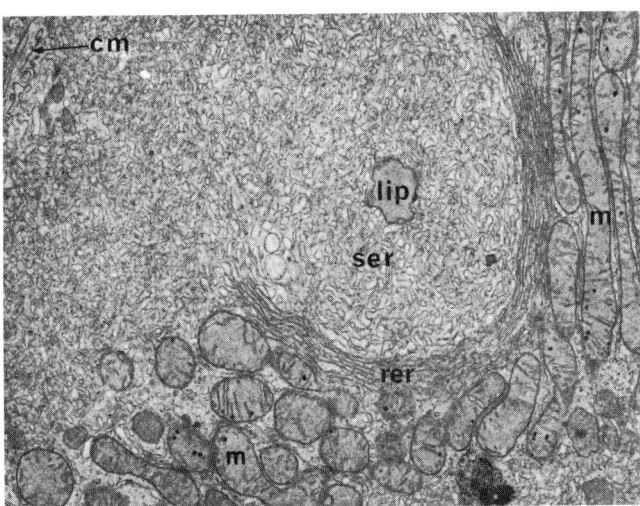

Fig. 4.3 Advanced proliferation of the smooth endoplasmic reticulum (ser) in the periphery of a rat hepatocyte following ethionine administration. The proliferated vesicles of the agranular reticulum are tightly packed and well demarcated from the rough endoplasmic reticulum (rer), which can be identified by the ribosomes studded on the membranes. Mitochondria (m) are elongated. cm—cell membrane; lip—lipid droplet. Lead hydroxide × 5500. (Photograph by courtesy of Dr. Katsumi Miyai, University of California at San Diego)

metabolism, it is not surprising that many cell functions are impaired. Thus ATP is required for the operation of the mechanism, or pump, regulating the concentration of ions in the cell. The sodium pump is impeded, and sodium and water accumulate in the cell, which in this way becomes progressively enlarged and waterlogged. The electrolytes can pass freely across the cell membrane, but the proteins within the cell cannot escape. When the sodium pump breaks down, there is therefore a *tendency* for the cell to become hypertonic. This is counteracted by the entry of water into the cell which thereupon swells. The breakdown of proteins into smaller molecules may further increase this tendency to hypertonicity. Mitochondrial swelling is commonly found in cells showing cloudy swelling.

Evidence of altered function. Changes may occur which indicate that the cell has acquired a new function; this is the basis of metaplasia.

Abnormal accumulation of substances in the cell. Lipid is an example, and has been described.

Degenerative changes. Localized areas of the cell may appear to become degenerate, and the term *focal cytoplasmic degeneration* has been applied. Sometimes cytoplasmic components, e.g. endoplasmic reticulum and mitochondria, are seen within vacuoles containing lysosomal enzymes. These are called *autophagocytic vacuoles*, *autophagosomes*, or *cytolysomes*, and an increase in their number is an indication of cell injury. Sometimes an area of cytoplasm degenerates and is actually cast off: damaged renal tubular cells can show loss of the brush border, which together with an area of the underlying cytoplasm is desquamated into the lumen. Such changes have been called necrosis of part of a cell.

Myelin figures. It is not uncommon to find intracellular whorls of laminated lipid material resembling the myelin of nerves. These are called *myelin figures*, and may either be artefacts or else represent real structures. It is well known that if hydrated lipid is allowed to remain undisturbed in vitro, myelin figures can form. Likewise, the prolonged fixation of lipid-containing tissue with glutaraldehyde (which fixes lipid slowly) will lead to the formation of myelin figures both within cells and in the extracellular spaces. Sometimes, however, myelin figures are present in membrane-bound structures containing lysosomal enzymes. These are called *myeloid bodies*, or *myelinoid bodies*, and are present whenever the secondary lysosomes are overloaded with lipid.

It should be appreciated that these various changes indicating hyperfunction, hypofunction, altered function, and focal degeneration can all occur within a single cell either simultaneously or sequentially. A damaged cell is not an inactive cell, and its reaction to injury may end in recovery. Parts injured beyond recovery are lysed or extruded, and the remaining structures reform the lost components. The cell may return to normal but some alterations may persist. Thus the retention of an abnormal function is seen in metaplasia and perhaps also neoplasia. The reaction of damaged cells is a highly complex and varied affair, but so far as routine human pathology is concerned it is rarely possible to obtain tissue fresh enough to detect these intracellular events even if time and equipment were available.

Not all the changes described above occur under any single circumstance. Cells subjected to adverse conditions show a complex reaction: some changes may be regarded as degenerative, while others are adaptive. A liver cell showing cloudy swelling due to carbon tetrachloride poisoning would therefore not be expected to show the same changes as one infected with a virus, or a kidney cell damaged by hypoxia.

Damage to DNA

Damage to DNA can occur in a variety of ways. An alteration in the sequence of nucleotides can occur as a result of a *mutation*. New nucleotides can be inserted as a result of *viral infection*. *Ultraviolet light* has the specific effect of causing damage to the bases without leading to a breakage of the polynucleotide chains. Dimers are formed between adjacent bases, especially thymine. This damage can be repaired by enzymatic action. First the chain is broken and the damaged segment is excised. A new section is then synthetized on the template provided by the undamaged chain. This is finally inserted into the chain by the action of a polynucleotide ligase. It follows that after the application of ultraviolet light to a tissue there is a burst of DNA synthesis which is not related to mitosis. This is termed *unscheduled DNA synthesis*. A defect in this repair mechanism occurs in xeroderma pigmentosum, and is related to the development of carcinoma.

Ionizing radiations also cause DNA damage. Both chains of the molecule can be broken and this may lead to chromosomal breaks. If only one strand of the double helix is broken, the lesion can be repaired by a process similar to that described for ultraviolet-light damage.

CELL DEATH AND NECROSIS

Cell death is difficult to define in precise terms, but in practice may be regarded as having occurred whenever a cell is incapable of further division or of continuing its normal synthetic functions.

The appearance of the dead cells varies according to the cause of the injury. If the cells are killed suddenly as the result of physical or chemical trauma, initially they show no changes other than those directly attributable to the agent concerned, e.g. disruption in electrical injuries, effects of freezing, burning, etc.

Cells less severely damaged, e.g. by poisons, may develop biochemical lesions which first result in degenerative or adaptive changes, e.g. fatty change. It will be recalled that the changes detectable by light microscopy are cytoplasmic, and in themselves do not indicate cell death.

In the dead cell, respiration ceases but glycolysis proceeds for a while and results in the production of lactic acid and therefore a drop in the pH. The synthetic activities of the cell stop, but the lytic destructive enzymes continue their work. These enzymes derived from lysosomes are most active at a low pH, and include a wide range of proteases, lipases, esterases, deoxyribonuclease, ribonuclease, etc. The cell undergoes a process of *self-digestion*, or *autolysis*, and within a few hours shows certain morphological changes (see below)

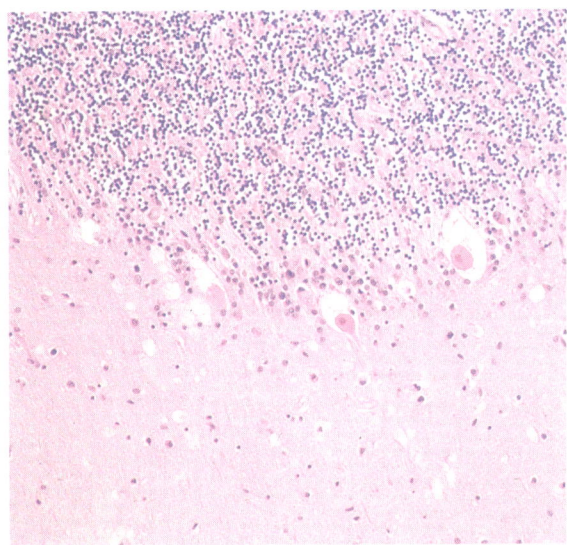

Fig. 4.4 Necrosis of Purkinji cells in the cerebellar cortex. The two large Purkinji cells in the centre of the field are surrounded by a clear space caused by marked shrinkage of the cytoplasm. There is also eosinophilia of the cytoplasm while the nuclei are pyknotic.

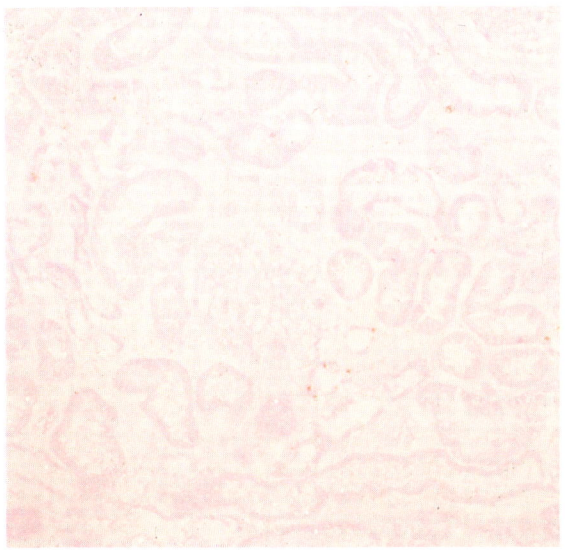

Fig. 4.5 Infarction of the kidney. There is good preservation of the general outline of the glomerulus in the centre of the field and the surrounding tubules, but nuclear staining is absent. All the cells are necrotic.

by which cell death can be recognized. This is called *necrosis* and it may be defined as the *circumscribed death of cells or tissues with structural evidence of their death.* Necrosis and cell death are therefore not synonymous.

The microscopic changes of necrosis affect the whole cell. The *cytoplasm* becomes homogeneous and often brightly eosinophilic; these early auto-lytic changes may resemble those seen in the degenerative lesions of living cells. Following cell death, however, the nucleus also shows autolytic changes, and it is these which are to be regarded as pathognomonic (absolutely diagnostic) of necrosis (Fig. 4.4).

Nuclear changes of necrosis

The nucleus becomes smaller, while the chro-matin loses its fine reticular pattern, becomes clumped, and stains intensely. This is termed *pyknosis*. The pyknotic nucleus either breaks up into fragments (*karyorrhexis*), or becomes indis-tinct as the nuclear material is digested (*karyo-lysis*).

Diagnosis of necrosis by biochemical means

A diagnosis of the occurrence of necrosis is frequently of great clinical importance. When areas of heart muscle, pancreas, liver, or brain are dying the patient's life is often in jeopardy. As necrosis occurs, various soluble substances, e.g. enzymes, diffuse out of the cells and are absorbed into the blood stream, and their detection is an aid to clinical diagnosis. Some examples may be cited. A raised plasma level of creatine phospho-kinase (CPK) is found after skeletal-muscle necrosis, and is also elevated in some types of myopathy (see also p. 283). Serum aspartate aminotransferase AST (previously called serum glutamate oxaloacetate transaminase (SGOT)), hydroxybutyrate dehydrogenase (HBD), CPK, and lactate dehydrogenase (LDH) are all raised after myocardial infarction. Increased serum alanine aminotransferase, ALT (previously called serum pyruvate transaminase (SGPT)) and LDH are found after liver-cell necrosis. Some enzymes can be separated into separate fractions by electro-phoresis, and particular fractions are in high concentration in certain tissues. Thus the MB isoenzyme of CPK is in high concentration in cardiac muscle, and a rise in its serum level is found in cases of myocardial infarction.

Types of necrosis

Coagulative necrosis

Necrotic tissue usually becomes firm and slightly swollen as its proteins are denatured. This causes the tissue to become opaque and firm, as does the white of an egg on boiling. It also becomes more reactive chemically, and side chains previ-ously saturated become exposed and are available for binding. This explains why the tissue initially binds dyes, e.g. eosin, more avidly than does normal tissue. Thus an increased eosinophilia of heart muscle fibres is a useful post-mortem indication of a recent myocardial infarct, and the magnitude of hypoxic brain damage can be judged by the extent and degree of the eosino-philia of the cortical neurons in patients who have died shortly after an episode of cerebral ischaemia, e.g. following cardiac arrest. The increased binding capacity of necrotic tissue might also be a factor in causing *dystrophic calcification* (p. 222).

A common cause of necrosis is sudden depri-vation of the blood supply to a part. This is called *infarction*, and is quite common in the heart and kidney when their supplying arteries are occlud-ed. These infarcts show the typical changes of coagulative necrosis. Microscopically, in addition to the nuclear changes, another feature is note-worthy: the general architecture of the tissue is still recognizable, even though its constituent cells are all dead. This is therefore called *struc-tured necrosis* (Fig. 4.5). In other examples of coagulative necrosis microscopic examination of the dead tissue fails to reveal any structure—this is *structureless necrosis*. The caseous necrosis of tuberculosis is an example of this (p. 164).

Necrosis in certain tissues presents special features. In adipose tissue, fat is liberated from the damaged cells, and is phagocytosed by macro-phages. These cells, distended with fat, are called *foam cells*. Deposition of cholesterol crystals, giant-cell formation, and fibrosis complete the microscopic picture of *traumatic fat necrosis*, as can occur in the breast following injury. Another type of fat necrosis occurs in the peritoneum whenever lipase escapes from the pancreas, as after its injury or inflammation (acute pancreatitis).

Colliquative necrosis

This is necrosis with softening, and rarely occurs as a primary event except in infarcts of the brain. Liquefaction is seen as a secondary event in suppuration (p. 59), and following caseation (p. 165).

Further changes in necrotic tissue

Necrotic tissue usually excites an acute inflammatory reaction followed by a phase of healing (Fig. 4.6): these events are considered in later chapters. Dystrophic calcification and gangrene are occasional complications.

Gangrene

Sometimes the dead tissue is invaded by saprophytic protein-splitting anaerobic bacteria, which cause its decomposition with the production of hydrogen sulphide and other foul-smelling substances. There is blackening of the area due to the formation of iron sulphide from the iron of decomposed haemoglobin. This *necrosis with superadded putrefaction* is called *gangrene*, an old clinical term which was applied to any black, foul-smelling area in continuity with the living.

Clostridial gangrene. The putrefactive bacteria are usually the clostridia of intestinal origin, and therefore necrosis of the bowel is often followed by gangrene. These putrefactive bacteria are of little importance in themselves, because they live on dead tissue and do not invade or harm the living tissue; nevertheless, gangrenous lesions always contain other bacteria which can cause further tissue destruction. It follows that gangrene is a very serious condition, and *unless treated expeditiously is fatal.*

Gangrene of the limbs. This is usually seen in the legs following arterial obstruction (p. 340). It is particularly common in diabetic patients. The limb becomes swollen and black ('wet gangrene'), and in addition to the putrefactive bacteria there are also pathogenic organisms present, which invade the adjacent living tissue. Gangrene of this type therefore steadily spreads (Fig. 4.7).

If the blood supply to a limb is *slowly* obstructed, the tips of the digits become black and necrotic, and at the same time undergo desiccation. This greatly impedes bacterial growth, and infection with pathogenic organisms is not a feature. The condition slowly extends until a point is reached where the blood supply to the tissue is adequate. A line of demarcation develops, and the dead tissue is discarded by a process of spontaneous amputation. This condition is called '*dry gangrene*', but since the amount of putrefaction is minimal, the term is somewhat of a misnomer. The process is in fact mummification of an infarcted portion of a limb.

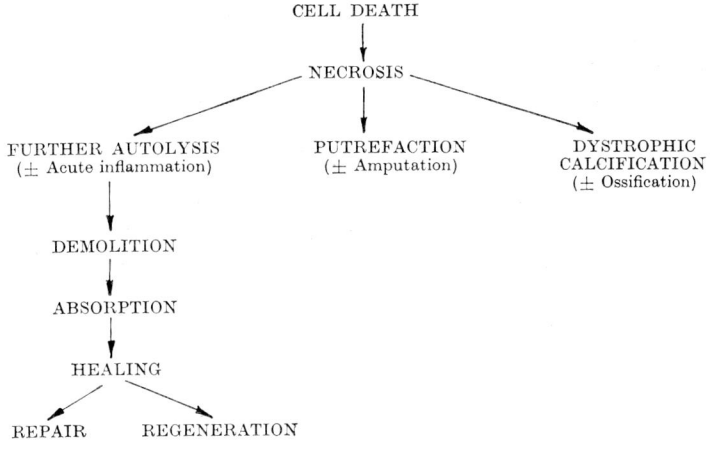

Fig. 4.6 The sequelae of cell death

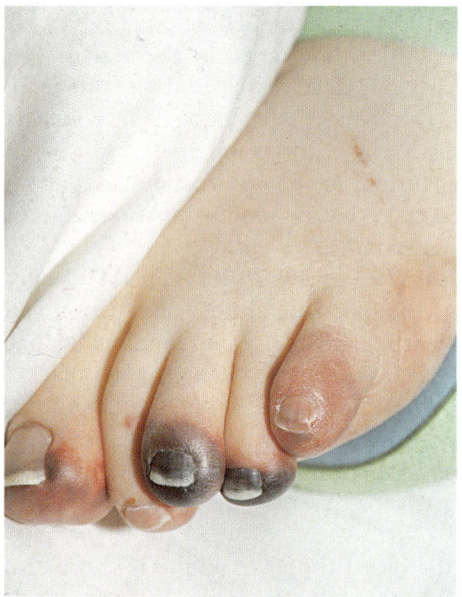

Fig. 4.7 Gangrene of the toes. All the toes show swelling and discolouration; the tips of two of them are black and gangrenous.

Gangrene due to other organisms. Some putrefactive bacteria are also pathogenic, e.g. certain strains of anaerobic streptococci (p. 155) and members of the family Bacteroidaceae. The latter includes the well-known member *Fusobacterium fusiforme*, which is often found in the company of *Borrelia vincenti* ('Vincent's organisms').

The putrefactive organisms mentioned are frequently associated with the common type of ulcerative gingivitis (Vincent's infection, or 'trench mouth'). It affects the free gingiva and the interdental papillae, and may be either acute or run a chronic relapsing course. A more severe gangrenous lesion which affects the soft tissues of the face, and may involve the bone is called *cancrum oris,* or *noma,* and occurs in malnourished debilitated children following an infectious disease, particularly measles. Extensive tissue destruction occurs. This condition is almost unknown in Britain and North America, but is not uncommon in developing countries.

Gangrene of the lung. A putrid lung abscess is an occasional complication of dental extraction under general anaesthesia, when the root of a tooth is inhaled and lodges in a bronchus. Once again organisms belonging to the family Bacteroidaceae are responsible for the putrefaction.

DAMAGE TO CONNECTIVE TISSUE

ABNORMALITIES OF COLLAGEN

The amount of collagen in a tissue is determined by a balance between collagen catabolism (presumably effected by collagenases) and the rate of collagen formation. Excessive catabolism, diminished synthesis, or a combination of the two lead to atrophy. The converse situation leads to fibrosis. It is unfortunate that in many human pathological conditions we are ignorant of the precise mechanisms involved and can only describe the end-results—either *atrophy* or *fibrosis.*

Collagen atrophy

There are many conditions in which collagen degradation exceeds collagen synthesis. *Glucocorticoids* inhibit collagen synthesis, and if administered in large doses over a prolonged period lead to generalized collagen atrophy. Thus the skin becomes paper-thin and bleeding follows mild injury. Osteoporosis (p. 405) poses a major threat. Local injections of glucocorticoids into the skin lead to dermal atrophy: this action is utilized in the treatment of keloids (p. 94) and hypertrophic scars.

Excessive production of collagenase is thought to be important in the pathogenesis of several diseases. In *rheumatoid arthritis* the destruction of the joint cartilage has been ascribed to the presence of collagenase produced by the synovium. The destruction of alveolar bone that leads to loss of teeth in *chronic periodontal disease* has likewise been attributed to collagenase activity.

Fibrosis

An increase in the amount of collagen, or *fibrosis,* is a common finding in chronic inflammation (see p. 102), and is a feature of any condition in which granulation tissue is formed. Thus myocardial fibrosis is the end-result of myocardial ischaemia as areas of necrotic muscle fibres are replaced by scar tissue.

In those organs where reticulin fibres are present the formation of type I collagen leads to production of histological collagen. This may explain fibrosis in organs like the spleen and lung.

Hyalinization

The term hyaline is used in a purely descriptive capacity—it literally means glassy, and is employed to describe any homogeneous eosinophilic material. Necrotic cells may take on this appearance, and under particular circumstances they have by tradition been described as hyalinized. Sometimes homogeneous areas in cells have been called hyaline. Thus eosinophilic areas in degenerating liver cells in the alcoholic patient have been called 'alcoholic hyaline' (Fig. 4.8).

Hyaline can also be used to describe extracellular material, and it is in relation to the connective tissues that the term is most commonly used. In collagen, with the passage of time, the fibres appear to fuse together to form a glassy, eosinophilic material. This hyalinization is very common in fibrous tissue which has been laid down as a replacement for lost parenchyma. Therefore it is very common in scars of any type and in chronic inflammatory lesions. Hyaline material is also seen in the intima of small blood vessels ('vascular hyaline'); it is a normal ageing process in the spleen, but in other organs, especially the kidneys, it is associated with hypertension.

Necrosis of collagen

Sometimes when connective tissue is damaged, its associated fibrocytes undergo necrosis and its fibres appear to degenerate. They break up, and are removed in the course of an inflammatory reaction. This necrosis of collagen differs from hyalinization in several important respects.

1 Hyaline material is extremely stable. Necrotic collagen, on the other hand, is either removed or organized.

2 Hyalinized collagen retains the staining characteristics of normal collagen. Necrotic collagen, on the other hand, is more eosinophilic and takes on many of the staining characteristics

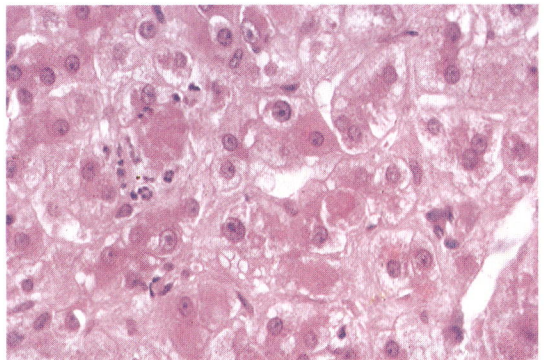

Fig. 4.8 Alcoholic hepatitis. The hepatocytes in this section of liver contain irregular clumps of eosinophilic material termed alcoholic hyaline. In addition some cells lack nuclei and are necrotic. A number of neutrophils are present in one area of the section.

of fibrin. The term *fibrinoid necrosis* is therefore often used. Fibrinoid necrosis is seen in the *walls of small blood vessels* in a variety of conditions: malignant hypertension (p. 326), the Arthus phenomenon (p. 139), and the generalized Shwartzman reaction (p. 78). The necrotic material may be degenerating collagen, damaged muscle, fibrin, or antigen–antibody complexes. Fibrinoid necrosis, like hyalinization, describes a particular microscopic appearance and does not imply a single morphological change or aetiological agent.

Fibrinoid necrosis occurs in collagen following severe injury, e.g. burning and exposure to ionizing radiation, and is also a feature of some collagen diseases (p. 145). It is particularly prominent in rheumatoid arthritis, and the degenerate material, which appears to be altered collagen, excites a chronic inflammatory reaction. This type of change is called necrobiosis; it excites a granulomatous reaction with epithelioid cells and sometimes giant cells.

CHANGES IN ELASTIC TISSUE

An increase in the number of fibres which stain black with orcein like elastic is a common finding in the dermis, and is a reaction to prolonged exposure to the ultraviolet light of sunshine.

CHANGES IN THE GROUND SUBSTANCE

Sometimes the connective tissue shows an excessive accumulation of ground substance, which appears as a basophilic pool of structureless material. This overhydration of the ground substance is sometimes a physiological event and appears to be under hormonal control: thus the colourful swelling of the sexual skin of the baboon is in large part due to this change. However, sometimes the associated connective tissue fibres undergo degeneration, and the condition is called *myxomatous degeneration*. A good example of this is seen in the aorta, where owing to the resulting weakness in the vessel its wall may rupture with dramatic effects (p. 346).

There is a group of genetically determined diseases involving an abnormality in the metabolism of mucopolysaccharide (*the mucopolysaccharidoses*). They are usually accompanied by skeletal deformities. The best known member of this uncommon group of diseases is *Hurler's syndrome*, which because of the grotesque appearance of the head is also known as *gargoylism*. Specialized texts should be consulted for details.

In this chapter some of the effects of cellular damage have been considered. Local injury is usually the prelude to inflammation and healing, and these are described in the chapters that follow. They are all local events, but it must not be forgotten that any injury, except the most trivial, is accompanied by a generalized response. This is considered in Chapter 25. Injury initiates changes which involve the whole individual, and it is a mistake to think of the reaction to injury solely in terms of local cellular degeneration or necrosis. Likewise at a clinical level, not only must the injuries be treated, but also the patient.

GENERAL READING

Dormandy T L 1983 An approach to free radicals. Lancet 2: 1010

Gelehrter T D 1976 Enzyme induction. New England Journal of Medicine 294: 522, 589, 646

Ghadially F N 1988 Ultrastructural pathology of the cell and matrix, 3rd edn. Butterworth, London

Halliwell B, Gutteridge J M C 1984 Lipid peroxidation, oxygen radicals, cell damage, and antioxident therapy. Lancet 1: 1396

Hayflick L 1976 The cell biology of human aging. New England Journal of Medicine 295: 1302

McCord J M 1985 Oxygen-derived free radicals in postischemic tissue injury. New England Journal of Medicine 312: 159

Naylor W G, Elz J S 1986 Reperfusion injury: laboratory artifact or clinical dilemma. Circulation 74: 215

5. The acute inflammatory reaction

Acute inflammation is one of the fundamental reactions of the body to injury, and although its pathogenesis is complex, the main features of the response are relatively simple and familiar to anyone who has ever experienced a boil. The area is *red*, *swollen*, *warmer* than the surrounding skin, and is *painful*. These four, *rubor*, *tumor*, *calor*, and *dolor*, are the *cardinal signs of inflammation* as described by Celsus (first century A.D.). Loss of function has been added subsequently but its origin is obscure. To attribute it to Galen is to perpetuate a misconception which has been handed down by many authors. Its Latin version *functio laesa* gives this origin an air of respectability but not truth.

The suffix *itis* is used to denote an inflammatory lesion, e.g. appendicitis or pulpitis. Unfortunately tradition sometimes demands that this rule be broken—e.g. osteitis fibrosa cystica is not an inflammatory lesion.

CAUSES OF ACUTE INFLAMMATION

Since the inflammatory reaction is a response to injury, its causes are those of cell damage. These may be enumerated briefly:

Physical agents. Trauma, e.g. mechanical injury such as cutting and crushing, heat, cold, and ionizing radiation.

Chemical agents. There are innumerable chemicals which injure cells either directly or by metabolism to toxic products.

Deprivation of blood supply. Infarction is described in Chapter 27.

Living organisms. Inflammation is often a feature of infection.

Immunological damage. This may be immunoglobulin mediated or T cell mediated.

CHANGES IN ACUTE INFLAMMATION

THE VASCULAR RESPONSE

Hyperaemia

Changes in the blood vessels are the most obvious manifestation of acute inflammation. Following trauma there may be an initial constriction of the blood vessels, but this is soon followed by a prolonged period of vasodilatation. It affects the arterioles, so that more blood passes into the area. Tissues near the skin surface are normally cooler than the arterial blood which supplies them, and, as the blood flow increases, so the area becomes warmer. This explains the *calor* of inflammation. The first result of arteriolar dilatation is that the blood flows by the most direct route to the veins through the *central*, or *thoroughfare, channels*. Subsequent opening of the precapillary sphincters allows blood to pass into the capillary bed, and vessels which were temporarily shut down become functional. The inflamed part therefore appears to contain an increased number of vessels. In addition, their calibre is increased. The whole area shows *hyperaemia*, i.e. it contains more blood and appears red (*rubor*). If incised it bleeds profusely.

Inflammation can be studied by examining fixed sections of tissue, but it is in the living animal that a truer picture of its ever-changing manifestations can be appreciated. Cohnheim based much of his classical description of inflammation on his observations on the tongue of the frog.

Changes in blood flow

In the arterioles of normal tissue the blood flow is so fast that the individual cells cannot be identified other than by the use of high-speed photography. In the venules the flow is considerably slower but it is still difficult to identify individual cells. However, they can be seen to travel in the central, or axial, part of the stream and leave a clear, cell-free *plasmatic zone* adjacent to the endothelium. In acutely inflamed tissue the velocity of the blood increases at first, but it soon diminishes. *Stasis* ensues, and coincidentally the clear plasmatic zone becomes occupied by innumerable colourless, glistening white blood cells. This is called *margination of the white cells*, and very soon the endothelium becomes covered, or *pavemented*, by them. This phenomenon is very characteristic of acute inflammation, and is due to changes in the white cells and the endothelium. White cells that strike the endothelium by chance, instead of bouncing off and passing on their way, stick to the endothelium and are retained. This adhesion between white cells and endothelium is believed to involve adhesion molecules. These substances are normally pre-

sent on the surface of both white cells and endothelial cells, but their number is increased by the action of certain chemical mediators that are formed during the inflammatory response. Thus chemotactic complement fragments increase the expression of leukocyte adhesion molecule LFA-1, while interleukin 1 causes an increase in the expression of endothelial intracellular adhesion molecule-1 (ICAM-1) which is a receptor for LFA-1. The adherent white cells, for the most part polymorphs, soon push pseudopodia between adjacent endothelial cells, penetrate the basement membrane, and emerge on the external surface of the venule. This remarkable process is called *emigration of the white cells*, and eventually large numbers of them accumulate in the extravascular space. The gap in the vessel wall closes up behind the emigrating white cells; a few red cells may, however, be forced out passively by the hydrostatic pressure of the blood. This is called *diapedesis of the red cells*, and must be distinguished from frank haemorrhage due to destruction of the vessel wall.

THE INFLAMMATORY EXUDATE

The most important feature of acute inflammation is the formation of the *inflammatory exudate*. This is a collection of fluid in the extravascular tissues and consist of a *fluid exudate* and a *cellular exudate*.

The fluid exudate

The really crucial factor in the formation of an inflammatory exudate is an *increased permeability of the vessel walls to plasma proteins*. If trypan blue is injected intravenously into an animal, the dye becomes bound to the plasma albumin and does not readily leave the circulation. When an inflammatory response is elicited, the tagged albumin can be seen to pass into the inflamed area as the exudate forms. A similar type of labelling may be done with radioactive iodine. In experimentally produced acute inflammation, it has been found that exudation of fluid occurs in several phases.

Immediate–transient phase. This lasts about 30 minutes, affects venules, and is largely mediated by histamine.

Immediate–prolonged phase. The exudation starts immediately but persists for days. It appears to be due to direct damage to vessels.

Delayed–prolonged phase. Capillaries and venules are affected both by direct injury of the agent and by chemical mediators. The reaction peaks at 4–24 hours after injury—an example of this is acute sunburn.

Mechanism of formation

As is described in detail in Chapter 27, the exchange of fluid between the blood vessel lumen and the interstitial tissues is related to the hydrostatic blood pressure within the vessel which drives the fluid out, and the effective, or colloidal, plasma osmotic pressure, also called the *plasma oncotic pressure*, which draws it into the blood vessel (Fig. 5.1). The effective osmotic pressure is due to the plasma proteins which are too large to pass through the vessel walls. Smaller molecules exchange with ease. In acute inflammation four mechanisms operate to cause fluid to leave the blood vessels and form the interstitial exudate.

1 There is an *increased vascular permeability* to plasma proteins. In this way the restraining colloidal osmotic pressure of the plasma is removed, and the hydrostatic pressure is free to drive a protein-rich fluid into the tissues. An exudate has virtually the same protein composition as plasma. This is the most important factor leading to the formation of inflammatory oedema.

2 There is an *increase in the capillary blood pressure* due to arteriolar dilatation.

3 There is *breakdown of large-molecule tissue proteins* into many small, osmotically active fragments.

4 There is an *increase in the fluidity of the tissue ground substance.* This has the effect of allowing exudate to diffuse more readily, thereby preventing an immediate rise in tissue tension. A rise in tissue tension is probably the important limiting factor in stopping the accumulation of tissue fluids both under normal conditions and those of acute inflammation. For this reason inflammatory oedema is a prominent feature of inflammation involving, or adjacent to, very lax tissues such as the eyelids and the scrotum. Swelling is not a feature of an infection involving a compact tissue such as the pulp of a finger.

Vascular permeability in normal tissues. Normally the walls of the capillaries and venules are freely permeable to water and electrolytes but not to proteins and other large molecules. Rapid exchange takes place between intravascular and extravascular water, and in fact about 70% of the water in the blood crosses the vessel wall every minute and is replaced by water from the interstitial space. The mechanism whereby this exchange takes place has been much debated. In most tissues the barriers which must be considered are:

1 The endothelial cell.
2 The basement membrane, which forms a complete sheath.
3 Pericytes, which form a discontinuous outer coat together with connective tissue fibres.

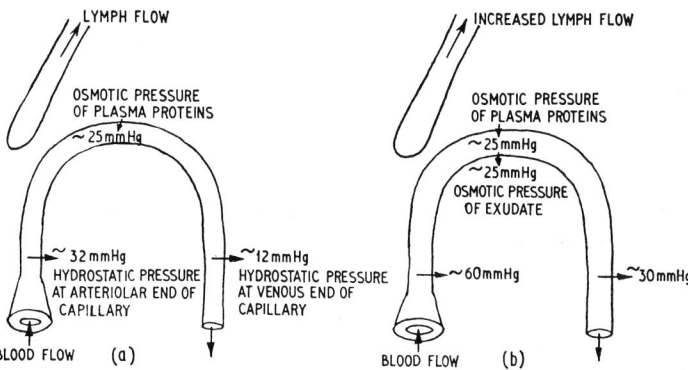

Fig. 5.1 Fluid exchange between blood and tissue spaces: (a) under normal conditions, (b) in acute inflammation.

The following possibilities have been suggested:

Direct transport through the cell by simple diffusion. The lipid (and presumably waterproof) nature of the cell membrane has led many authorities to regard this as an unlikely mechanism.

Transport across the endothelial cell by cytopempsis (p. 10). This process probably does take place, but it seems unlikely that it could explain the large volume of fluid which is known to leave the vessels. Furthermore, the vesicles formed by micropinocytosis would be expected to contain protein, but the fluid which escapes from the blood vessels has a low plasma protein content.

Passage through pores in the endothelial cells. Pores are present in the sinusoids of the liver; in certain other sites, e.g. kidney and intestine, there are fenestrations which are covered by a very thin membrane. In other areas no pores or fenestrations can be seen on electron microscopy.

Passage through spaces between the endothelial cells. The endothelial cells closely adjoin each other and the gap between them is about 15 nm wide. Junctional complexes are present, and in the zonula adherens (Fig. 2.4) the central fused membrane is about 4 nm thick.

The relative importance of these possible methods of transport is not clear at the present time.

A final consideration concerns the basement membrane, since all substances leaving or entering the vessel must cross it. The membrane appears to have no holes nor does it seem to be a barrier to the passage of water or electrolytes. Cells, large particles, and perhaps the plasma proteins are held back and their passage delayed.

Vascular permeability in inflamed tissue. Examination of the endothelial cells of capillaries in acutely inflamed tissue has revealed several changes—increase in the number and size of the micropinocytotic vesicles, blebs under the luminal cell membrane, and projection or spikes arising from the membrane. The changes are, however, inconstant and seem inadequate to explain the great increase in vascular permeability. On the other hand, important changes occur in the venules. Gaps (0.1–0.4 μm in diameter) appear in the endothelial lining due to the separation of adjacent endothelial cells.

If an animal is first given an intravenous injection of mercuric sulphide suspension, the particles, which are 10–15 nm in diameter, are found to be situated between the endothelial cell and the basement membrane. It appears therefore that in acute inflammation, endothelial cells contract and the gaps between them widen, thereby allowing plasma to reach the basement membrane and escape to the extravascular spaces. The particles of mercuric sulphide being unable to penetrate the intact basement membrane accumulate between it and the endothelial cell (Fig. 5.2). Whether other changes occur, for instance in the basement membrane, and whether the prolonged phase of exudation is associated with other features, is not yet clear.

As plasma escapes from the vessels, the plasmatic zone becomes reduced in size. This zone has great functional importance, for the viscosity of plasma is much lower than that of whole blood, and therefore the peripheral resistance is lower than it would be if the blood components were intimately mixed. In inflammation the lubricating action of this zone is impaired or lost and the blood stream slows. This is the explanation of the *stasis* of inflammation, and it may be so marked that thrombosis sometimes supervenes. This may cause further tissue damage.

Function of the fluid exudate

All the constituents of the plasma are poured into the area of inflammation. These include natural antibacterial substances, like complement, as well as specific antibodies. Drugs and antibiotics, if present in the plasma, will also appear in the exudate. The importance of the early administration of therapeutic agents is obvious when it is remembered that they are merely carried to the inflamed area in the exudate, and are in no way concentrated there. The fluid of the exudate (*inflammatory oedema*) has the effect of diluting any irritant substance causing the inflammation. The fibrinogen in it is converted into fibrin by activation of the clotting mechanism and a *fibrin clot* forms.

This fibrin has three main functions:

1. It forms a *union between severed tissues*, as in a cut.

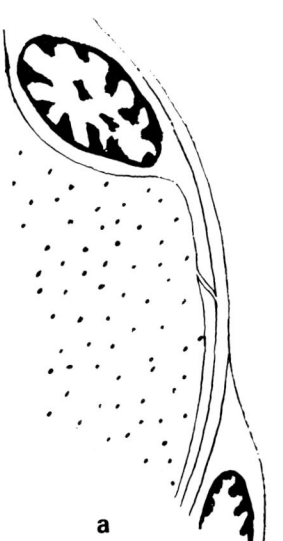
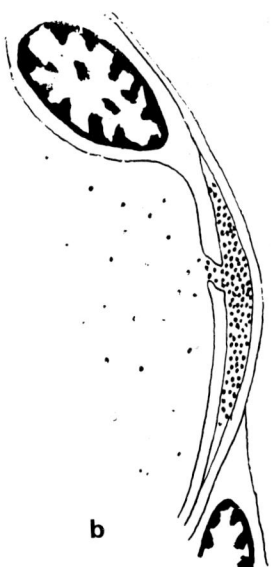

Fig. 5.2 Diagrammatic representation of the changes in a venule following the intravenous injection of a suspension of mercuric sulphide (particle size 10–15 nm). (a) Shows the wall of normal venule with the particles distributed in the plasma. (b) After the local application of histamine. The appearances suggest that the plasma has leaked through the gap between the endothelial cells, and that the basement membrane has held back the particles but allowed the fluid exudate to pass through.

2. It may form a *barrier against bacterial invasion* (p. 81).
3. It aids phagocytosis (p. 57).

The exudate accounts for the remaining cardinal signs of inflammation. It causes swelling (*tumor*), and the increased tissue tension is an important factor in the causation of pain (*dolor*), which is particularly severe in tissues that cannot swell readily, e.g. the pulp space of a finger, the pulp of a tooth (where pain is the only symptom), and the medullary cavity of a bone. Pain limits activity, and this explains the loss of function.

Changes in the lymphatics

The small lymphatics of a tissue form a blind-ended system of vessels, which closely resemble the vascular capillaries except that a basement membrane is incomplete or absent and their walls are permeable to proteins. Normally there is contraction of the lymphatics and this, in conjunction with the presence of valves in the vessels, assists the drainage of lymph so that it ultimately reaches the blood stream. In acute inflammation the permeability of the vessels is increased, they are held widely open and the flow of lymph containing excess protein is augmented. However, contraction of the vessels is inhibited and drainage is impaired, thereby favouring the formation of oedema.

The cellular exudate

The emigration of the white cells and their accumulation in the extravascular space has already been described (p. 52). These cells accumulate at the same time as the fluid exudate forms; they constitute the cellular component of the exudate (Fig. 5.3). At first the majority of the cells are neutrophil polymorphonuclear leucocytes, but later monocytes predominate. Within a few days the polymorphs undergo necrosis but the mononuclears remain. It therefore follows that *the cellular exudate changes from polymorphonuclear initially to mononuclear at a later stage.*

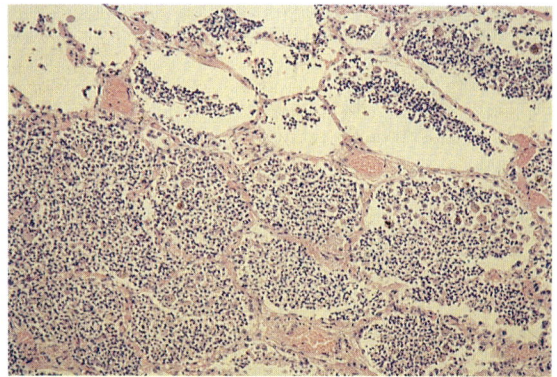

Fig. 5.3 Bronchopneumonia. Some alveoli are filled with inflammatory exudate containing densely packed neutrophils and scattered macrophage—cells with more abundant, eosinophilic cytoplasm. Adjacent alveoli contain scattered inflammatory cells only. The picture differs from lobar pneumonia in which the affected lung is uniformly affected.

Mechanism of formation

The stimulus which impels the white cells to force their way through the vascular wall and move to the area of tissue damage is generally thought to be the attraction of some chemical substance. Such directional movement in response to a chemical gradient is well known in biology, and is called *chemotaxis*. The *Boyden chamber* has facilitated the study of the possible mediators. Polymorphs are placed in the upper of a double tissue-culture chamber; the chambers are separated by a membrane of 3 μm pore size. Test substances are placed in the lower chamber, and the number of cells migrating to the lower side of the filter is a measure of the chemotactic effect.

Both neutrophil polymorphs and monocytes have been shown to be attracted in vitro to a number of agents; these include starch and certain bacteria. Antigen–antibody complexes and dead tissue are chemotactic, but only if complement is activated. The anaphylatoxins C3a and C5a, and leukotriene B_4 are the most important chemotactic agents. Kallikrein and some fibrinopeptides have also been claimed as chemotactic agents.

Chemotaxis has also been demonstrated with monocytes which appear to react to many of the substances which attract polymorphs. The change in the cell population of the exudate from neutrophils in the early stage of acute inflammation to monocytes later on has been the topic of frequent speculation. One explanation is that the polymorphs which have short life-span (3–4 days at most), soon die and disappear. The long-lived monocytes remain, an effect that could be accentuated by the presence of the migration-inhibition factor (p. 119), thus the relative number of monocytes would steadily increase. Another possibility is that the monocytes undergo division before assuming macrophage activity.

A number of observations now suggest that some chemotactic agents are selective in their action. Thus, when lymphocytes with specific receptors react with antigen, factors called lymphokines are released (p. 117). Some of these are chemotactic agents, and separate agents affect neutrophils, monocytes, eosinophils and lymphocytes. The reaction of antigen with mast cells sensitized by IgE causes the release of an agent that is chemotactic for eosinophils (see ECF-A, p. 139). This could well explain why these cells are prominent in some of the inflammatory lesions associated with atopy and also in many parasitic infections. Lymphocytes are found in certain inflammations, particularly viral infections and acute dermatitis. Chemotactic agents for these cells are poorly defined.

The varied and changing population of inflammatory cells found in inflammatory disease would be more easily understood if selective chemotaxis were the mechanism. Precisely how the phagocytes sense the presence of a chemical gradient and respond to it is not known. Movement is presumed to involve the actin–myosin contractible elements associated with the microfilaments of the cell. The energy needed is derived from the hexose monophosphate shunt.

Function of the cellular exudate:

Phagocytosis. The major function of neutrophils and macrophages is phagocytosis. They ingest foreign particles as well as bacteria.

Phagocytosis is aided by various mechanisms. *Fibronectin* aids phagocytosis by monocytes; there are other proteins present in the blood that also favour phagocytosis both by neutrophils and monocytes. One such protein, termed *non-specific opsonin*, coats bacteria and in association with complement aids phagocytosis. *Immune opsonins* are especially important in phagocytosis of virulent encapsulated organisms. The specific antibodies attach to the organism and leave their Fc component exposed. Neutrophils and monocytes have Fc receptors and their attachment to the organisms is the first step to phagocytosis. Immune opsonins are therefore an important defence mechanism in the immune individual. Complement activation is also important in aiding phagocytosis because phagocytes also have C3b receptors.

Surface phagocytosis. Phagocytes can ingest organisms even in the absence of opsonins, if a suitable framework is provided in which they can trap the organism. Fibrin provides such a surface, and the process is called surface phagocytosis.

The energy for phagocytosis both by polymorphs and macrophages is derived mainly from anaerobic glycolysis. Phagocytosis of a particle is accompanied by the production of lactic acid (p. 80). Following phagocytosis a series of metabolic events occur that have been called the *respiratory burst*, since they result in a dramatic increase in glucose utilization through the hexose monophosphate shunt. This burst of oxidative metabolism results in the formation of powerful oxidizing agents, such as H_2O_2, which are essential for the intracellular destruction of bacteria (p. 81).

Fate of ingested particles. Material ingested by neutrophils is enclosed in phagocytic vacuoles, the membrane of which fuses with that of the granules—both the specific ones and the azurophil granules. The lysosomal enzymes thus enter the phagosomes, and as digestion vacuoles are formed the neutrophils undergo degranulation.

Fate of ingested bacteria. The mechanisms whereby intracellular organisms are destroyed are described on pages 80–81.

Macrophages

These cells are highly phagocytic and play an important role in the destruction of microorganisms, particularly intracellular organisms such as mycobacteria and fungi. In addition to intracellular destruction, the mechanism of antibody-dependent cytotoxicity is involved. The macrophages also play an important role in the *demolition phase* of acute inflammation. They also have a *secretor function* and release a variety of agents termed *monokines*. These include lysosomal enzymes, lysozyme, plasminogen activators, collagenase, elastase, complement components, and members of a group of polypeptide termed *cytokines*. These include platelet activating factor, fibroblast stimulating factor, angiogenic factor and interleukin-1. *Interleukin-1* stimulates T helper cells, and acts as a pyrogen by acting on the hypothalamus to cause fever. Finally the macrophages play a part in the initiation of the immune response, by processing antigen and presenting it to T cells. In turn, their activity as effector cells is modified and stimulated by lymphokines released by sensitized lymphocytes.

Eosinophils

These cells are found instead of the usual neutrophil leucocytes in inflammation produced by many helminthic parasites and also in some allergic conditions (asthma and hay fever) which are accompanied by a high plasma level of IgE. Eosinophils are motile, but unlike neutrophils are poorly phagocytic. Their role in inflammation is poorly understood, but they may play a moderating part in allergic processes. Thus several of their granule constituents may alter the hypersensitivity reaction by inhibiting or promoting the action of mediators of inflammation, and arylsulphatase, preferentially present in eosinophils, inactivates slow-reacting substance of anaphylaxis (SRS-A). Stimulated eosinophils produce an inhibitor of histamine release which acts through the cyclic-AMP system.

Lymphocytes

The lymphocyte is a key cell in the immune response; this is considered in later chapters.

LOCAL SEQUELAE OF ACUTE INFLAMMATION

The changes which follow the formation of an acute inflammatory exudate depend upon two major factors (Fig. 5.4):

1. The amount of tissue damage sustained
2. Whether or not the causative agent remains.

Assuming that the causative agent is removed or destroyed, the initial polymorphonuclear exudate is replaced by a mononuclear one. Their appearance heralds the onset of the demolition phase. The mononuclear cells are phagocytic, and regardless of their origin are called *macrophages*.

Origin of macrophages. The macrophages which accumulate in areas subjected to injury in lower forms of life appear to be derived from histiocytes, which are resting tissue representatives of the *mononuclear phagocyte system* (MPS). In mammals tissue histiocytes may also perform a similar function, but the current evidence suggests that the majority of macrophages present in the stage of demolition are of bone marrow origin and the progeny of monocytes that emigrated from the blood stream.

Demolition phase

Macrophages engulf fibrin, red cells, degenerate polymorphs, bacteria, etc., and thereby perform a scavenger function. They therefore contain a variety of intracellular structures—fat, haemosiderin, cholesterol, and foreign material. Sometimes they fuse together to form giant cells. If the macrophages ingest large quantities of fat they become swollen and are called *foam cells*.

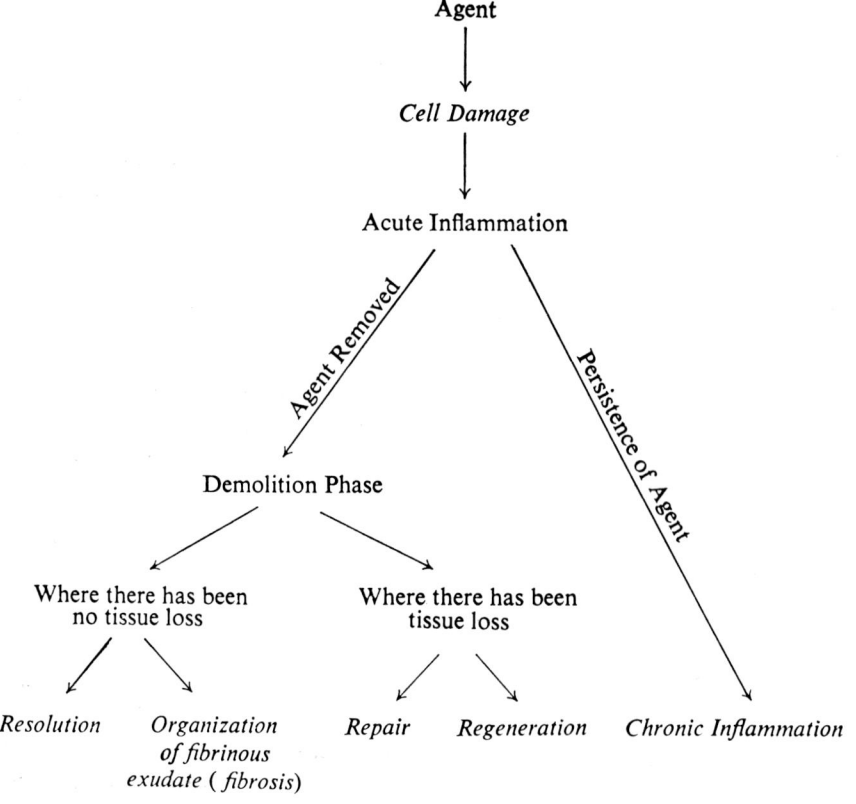

Fig. 5.4   The sequence of events following tissue damage.

Resolution

In acutely inflamed tissue in which cellular damage has been relatively slight, the cellular and tissue changes are reversible, and necrosis does not occur. The demolition phase results in the removal of the exudate, and the organ returns to normal. To this process the term *resolution* is applied, and one of the best examples is found in lobar pneumonia (p. 367). *Resolution thus means the complete return to normal following acute inflammation.*

It should be noted that while demolition is proceeding there is a reverse flow of exudate back into the blood vessels. Most of the exudate, however, is carried away by the lymphatics.

Sometimes removal of the exudate appears to be delayed, and invaded by granulation tissue. In this way fibrous adhesions, e.g. pleural and peritoneal, are produced.

Suppuration

When the noxious agent produces much necrosis, resolution is impossible and the process frequently proceeds to *suppuration*. This is typical of pyogenic infection, e.g. boils, but can also occur when the agent is a chemical substance, e.g. turpentine.

The first reaction is circumscribed necrosis accompanied by a profuse polymorph infiltration. The agent kills many of these leucocytes—which are often called 'pus cells'. The necrotic material undergoes softening by virtue of the proteolytic enzymes released from the granules (lysosomes) of the dead leucocytes as well as through the autolysis mediated by the tissue's own lysosomal enzymes. The resulting creamy fluid material is called *pus*, and is contained within a cavity to form an *abscess*. This is lined by a *pyogenic membrane*, which at this stage consists of inflamed and necrotic tissue with much fibrinous exudate and polymorphs. This soon undergoes organization into granulation tissue.

The pus itself is made up of:

1. *Leucocytes*, some of which are dead.
2. *Other components of the inflammatory exudate*—oedema fluid and fibrin.
3. *Organisms*, many of which are living and can therefore be cultured; if the pus is chemically induced it is sterile.
4. *Tissue debris*, e.g. nucleic acids and lipids.

The pus tends to track in the line of least resistance until a free surface is reached. Then the abscess bursts and discharges its contents spontaneously—in clinical practice this is usually anticipated by surgical drainage. An abscess when drained heals by granulation tissue, but sometimes chronic inflammation ensues.

If, as occasionally happens, the abscess is not drained but remains isolated, or sequestered in the tissue, its walls become further organized and converted into dense fibrous tissue and the pus undergoes thickening, or *inspissation*, as its fluid component is gradually absorbed. In due course it develops a porridge-like consistency, and may eventually become *calcified*.

When an acute suppurative inflammation involves an epithelial surface, the covering is destroyed; such a defect is called an ulcer. The floor is composed of necrotic tissue and acute inflammatory exudate; this layer of dead tissue forms a *slough*, and is at first adherent because the dead material has not been liquefied. Eventually, however, the slough becomes detached, and the ulcer heals by the process of repair and regeneration, as described in Chapter 8.

Chronic inflammation

The other sequel of acute inflammation is progression to a state of chronic inflammation in which the inflammatory and healing processes proceed side by side. This is described in Chapter 9.

CONCLUSION

Inflammation may be defined as *the reaction of the vascular and supporting elements of a tissue to injury, and results in the formation of a protein-rich exudate provided the injury has not been so severe as to destroy the area.* Acute inflammation is thus essentially a vascular phenomenon, and cannot occur in an avascular tissue like the cornea or cartilage. The reaction is usually beneficial, but this is not necessarily so under all conditions. The inflammatory cells may themselves spread infection (see Tuberculosis, p. 165) and the inflammatory oedema may, in a situation like the larynx, actually endanger life. The relationship between inflammation and infection is further considered in Chapter 7.

The term *subacute inflammation* is used by some authorities; it appears to mean a mild acute inflammation, but since no exact definition is possible, there seems no good reason for retaining the term.

THE CHEMICAL MEDIATORS OF ACUTE INFLAMMATION

The apparent uniformity of the inflammatory response irrespective of its cause has led many investigators to presume that the changes are mediated by chemical agents which are formed when tissue is damaged, rather than being caused directly by the damage itself. The search for these mediators has a practical as well as a theoretical objective. If they could be identified, antagonistic drugs might be designed and administered to prevent or modify the acute inflammatory response.

Many mediators have been identified and the list seems to be never-ending; only a brief account will be given with emphasis on those agents that seem to be of importance in human pathology. The mediators may be classified as follows:

I.   Amines
      (a) histamine
      (b) 5-hydroxytryptamine (5-HT)
II.   The kinins
III. Kinin-forming enzymes
      (a) kallikrein
      (b) plasmin
IV.   Biologically active products of the complement system
V.   Biologically active components of the polymorphs
VI.   Arachidonic acid derivatives
      (a) prostaglandins
      (b) leukotrienes
VII. Others.

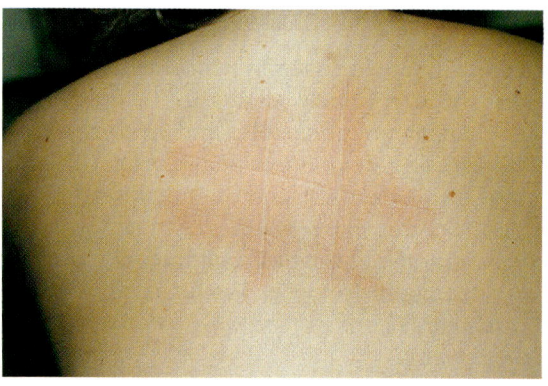

Fig 5.5 Dermographism. The back of this patient illustrates the triple response obtained by applying firm pressure with a blunt instrument about 3 min before the photograph was taken. Each line shows a central pale weal surrounded by an erythematous ill-defined flare.

The amines

Histamine

The classical experiments of Lewis on the triple response showed that injury to the skin produced a type of inflammation which had many features in common with the effect of an injection of histamine. Lewis showed that injured skin released some substance ('H' substance) which behaved like histamine (Fig. 5.5).

There is good evidence that histamine is liberated in acute inflammation, and that it can mimic some of the vascular events. It seems likely that it is important during the early phase and in certain immune mediated responses (see p. 138).

Histamine is contained in the granules of mast cells. It can be released by injury, by the action of various histamine-releasing agents (including the anaphylatoxins C3a and C5a), and by antigen if the cells have been previously sensitized by IgE (see later).

5-Hydroxytryptamine (5-HT, or serotonin)

5-HT rather than histamine is liberated in rats during the early phase of acute inflammation; it is liberated from mast cells or platelets.

The kinins

The name kinin has been applied to a variety of

physiologically active polypeptides which cause contraction of smooth muscle. *Bradykinin* is the most important, and was so named because of the slow contraction which it induces in vitro in the muscle of the guinea-pig ileum; it appears to be the active agent in producing the effects of poisoning due to certain snakebites. It may also be concerned in the regulation of blood flow in the salivary glands.

The kinins are formed from precursor kininogens by the action of the enzymes *kallikrein* or *plasmin* (Fig. 5.6). Two groups of kininogens are

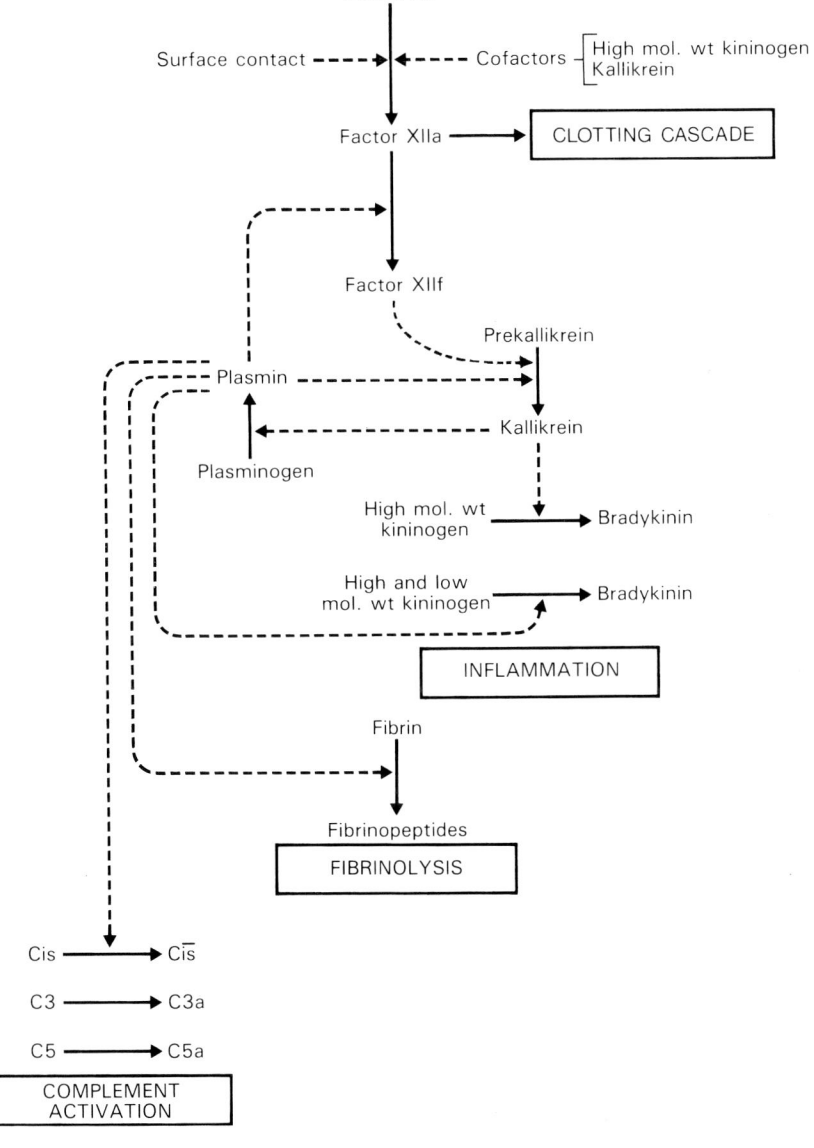

Fig. 5.6 The current hypothesis for the activation of the kinin system. Note the central role of Hageman-factor (factor XII) activation which initiates clotting, fibrinolysis, and kinin formation. Factor XIIa has a major role in initiating the clotting cascade but a minor one in activating prekallikrein. Factor XIIf, on the other hand, has as its major action the activation of prekallikrein to kallikrein. Transformations are depicted as solid lines, while enzymatic actions are shown as interrupted lines. Inhibitors are not shown. They include α_1-macroglobulin, α_2-antiplasmin, antithrombin III, and C_1 inactivator (also called C_1-esterase inhibitor).

known. The *low-molecular-weight kininogens* are acted upon by plasmin only, while the *high-molecular-weight kininogens* are the substrate for both kallikrein and plasmin.

Bradykinin, a nonapeptide, has been synthetized, and is ten times more active as a vasodilator than is histamine (on a molar basis). It produces pain when applied to tissue. Bradykinin also causes an increase in vascular permeability and stimulates the contraction of smooth muscle, but is not chemotactic to white cells; and it has been suggested that it acts as a mediator during the early phases of acute inflammation.

Kallikrein*

Kallikrein is an enzyme that can form bradykinin from high-molecular-weight kininogen of the blood. It can also activate Hageman factor (Factor XII) to Factor XIIa, and is chemotactic to white cells. The enzyme exists as an inactive precursor (*prekallikrein*), which can itself be activated by Factor XIIf. Plasma kallikrein is one member of a group of enzymes that can form kinins from plasma. Others occur in urine, pancreas and snake venom.

Plasmin

Plasminogen is a normal component of the plasma proteins. It can be converted into plasmin by the action of kallikrein (previously called plasminogen activator). Plasmin itself is a proteolytic enzyme, and digests fibrin as well as other plasma proteins. The breakdown of fibrin leads to the formation of a variety of polypeptides (*fibrinopeptides*) that have a number of properties, including anticoagulant activity, the ability to increase vascular permeability, and being chemotactic to white cells.

Plasmin can increase vascular permeability in many ways. It can act directly on kininogen to liberate kinin; this action is slow compared with that of kallikrein. Secondly, it can activate prekallikrein to kallikrein. Finally, it can act on the third component of complement to produce C3a

---

*Kallikrein is so called because it is found in high concentrations in pancreas. Kallikreas is Greek for pancreas.

and on Factor XIIa to produce Factor XIIf.

Other proteolytic enzymes have been described. One is present in skin, and another, present in white blood cells, leads to the formation of leucokinin.

Biologically active cleavage products of complement

Activation of the complement system leads to the formation of two anaphylatoxins, C3a and C5a, which cause the release of histamine from mast cells. They also exert a chemotactic influence. These components are important in the pathogenesis of the inflammation present in some lesions of immune-complex disease (p. 139). The alternate pathway of complement activation explains how vasoactive complement components can be formed following tissue damage which is not immunologically mediated. Necrotic tissue, e.g. heart muscle, can release enzymes capable of activating C3, and so also can the lysosomal enzymes released from polymorphs. What part they play in inflammation in the non-immune animal and that due to trauma is not known.

Biologically active components of polymorphs

Neutrophils release a variety of agents in acute inflammation. The following agents have been described:

Cationic proteins. These have various actions, including direct action on blood vessels to increase permeability, histamine-releasing factors, neutrophil-immobilizing factor, and a chemotactic factor for monocytes.

Acid proteases. These act on a kininogen to produce a kinin (leucokinin).

Neutral proteases. These have been credited with many activities: they degrade collagen, basement-membrane material, fibrin, etc., they cleave C3 and C5 to form active products, they activate kininogen to kinin, and they have a direct effect on blood vessels to increase their permeability. These actions are inhibited by α_1-antitrypsin.

The release of these various neutrophil substances may occur by a type of secretion, as the contents of granules are discharged by exocytoxis—particularly during phagocytosis. They are also released when the cell dies and undergoes autolysis.

It is evident that the role of polymorphs in acute inflammation is very complex. Under some circumstances they provide protection against microorganisms, since infection introduced into animals rendered leucopenic can be spreading and lethal, while a similar infection in a normal animal would lead merely to a local acute inflammation. On the other hand, the damage seen in the lesions of the Shwartzman reaction and in the vasculitis of immune-complex disease appears to be produced by agents released by the polymorphs.

Arachidonic acid derivatives

When cells are disturbed or damaged, phospholipid in the cell membrane is acted upon by phospholipase A_2 to form arachidonic acid. This is further metabolized to form two important groups of substances—the *prostaglandins* (PG) and the *leukotrienes* (LT) (Fig. 27.3). These are regarded as secondary mediators because they are formed in cells, e.g. mast cells, rather than being released from preformed products stored in granules.

The leukotrienes (LT)

This group of long chained fatty acids includes LTB_4 which is the most potent chemotactic factor known for both polymorphs and monocytes. A mixture of LTC_4, LTD_4 and LTE_4 is a vasoactive mixture with a histamine-like action but far more potent; it was previously known as *slow-reacting substance of anaphylaxis (SRS-A)*, and is released from mast cells. It is believed to be a mediator of the inflammatory reaction and also important in the pathogenesis of bronchial asthma.

The prostaglandins

The name prostaglandin was given to a substance found in human seminal fluid by von Euler. Prostaglandins have been isolated from virtually every tissue of the body, and have been grouped on the basis of their chemical structure. They are derivatives of prostanoic acid, the 20-carbon parent substance. They are credited with many diverse functions—from acting as chemical transmitters in the nervous system to playing an important role in parturition. Their role in thrombosis is described on page 331. They have been isolated in the tissues of human skin in allergic contact dermatitis, and are released from polymorphs during phagocytosis.

Some, e.g. PGE_1 and PGE_2, produce vasodilatation, increase vascular permeability, and cause pain; others have converse effects, protecting tissues from these actions. An effect of some prostaglandins that may be of importance is their potentiation of the action of kinins in increasing vascular permeability. The prostaglandins may therefore be significant mediators of acute inflammation either by a direct action or, more likely, by regulating or *modulating* the action of other mediators.

One important source of prostaglandin is the platelet, which contains prostaglandin-forming enzymes. It is significant that aspirin and indomethacin both inhibit the formation of prostaglandins from the substrate arachidonic acid, and thereby have an anti-inflammatory action. The release of prostaglandins from platelets is inhibited by glucocorticoids.

Other possible mediators

Many other possible mediators of acute inflammation have been described. Platelet activating factor (PAF) is a lipid that is released from mast cells that in addition to causing aggregation of platelets, is chemotactic to white cells, increases vascular permeability and causes vasodilatation. *Lactic acid* is present in inflamed tissue, and may play a part in the vasodilatation and change in vascular permeability. The *lymphokines*, which are described in Chapter 11, are undoubtedly liberated in certain types of inflammation in which immune mechanisms are involved.

It is possible that some *bacterial toxins* are capable of directly initiating or modifying the inflammatory response. The gas-gangrene organisms, in particular *C. novyi*, produce toxins which appear to act directly upon blood vessels and increase their permeability.

It is instructive to summarize the role of the mast cells and platelets at this point.

ROLE OF THE MAST CELL

The mast cells can release the contents of their granules when directly injured, and also in response to a number of other stimuli. C5a is a cleavage product of C5 (p. 125), and has such an action; it is the classical anaphylatoxin, so named because its formation, by causing the release of histamine, can produce a state resembling acute anaphylactic shock. C3a is another anaphylatoxin, but is less potent. Another agent is one of the cationic proteins of polymorphs. Mast-cell degranulation can be mediated immunologically; if the cells are coated with IgE, contact with antigen causes degranulation.

Mast cells release many substances including: histamine, 5-HT, heparin, eosinophil-chemotactic factor of anaphylaxis, and platelet-activating factor. In addition secondary mediators derived from arachidonic acid, such as SRS-A, are formed.

ROLE OF THE PLATELETS

Platelets become adherent to areas of vascular damage, and undergo a release reaction whereby the contents of their granules are liberated. The dense granules contain vasoactive amines (histamine or 5-HT according to species), while the α granules contain lysosomal enzymes.

SUMMARY

The number of chemicals that have been suggested as mediators of acute inflammation is now so large, and their inter-relationship is so complex, that it is not possible to give any clear account of their role in acute inflammation. Indeed, as noted by Ryan and Majno, the inflammatory 'soup' is so complicated that no single individual can claim to know how the dozens of components relate to each other or how they change during the evolution of an inflammatory response.

It is generally agreed that the exudation of acute inflammation involves both capillaries and venules. The capillaries are so narrow that any marked increase in their permeability would bring about their blockage; the resulting ischaemia would lead to a cessation of the inflammatory process and necrosis of the area involved. It is doubtful whether any such mechanism would be evolved. In support of this contention is the observation that capillaries do not respond to the action of vasoactive drugs. Hence it is unlikely that any mediator acts directly on the capillaries. On the other hand, capillaries do appear to respond to direct injury.

The present evidence suggests that the capillary changes in acute inflammation are due to a direct effect of the injuring agent—trauma or chemical or microbial toxin.

The venules, on the other hand, react to vasoactive drugs and mediators. Histamine is an accepted mediator of the early exudation of acute inflammation, and the kinins are probably important also. The prostaglandins probably modulate their actions. The mediators of the late and prolonged phases of inflammation remain enigmatic; every mediator mentioned in this chapter has at some time or another been proposed as a candidate.

The accumulation of inflammatory cells in inflammation is believed to be due to chemotaxis, and the most likely agents are the activated components of complement and LTB$_4$. The change in cell population from polymorph to macrophage, and the appearance of eosinophils in some inflammations, are related largely to the actions of different chemotactic agents that attract the particular cell in question.

Although much stress has been placed upon the uniformity of the inflammatory reaction regardless of its cause, it must not be forgotten that there is, in fact, also very considerable individual diversity, both in the amount of exudate and in the type of cell involved. This individuality of an inflammatory reaction is a reflection of the individuality of the agent causing it. It would be hard to deny the importance of many bacterial products; the leucocidins, haemolysins, kinases, permeability factors, etc., must all influence the final outcome. Products of tissue damage and mediators generated from plasma and cellular constituents, are not the only agents present in the inflammation of infection. So far, much research has been done on the vasodilatation and increased vascular permeability of acute inflammation caused by trauma or chemical agents. The complex cellular changes and the intricacies of infection have been largely neglected. Until we have much more reliable information, the role of the individual chemical mediators in acute inflammation will remain ambiguous.

GENERAL READING

Babior B M 1984 The respiratory burst of phagocytosis. Journal of Clinical Investigation 73: 599

Benveniste J 1985 PAF-acether (platelet activating factor). Advances in ProstaglandinThromboxane Leukotriene Research 13:11

Butterworth A F, David J R 1981 Eosinophil function. New England Journal of Medicine 304: 154

Demers L M 1984 Prostaglandins in human disease. Clinical Laboratory Medicine 4: 889

Ford-Hutchinson A W 1985 Leukotrienes: their formation and role as inflammatory mediators. Federation Proceedings 44:25

Harlan J M 1985 Leukocyte–endothelial interactions. Blood 65: 513

Hurley J 1983 Acute inflammation, 2nd edn. Churchill Livingstone, New York

Lewis G P 1986 Mediators of inflammation, John Wright, Bristol

Majno G, Cotran R S (eds) 1982 Current topics in inflammation and infection. Williams and Wilkins, Baltimore

Nathan C F, Murray H W, Cohn Z A 1980 The macrophage as an effector cell. New England Journal of Medicine 303: 622

Panush R S 1983 Modulation of human mononuclear cell responses by neutrophil-derived factors. Inflammation 7: 35

Pierce C W 1980 Macrophages: modulators of immunity. American Journal of Pathology 98:10

Smith M J H 1982 Biological activities of leukotriene B4. In: Sammuelsson B, R, Poaletti R (eds) Leukotrienes and other Lipoxygenase Products. Raven Press, New York

Stossel T P 1974 Phagocytosis. New England Journal of Medicine 290: 717, 774, 883

6. The body's defences against infection

Microorganisms can cause disease in two ways. Either they gain access to tissues of the host, multiply, and cause *infection*, or they manufacture powerful toxins which are subsequently introduced into the body and produce an *intoxication*.

Staphylococcal enterotoxic food-poisoning and botulism provide typical examples of an *intoxication*.

By far the most important method whereby microorganisms cause disease is by their *invasion of and multiplication in the living tissues of the host*. This is the definition of *infection*, and organisms capable of producing it are termed *pathogens*.

Organisms may reach the fetus by *transplacental spread* from the mother. This is uncommon. *Postnatal infection* may arise by spread of organisms from a site within the body. This is termed *endogenous* infection in contrast to *exogenous* infection in which the organisms are derived from the external environment.

TRANSPLACENTAL SPREAD

During the early stages of pregnancy the fetus is particularly susceptible to the damaging effect of infection transmitted from the mother. Syphilis is the classical but now uncommon example. Rubella (German measles) is a serious hazard and can give rise to serious fetal infection as well as congenital malformations. Other viral infections include cytomegalovirus, coxsackieviruses and herpes simplex virus. Fetal infection with the protozoal disease toxoplasmosis may result in hydrocephalus, mental defect, and blindness.

POSTNATAL INFECTIONS

Endogenous infections

Many surfaces of the body are contaminated with organisms that constitute the resident flora and cause little trouble—indeed they are beneficial. When they reach other sites serious infection can result. Examples include bronchopneumonia, when organisms of the oral and pharyngeal mucosa reach the lung in a debilitated subject. The intestinal organisms are a common cause of peritonitis if the bowel wall is perforated; and may also cause urinary tract infection.

Exogenous infections

Organisms from the external environment may reach the tissues of the host by several routes. They may be injected into the host. The agent may be an arthropod whose bite transmits pathogenic organisms, e.g. arboviruses, *Yersinia pestis* (causing plague), and rickettsiae. Hepatitis B virus is caused by introduction of blood containing virus by means of a contaminated needle or instrument.

A second route of infection involves transmission of the organisms to a body surface which thereby becomes contaminated. If the organisms are not destroyed they may gain access to the tissues and cause infection.

The following modes of transmission are important.

Ingestion of contaminated food

Food may be contaminated directly by a human carrier or indirectly by flies. Diseases transmitted by food include typhoid fever, bacillary dysentery, and amoebiasis. Poliomyelitis is acquired by ingestion. Milk and eggs may contain bacteria because the animal itself is diseased, e.g. bovine tuberculosis and brucellosis, and *Salmonella* infections of fowls.

Direct skin contact

Wound infection may result from contact with a staphylococcal carrier or by contamination with soil containing clostridia. Contaminated air is important in causing wound infection in hospitals. The venereal diseases, e.g. syphilis and gonorrhoea, are also transmitted by direct contact.

Spread by droplets and dust

Droplets are produced when air, passing rapidly over a mucous membrane, causes atomization of the secretion which covers it. A few of these droplets are large, and due to the effect of gravity have a limited range. The vast majority are smaller than 100 μm in diameter, and dry up almost instantaneously to form *droplet nuclei* which stay suspended in the air for many hours.

Droplet formation occurs during talking, coughing, and particularly sneezing; the main source is from the *saliva in the front of the mouth*. It is possible for aerosols from highspeed dental handpieces to spread infection from the patient to the dentist; precautionary measures, such as wearing a mask and spectacles, or goggles, are recommended. The viruses of mumps, measles, smallpox, and chickenpox are found in the saliva, and these diseases may well be spread in this way.

Bacteria residing in the nose (*S. aureus*), nasopharynx (*Streptococcus pyogenes*), or lung (tubercle bacilli) do not commonly reach the front of the mouth, and it is very unlikely that droplets are an important vehicle of their spread. Some may be spat out as sputum, but the most important means of dissemination is by the fingers and handkerchief. Using fluorescein or test organisms as markers, it has been found that normal human beings frequently dispense nasal secretions and saliva to their hands, face, and clothing, and to every object that is touched. After desiccation the organisms are readily disseminated in the form of dust particles, and it is these which are important in the transmission of many infections.

Hospital (nosocomial) infection

Whenever human beings live together in confined quarters, there is always the danger that in the group there will be carriers of pathogenic organisms. Although not suffering from clinical illness themselves, they may pass on the organisms to others who, having little resistance, succumb to the infection. In turn they further transmit the disease. This is called *cross-infection*. In the past there have been many examples of epidemics of meningococcal meningitis and dysentery occurring in nurses' homes, army camps, and other places housing large numbers of people. In hospitals it is not uncommon for patients to acquire severe infections from their environment; this is hardly surprising, because many patients are debilitated and their resistance to infection is lowered. Furthermore, surgical incisions provide a ready avenue for the invading bacteria.

A particular feature in hospitals is that the staff acquire pathogenic organisms from their patients, become carriers, and further disseminate the bacteria. Often the strain is one that is resistant to the antibiotics which are in common use in that particular hospital. The infection is therefore all the more serious.

In the past *streptococcal infections* were serious,

particularly in labour words. However, penicillin therapy is very effective in streptococcal infections, since resistant organisms do not occur. It follows that outbreaks of streptococcal hospital infection are not a problem at the present time.

The staphylococcus has, on the other hand, attained a much more prominent position. Outbreaks of postoperative wound infection are not uncommon, and the methods of control which proved effective with streptococcal outbreaks are quite inadequate. Often the majority of the staff are found to be carriers, and in addition the hospital itself—the floors, air-conditioning plant, bedclothes, etc.—is also contaminated with a virulent strain of staphylococcus. Although human carriers provide the reservoir, the hardy staphylococcus often infects patients by indirect means, for instance in airborne dust particles. The problem of control is not easy; indeed there is no simple answer to an outbreak of staphylococcal wound infection.

Other organisms which sometimes cause hospital infection are the coliform group, *Proteus* species, and *Pseudomonas aeruginosa*. As with the staphylococcus, the transfer of these organisms is usually indirect, via dust, contaminated articles, and fomites.* The source of organisms is often a patient with urinary tract infection who contaminates the immediate environment—bedclothing, urine bottle, and other articles with which contact can be made.

DEFENCES OF INDIVIDUAL BODY SURFACES

It is evident that there may be contamination of the body, both externally on the skin and internally in the intestinal, respiratory, and other tracts. Contamination with virulent organisms is a common event, but infection is rare. Whether contamination is followed by infection is dependent upon two factors: the *mechanical integrity* of the body surface, which is only of importance in the skin, and its *powers of decontamination.*

The mechanisms involved in decontamination of a surface can be considered under three headings:

Mechanical mechanisms. Desquamation of surface cells and a steady washing effect of secretion are commonly involved.

Biological mechanisms. Most surfaces are colonized by organisms of low resistance that constitute the resident flora. They may flourish on a surface because their pili or fimbriae contain substances (*adhesins*) for which the epithelial cell surfaces have specific receptors. The organisms of the flora are beneficial in many ways; thus they produce antibiotic substances* and compete with other more pathogenic organisms for foodstuffs. It follows that if the flora is upset by the administration of a broad spectrum antibiotic infection may occur, e.g. candidal vaginitis related to tetracycline therapy.

Chemical mechanisms. The secretions of the body contains a variety of chemicals that destroy some organisms. Antibodies of the IgA class are secreted locally as dimers. Epithelial receptor analogues (such as bloodgroup-reactive glycoproteins) neutralize bacterial adhesins. *Lysozyme (muraminidase)* is an enzyme, a polysaccharidase, capable of lysing some organisms and inhibiting the growth of others. It acts on the muramic acid of bacterial cell walls, but with many organisms the outer coat must first be damaged by other means, e.g. complement activation or the action of peroxide, before the organism is killed.

These protective mechanisms vary greatly from one tissue to another, and each will therefore be considered separately.

THE SKIN

The skin is frequently contaminated, and its exposed position renders it liable to both major and minor physical trauma. Its protective function is carried out mainly by the epithelial cells, and indeed the inability of the subcutaneous tissues to resist infection was one of the limiting

---

*Fomites are articles, such as bedding or clothing, capable of acting as a medium for the transmission of organisms which may give rise to infection.

*An antibiotic is a substance produced by one organism which is inimical to the growth of another. Thus *penicillin* is produced by the mould *Penicillium notatum.*

factors in pre-Listerian surgery. Its defences are:

Mechanical strength

The many layers of epithelial cells, the tough outer layer of keratin, and the distinct basement membrane all play a part in the formation of a mechanical barrier, which if impaired, may result in infection. For example, excessive sweating softens the keratin layer; for this reason skin infections are very common in the tropics, and boils are frequently seen in moist areas like the axillae and groins.

The skin when intact appears to be completely impervious to invasion by organisms, but following trauma it becomes the portal of entry for staphylococci, streptococci, and the clostridia. In the tropics insect bites penetrate the skin barrier, and serve to introduce the causative agents of plague, typhus, yellow fever, malaria, dengue fever, etc.

Decontamination

The powers of decontamination of the skin may be demonstrated by deliberately contaminating the hands with haemolytic streptococci, and subsequently estimating their rate of disappearance by taking swabs at regular intervals. The organisms are often removed or destroyed within 2–3 hr. The mechanisms involved may be considered under three headings—mechanical, biological, and chemical:

Mechanical. The *desquamation* of surface squames removes some of the superficial organisms. *Desiccation* is probably of some importance in destroying organisms on the surface of the skin.

Biological. It is probable that the resident flora plays an important part in the decontamination mechanism. It includes *Staphylococcus epidermidis*, corynebacteria and propionibacteria. In addition about 25% of people harbour *Staph. aureus* particularly on the hands, face, and perineum. It is impossible to remove all the resident organisms from the skin; they survive in the gland ducts, and though the surface may be disinfected, the organisms are soon replaced. It is for this reason that sterile rubber gloves must always be worn while performing any surgical procedure.

Chemical. The sweat is normally acid and is unsuitable for the growth of most pathogens. This bactericidal activity is probably due to its lactic acid content. There are certain gaps in this acid coat; these are the alkaline areas where infection is quite common, e.g. axillae, groins, and interdigital clefts of the toes. *Unsaturated fatty acids* are present in the sebaceous secretion and are bactericidal; it is interesting that some of the corynebacteria grow only in the presence of these fatty acids, so well are they adapted to their environment.

There is no doubt that the mechanical strength together with the decontaminating mechanisms are of great importance in maintaining the integrity of the skin. When one remembers how often it must be contaminated with all types of organisms, and, apart from staphylococci how rarely it is invaded, one appreciates its efficiency as a protective coat.

THE ALIMENTARY TRACT

The mouth and throat

Mechanical strength

The toughness and integrity of the mucous membrane is important; this mechanical barrier is weakest at two points:

The *gingival margin* has only a thin epithelium, and is therefore easily traumatized. This is particularly so in the interdental region, where it is believed that a covering epithelium is present only in young healthy adults.

The *tonsillar crypts*. Here the epithelium is very thin; it has been shown that carmine powder dusted on to the tonsils appears in the underlying cells and connective tissue within 20 min. Probably the dye is transported there by phagocytes which are normally resident on the surface. Organisms may similarly reach the subepithelial tissue. It is therefore no wonder that these two sites, the tonsils and the gingivae, are the places where infection occurs when the general body defences are impaired, e.g. in acute leukaemia and agranulocytosis. Nevertheless, it is remarkable how the tissues of the mouth, including the bone, can resist infection even with the contamination that follows injuries or dental extraction. On the other hand, skin wounds caused by human bites often become infected, and they heal very badly. Some form of 'tissue immunity' in the oral cavity must be postulated, but its nature is obscure.

Decontamination

Mechanical. A regular flow of saliva is of importance for its mechanical action in keeping the mouth clean.

The continual backward flow of saliva traps organisms, which are then swallowed. Carbon particles placed on the mucosa are removed from the mouth in 15 to 30 min.[4]

Biological. As in the skin the resident flora is important. These organisms are α-haemolytic streptococci (*Streptococcus viridans*), *Branhamella catarrhalis*, *Streptococcus pneumoniae*, diphtheroids, lactobacilli, *Borrelia vincenti*, actinomyces organisms, *Candida albicans*, and various Bacteroidaceae. Many strains of α-haemolytic streptococci produce hydrogen peroxide, and this has been thought to play some part in the decontaminating mechanism.*

Chemical. The saliva inhibits many pathogens: this may be due to its mucin, lysozyme, or IgA content.

The secretion of saliva is therefore of importance, as can be appreciated when its secretion is suppressed for example in shock, dehydration, and fever, or as a result of infective processes, neoplasia, or irradiation. Under these circumstances the lips, tongue, teeth, and remainder of the mouth become coated with a mixture of food particles and dead epithelial cells, which if not actively removed, become the site of bacterial colonization and a source of infection. Thus there may be an ascending infection of the salivary glands terminating in suppurative sialadenitis.

In spite of the defence mechanisms of the mouth potent pathogens can adapt themselves to the mouth and throat, e.g. meningococci, diphtheria bacilli, *Haemophilus influenzae*, and *S. pyogenes*. These may lead to infection, but if the person has considerable immunity, they may remain as 'transients' for a period of time. Such carriers are of great importance in the spread of streptococcal infections, diphtheria, and meningococcal meningitis.

The stomach

The stomach stands guard over the intestines and deals not only with food, but also with the secretions of the mouth and swallowed sputum. Its major defence mechanism is the bactericidal activity of gastric juice due to its hydrochloric acid content.

Coliform organisms and tubercle bacilli can withstand the acidity of the stomach, and are able to reach, and occasionally infect, the lower intestinal tract. Other organisms, e.g. salmonellae, brucellae and enteroviruses will pass through the stomach, particularly if ingested with food or large quantities of fluid.

The intestine

The intestine undoubtedly relies upon the stomach's protective action. The minor intestinal upsets of infancy may in part be related to the low gastric acidity in this age-group. The intestine has, however, its own defence mechanism. The presence of IgA in the intestinal secretions is one factor and the bacterial flora is of great importance. The small intestine generally contains few organisms, while the colon is heavily contaminated with coliforms, *Bacteroides* organisms, *Streptococcus faecalis*, and clostridia. When the flora is altered by the ingestion of broad-spectrum antibiotics, infection with *Clostridium difficile* may cause fatal pseudomembranous colitis. *Candida albicans* can likewise cause a troublesome stomatitis and pruritus ani.

The appendix is one of the weakest links in the alimentary tract, the reason for which is not known. Possibly damage by hard concretions and the ease with which its lumen can be obstructed play a part, but it is humiliating to admit how little we know about the cause of such a common disease as acute appendicitis.

---

*In this connexion the rare Japanese hereditary disorder of *acatalasia* is of interest. The enzyme catalase which normally breaks down H_2O_2 is absent from the blood, and peroxide formed in the mouth produces sufficient damage to cause ulcerating gangrenous lesions in the mouth.

THE CONJUNCTIVAL SAC OF THE EYE

Large particles are prevented from contaminating the eye by the action of blinking. This also is important as it ensures that the conjunctiva and cornea are always covered by a thin protective layer of lacrimal secretion.

In the absence of the *blink reflex* the cornea desiccates, and repeated trauma leads to its ulceration and infection. Impairment of this reflex occurs under two circumstances:

1. Motor loss—in facial nerve paralysis, e.g. Bell's palsy
2. Sensory loss—with trigeminal nerve lesions, e.g. following zoster.

In order to prevent corneal ulceration and ocular infection, the eye should either be covered with a pad or else the lids should be sutured together.

The lacrimal secretions have other important functions, for if the cornea is irritated the volume of secretion is increased. The tears so produced mechanically wash away the irritant. The other important protective function of tears is due to their content of *lysozyme*: they contain the highest concentration of lysozyme of any body fluid.

THE RESPIRATORY TRACT

The respiratory tract acts as a whole, the upper part functioning as an air-conditioner for the lungs. The vibrissae filter off large particles, but the main filter is the nasal mucosa itself, covering as it does the complicated ramification of the turbinates. Not only is the inspired air warmed and humidifed, but the mucus-covered surface traps organisms and particles just as flies are trapped on fly-paper. The anterior nares are distinct from the remainder of the respiratory tract, because their epithelium and bacterial flora resemble that of the skin. Their great importance lies in their frequent colonization by *Staph. aureus*.

The nose and nasopharynx

The epithelium of the respiratory tract does not provide an adequate barrier against local infection. This is well demonstrated by the ease with which rhinoviruses and adenoviruses cause acute upper respiratory tract infection. Meningococci are apparently able to penetrate the mucosa of the nasopharynx without much difficulty.

Irritants are expelled by the act of sneezing. If organisms are deliberately implanted in the nose, they disappear within 15 min. One of the main mechanisms involved is the continuous flow of mucus backwards to the nasopharynx. The nasal secretion contains lysozyme, lactoferrin, and IgA. Nevertheless, pathogens like meningococci and diphtheria bacilli can colonize the nose, and carriers of these constitute an important reservoir of human infection. The fact that the olfactory mucosa is non-ciliated and has beneath it much lymphoid tissue has been held to explain why some organisms gain entry through this area. Experimentally dye, proteins, and viruses can be shown to penetrate the olfactory mucosa and enter the underlying lymphoid tissue.

The nasopharynx has a resident bacterial flora similar to that of the throat (especially *Strep. viridans* and *Branhamella pharyngis*), and this has a biological decontaminating function.

The trachea and lower respiratory tract

Below the larynx the respiratory tract should normally be sterile. The mucosa itself forms a poor mechanical barrier as in the nose, and is easily infected by a number of viruses, e.g. the influenza virus.

The cough reflex initiated by stimulating the larynx or upper trachea expels irritants, but may also disseminate organisms within the lung. Although the diameter of the air passages decreases steadily with each division from the trachea downwards, the total cross-sectional area of all the respiratory bronchioles is over a hundred times that of the trachea. It follows that the velocity of the inspired air steadily decreases as it passes down the air passages, and this allows particles to fall out of the stream and adhere to the mucus-covered walls. The film of fluid which covers the mucosa is derived partly by transudation, partly from the secretion of surface goblet cells but mainly from the secretions of the underlying mucous glands. By its chemical composition it protects the epithelial cells from dangerous gases, e.g. SO_2, and its proper consistency allows the cilia to move it on as a continuous sheet. The sheet of mucus ever moving upwards by ciliary activity is an important decontaminating mechanism, and any obstruction to it impairs the defences of the respiratory tract. This frequently leads to infection, and is well seen in the bronchopneumonia which follows the obstruction caused by carcinoma or a foreign body, e.g. an inhaled tooth or root.

In the respiratory bronchioles and alveoli, mucociliary streams play little part in the defence of the lung, and it is here that the macrophages, or *septal cells*, are important. Bacteria are phagocytosed by these mononuclear phagocytic cells and killed in their cytoplasm.

The bronchial mucus contains lactoferrin, lysozyme, and IgA. Although IgA is regarded as an important protective antibody, patients with a low IgA do not seem, curiously enough, to be particularly prone to respiratory infections.

SUMMARY

An important aspect of the defence mechanism against infection is the manner whereby the various body surfaces are able to rid themselves of contaminating bacteria. But apart from this it appears that each surface has an intrinsic ability to resist infection which cannot easily be explained. Thus the skin is frequently colonized by *Staph. aureus*, and yet infection is relatively uncommon. These organisms when introduced into the subcutaneous tissues readily cause infection. The skin itself is able to resist infection, and therefore exhibits some type of local tissue immunity. The nature of this is unknown. Nowhere is this type of immunity more important than in the mouth. Subepithelial tissues, muscle, and bone may be exposed and contaminated, and yet no infection ensues. Were it not for this defence mechanism dental extraction and oral surgery would be impossible.

GENERAL READING

Eikoff T C 1982 Nosocomial infections, New England Journal of Medicine 306: 1514

Källenius G, et al 1981 Structure of carbohydrate part of receptor on human uroepithelial cells for pyelonephritogenic *Escherichia coli*. Lancet 2: 604

Leading Article, 1976 In defence of the lungs. British Medical Journal 1: 773

Leading Article 1982 Pulmonary mucociliary clearance. Lancet 1: 203

Lomberg H, et al 1983 Correlation of P blood group, vesicoureteral reflux, and bacterial attachment in patients with recurrent pyelonephritis New England Journal of Medicine 308: 1189

Lowbury E J L, et al 1975 Control of hospital infection. Chapman and Hall, London

Mackowiak P A 1982 The normal microbial flora. New England Journal of Medicine 307: 83

Mason D Y, Taylor C R 1975 The distribution of muramidase (lysozyme) in human tissues. Journal of Clinical Pathology 28: 124,

Newhouse M, Sanchis J, Bienenstock J 1976 Lung defense mechanisms. New England Journal of Medicine 295: 990, 1045

Osserman E F 1975 Lysozyme. New England Journal of Medicine 292: 424

7. The body's response to infection

When organisms gain access to the tissues of the body, their fate depends on the *immunity* of the host and the *virulence* of the organism. Immunity and virulence are in effect two descriptive approaches to the encounter between an organism and its host. The possible end-results of such an encounter are:

1. Rapid destruction of the organisms, e.g. with non-pathogens.
2. The organisms grow for a time, but are soon destroyed, e.g. minor or subclinical infection.
3. The organisms enter into a symbiotic state with their host, e.g. herpes simplex virus and adenovirus.
4. There is a local proliferation of organisms to produce tissue damage, but there is little spread of the infection, e.g. a boil due to *Staph. aureus*.
5. Organisms may proliferate locally and produce severe damage to distant tissues by means of an exotoxin. The local lesion may be insignificant, as in tetanus, or severe as in diphtheria.
6. A local lesion is produced, but rapid spread of organisms follows, so that a diffuse, ill-defined inflammation results. This is called *cellulitis*, *Streptococcus pyogenes* can be a cause.
7. No local lesion forms but the organism spreads rapidly, e.g. European typhus due to *Rickettsia prowazeki*.
8. No local lesion forms initially, but the organisms spread rapidly and later a lesion develops at the portal of entry, e.g. syphilis, typhoid fever, and scrub typhus due to *Rickettsia tsutsugamushi*.
9. The organisms induce cellular proliferation, e.g. Rous's sarcoma.

This list is by no means complete. Thus, the slow viruses produce a type of infection which appears to be unique, but is not well understood. Cholera is peculiar in that the organisms multiply in the gut, produce a toxin which damages the epithelium, but yet never penetrate beyond the basement membrane. It is obvious in this example how difficult it is to separate true infection from intoxication.

Pathogenicity of organisms—virulence

An organism is described as *non-pathogenic* if it is unable to multiply in the tissues and produce disease. Such an organism is usually phagocytosed by the polymorphonuclear leucocytes and macrophages, and destroyed in the cytoplasm of these cells. Specific receptors are required for cells to be susceptible to certain infections. Thus the Duffy blood-group antigens are necessary for the parasitization of human red cells by the protozoon (*Plasmodium vivax*) that causes benign tertian malaria. A factor is present on chromosome 19 that determines human susceptibility to poliovirus.

Some organisms, on the other hand, are capable of causing disease (i.e. are *pathogenic*) and have the ability to grow in the tissues where they produce *infection*. Disregarding for the moment the immune state of the host, the severity of this infection depends on the intrinsic nature of the organism, and the factor concerned is generally described as its *virulence*. This may be manifest in two ways:

1. The ability of the organism to spread throughout the tissue
2. The ability of the organism to cause tissue damage, for instance by the production of toxins.

The ability to spread, in respect of many organisms, is inversely proportional to the tendency to produce initial local damage and a subsequent inflammatory reaction. Thus an organism like *Staph. aureus* produces severe tissue damage, a marked inflammatory response, and usually has little tendency to spread. On the other hand, some organisms, e.g. many viruses, *Mycobacterium leprae*, etc., excite little immediate inflammatory reaction, and are able to spread widely without leaving any trace of the site of entry. Other organisms, although behaving essentially in the same manner, produce diseases in which a lesion develops later at the site of entry. Syphilis is an excellent example of this, and it should be noted that the local lesion (chancre) occurs *long after the organisms have spread throughout the body*.

Sometimes an organism may live in a symbiotic state with its host and produce no damage. Such a relationship exists between humans and the virus of herpes simplex. The virus lives harmlessly in the sensory nerve cells until the subject develops a fever. Then it multiplies and produces the familiar fever blister (cold sore), or herpes febrilis. Such latent virus infections are probably quite common—probably many tumour-producing viruses behave in a similar manner. This is considered in Chapter 21.

The existence of L-forms raises many possibilities. They are generally considered to be non-pathogenic, but following an overt infection they might remain in the tissues in a dormant form and provide sufficient antigen to sustain an immunological response. Rheumatic carditis and chronic post-streptococcal glomerulonephritis are obvious candidates for such a pathogenesis. L-Forms might also revert to type; this could explain recurrent infections, e.g. chronic pyelonephritis and infective endocarditis.

From this brief review it is evident that microorganisms are capable of initiating a great number of disease patterns, and that no simple generalization will suffice to describe the types of host response that occur with infection.

Manner by which organisms produce damage

Some organisms produce damage by elaborating powerful *exotoxins*. Exotoxins are freely diffusible and therefore found in the medium of a bacterial culture. They can be purified, identified, and estimated with relative ease. Their mode of action is known in many cases, and it is very specific. On a quantitative basis exotoxins are very potent; thus botulinum toxin is the most poisonous substance known. Bacteria whose main offensive weapon is an exotoxin are called *toxic organisms*. Examples of these are the causative organisms of *diphtheria*, *tetanus*, *gas-gangrene*, and *scarlet fever*. Although the infection which they produce remains localized, distant tissues of the host are damaged as a result of circulating toxins.

With most other organisms no powerful exotoxins are produced. Some substances are released during growth, such as hyaluronidase, haemolysins and leukocidins, but they lack the potency of the classical exotoxins. Some substances, sometimes called *endotoxins*, appear to be components of the bacterial cell, e.g. the lipoproteins of the gram negative bacilli. Organisms which do not secrete exotoxins are termed *invasive* and damage is inflicted only where organisms are actually present. An exception to this is when lesions are produced by an immune mechanism, as appears to be the case in acute rheumatic fever and post-streptococcal glomerulonephritis.

The manner whereby the invasive organisms produce damage is not clearly understood. Some seem to have a direct action on the tissues, and produce necrosis and acute inflammation. The pyogenic organisms fall into this group. In infections with some organisms it seems that damage is caused by an immune mechanism either of cell-mediated delayed hypersensitivity type or a reaction involving specific immunoglobulins, with either IgE sensitizing mast cells or IgG leading to immune complex formation. Tuberculosis provides a good example of this situation. It is also well-documented in measles and respiratory-syncytial-virus infections that the disease can be more severe in the partially immunized individual than in the non-immune. In infection with other organisms the situation is much more complicated. *Typhoid fever* illustrates this particularly well.

Typhoid fever. The pathogenesis of mouse typhoid (infection with *Salmonella typhimurium*) has been studied in considerable detail, and by analogy the sequence of events in humans is probably as follows:

Typhoid fever is contracted by the ingestion of food contaminated with *Salm. typhi*. The organisms reach the lumen of the small intestine, and on its mucosal surface they are taken up by phagocytes. They are carried into the mucosa itself and thence to the local lymphoid tissue (Peyer's patches). Scarcely any local damage occurs, and little or no inflammation results. The organisms multiply, and some pass into the lymphatics to the mesenteric nodes and finally reach the blood stream via the thoracic duct. In this way there develops a *bacteraemia, which is defined as the transient presence of organisms in the blood stream*. The phagocytic cells of the MPS are well able to deal with this, and the organisms are engulfed by them. However, the organisms are able to live and multiply in these cells. By about the tenth day the parasitized cells undergo necrosis, and the blood stream is flooded with large numbers of bacilli. This is the end of the incubation period (usually 10–14 days), and the patient becomes seriously ill with *septicaemia, which is defined as the presence of organisms in the blood stream which are causally associated with severe constitutional upset*. This differs from *bacteraemia* in that it is associated with severe clinical symptoms, there are more organisms in the blood, and it indicates that the host's resistance to the organism is very inadequate. The septicaemic phase lasts about 1 week and is characterized clinically by a progressive rise in temperature (step-ladder pattern) and severe constitutional symptoms. Death may occur at this stage.

The next phase of the disease is marked by the onset of diarrhoea, ulceration of the small intestine, and the appearance of organisms in the faeces. The bacilli reach the gut via the bile, which is heavily contaminated as a result of the passage of the bacteria from the Kupffer cells of the liver. The ulceration occurs over the inflamed Peyer's patches, and is associated with mesenteric adenitis. In both the ulcers and the lymph nodes there is an accumulation of macrophages, while polymorphs are not present. The most likely explanation of these events is that the local lymphoid tissue of the gut has become sensitized to the organism, and that subsequent contact with it produces damage. A local sensitizing immune reaction must be postulated, and the blood level of detectable antibodies (agglutinins) does not rise till later in the course of the disease. During the second week diagnosis depends upon finding the organism in the faeces. By the third week the level of antibodies in the serum rises (Widal reaction), and the patient gradually recovers (Fig. 7.1). Many viruses, e.g. measles, behave in a similar manner, gaining entry into the body through the upper respiratory tract, proliferating in the cells of the mononuclear phagocyte system, and followed by the appearance of a widespread skin rash on the 14th day as effector immune mechanisms lead to viral destruction. Such a mechanism should always be suspected in an infective disease that has an incubation period exceeding 7–10 days.

Septicaemia

The cause of death in septicaemia is poorly understood. It has been most extensively studied in anthrax. *Bacillus anthracis* infection in animals leads to fatal septicaemia, and the animals die with vast numbers of organisms in the blood. The organism, although a typically invasive one, has been found to produce a number of factors (anthrax toxic complex) both in vitro and in vivo that act to increase the permeability of blood vessels. A state of hypovolaemic shock develops. Early treatment with antibiotics will save infected animals, but there is a critical time after which treatment is of no avail. Although the organisms may be destroyed, the animal still dies as shock passes into an irreversible phase.

In septicaemia due to streptococci and staphylococci, death can reasonably be attributed to

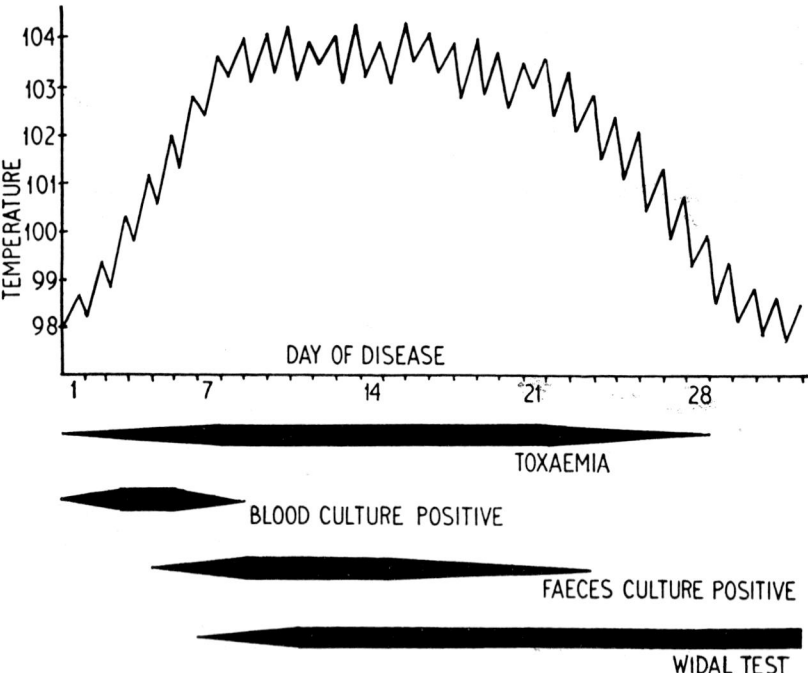

Fig. 7.1   Chart correlating the clinical course of a typical case of typhoid fever with the principal methods of bacteriological diagnosis (After Harries E H R, Mitman M 1947 *Clinical practice in infectious disease*, 3rd edn. Livingstone, Edinburgh, p 464)

intense toxaemia consequent on the release of toxins. However, with other organisms, e.g. pneumococci, the symptoms are less easily explicable, because these organisms do not appear to produce toxic substances.

The generalized Shwartzman phenomenon

Gram-negative bacilli, e.g. *Salm. typhi* and coliform organisms, produce an ill-defined endotoxin of lipoprotein nature. Experimentally it has been shown that this substance can produce shock if injected intravenously, especially if the dose is repeated *twenty-four hours later*. This

enhancing effect of a previous dose is known as the *generalized Shwartzman phenomenon,*[*] and may be the experimental counterpart of the shock which is seen in some human cases of coliform septicaemia. The mechanism of the Shwartzman phenomenon is not well understood. It is probable that the endotoxin causes endothelial cell damage and that this initiates intravascular clotting. The occlusion of the vessels in the kidney leads to cortical necrosis with subsequent acute renal failure. The effect of the first injection of endotoxin is probably to block the MPS so that the second injection of endotoxin is less quickly removed. The generalized Shwartzman reaction is not immunologically mediated.

TYPES OF ACUTE INFLAMMATION

Although all examples of acute inflammation have many features in common, certain types have been categorized, depending upon some

---

[*]This should no be confused with the *localized Shwartzman phenomenon*. To demonstrate this, a quantity of Gram-negative bacterial endotoxin is injected into the skin of an animal and 24 hrs later an intravenous dose is given. The site of the skin injected then undergoes necrosis. The pathogenesis is not understood, and there is little evidence that a similar reaction ever occurs in any human disease.

particular feature. The terms are useful for descriptive purposes but are of no fundamental significance.

Suppurative inflammation. Certain organisms, termed the pyogenic organisms, as well as some chemicals, produce considerable tissue destruction. This is associated with a marked neutrophil infiltration, and the disintegrating phagocytes liberate proteolytic enzymes which cause liquefaction of the dead area. The fluid produced is *pus*, and the inflammation is called *suppurative*. Suppuration occurring in infection generally indicates that localization is becoming established, and therefore in the days before chemotherapy it was regarded as a favourable sign; hence the origin of the term 'laudable pus'. The presence of pus in a natural cavity is called an *empyema*.

While suppuration is usually localized, pus formation may occasionally occur in a spreading cellulitis (Fig. 7.2). Such a diffuse suppurative process is generally caused by *Strep. pyogenes*, and this type of inflammation is called *phlegmonous*.

Serous inflammation. In inflammation of loose tissues and in serous sacs the fluid component of the inflammatory exudate exceeds the cellular one, because the limiting factor of increased tissue tension (p. 53) is absent. There results a large accumulation of inflammatory oedema, and this is termed *serous inflammation*. Gas-gangrene provides another example. The invading organisms (particularly *Clostridium novyi*) produce toxins that directly act on blood vessels to increase their permeability.

Fibrinous inflammation. Fibrin formation is a feature of inflammation in serous sacs and in the lungs. It is well marked in most forms of pericarditis and peritonitis (Figs 7.3 and 7.4). It is also frequent in pneumococcal and staphylococcal infections. Often there is considerable serous exudate, and the inflammation is then termed *sero-fibrinous*.

Haemorrhagic inflammation. A blood-stained exudate indicates that the irritant has caused severe vascular damage. It is seen in the lungs in phosgene poisoning and acute influenzal pneumonia.

Catarrhal inflammation. This type is seen when a mucous membrane is involved in an acute inflammatory reaction. There is some destruction of the epithelial cells, and a profuse mucus secretion from those that remain as well as from the underlying glands. The common cold provides an excellent example.

Membranous inflammation. A membrane of mucus and fibrinous exudate covering an inflamed area of mucosa is seen in *membranous bronchitis*. It may be coughed up as a cast.

Pseudomembranous inflammation. This type differs from membranous inflammation in that the membrane contains necrotic epithelium as well as fibrin and inflammatory cells. It is seen typically in diphtheria and in pseudomembranous enterocolitis.

Gangrenous inflammation. Gangrene occurs in inflammation when the dead tissue is invaded by putrefactive organisms (p. 47).

Variability of the cellular exudate

Certain inflammations do not show the usual neutrophil polymorph response. In typhoid the inflammatory reaction has virtually no polymorphs, but instead is characterized by macrophages. Eosinophils are usually plentiful in inflammations produced by parasitic worms, and also in some allergic conditions, e.g. hay fever. Lymphocytic infiltration is frequent in inflammatory lesions produced by viruses, even in the early stages. It is also a feature of acute inflammation in many skin diseases. This variation in cellular response is presumably related to the nature of the causative irritant which, in a variety of ways, leads to the release of specific chemotactic factors. This is discussed in greater detail in Chapter 5.

MODE OF DESTRUCTION OF ORGANISMS

Although a completely teleological view of the inflammatory reaction is unjustifiable, it is generally accepted that the reaction is an adaptive response having survival value for the species. It creates around the invading organisms a micro-environment unfavourable for their multiplication and survival. *Local inflammation is therefore the first line of defence against the spread of infection.* An inhibition of the inflammatory re-

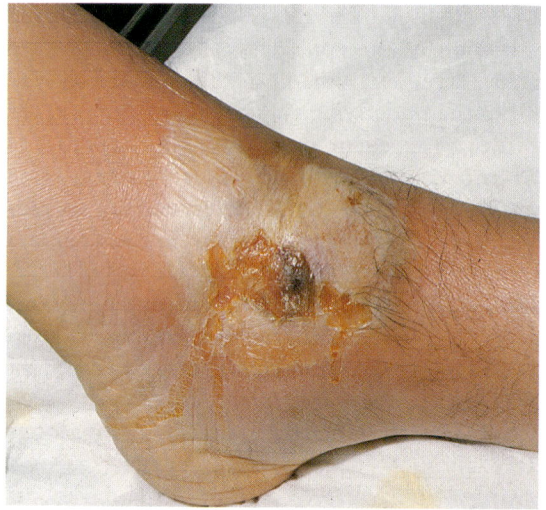

Fig. 7.2 Cellulitis of ankle. The soft tissues of the ankle are swollen and erythematous. The central white area is covered by necrotic epidermis caused by the formation of a subepidermal bulla.

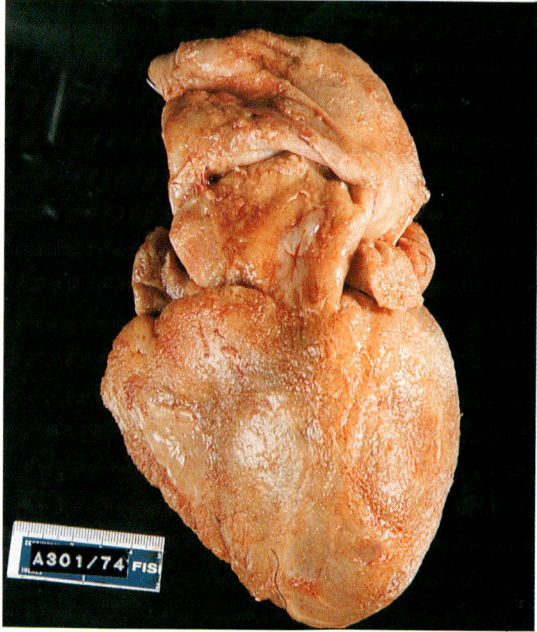

Fig. 7.3 Acute pericarditis. The whole of the pericardial surface is covered by a fibrinous acute inflammatory exudate that gives it a shaggy dull appearance.

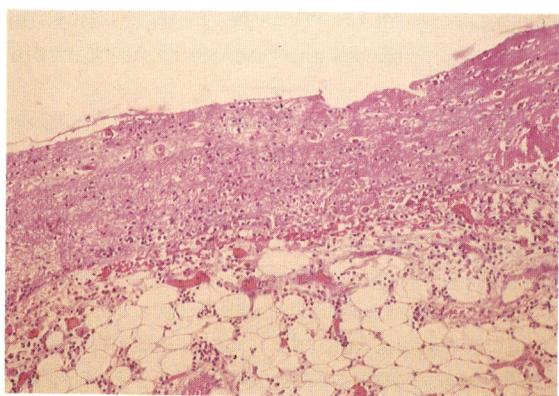

Fig. 7.4 The normal, flattened mesothelial cells covering the epicardial fat have been replaced, by a thick zone of fibrinous inflammatory exudate.

Part played by phagocytes

The polymorphonuclear leucocytes. Although many pathogenic organisms can multiply in the cytoplasm of the polymorphonuclear leucocytes and even be spread by them, the ultimate destruction of the organism often takes place within these cells. The precise mechanism involved probably varies from one organism to another. The following intracellular antimicrobial agents may be involved:

Lysosomal enzymes. Although these acid-hydrolytic enzymes digest dead bacteria, it is unlikely that they can kill living organisms.

Lysozyme. This enzyme is released by both the specific and the azurophil granules of the polymorphs.

Acidity. The low pH may destroy some organisms. Lactic acid is bactericidal, and is produced as a consequence of the glycolysis but accompanies phagocytosis.

Lactoferrin. This protein inhibits bacterial growth by binding iron which is an essential growth requirement for microorganisms.

Cationic lysosomal proteins. At least seven antimicrobial proteins of this type are found in neutrophils. One of these is called *phagocytin*.

Oxidizing agents. A number of bactericidal oxidizing agents are formed as a result of the hexose-monophosphate shunt activity that follows phagocytosis. The *superoxide anion* O_2^- and *singlet oxygen* are thought to be important. Also

action generally increases the tendency of an infection to spread.

The manner in which organisms are killed in the exudate must now be considered:

important is H_2O_2 which acts on bacteria in the presence of a halide and the enzyme myeloperoxidase that granulocytes contain.

Mononuclear phagocytes. These phagocytic members of the MPS are particularly important in providing a defence against acid-fast bacilli, fungi, and viruses. General conditions, like shock and haemorrhage, impair the MPS's phagocytic activity. This may well explain the lowered resistance under these circumstances.

Part played by the fluid exudate

The inflammatory oedema contains complement and other antibacterial substances present normally in the plasma. It contains lactic acid in considerable quantities. This may be a factor in the destruction of invading organisms. Indeed, the conditions may be so unfavourable that some of the host cells as well as the bacteria are destroyed. To some extent this may actually be beneficial, because necrotic tissue has been shown to contain bactericidal substances.

Part played by acquired immunity

Antibodies, e.g. opsonins, are present in the inflammatory exudate and aid phagocytosis. Antibody-dependent cell-mediated cytotoxicity is further described on page. 116. Activation of complement is another important mechanism whereby antibodies assist in the destruction of organisms.

Cellular immunity also plays an important part. In the immune individual macrophages are activated and more adept at destroying organisms. Delayed-type hypersensitivity reactions cause tissue destruction and with it destruction of organisms.

SPREAD OF INFECTION

Local spread

The natural cohesion of tissues tends to prevent the spread of organisms. The tissue fluids are, however, in constant motion under normal conditions. Organisms are carried in any stream of fluid which may be present. The activity of muscles causes considerable movement of tissue fluids, and it is for this reason that the time-honoured treatment of inflammation is to rest the part. It should be noted that the motility of the organism itself appears to play no part in its spread. There is no correlation between the motility of the organism and the rapidity with which it spreads. Thus, *Clostridium tetani* is a motile organism but tetanus is a localized infection, where *Clostridium perfringens* is non-motile and yet produces the rapidly spreading gas-gangrene.

Local spread may also occur in an entirely different way. Organisms ingested by phagocytes may be transported by these cells. This is an important means of spread in tuberculosis, and almost certainly occurs in many other infections.

The local defence mechanism. The acute inflammatory reaction must be regarded as a defence mechanism, although as we have seen, it is called forth only in the case of certain infections. With these infections the acute inflammatory reaction, including the laying down of fibrin, plays an important part in the destruction of the organism. It has been thought that the fibrin forms a barrier and is important in limiting the spread of infection. However, it seems much more likely that it is the whole inflammatory response which is important rather than the fibrin itself. The presence of a fibrin barrier around the zone of infection is thus indicative of a severe inflammatory response which causes destruction of the organism, and is probably not the prime mover in the destruction itself.

Spread by natural channels

If local spread implicates a natural passage, infection may spread by this route. The following examples are important: *peritoneum*— Infection may spread rapidly throughout the peritoneal space from localized lesions; it is for this reason that acute appendicitis is serious. Following perforation of the organ, the whole peritoneal cavity becomes infected, and as a large surface is involved, there is a rapid absorption of toxic substances. Infection may likewise spread through the *pleura, subarachnoid space, pericardium,* and *joint spaces*.

Infection may also spread along tubes, like the *bronchi* (in bronchopneumonia and pulmonary tuberculosis), the *ureter*, and the *gut*.

Spread by lymphatics

In acute inflammation lymphatic vessels are held open by the increase in tissue tension. The permeability of their walls is increased, as is also the flow of lymph. Invading organisms frequently gain access to the lymphatics, and are carried to the nearest lymph node. Phagocytes which have ingested the organisms but which are unable to destroy them, also travel by the same route. Here the MPS cells lining the sinuses phagocytose the organisms and prevent their further spread. The lymph nodes may be regarded as the *second line of defence* against the spread of infection. Toxins may also be absorbed by the lymphatics. *Lymphangitis* is therefore a common event in spreading lesions, and when the vessels are superficial, as in the forearm, they appear as bright red streaks. Organisms may become arrested in the lymph nodes and yet not be destroyed. In this way *lymphadenitis* arises; the filter will have protected the individual, but at the expense of the node. If organisms pass through the lymphatic barrier, they then enter the blood stream.

Spread by the blood stream

The blood stream forms the *third and last line of defence* against the spread of infection. It has two main defence mechanisms.

1.   The circulating blood itself contains a wide array of antibacterial substances. These include complement, properdin, and opsonins, as well as antibodies of specific acquired immunity.

2.   The MPS, especially the sinus-lining cells of the liver (Kupffer cells), bone marrow, and spleen, forms the main defence against generalized infection. Organisms injected experimentally into the blood stream are rapidly removed. In natural infections with highly invasive organisms like the typhoid bacillus early invasion of the blood stream occurs, and the circulating organisms are rapidly taken up by the MPS. This is the first step in the general immune response (p. 110).

The presence of organisms in the blood stream is a common event. It occurs under several conditions.

Direct invasion of blood vessels. A few organisms may invade blood vessels in the course of any local infection, e.g. a boil. The infection is often quite trivial, but the adjacent blood vessels may be ruptured by trauma, thereby allowing organisms to enter. Gingival infection or abscesses related to the apices of the roots of teeth are common lesions in which this is thought to occur, e.g. following dental extraction, scaling of teeth, or even chewing hard food. When small numbers of organisms enter the blood stream in this way, they are rapidly removed by the cells of the MPS and are destroyed. Bacteraemia usually causes few symptoms, but rigors may occur in the Gram-negative bacteraemia which follows catheterization. Its real importance, however, is that under certain conditions it may lead to serious sequelae.

Metastatic lesions. Experimentally it has been shown that when an animal has a bacteraemia, histamine injected at any site will precipitate a local infection with the organism concerned. Trauma has a similar effect. Staphylococci may be localized in a bone in this way and set up osteomyelitis (p. 105). Another danger is that the organisms are filtered off by the kidneys, and if there is a coincidental obstruction to the outflow of urine, pyelonephritis may result. A further hazard of bacteraemia is that the organisms may colonize a damaged heart valve and cause endocarditis (p. 358).

Transplacental spread. If the patient is pregnant, organisms may cross the placenta and reach the fetus (p. 67).

Septic thrombophlebitis. When infection spreads to a vein, its wall becomes inflamed and thrombosis may occur, a condition called thrombophlebitis. With pyogenic organisms pyaemia results as the thrombus softens, breaks up and embolises.

Pyaemia is the presence in the circulation of infected thrombi which are carried to various organs where they produce metastatic abscesses or septic infarcts. Which of these occurs depends on the vascular arrangements of the organ in which the emboli become lodged. Involvement of an artery can so weaken the vessel wall that a *mycotic aneurysm* results. Pyaemia was a common complication of staphylococcal osteomyelitis before the days of chemotherapy. It is now much less frequent. It sometimes follows suppuration of the gastrointestinal tract, e.g. acute appendicitis and infected piles, and the *portal pyaemia* produces multiple abscesses in the liver.

Spread from the lymphatics. Organisms which are not held up in the tissues at the site of entry or in the lymph nodes, reach the venous circulation via the lymphatic ducts. Bacteraemia produced in this way is a common event with many invasive organisms, e.g. *S. typhi*. If the cells of the MPS having phagocytosed the organisms, are unable to destroy them, the bacteria proliferate and are subsequently liberated into the circulation which is flooded with them. The patient becomes gravely ill with septicaemia.

Spread along nerves

Some viruses, e.g. rabies virus, are believed to travel up the nerves to reach the central nervous system. Whether they pass up the axoplasm or in the periaxonal space is uncertain.

FACTORS DETERMINING THE LOCALIZATION OR SPREAD OF INFECTION

It is convenient at this point to summarize the factors which determine whether a particular organism is likely to spread from the site of infection or remain localized.

Factors involving the organisms

Virulence. It should be appreciated that within each species of organism there are many strains, each with differing degrees of virulence. Thus certain staphylococci produce severe infection, while others produce trivial skin lesions.

Dose. With many organisms a large dose produces a severe spreading lesion while a small one leads to a minor lesion which heals. This can be demonstrated experimentally in tuberculosis produced in animals. It is probably less true of viral infections.

Portal of entry. Some organisms will cause infection only if administered by a particular route, e.g. *Vibrio cholerae* is non-pathogenic if injected, but may cause cholera if swallowed.

Synergism. The combined effect of two infecting organisms may be greater than either one alone. The best known example is Vincent's infection, which is a common cause of gingivitis and in which two organisms, the *Fusobacterium fusiforme* and the *Borrelia vincenti*, are in association (See also clostridial infections, p. 158).

Products of the organisms. Certain organisms produce factors which may aid their spread; streptococci produce an enzyme *hyaluronidase* which acts by depolymerizing the ground substance, and probably aids in spreading the infection. *Strep. pyogenes* also produces the enzyme *streptokinase* which aids in the lysis of the fibrin barrier by activating the plasmin system (p. 319).

Factors involving the host

General factors. The general state of health is important. Starvation and haemorrhagic shock have been shown experimentally to render animals more liable to infection. It is frequently observed that patients with chronic debilitating diseases, e.g. renal failure and diabetes mellitus, are less capable of resisting infection. The factors involved are complex, and probably involve both humoral factors, e.g. a low complement level, and an impaired activity of the phagocytes.

The immune state. This involves both non-specific factors like complement and the specific antibodies of acquired immunity. Primary infections tend to spread much more widely than do subsequent ones due to the absence of active immunity (see tuberculosis, p. 168).

Low white-cell count. Infections tend to spread whenever the neutrophil polymorphonuclear leucocytes count is low, e.g. in agranulocytosis or acute leukaemia.

Defects in the polymorphs. The importance of polymorphs in the defences against infection is highlighted by a number of conditions of genetic origin in which polymorph function is impaired. In *chronic granulomatous disease*, inherited as an X-linked recessive trait, there are repeated episodes, often staphylococcal, of infection of skin, lymph nodes, lungs and other organs. Phagocytosis is normal but ingested organisms, particularly *S. aureus*, cannot be killed because of a defect in the mechanism that generates superoxide and H_2O_2. Other diseases are known in which chemotaxis, phagocytosis or other function is impaired. For instance, there may be a deficiency of one of the adhesion molecules. Polymorph function can be investigated in vitro and testing is advisable in any child who suffers from repeated or unusual infections.

Local factors. The local blood supply is important. Ischaemia from whatever cause, e.g. injection of adrenaline, peripheral vascular disease, etc., adversely affects the inflammatory response designed to destroy the organism. Similarly, foreign bodies and chemicals which cause necrosis are harmful. Thus silica potentiates the pathogenic action of the tubercle bacillus, and ionic calcium aids the inception of anaerobic infections in wounds.

It is evident from this account of the various patterns of infection that the relationship between the host and the infecting organism is extremely complex. This is well illustrated in the case of the human subject and the *Brucella* organism. The infection can vary from an acute illness to a chronic disease, or even a symptomless carrier state in which a symbiotic relationship has been established. Only in the case of the exotoxin-producing organisms is the pathogenesis of the disease which they cause at all clearly understood. It is not surprising therefore that it is in this group of infections that our understanding of immunity is also most complete.

GENERAL READING

Braude A I 1981 Medical microbiology and infectious diseases. Saunders, Philadelphia
Heggie A D (1971). Pathogenesis of the rubella exanthem. New England Journal of Medicine 285: 664
Leading Article 1989 Immunology of measles. Lancet 2: 780
Miller D A 1974 Human chromosome 19 carries a poliovirus receptor gene. Cell 1:167
Quie P G, Hetherington S V 1984 Patients with disorders of phagocytic cell function. Pediatric Infectious Disease 3: 272
Youmans G P, Paterson P Y, Sommers H M 1980 The biologic and clinical basis of infectious diseases, 2nd edn. Saunders, Philadelphia

8. Healing: repair and regeneration

The word *healing*, used in a pathological context, refers to the body's replacement of destroyed tissue by living tissue. It is therefore useful, at the outset, to enumerate the causes of tissue loss or destruction.

Traumatic excision, whether accidental or surgical.

Physical, chemical, and microbial agents.

Ischaemia, which leads to infarction.

Hypersensitivity reactions to foreign proteins, or to products of organisms, are instances when the body's response to external agents can itself engender necrosis (see Arthus phenomenon, p 139, caseation in tuberculosis, p. 165).

In insects, amphibians, and crustaceans the ability to replace lost parts is truly remarkable. Thus, if the lens of the eye of a salamander is removed a new lens develops from the adjacent iris; even the complex neural part of the retina, if destroyed, can be reformed from the outer pigmented layer of the retina. Other well-known examples of regeneration are the reformation of the amputated limbs of insects and newts, and of the claws of lobsters. The process whereby whole limbs are reformed is well developed in lower forms of life: it is complex, and resembles embryonic development or asexual reproduction. The process is termed *axial regeneration* by zoologists, but the term *reconstitution* is also used by pathologists. One would think that the ability to reform a lost limb or organ was so useful to survival that it would have been retained during evolution Such has not been the case. The higher animals—including humans—do not have the ability to replace lost limbs following their amputation. Perhaps this is because sexual reproduction has been evolved and preserved at all costs as a means of improving and remoulding the species. 'If there were no regeneration there could be no life. If everything regenerated there would be no death. All organisms exist between these two extremes. Other things being equal, they tend towards the latter end of the spectrum, never quite achieving immortality because this would be incompatible with reproduction.'[*]

The regeneration of the amputated arm of the newt has been extensively studied. The stump

---

[*]Quoted from Goss R J 1969 *Principles of Regeneration*. Academic Press, New York.

rapidly becomes covered by a layer of epidermal cells that slide in from the adjacent skin. The cells multiply to form an *apical cap*, and intimate contact of these cells with the stump, particularly its nerves, is an essential step in the regeneration process. After a brief inflammatory reaction the cells of the stump—fibroblasts, muscle cells, osteoblasts and other cell types—appear to revert from their differentiated form into a primitive cell type by a process termed *dedifferentiation*. Connective tissue fibres—collagen, muscle, and bone— break down, and the cells of regeneration lie in an oedematous stroma that resembles the mesenchyme of the developing embryo. This mass of cells is termed the *blastema*. Its cells multiply rapidly in an avascular field in the first instance. Later there is vascularization and differentiation: bone, muscle, tendon, nerves, and blood vessels are produced in a coordinated manner such that there is accurate replacement of the parts of the limb that were lost. No matter what the level of the original amputation, only the distal parts are replaced. Thus with a forearm amputation, a wrist and hand are formed but never an elbow. This rule of *distal transformation* has been summed up by the trite description of 'hands from elbows, but never elbows from hands'.

In humans the cells adjacent to the area of damage fail to dedifferentiate, and no blastema comparable to that described above is formed. The healing process has two aspects:

Contraction, a mechanical reduction in the size of the defect occurring in the first few weeks (see below).

Replacement of lost tissue, which is brought about by migration of cells as well as division of adjacent cells to provide extra tissue to fill the gap. This can be accomplished in two ways:

Repair, the replacement of lost tissue by granulation tissue which matures to form scar tissue. This is inevitable when the surrounding specialized cells do not possess the capacity to proliferate, e.g. muscle and neurons.

Regeneration, the replacement of lost tissue by tissue similar in type. There is a proliferation of surrounding undamaged specialized cells. Regeneration is predominant when the cells comprising the tissue are capable of multiplication, and is well illustrated by the healing of a damaged epidermis.

HEALING BY REPAIR

WOUND CONTRACTION

Measurement is conveniently studied by excising a small, circular, full-thickness disc of skin from the back or flank of an animal. Figures 8.1 and 8.2 show the results of such an experiment. The size of the wound is measured at regular intervals, and it can be seen that after an initial period of 2–3 days there follows a period of rapid contraction which is largely completed by the 14th day. The contribution by newly formed granulation tissue and epithelium is not included, since the measurements are made from the original wound edges. The wound is reduced by approximately 80% of its original size in the rat, but the actual extent of the contraction varies with the species of animal, and with the shape, size, and site of the wound. Contraction results in much faster healing, as less new tissue has to be formed. If contraction is prevented, healing is slow and a large ugly scar the result.

Contraction probably plays a similar role in the healing of wounds of the oral mucosa. In the nonkeratinized mucosa scarring persists as on the skin, but in wounds of the keratinized mucosa of the

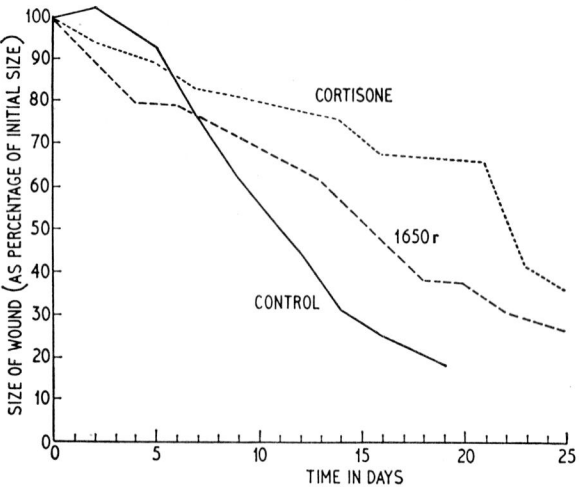

Fig 8.1 Wound contraction in the rat. Daily administration of cortisone acetate causes considerable delay in the process. Irradiation with 1650 r immediately after inflicting the wounds has a similar delaying effect.

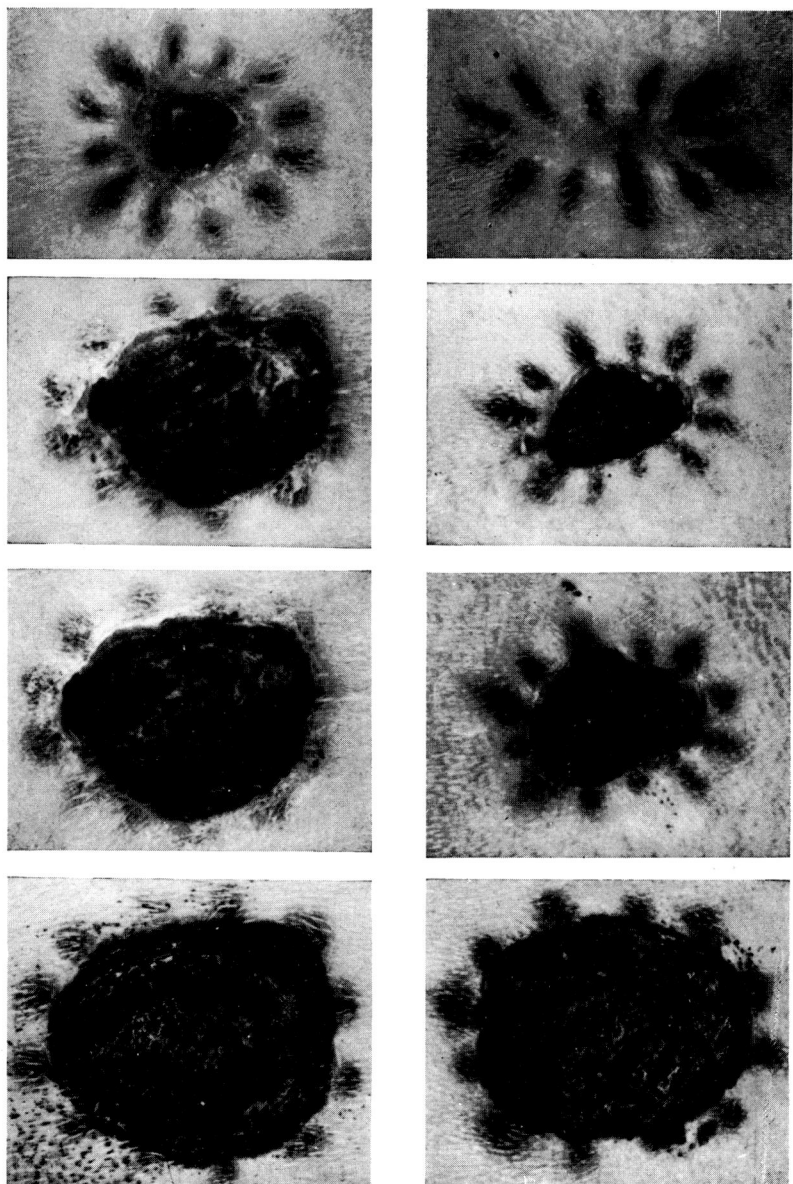

Fig. 8.2 Wound contraction in the rat and the effect of x-irradiation. The edges of the skin wounds have been tattooed with carbon so as to render them easily visible. Note how the delivery of 1650 rads to the wound on the right has delayed the contraction process. (From Blair G H, Slome D, Walter J B 1961 *Review of experimental investigations on wound healing, British surgical practice: Surgical progress*, Ross J P (ed.). Butterworth, London.)

gingiva, edentulous ridge, and the palate, only a small amount of scar tissue forms during healing and it soon becomes so inconspicuous that the actual site of the wound can no longer be found.

Contraction occurs in wounds at a time when granulation tissue is being actively formed, and it is generally agreed that the granulation tissue at the edge of the wound is effected by contraction of myofibroblasts in the granulation tissue at the edge of the wound (the *'picture-frame area'*).

These cells resemble ordinary fibroblasts but their cytoplasm contains fibrillar components similar to those found in smooth muscle cells; furthermore they can contract.

Interference with the formation of granulation tissue, e.g. by *irradiating the wounded area* or the administration of *glucocorticoids*, causes considerable delay in wound contraction (Fig. 8.1). Interference with the formation of collagen, on the other hand, as in the vitamin-C-deficient animal, has no such effect. The contraction of wounds may also be impaired following burns, and also if the raw area of the wound is skin-grafted.

Healing by repair

Organization

Organization is one of the fundamental processes in pathology, and can be defined as *the ingrowth of fibroblasts and vascular endothelial cells into a blood clot, dead tissue or a fibrinous exudate*, which are thereby replaced by living granulation tissue.

The situations where organization is encountered are in an *inflammatory exudate* (this is especially important in chronic inflammation), a *haematoma*, a *thrombus*, and an *infarct*. A type of granulation tissue grows around tumour cells and forms the stroma.

The growth of granulation tissue into a wound involves four phases.

Haematoma formation

A clot forms.

Inflammation

The damage caused by the injury sets in motion the phenomenon of acute inflammation in the surrounding tissue. An exudate containing fibrin and polymorphs therefore accumulates.

Demolition

The dead tissue cells liberate their autolytic enzymes, and other proteolytic enzymes come from disintegrating polymorphs. There is an associated mononuclear infiltration with macrophages. These are mostly derived from the blood monocytes, and their function is to ingest particulate matter, which they either digest or remove (p. 56).

Granulation tissue formation

Granulation tissue is formed by the proliferation and migration of surrounding connective-tissue elements. It is composed, in the first instance, of *capillary loops* and *fibroblasts* together with a variable number of inflammatory cells (Fig. 8.3). Initially this is a highly vascular tissue, but with the passage of time it develops into avascular scar tissue. Two stages may be recognized: there is first a stage of *vascularization*, and this is subsequently followed by *devascularization*.

Buds of endothelial cells grow out from the existing blood vessels at the wound margin, undergo canalization, and by joining with their neighbours form a series of vascular arcades. At first the newly-formed vessels all appear similar; the electron microscope shows gaps between the endothelial cells and a poorly-formed basement membrane. Protein escapes from these newly-formed vessels, and it is easy to imagine that the tissue fluid around them forms a very suitable medium for cellular growth. Very soon differentiation occurs. Some vessels acquire a muscular coat and become arterioles, while others form thin-walled venules. The remainder either disappear, or persist as part of the capillary bed.

As the blood vessels grow into the clot, the myofibroblasts at the wound edge multiply and accompany the vascular invasion. Thus the clot is converted into a living vascular granulation tissue, and the process is known as *organization*. The myofibroblasts which accompany the capillary loops are large and plump, but gradually, as collagen fibrils form around them, the cells become elongated fibrocytes. In the early stages of fibroplasia, type III collagen is formed and its thin fibres, called reticulin, can be demonstrated by silver impregnation methods. As the granulation tissue matures, type I collagen is formed and appears as thick eosinophilic fibres on light microscopy that also stain by the conventional collagen stains (van Gieson's, Mallory's trichrome, etc.). The myofibroblasts are also responsible for the formation of the proteoglycans of the ground substance. Fibronectin is formed by these cells as well as other cell types. Lymphatic vessels grow into the maturing granulation tissue in much the same

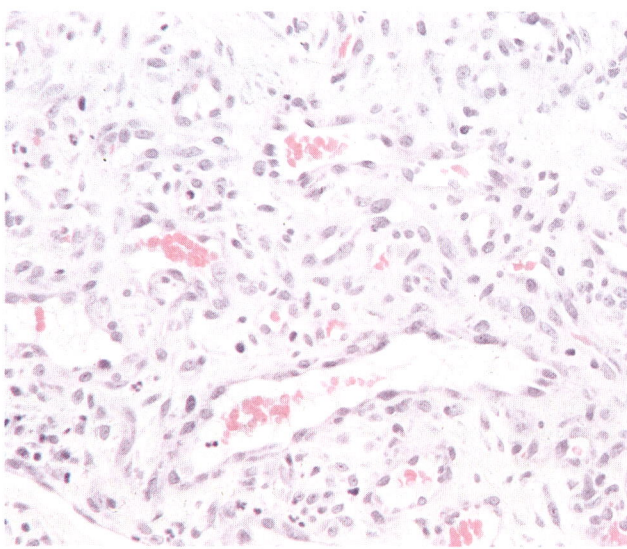

Fig. 8.3 Early granulation tissue. The tissue is vascular, being composed of thin-walled capillary blood vessels, and between them loose tissue, plump fibroblast-type cells and scattered inflammatory cells — lymphocytes and neutrophils. Collagen formation is not marked at this stage.

manner as do the blood vessels, only later. The two sets of vessels do not anastomose. At the same time there is an ingrowth of nerve fibres to supply the arterioles, which are then capable of exhibiting contraction.

As maturation proceeds, so some vessels undergo atrophy and disappear. Others show thickening of their intimal coats and eventual obliteration of the lumen (*endarteritis obliterans*). This process of devascularization results in the formation of a pale avascular scar. Coincident with the devascularization there is often *cicatrization* of scar tissue with much local tissue distortion. This process must be clearly distinguished from contraction. *Cicatrization* (or *contracture*, as it is sometimes called) is a diminution in the size of a *scar* and is a late event; *contraction* is a diminution in the size of a *wound* and is an early event.

Tensile strength. Another method of examining a wound is the estimation of its tensile strength. The strength of the wound is of great practical importance because it is the main safeguard against *wound disruption*, or *dehiscence*. Three stages may be recognized.

At first the strength of a skin wound is only that of the fibrin cementing the cut surfaces together. It is for this reason that skin wounds are held together by sutures, clips, or tapes. There then follows a period of increasing tensile strength which corresponds to the amount of collagen produced by the granulation tissue uniting the cut wound edges. Thus the increase in tensile strength parallels the increase of hydroxyproline in the wound area, since this is a reflection of the amount of collagen present. Finally as the months go by the strength of a wound increases further.

The steady development of cross-linkages between collagen fibres is responsible for this steady increase in tensile strength. Collagen synthesis continues for many weeks but there is no increase in the total amount because it is accompanied by collagen breakdown. The balanced state of collagen synthesis and collagen degradation brings about a remodelling of the scar so that it reaches an optimum state. An imbalance could result in a weak scar (see scurvy and wound dehiscence) on the one hand, and keloid formation on the other.

Thus many factors influence the rate of increase of tensile strength. These are both local

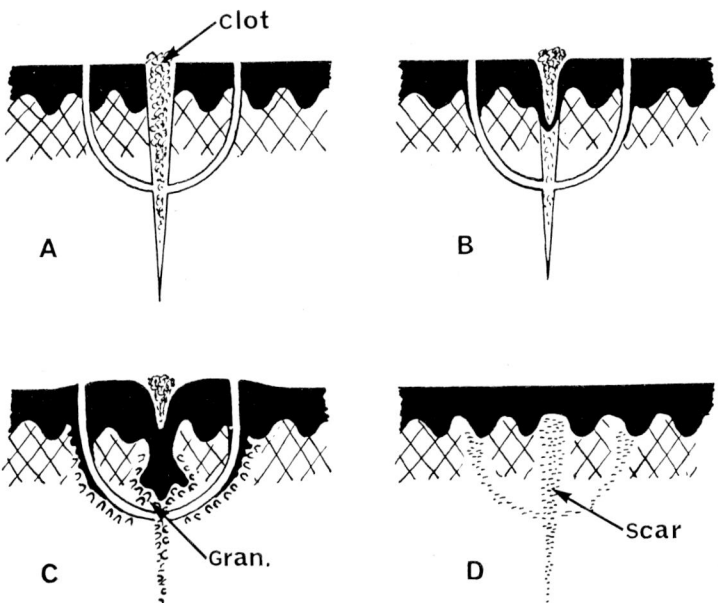

Fig. 8.4 Diagrammatic representation of the healing of an incised wound held together by a suture, the track of which alone is shown. The wound rapidly fills with clot (A) and shortly afterwards the epithelium migrates into the wound and down the suture tracks (B). Epithelial spurs are formed, and granulation-tissue (Gran) formation proceeds (C). In D the suture has been removed, and scar tissue remains to mark the site of the incision and the suture tracks. The epithelial ingrowths have degenerated.

and general, and in the main are related to granulation-tissue and collagen formation.

HEALING OF SKIN WOUNDS

Healing of wounds differs depending on whether the edges are accurately opposed or widely separated.

Healing of a clean incised wound with edges in apposition

This process is described as *healing by primary intention*, and is the desired result in all surgical incisions. The following changes occur:

Initial haemorrhage results in the formation of fibrin-rich haematoma.

An acute inflammatory reaction occurs, and the fibrinous exudate helps to cement the cut margins of the wound together.

Epithelial changes. Within 24 h of injury epithelial cells from the adjacent epidermis migrate into the wound and insinuate themselves between the inert dermis and the clot (Fig. 8.4(B)). With well-approximated wounds by 24 h a continuous layer of epidermal cells covers the surface. Overlying the area there is a crust or scab of dried clot. During the next 24–48 h the epidermal cells invade the space where connective tissue will eventually develop; in this way a spur is formed (Fig. 8.4(C)). Mitotic activity occurs in the basal cells a short distance from the edge of the wound, but not in the epidermal cells that are migrating. Epidermal cells also migrate along suture tracks, and where the suture or the incision encounters a sweat gland or other skin appendage, epithelial cells are contributed from this source. (Fig. 8.4 (C)).

A *demolition phase* follows the acute inflammatory reaction in the area of the wound.

Organization. By about the third day the wound area is filled with fibroblasts (myofibroblasts) and capillary buds growing in from the cut surfaces. This ingrowth occurs mainly from the subcutaneous tissues, with little or no contribution from the inert reticular layer of the dermis. There may be some contribution from the papillary layer of the dermis. Collagen appears a day or two later. This granulation tissue appears to prevent excessive epithelial migration into the wound, and the epithelial cells which form the spurs and the lining of suture tracks degenerate and are replaced by granulation tissue. Only the surface epithelial cells persist, and these divide and differentiate so that a multilayered covering of epidermis is reformed. It first covers a vascular granulation tissue, but as devascularization proceeds the scar shrinks in size and changes in colour from red to white.

Epithelial cells are thus the first cells to be stimulated, and their presence excites a connective tissue response which in its turn inhibits the epithelial growth. The early role that epithelium plays in the process of wound healing explains the ugly punctate scars which appear if sutures are left in position for any length of time. Punctured wounds due to injections do not form such scars, because the wound is not held open and therefore no epithelial 'invasion' occurs. The use of adhesive tapes instead of sutures for closing wounds avoids these marks and produces a better cosmetic result.

Healing of a wound with separated edges
(*healing by secondary intention*)

Although stress is sometimes laid on the difference between healing by primary intention and secondary intention, the pathological changes in both are very similar. When there is extensive tissue loss, either by direct trauma, necrosis secondary to inflammation or hypersensitivity, or simply failure to approximate the wound edges, a large defect is present which must be made good. The main bulk of tissue which performs this service is granulation tissue, and this type of healing is therefore sometimes known as *healing by granulation*.

In *healing by secondary intention* the wound edges are widely separated, so that healing has to progress from the base upwards as well as from the edges inwards. From the clinical point of view healing of a well-approximated incised wound (primary intention) is fast and leaves a small, neat scar. Healing by secondary intention is slow and results in a large, distorted scar. The difference lies in the type of wound and not in the type of healing.

The following account of the healing of a large uninfected wound is illustrated in Fig. 8.5.

1. There is an initial inflammatory phase affecting the surrounding tissues. The wound is filled with coagulum, as described in simple incisions. This coagulum dries on its surface, and forms a scab in some wounds.

2. An important feature is *wound contraction*, which has already been fully described (see p 86). Fig. 8.2 shows the changes in size of full-thickness skin loss.

3. As with incised wounds, the epidermis adjacent to the wound shows hyperplasia, and epithelial cells migrate into the wound. They form a thin tongue which grows between pre-existing viable connective tissue and the surface clot with necrotic material. The epithelial cells secrete a collagenase which probably aids their penetration between living and dead connective tissue.

4. Demolition follows acute inflammation, and the clot in the centre of the wound is invaded and replaced by granulation tissue. This grows from the subcutaneous tissues at the wound edge, and is important in causing wound contraction. Granulation tissue is also formed from the base of the wound, the amount from this source depending upon the nature and vascularity of the bed.

When the wound is viewed with a magnifying glass, the surface (under the scab) is deep red and granular, the capillary loops forming elevated mounds (Fig. 8.6). It is very fragile, and the slightest trauma causes bleeding. It was this granularity which was responsible for the name 'granulation tissue'. The covering of the wound by granulation tissue serves an important protective role. If organisms are introduced into a recent wound, infection is likely to result, but not, however, if the wound is first allowed to granulate. Thus granulation tissue forms a temporary protective layer until the surface is covered by epithelium.

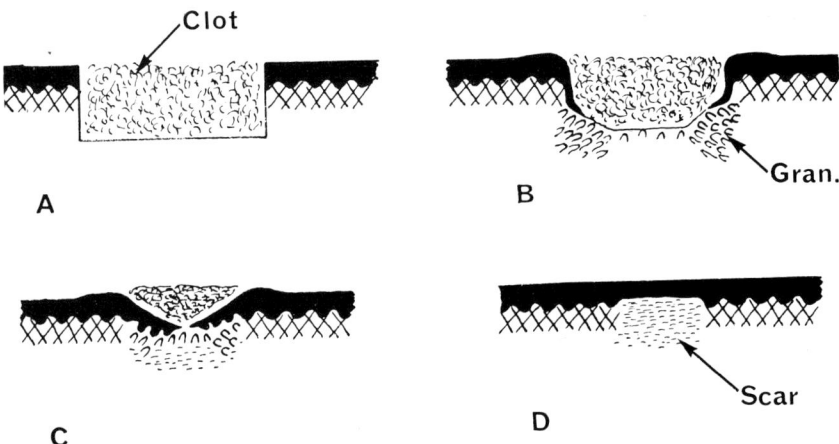

Fig. 8.5   Diagram to illustrate the healing of an incised wound. The wound is rapidly filled with clot (A). Epithelium soon migrates in from the margins to undermine the clot, which dries to form a crust. Granulation tissue (Gran) grows into the wounded area, and is most profuse around the circumference where it is derived from the subcutaneous fat (B). Epithelial ingrowth continues and spurs are produced (C); these, however, do not persist, and the end-result (D) is a scar covered by epidermis which lacks rete ridges. During the healing process contraction has taken place so that the final scar is considerably smaller than the original wound.

5. The migrating epidermis covers the granulation tissue, and in this way a mushroom-shaped scab is formed with a central attachment, which finally becomes nipped off. (Fig. 8.5(C)).

6. The regenerated epidermis becomes thicker, and sends short processes into the underlying tissue. These are transient structures and do not persist as rete ridges, for neither these nor the skin appendages are reformed in the human subject. The epidermal incursions appear to stimulate the formation of granulation tissue, so that the scar gains thickness and is eventually level with the surface of the skin. The scar is at first pink, but the subsequent devascularization leaves it white.

It can be seen that with full thickness skin loss, part of the clot occupying the wound is organized but much of it is cast off. With partial thickness skin loss, as many occur following burns or at the donor site of a Thiersch graft, the area of the wound is covered by epithelium both from the wound edges and from the cut remains of hair follicles and sweat glands. Epithelialization is therefore very fast, and the granulation tissue which is formed is produced beneath the new epithelium.

FACTORS INFLUENCING REPAIR

Although it would be desirable to analyse the factors which influence repair according to whether they affect granulation tissue formation, collagen production, contraction, etc., it must be admitted that in many instances we have insufficient information to adopt this policy. In practice, the factors which affect wound healing may be divided into two groups—those which act locally, and those whose influence is general or systemic. There are many factors which delay wound healing, but few are known which accelerate it. The following account consists therefore largely of the causes of delayed wound healing.

Local factors

Blood supply

Wounds in an area such as the lower leg where there is a poor blood supply heal slowly in comparison with the face and oral mucosa which have a good blood supply. Healing is particularly slow in the legs if there is venous stasis related to varicose veins, or in patients with peripheral vascular disease. Likewise there is slow healing in an area of

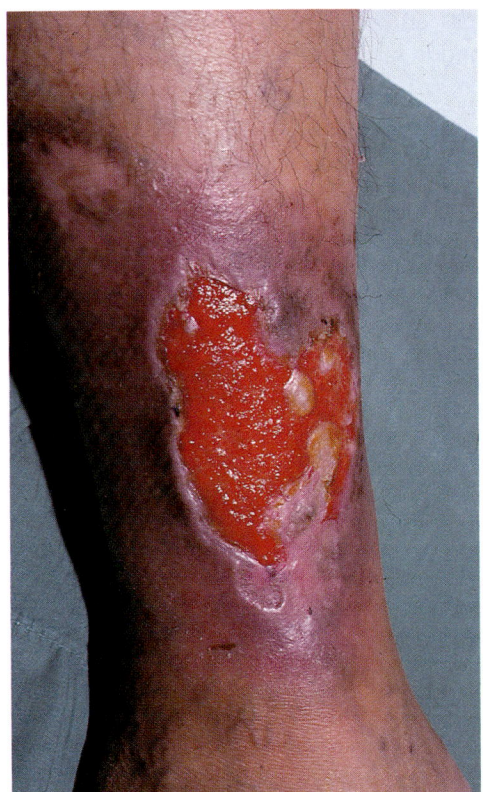

Fig. 8.6 Granulating leg ulcer. The skin shows the changes of stasis dermatitis, and a large stasis ulcer. The bed of the ulcer consists of vasular granulation tissue; in places there are areas of regenerating epidermis.

chronic radiodermatitis, or indeed if there is chronic inflammation from any cause.

Continued tissue breakdown and inflammation

Any condition causing continued tissue breakdown leads to persistent inflammation, and therefore delays completion of the healing process.

The most important examples are infection, the presence of a foreign body or irritant chemical, and excessive movement.

Infection

In an infected skin wound a scab does not form, and often the base is composed of dead tissue and inflammatory exudate forming a slough. Underlying this there is chronic inflammatory granulation tissue.

Foreign bodies and other irritants

The presence of a foreign body in a wound, even in the absence of infection, may delay healing. The over-enthusiastic use of irritating disinfectants may cause considerable delay in the healing of skin ulcers, and indeed, if hypersensitivity develops, may lead to extensive necrosis.

Movement

This delays healing by submitting the delicate granulation tissue to repeated trauma.

Poor apposition of the wound edges

This will obviously delay the healing of the wound. If the wound is adherent to a bony surface, this, by anchoring the wound edges, will tend to prevent contraction. This is well seen in wounds over the tibia, and also in chronic stasis ulcers of the legs.

Direction of the wound

Skin wounds made in a direction parallel to the lines of Langer heal faster than those made at right angles to them. *The lines of Langer*, first described in fact by Dupuytren in 1832, are due to the orientation of the collagen bundles in the dermis. The skin is less tensile in the direction of the lines than at right angles to them. In general they correspond to the direction of the crease lines, although the latter are in fact related also to the movements of the underlying muscles and joints. Skin incisions made across the crease lines tend to gape, and their healing is delayed. Therefore, when planning a surgical incision these should be taken into consideration. Wounds parallel to or in the crease lines are more satisfactory and the resulting scars less visible.

General factors

Age

Wound healing is fast in the young, but is not prolonged in old age unless there is some associated debilitating disease or ischaemia.

Nutrition.

Protein deficiency. Animals starved of protein show poor wound healing and deficient collagen formation. This abnormality may be corrected by administering proteins containing methionine or cystine, or by supplementing the diet with these amino acids only. Although cystine is not present in mature collagen, it is necessary for normal wound healing and collagen formation (see p. 26)

Vitamin-C deficiency. Experimentally in guinea-pigs (scurvy does not occur in other rodents because they can synthetize vitamin C), wound contraction and epithelial regeneration proceed normally. Granulation tissue is produced, but is abnormal; the fibroblasts are arranged in an irregular manner and although they produce a little reticulin, normal collagen fibres are not formed. The wound is therefore very weak. Capillaries are unduly fragile and haemorrhages occur. In those who have teeth, swelling of and bleeding from the gingivae are characteristic. Vitamin C is necessary for the hydroxylation of proline prior to its incorporation into the collagen molecule (p. 26).

Although frank scurvy is uncommon, minor degrees of vitamin-C deficiency are not infrequent in patients who are on a marginal intake and who are in other ways stressed.

The role of zinc. The addition of zinc to the diet of rats has been shown to promote the healing of thermal burns and excised wounds. The mechanism is not known, but the fact that zinc is an important component of several enzymes may be related. The oral administration of zinc sulphate has been tried in humans, and a beneficial effect on wound healing claimed.

Glucocorticoids

In excessive amounts these inhibit the formation of granulation tissue and also delay wound contraction.

Temperature

It is the general experience that wounds of the exposed parts heal much more slowly in cold weather, and experiments on animals during hibernation have supported this observation.

COMPLICATIONS OF WOUND HEALING

Wound dehiscence

The bursting open of a wound is described as dehiscence, and it occurs when stress is applied before the wound has healed sufficiently. It is particularly serious in abdominal incisions, because it results in the exposure of the abdominal contents to the atmosphere outside. Increased intra-abdominal pressure combines with poor wound healing to precipitate this catastrophic event.

Cicatrization

This is a frequent complication of extensive burning of skin, and may produce great deformity. Cicatrization involving hollow viscera, e.g. the intestine or the urethra, is an important cause of narrowing (stenosis) of the lumen.

Keloid formation

Occasionally an excessive formation of collagenous tissue results in the appearance of a raised nodule of scar tissue called a keloid (Fig. 8.7). The cause of this is unknown but there seems to be a genetic factor in some families. Repeated trauma and irritation caused by foreign bodies, hair, keratin, etc., may play a part. Keloids are more common in adolescence, especially in girls, in black people, and during pregnancy. They are found most commonly in the earlobes, neck and shoulders and are especially frequent after burns.

Weak scars

If scar tissue is subjected to continuous strain, stretching may result. In elderly people the abdominal viscera may bulge through a weak scar to produce a local protrusion, or *incisional hernia*.

Painful scars

Pain either local or referred may be experienced if a nerve is included in the scar tissue.

Pigmentary changes

Coloured particles introduced into the wound may persist and cause colouring or tattooing. Healed chronic ulcers sometimes have a russet colour due to staining with haemosiderin.

HEALING IN OTHER SPECIALIZED TISSUES

It is generally stated that the greater the degree of specialization of a tissue, the less well developed are its powers of regeneration. Certainly neurons are highly specialized and incapable of division, but degrees of specialization in cells are as difficult to define as they are amongst human beings. Is a liver cell more or less specialized than a simple unstriped muscle fibre? Liver cells show remarkable powers of proliferation, yet perform functions of which they alone are capable. Similarly, it is impossible to compare the degrees of specialization of the different types of epithelium, each of which has its own peculiar characteristics. It seems more likely that the power of regeneration is best developed in those organs and tissues which are most liable to injury, and the replacement of which has survival value for the individual and species.

EPITHELIAL TISSUES

All covering epithelia show good regenerative power. This is hardly surprising because they are being continuously subjected to trauma, and their integrity depends upon their ability to replace the lost cells. Grandular epithelia, on the other hand, show erratic regenerative capacity.

Covering epithelia

As described previously, *epidermis* shows good regeneration, although specialized structures like the rete ridges, hair follicles, sweat glands and sebaceous glands are not replaced.

With *oral epithelium*, complete regeneration occurs. The lamina propria and submucosa heal by repair, and scar tissue may remain in the lining mucosa but not in the masticatory mucosa.

Regeneration of *intestinal epithelium* and *respiratory epithelium* is excellent. Likewise in the stomach epithelial regeneration is good, although the regenerated epithelium that covers a healed chronic gastric ulcer may be of intestinal rather than gastric type.

Glandular epithelium

Liver

The liver has remarkable powers of regeneration. In the rat, resection of three-quarters of the organ results in such active division of the remaining cells that within two weeks the organ is restored to its orginal weight.

In the human, regeneration of liver cells is seen following any type of necrosis, provided the patient survives. The end-results of this regeneration vary so widely, depending upon the type of hepatic necrosis, that this important subject will be considered in Chapter 32.

Kidney

The renal tubular epithelium has considerable powers of regeneration; thus in acute tubular necrosis, in spite of extensive damage, complete return to normal may occur. This type of lesion is therefore most eligible for treatment with dialysis, since recovery is quite possible. When damage to the kidney results in destruction of a complete nephron, regeneration does not occur. Glomeruli once destroyed cannot be replaced.

CONNECTIVE TISSUES

When conditions are favourable many of the specialized connective tissues show excellent regeneration. However, not infrequently adverse factors operate and these result in healing by repair.

Mesothelium

Lost mesothelial cells of the peritoneum and other serous cavities are replaced from underlying connective tissue cells, which take on the appearance of flattened mesothelium.

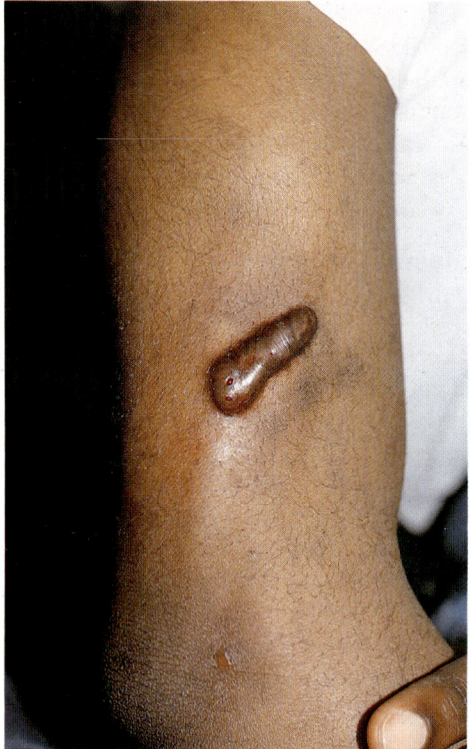

Fig. 8.7 Keloid. Following the removal of a melanocytic naevus this smooth keloidal mass of dense collagen developed. The overlying epidermis is deeply pigmented, a change that commonly occurs following inflammation in dark coloured skin.

Synovium

Synovial lining cells are also replaced from underlying connective tissue. The adjacent un-injured synovial cells are inert, and play no part in the process of healing.

Vascular endothelium

In large arteries, e.g. the aorta, new endothelial cells arise by mitotic division of pre-existing ones, and slowly spread over the denuded area.

Fat

Although fat cells may appear in fully mature granulation tissue, defects in fatty tissue are usually made good by fibrous tissue. The process of repair shows a characteristic feature during the demolition phase; the macrophages ingest large quantities of fat, becoming greatly swollen in the process. These *foam cells* form a prominent feature of traumatic fat necrosis (p. 46).

Cartilage

Regeneration in cartilage is generally poor. In the case of the hyaline cartilage of joint surfaces small defects are made good by regeneration. With large injuries which involve damage to the underlying vascular bone, a haematoma forms, becomes vascularized and converted either into fibrous tissue or bone.

Tendon

Regeneration in tendon is good, but the process is slow. It is said that the tendon ends should be accurately opposed and under some tension, otherwise union is by scar tissue.

Muscle

It is generally taught that damaged muscle is not replaced, and that union is by scar tissue. In large destructive lesions of smooth muscle, a permanent scar remains to mark the site of the original injury, and this is well illustrated by the appearance of a healed chronic gastric ulcer. Although smooth muscle cells appear incapable of division in postuterine life, the arterioles of granulation tissue acquire a muscular coat; the origin of these fibres is not known.

In respect of striated muscle, when part of an individual muscle fibre is damaged, there may be limited regeneration with the production of new myocytes which later fuse to form a syncytial mass. In a clean surgical wound of voluntary muscle, the sarcolemmal masses on either side of the incision may unite, so that the continuity of the muscle is restored, and in time no indication of the site of injury can be found. However, with extensive damage to muscle the architecture is destroyed, and healing is by scar tissue; this is seen following infarction.

Cardiac muscle shows no regenerative capacity, and once necrosis has occurred, as in infarction, a permanent scar remains.

Bone marrow

Bone marrow provides an excellent example of tissue in which regeneration is complete.

Bone

The regeneration of bone as seen in the healing of a fracture is described in Chapter 34.

Nervous tissue

Adult nerve cells are unable to divide and therefore when a part of the brain or spinal cord is destroyed, new neurons are not produced.

Peripheral nervous system

Following section of axis cylinder the neuron shows changes described as *chromatolysis*. The cell swells and its Nissl granules disappear. These bodies are zones of endoplasmic reticulum studded plentifully with ribosomes, and their disappearance reflects dysfunction in the protein synthetizing system of the nerve cell. The axis cylinder becomes irregular and varicose, and by 48 h has broken up. The surrounding myelin shows splitting of the laminae, and later fragmentation. The Schwann cells enlarge, proliferate, and become filled with lipid droplets from the degenerated myelin. These changes were originally described as *Wallerian degeneration*. They affect the nerve fibre distal to the point of section and also, in myelinated fibres, a short area proximally up to the first node of Ranvier. The next stage is described as regeneration. From the proximal portion of the cut axon numerous neurofibrils sprout out, and are seen to lie invaginated into the cytoplasm of the Schwann cells. They push their way distally through the Schwann cells at the rate of about 1 mm/day. Many of the fibrils lose their way and degenerate, but some reach an appropriate end-organ, and persist to form the definitive replacement axon. It is evident that accurate apposition of the cut ends of the nerve is of great importance in facilitating this process. The final process involves the reformation of the myeline sheath as the regeneration axon matures and increases in diameter.

The functional end-result of nerve damage depends on various factors: if the axons are damaged but the nerve trunk itself is not severed, an excellent result may be expected. When the nerve is severed, careful suturing and absence of infection are important. Functional recovery is more complete when a pure motor or sensory nerve is cut. Recovery from a lesion of a mixed nerve, like the median nerve of the forearm, is often poor.

Central nervous system

Here oligodendroglia take the place of the Schwann cells in relation to nerve fibres. It is often stated that regeneration of central nerve fibres does not occur. The affected nerve cells show chromatolysis often followed by necrosis, and the destroyed tissue is replaced by proliferating neuroglia to form a dense glial scar. Nevertheless, there is considerable evidence that some regeneration is possible. In the clinical field it is noticeable that in patients with partial spinal-cord lesions, voluntary muscle strength seems to increase steadily for 9–12 months. This is generally attributed to improved utilization of residual undamaged pathways. In the lower animals regeneration of the long-tract axons in the spinal cord is a usual feature, and it is possible that some regeneration may occur in the higher animals, including the human being.

MECHANISM OF HEALING

When one considers that in a healing wound there is cell and tissue production proceeding at a rate which exceeds that seen in the most malignant tumours, it is humiliating to admit how little we know of the mechanisms involved. A number of growth stimulating factors have been described. These include insulin-like substances (somatomedins) epidermal growth factor, and macrophage derived factors which stimulate fibroblastic proliferation and induce new blood-vessel formation (angiogenic factor). The platelet derived growth factor stimulates the division of fibroblasts and smooth muscle cells. It is of great interest that these growth factors appear to be formed as the products of cellular oncogene activity. These genes are present in normal cells and their products are involved in normal cellular growth and differentiation. Precisely how they are regulated is not clear. Nevertheless the chemical nature of these growth factors and their receptors is now being unravelled, and it is to be hoped that in the future they can be used to stimulate the rate of wound healing.

Alternatively it has been postulated that removal of an inhibiting substance (*chalone*), normally present, is responsible for stimulating cell division. No pure substance with this effect has been isolated.

Physical factors may play some part; for instance epithelial cells tend to maintain contact with each other and spread over surfaces. The migration of squamous epithelium in wound healing can be easily understood. When cells establish contact with similar cells movement stops.

This is termed *contact inhibition*. In tissue culture, cells multiply until a particular concentration of cells is reached, and at this point division ceases. This is termed *density dependent regulation of growth*. The precise mechanism involved in these processes is not understood, but it appears to involve direct cell-to-cell contact and production of regulatory peptides or cytokines whereby one cell influences another. The remarkable relationship between epidermis and dermis in wound healing is another example of how the growth of one cell is influenced by the presence of another type. Although some general factors, such as food supply and hormones, affect the processes of healing, in the control of cell division and maturation local factors are most likely to play the dominant role.

GENERAL READING

Forrester L 1983 Current concepts in soft connective tissue wound healing. British Journal of Surgery 70: 133
Green A R 1989 Peptide regulatory factors: multifunctional mediators of cellular growth and differentiation. Lancet 1: 705
Hunt T K (ed) 1980 Wound healing and wound infection. Appleton–Century–Crofts, New York
Leading Article 1978 The myofibroblast. Lancet 2: 1290

Leibovich S J, Ross R 1975 The role of the macrophage in wound repair. American Journal of Pathology 78: 71
Ross R 1989 Platelet-derived growth factor. Lancet 1: 1179
Rytomaa T 1976 The chalone concept. International Review of Experimental Pathology 16: 155
Sibbit W L 1988 Oncogenes, normal cell growth, and connective tissue disease. Ann Review of Medicine 39: 123

9. Chronic inflammation

Although the concept of chronic inflammation is in part a clinical one implying that the inflammatory process persists for a long period, pathologically it is best defined as *a process in which destruction and inflammation are proceeding at the same time as attempts at healing.*

The tissue response to injury has been divided into three phases: the initial vascular and exudative phenomena of *acute inflammation* are followed by a second phase of *demolition* which is accomplished by macrophage activity. The third and final phase is one of *healing*, by which lost tissue is replaced by the processes of *repair* and *regeneration*.

It is evident that complete healing can occur only when the acute inflammation and demolition phases are themselves completed. Since these are the consequences of the initial damage, it follows that healing results only when the cause of the inflammation is itself removed. If tissue damage continues, a disease process develops in which there is present a mixture of the phenomena of acute inflammation, demolition, repair, and regeneration. To such a lesion the term chronic inflammation is applied.

CAUSES OF CHRONIC INFLAMMATION

Any cause of tissue damage can, if it persists, lead to chronic inflammation. Three main groups can be recognized.

INFECTIONS

The body has a limited ability to destroy certain organisms, e.g. the tubercle bacillus and *Treponema pallidum*. Infection with these agents therefore commonly leads to chronic inflammation. Moreover, if local or general conditions impair the body's defences, an organism that usually produces a self-limiting acute inflammation may persist to cause a chronic one. Thus, *Staph. aureus*, which can produce a boil that generally heals rapidly, can also produce chronic inflammation in some situations, such as in the bone marrow (see *chronic osteomyelitis*, p. 105). Any of the causes of delayed healing may so turn the scales against the host that there develops the 'frustrated healing' that chronic inflammation has so aptly been called.

INSOLUBLE PARTICULATE IRRITANTS

Silica and asbestos are examples of irritant particles that the body cannot easily remove. Inhalation of such substances leads to persistent chronic inflammation of the lungs (see *pneumoconiosis*, Ch. 30).

IMMUNE-MEDIATED DAMAGE

The development of delayed type hypersensitivity is an important factor in the continuing tissue that accompanies perpetuation of chronic infective diseases, of which tuberculosis is the prototype. Damaging immune complexes are involved under other circumstances. This is thought to occur in lupus erythematosus.

TYPES OF CHRONIC INFLAMMATION

Although chronic inflammation may follow obvious acute inflammation, some agents, e.g. the tubercle bacillus, cause only a mild fleeting acute reaction but persists and by causing continued damage lead to the development of chronic disease. The initial acute phase is often inconspicuous and completely missed clinically. Chronic inflammation may therefore follow an obvious acute inflammation or it may appear to start de novo.

The histological features of a chronic inflammatory lesion may be used in a descriptive classification. Any of the components of the chronic inflammatory reaction may predominate, and it is convenient to use this as the basis of classification (Table 9.1).

Table 9.1 Components of chronic inflammation

Component	Tissue response
Acute inflammation	Polymorph infiltration
	Oedema
	Fibrin
Demolition	Macrophage formation
	Epithelioid-cell formation
	Giant-cell formation
Healing	
Repair	Granulation tissue
	Blood vessels
	Fibroblasts
	Collagen
	Neuroglia in CNS
Regeneration	Epithelial overgrowth
	Specialized connective-tissue overgrowth
Immune response	Lymphocytes
	Plasma cells
	Eosinophils

CHRONIC INFLAMMATION WITH FEATURES OF ACUTE INFLAMMATION

This type of chronic inflammation is characterized by tissue necrosis and the formation of inflammatory exudate containing fluid and numerous neutrophils. Pus is therefore formed and this type of reaction is termed *chronic suppurative inflammation*. It is seen in a chronic abscess (Fig. 9.1) or staphylococcal osteomyelitis. Sometimes fluid exudation is marked as in a chronic empyema.

Pus, rich in polymorphonuclear leucocytes, is very evident, and fibrin may not only be seen microscopically, but on occasions forms large masses easily visible to the naked eye (Fig. 9.1). Fluid exudation is also a feature of chronic suppurative disease, and if drained the continued protein loss may lead to hypoalbuminaemia (p. 330). Accumulations of protein-rich fluid are frequent in chronic inflammation of the serous sacs, e.g. tuberculous peritonitis.

Eosinophils are sometimes present in large numbers in the exudate in chronic inflammation. Whether this is a manifestation of hypersensitivity is not known.

CHRONIC INFLAMMATION WITH FEATURES OF DEMOLITION PREDOMINATING

A heavy macrophage infiltration is characteristic of certain types of chronic inflammation. Often the accumulation of cells produces a tumour-like mass and by tradition this type of inflammation is termed *granulomatous*. The macrophages are derived from emigrating monocytes of bone-marrow origin, and they constitute the bulk of granulomatous lesions. In some granulomata the monocytes are soon destroyed, but are replaced by new cells from the blood stream. This type constitutes the *high-turnover granulomata*. In other circumstances (*low-turnover granulomata*) the monocytes remain for many weeks in the tissues, and may undergo mitosis before entering a resting phase and subsequently developing into phagocytic cells. In these low-turnover granulomata the proliferation of local histiocytes probably contributes to the macrophage population, and a constant

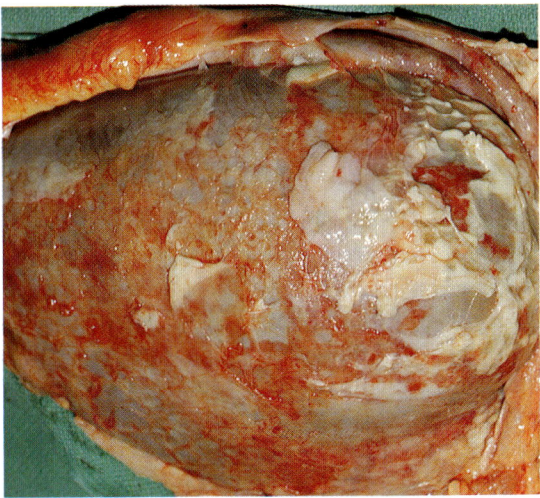

Fig. 9.1 Subphrenic abscess. In this necropsy specimen the diaphragm has been incised and turned back to reveal the superior surface of the liver. The liver is covered by thick purulent exudate. The abscess was formed as the result of a perforated duodenal ulcer.

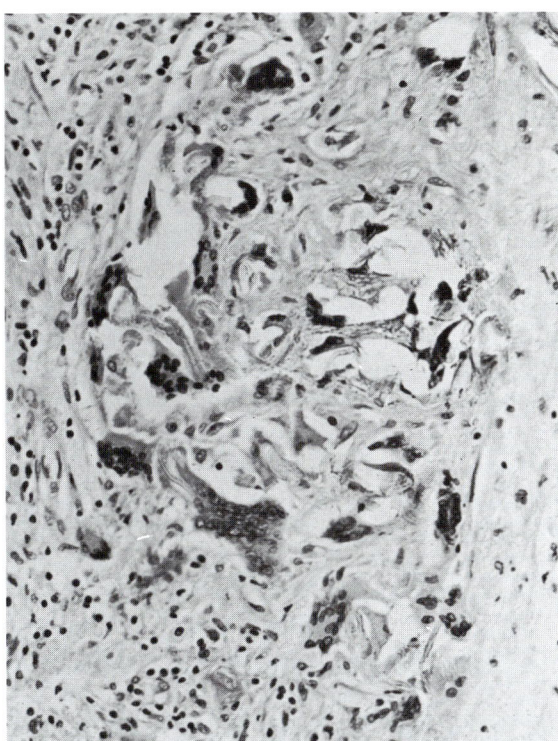

Fig. 9.2 Foreign-body reaction. This is a section through an old operation scar at the site of an unabsorbed nylon suture, which is not recognizable in the figure. There is a heavy accumulation of foreign-body giant cells, around which there are empty spaces. The whole is enclosed in dense fibrous tissue in which there is a moderate lymphocytic infiltration. × 100.

recruitment for monocytes of bone-marrow origin is not required.

The macrophage infiltration in chronic inflammation may be diffuse (*diffuse granulomatous inflammation*), but this is an uncommon reaction; it is characteristic of lepromatous leprosy. More commonly the macrophages lose their phagocytic function, enlarge and develop abundant eosinophilic cytoplasm. They are called *epithelioid cells* because of their resemblance to the epithelial cells of the epidermis. Under these circumstances the cells tend to be arranged in discrete groups termed tubercles, so called because this type of reaction is typical of the reaction to the tubercle bacillus (*tuberculoid granulomatous inflammation*) (see Figs 15.1 and 15.2). The cell membranes are so interdigitated that on light microscopy it is difficult to delineate each cell from its neighbours. Although epithelioid cells are not phagocytic they can take up material by pinocytosis. They have well-developed endoplasmic reticulum and a prominent Golgi complex, suggesting that they have a secretory function. Indeed, they secrete many polypeptide substances or cytokines. One such substance is cachexin which is probably identical to tumour necrosis factor (see later).

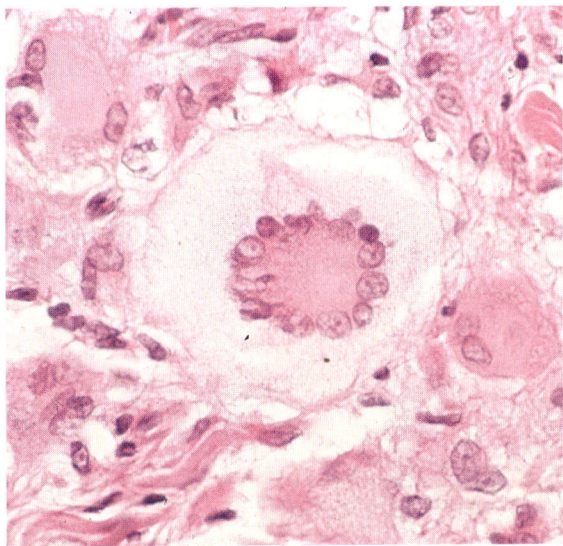

Fig. 9.3 Touton giant cell. The giant cell shows a central area of eosinophilic cytoplasm surrounded by a circle of nuclei forming a wreath. External to this the cytoplasm is pale and vacuolated because of its high lipid content.

Precisely why macrophages differentiate into epithelioid cells is not clear, but they do so under a number of circumstances. Thus they do so when they have completely digested phagocytosed material, or have successfully extruded phagocytosed material by exocytosis. Epithelioid-cell formation is inhibited if phagocytosed material can neither be digested nor extruded. Thus lepra cells stuffed with lepra bacilli do not become epithelioid cells. In a tuberculous granuloma, bacilli are very scanty and epithelioid cells are formed. It follows that in any chronic inflammation with a well-developed tuberculoid granulomatous reaction, the causative organism is very difficult to find. It should be noted that when epithelioid-cell formation is marked, the cells tend to be grouped into follicles or tubercles. This contrasts with the more diffuse infiltration of phagocytic macrophages that do not differentiate into epithelioid cells.

When macrophages encounter insoluble material they frequently fuse together to form *giant cells*. This occurs around exogenous foreign bodies like silk and talc, as well as around endogenous debris such as pieces of dead bone (sequestra), keratin, cholesterol crystals, and uric acid crystals. They are also formed in response to certain organisms such as the tubercle bacillus and many fungi. Three forms of these giant cells have been described.

Langhan's giant cells. The nuclei are disposed around the periphery of the cell in the form of a horseshoe or a ring. These cells are particularly frequent in tuberculous lesions.

Foreign-body giant cells. (Fig. 9.2). In this type the nuclei are scattered haphazardly throughout the cytoplasm. In many lesions giant cells of both Langhan's and foreign-body type are present, and the two should not be regarded as distinct types.

Touton giant cells. This type of giant cell is found in xanthomata (Fig. 9.3). Its peripheral cytoplasm has a foamy appearance, and the nuclei surround a central area of clear eosinophilic cytoplasm.

CHRONIC INFLAMMATION WITH FEATURES OF HEALING

Repair

Granulation tissue is prominent in many chronic inflammatory lesions. It contains:

1. Endothelial cells forming blood and lymphatic vessels
2. Fibroblasts or myofibroblasts forming collagen and proteoglycans.

The vascularity of the granulation tissue may give rise to haemorrhage. Thus bleeding occurs from the base of chronic peptic ulcers, the inflamed dilated bronchi in bronchiectasis, and in chronic gingivitis.

In chronic suppuration, the pus-filled cavity is lined by acutely inflamed granulation tissue which forms a pyogenic membrane.

Fibroblasts are prominent in most chronic inflammations. They lay down collagen, and the resulting scar formation is characteristic of many chronic inflammatory lesions. The proliferation of fibroblasts and their synthesis of collagen appears to be stimulated by cytokines released from macrophages and platelets. Fibrosis is especially well seen in fibroid tuberculosis, Crohn's disease, deep in the base of a chronic peptic ulcer, and in the wall of an abscess. If fibrin is the hallmark of acute inflammation, fibrosis can be considered the salient feature of chronic inflammation. As scarring proceeds, so the lumina of small arteries and arterioles are gradually obliterated by thickening of the tunica intima. This process is called *endarteritis obliterans*. Ultimately a mass of dense avascular scar tissue is formed. Cicatrization may ensue and produce serious effects. For instance a chronic ulcer of the pylorus may lead to narrowing and obstruction of the lumen (pyloric stenosis).

Regeneration

When the tissue destroyed in chronic inflammation is of a type capable of division, regeneration rather than repair takes place. This is particularly obvious in surface epithelia. Indeed, regeneration may become so exuberant that the line of demarcation between it, hyperplasia, and neoplasia may be difficult to define.

The epithelial overgrowth at the edge of a chronic ulcer is sometimes quite remarkable, and may be misinterpreted by the unwary as cancer. The greatly divergent views expressed in the past on the frequency of malignant change in chronic peptic ulcer are largely due to the difficulties in interpreting the microscopic appearances at the edge of the ulcer.

The position is complicated by the fact that malignancy may indeed supervene on the exuberant regeneration of chronic inflammation. This is sometimes seen in chronic ulcerative colitis and in chronic sinuses, e.g. in chronic osteomyelitis.

CHRONIC INFLAMMATION WITH EVIDENCE OF AN IMMUNE REACTION

Although a few lymphocytes and plasma cells are found in uninflamed granulation tissue, many examples of chronic inflammation are characterized by a heavy infiltration by the cells (Fig. 9.4). Because of the difficulty in distinguishing lymphocytes from developing plasma cells they are conveniently grouped together as 'small round cells'. Some of the lymphocytes are of T-cell lineage while others are B lymphocytes and differentiate into plasma cells. Plasma cells are a feature of some chronically inflamed tissues (Fig. 9.5). They are particularly prominent in lesions involving mucous membranes and in the skin adjacent to a mucocutaneous junction such as the lips. Chronic gingivitis is characterized by a massive plasma-cell infiltration. In contrast the inflammatory infiltrate of lichen planus is predominantly lymphocytic. The lesions of syphilis also contain many plasma cells. Occasionally the plasma cells contain one or more spherical, eosinophilic, PAS-positive, hyaline structures called Russell bodies (see Fig. 2.7). When the cell dies these structures are released into the stroma. They are of no great significance, but should not be mistaken for fungi.

Eosinophils are also involved in the immune response, but their role is complex (p. 57).

GENERAL EFFECTS OF CHRONIC INFLAMMATION

The general effects of chronic inflammation depend upon the nature of the responsible agent and the extent of the lesion. In a localized foreign-body reaction there is no noteworthy response at all. On the other hand, in chronic infective disease like tuberculosis or actinomycosis there may be widespread changes in the mononuclear phagocyte system (MPS) and in the blood stream.

CHANGES IN THE MONONUCLEAR PHAGOCYTE SYSTEM (MPS)

Apart from the local accumulation of MP macrophages already described, the lymph nodes draining a chronic inflammatory lesion show hyperplasia. This may sometimes affect the sinus-lining cells ('sinus catarrh'), while at other times there is a marked increased in the number of germinal centres of B lymphocytes. These changes are related to the development of an immune response.

If organisms or their toxins gain access to the blood stream there may be a more generalized hyperplasia of the MP cells, producing enlargement of the spleen (splenomegaly) and lymph nodes (lymphadenopathy). Sometimes this is related to formation of antigen-antibody complexes in the blood stream, which are subsequently removed by the MP system. In other instances, e.g. leishmaniasis, there is a widespread parasitization of the MP cells.

An immune response including both B and T cells is a prominent feature of most chronic inflammatory diseases. It may be reflected in definite morphological changes, and is an additional factor in the production of splenomegaly and generalized lymphadenopathy. Polyclonal gammopathy may occur, and finally the long continued stress on the antibody-producing mechanism can lead to amyloid disease (p. 288).

CHANGES IN THE BLOOD

The white cells frequently show changes which are related to the causative agent and to the extent of infection. These are considered later (p. 311). *Anaemia* is frequent, and is usually of the normochromic normocytic type. Repeated haemorrhages may lead to a hypochromic microcytic anaemia.

A rise in the erythrocyte sedimentation rate (ESR) occurs in many chronic inflammatory diseases, and is commonly used as an aid both to diagnosis and in assessing progress, e.g. in tuberculosis and rheumatoid arthritis (p. 300).

OTHER CHANGES

Tiredness, loss of appetite, loss of weight, fever, malaise, and headaches are common in chronic infections, and although 'toxaemia' is often described in chronic infection it is unlikely to be due to the direct effects of the toxins of bacteria. The endotoxins of the Gram-negative bacilli have been most studied and are important under some circumstances, but no such toxins have been identified with other organisms. The action of cytokines, released from stimulated monocytes, has helped to explain some of the general effects of chronic infection. *Interleukin-1* acts on the hypothalamus to cause a rise in body temperature (see Ch. 23); another important action is to increase protein catabolism in muscle. Another cytokine, *cachexin* (also known as tumour

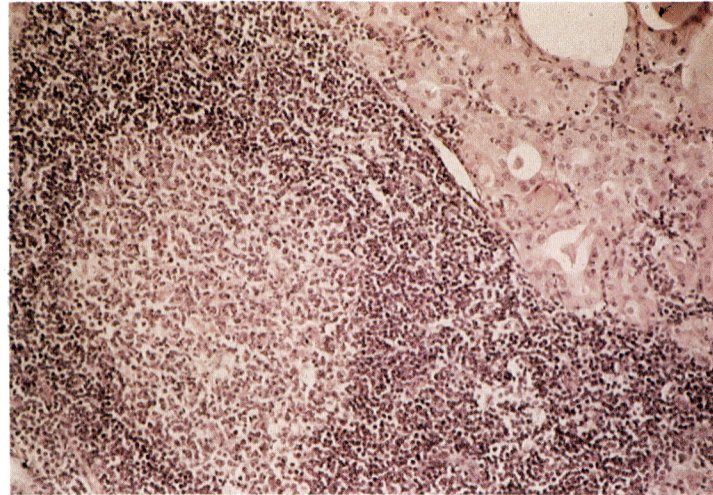

Fig. 9.4   Chronic inflammation. Hashimoto's disease. Remnant of thyroid acini are present (right) but the remainder of the section shows densely packed lymphocytes surrounding one well-defined germinal centre.

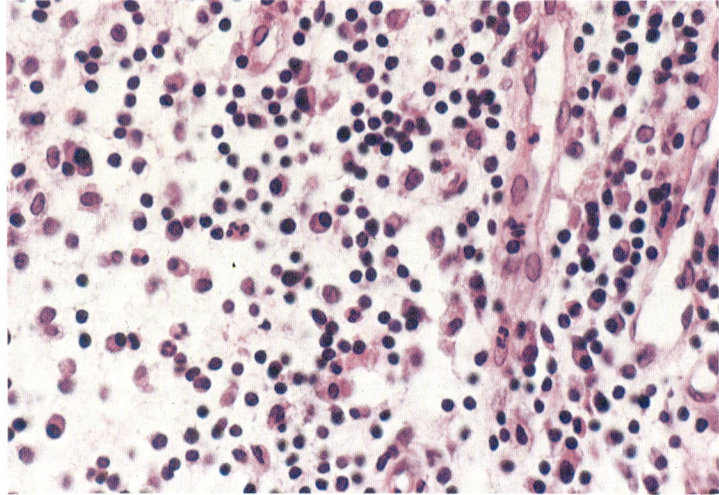

Fig. 9.5   Plasma cells. The section of granulation tissue shows several capillaries lined by plump endothelial cells. In the interstitial tissue there is an infiltrate of lymphocytes, neutrophils and plasma cells. A plasma cell is easily recognized by the eccentric position of its nucleus and the clear space (negative Golgi) adjacent to this.

necrosis factor-alpha) also acts as a pyrogen, but has a major action on adipose tissue to cause breakdown of lipid. The combined action of these cytokines is to lead to increased fat and protein catabolism; in addition, pyrexia, which they induce, increases the metabolic rate and this contributes to tissue breakdown and weight loss.

EXAMPLES OF CHRONIC INFLAMMATION

The types of chronic inflammation can be grouped as those due to:

1. Non-specific, pyogenic bacterial agents like *Staph. aureus* and *Escherichia coli*
2. Inanimate foreign bodies
3. Organisms like *Mycobacterium tuberculosis* that regularly cause chronic inflammation. This third group is so important that it is dealt with separately in Chapter 15
4. Ionizing radiation. This is described in Chapter 22
5. Hypersensitivity. This is discussed in Chapter 13. The collagen vascular diseases can be conveniently included in this group, though their aetiology is obscure.

The first group embraces a wide collection of conditions which are very commonly encountered in clinical practice. For the purpose of this discussion one important example has been selected.

OSTEOMYELITIS

Acute osteomyelitis occurs most often in children at the metaphysis of one of the long bones of the lower limbs. This is the area which is most easily traumatized, and should this occur during the course of a *S. aureus* bacteraemia, the organisms become lodged in a haematoma and produce a metastatic lesion. A typical acute inflammatory reaction occurs, and owing to the rigidity of the bone the increased tension produced by the exudation causes compression of the blood vessels and subsequent ischaemia. Necrosis of marrow and bone therefore follows: pus is formed, and it tracks under the periosteum, thereby further

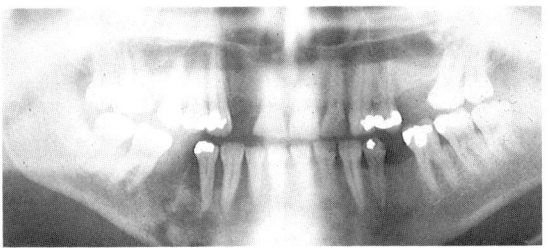

Fig. 9.6   Panoramic radiograph of a 28-year-old male patient who developed osteomyelitis following extraction of the lower right second premolar. The sequestrum is radio-opaque and is surrounded by an area of the infection which is radiolucent. (Radiograph by courtesy of the Professor H D Edmondsen and Dr J D G Rout, Birmingham University.)

imperilling the blood supply to the cortex. In this way quite extensive necrosis may occur, sometimes involving the whole shaft. This dead bone is called a sequestrum and acts as a foreign body; it cannot be easily removed, and it not only provides a focus for the growth of organisms but also prevents the adequate drainage of pus. Conditions are ideal for the development of chronic infection (Fig. 9.6).

Pus ruptures through the periosteum into the muscular and subcutaneous compartments. Usually it is discharged on to the skin surface through sinuses.[*] The vascular periosteum attempts to reform the shaft of the bone by producing bone. This encases the sequestered shaft, and is called the involucrum (Fig. 9.7). The shaft is bathed in pus which escapes through holes, or cloacae, in the involucrum, and is then discharged to the surface. Osteoclasts slowly erode the sequestrum, detaching it at each end from living bone and slowly destroying it. This must be completed before healing can be accomplished. In practice, this is seldom possible without elaborate surgical intervention. If nothing is done, the condition may lead to death as the result of pyaemia, 'toxaemia', or amyloid disease.

Chronic osteomyelitis is fortunately uncommon nowadays since the advent of antibiotic therapy, which is used in combination with early surgical drainage in the acute stage.

From a pathological point of view the disease illustrates many points. It shows how an acute

---

[*] A *sinus* is an abnormal channel, often lined by epithelium, which leads from the interior of the body to a free surface.

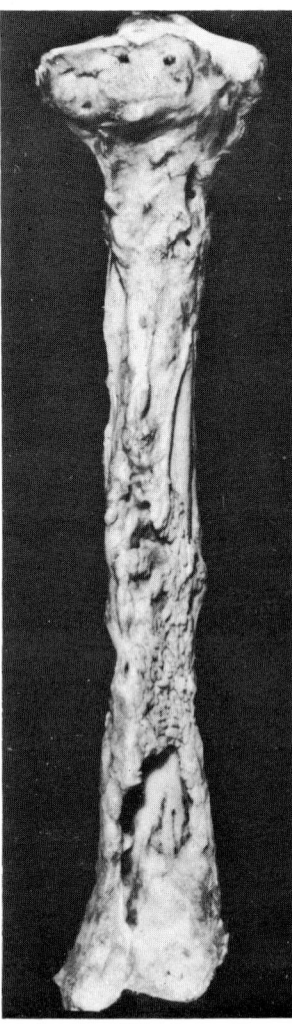

Fig. 9.7 Osteomyelitis of tibia. The extensive central sequestrum is largely encased in an exuberant involucrum formed from the detached periosteum. There is a cloaca at the base of the shaft, and through it the pitted sequestrum is clearly visible. (HS44.1. Reproduced by permission of the President and Council of the Royal College of Surgeons of England.)

infection can become chronic due to inadequate drainage of pus, as well as to the presence of a foreign body, in this case the sequestrum. Moreover, all the features of chronic inflammation are present. Acute inflammation is evident by the polymorphonuclear and fluid exudate, demolition by macrophages and osteoclastic activity, regeneration by bone formation, and repair by the surrounding scarring.

TISSUE RESPONSE TO INSOLUBLE INANIMATE FOREIGN MATERIALS

The tissue response to these substances is very complex, but with the increasing use of metals and plastics in reconstructive surgery, it is a matter of considerable importance. In the root treatment of non-vital teeth a variety of compounds have been used. As they are in contact with vital tissues in the apical region, it is important that they should be non-irritant. Research on some of these compounds shows that, although most of them cause an inflammatory response when first inserted, this usually subsides within a few weeks. It is probably true to state that all foreign materials are capable of producing an inflammatory response under certain circumstances. Nothing is truly inert. The factors which determine the severity of the inflammatory response are not completely understood, but the following are important:

Chemical nature of the material. The chemical stability and solubility are of great importance; thus stainless steel is more inert than ordinary steel.

Physical state of substance. Smooth, highly-polished surfaces provoke much less reaction than do rough, irregular surfaces. It is important to bear this in mind when inserting metal prostheses or pins. Finely divided or colloidal substances are particularly irritating. Nylon has been used in joint reconstruction, but the scratching and powdering which occur during use lead to a brisk foreign body reaction.

Electro-chemical potentials. These are set up by the close proximity of dissimilar metals, and cause tissue damage. This is particularly important in orthopaedic and traumatic surgery. Plates and screws must all be of exactly the same composition, otherwise there is sufficient reaction to cause loosening of the screws. Even the metal scraped off the screwdriver may be enough to produce this effect.

The relatively insoluble foreign materials cannot be removed by the inflammatory reaction which they excite, and it follows that the lesions induced are typically chronic in character. Giant cells abound, and while most of these are of the foreign-body type, Langhan's giant cells are also seen.

The extent of the reaction to foreign material depends on the nature of the material itself. A few important examples will be cited.

Examples of foreign-body reaction

Carbon. Tattooing consists of introducing carbon or cinnabar into the dermis. It excites a mild inflammatory response and is soon taken up by macrophages, in which it remains in the tissues indefinitely. The small amount of carbon which is deposited in the lungs of city-dwellers likewise causes little damage.

Metals. Vitallium and stainless steel cause little reaction when used in the form of polished plates, pins, arthroplasty cups, dental implants, etc. Tantalum, titanium, and zirconium are also used for their inertness. Other metals, e.g. iron, produce much more reaction, and in certain situations, e.g. the eye, can lead to serious damage.

Dental implants. The idea of embedding foreign materials into the jaw bones is not a new one. Different materials and designs have been used for the past 40–50 years in an attempt to support crowns, bridges and dentures, many of which have been rejected as foreign bodies. However, after a decade of experimental research Brånemark in Sweden has shown that osseo-integration occurs between pure titanium and bone. Cellular attachment takes place by growth of bone cells onto the surface of the titanium without any intervening fibrous tissue. The first osseointe-grated implant was performed in 1965, and the success of the system has been recognized world-wide. The technique has now been extended for the prosthetic replacement of ears, noses and eyes which have either failed to form or have been lost as a result of trauma.

Suture material. Catgut excites a brisk acute inflammatory reaction which is soon followed by an infiltration of macrophages and giant cells. The strength of the plain catgut is reduced to half within 2 days, while for chromic catgut the time is 10 days. Plain catgut is therefore unreliable, and should be discarded from general use. Fine chromic catgut should be used whenever absorbable material is indicated. The tissue reaction to nylon, linen, etc. does not readily remove the material, which therefore persists for a long period (Fig. 9.2).

Silica. Small particles of silica are inhaled during the course of certain occupations like mining. An inflammatory response ensues in the interstitial tissues of the lungs, and this is later followed by dense nodular fibrosis. The precise manner by which silica causes such extensive destruction of lung is not known. The silica particles are phagocytosed by macrophages and being toxic destroy these cells. Lysosomal and other factors are released and these attract more macrophages to the area and also stimulate fibrogenesis (p. 102).

Many other dusts when inhaled into the lungs induce an inflammatory response which terminates in fibrosis. Such diseases are called the *pneumoconioses*. Silicosis and asbestosis are the most important.

GENERAL READING

Adams D O 1976 The granulomatous inflammatory response. Journal of Pathology 84: 164

Allison A C, Clark J A, Davies P 1977 Cellular interactions in fibrogenesis. Annals of the Rheumatic Diseases 36 (suppl): 27

Boros D L 1978 Granulomatous inflammation. Progress in Allergy 24: 183

Brånemark P-I, Hansson B O, Adell R et al 1977 Osseointegrated implants in the treatment of the edentulous jaw—experience from a ten-year period (monograph). Almquist and Wiksell, Stockholm

Epstein W L 1977 Granuloma formation in man. Pathology Annual 7: 1

10.   The immune response

Immune reactions plays an important and complex role in many pathological processes, and this chapter will describe the general features of the immune response.

One of the characteristic features of the adult vertebrate is its ability to distinguish between its own normal constituents ('self') and those of external or foreign origin ('non-self'). Encounters with foreign biological materials (e.g. microbes or their products) result in the recognition of the foreign components (called antigens) by cells bearing specific antigen receptors.

Antigens are high-molecular-weight substances, generally proteins, the specificity of which is determined by specific sites, called *antigenic determinants* or *epitopes*. New epitopes can be added to a protein either in vivo or in vitro. This new epitope or *hapten* needs be neither protein nor antigenic, but when combined with a carrier protein it becomes antigenic and able to stimulate an immune response that is specific to itself as well as to the carrier protein. In this way small molecular substances acquire antigenic properties. Examples include drugs and their metabolites, and chemicals which when applied to skin cause acute 'allergic' dermatitis.

Two types of immune response follow the introduction of an antigen. There may be a *positive response* in which cells and antibodies are generated that facilitate the elimination of the antigen. This is an important mechanism which has been adapted during evolution as a protection against infection. Alternatively there may be a *negative response* for that particular antigen, and subsequent encounter with the antigen leads to no response; this is termed *specific immunological tolerance* and has been evolved to prevent rejection of self proteins. In either case, the initial response to the encounter with an antigen induces a change such that there will be an altered response to that particular substance in the future. The immune response is therefore *specific* and displays *memory*.

The key cells in the immune system are the lymphocytes. During development their precursor cells have the potential to make millions of different antigen-specific receptors, but by irreversible gene arrangement and mutation, each cell randomly selects a unique DNA arrangement that encodes a unique receptor (see later). All mature daughter lymphocytes derived from it inherit this unique DNA arrangement and produce the same antigen-specific receptor. Each mature lymphocyte is a member of a clone, i.e. a set of cells derived asexually from a single precursor cell. All members of a clone have an identical specificity for binding antigen, and the specificity is distinct from that of all other clones. This specificity is a property of an antigen-specific receptor protein. Thus there is one, and only one, specificity for each clone. The irreversible gene rearrangement takes place either in the thymus or, in birds, the bursa of Fabricius. In the thymus the pre-T cells mature to form T cells which then migrate in the blood stream to populate the T cell areas of the lymph nodes and other lymphoid tissues. In the bursa the pre-B cells mature and similarly populate the B cell areas of the peripheral lymphoid tissues. Humans do not have a bursa and it is thought that maturation occurs in the bone marrow itself.

The lymphoid system is made up of many thousands of unique clones. When antigen is encountered, it reacts with those clones to which it can bind specifically with high affinity. With appropriate signals from other cells (see interleukins) this event of antigen binding results in the stimulation and proliferation of those clones. Since antigen selects the antigen-specific clones, the process is known as *clonal selection*.

Lymphocytes are of two principal classes: B and T lymphocytes. *B lymphocytes* have an immunoglobulin antibody of a unique specificity as their surface antigen-specific receptor. The function of each B lymphocyte is to synthesize immunoglobulin of the same specificity as the receptor.

T lymphocytes have a specific T cell receptor composed of an α and a β chain. The role of the T lymphocyte is to become either an effector cell of cell-mediated immunity or a regulatory cell.

The introduction of antigen into an organism by whatever route frequently involves much of the antigen being taken up on the mononuclear phagocyte system (MPS). The eventual fate of a small portion of the antigen is to bind to lymphocytes bearing receptors for the antigen. Such lymphocytes, at the time of first exposure to antigen, form a small minority of the lymphocytes present in the body. B cells bind antigen directly, independently of macrophages. However, T cells recognize antigen in a more complex way. Antigen must be degraded to short polypeptides (*antigen processing*). The processed antigen is then expressed on the surface of specialized cells, usually macrophages of the MPS or similar marrow-derived cells, for T-cell recognition (*antigen presentation*). Furthermore, T cells only recognize antigen when it is associated with antigens of the *major histocompatibility complex* (MHC) on the surface of the presenting cells. This phenomenon is known as the *MHC restriction of T-cell recognition*.

When the immunologically competent cells (B and T) are exposed to antigen, those with a specific receptor capable of binding to some portion of the antigen are ready to undergo *activation, differentiation,* and *proliferation* (Fig. 10.1). Antigen alone is often not a sufficient signal for triggering B cells; usually a second signal (an interleukin from a helper T cell) is required. Assuming that conditions are right, the B cells are triggered to become antibody-producing lymphocytes or plasma cells.

The relatively simple process of immunoglobulin production by the B cells is in contrast to the complexity of the T-cell response in which either *regulatory* or *effector* cells are generated. The regulatory cells are either *helpers* or *suppressors*. They can regulate every aspect of the immune response, including one another, by way of a complicated series of circuits designed to prevent runaway responses, while facilitating the rapid mobilization of specific immune products in the event of an exposure to a pathogen. It is a life-and-death balance: too little and the individual may perish of infection, too much and there may be the development of uncontrolled lymphoproliferation, autoimmunity, or unnecessary tissue injury. Regulation is a key feature of the immune system.

LYMPHOCYTE ACTIVATION

Lymphocytes may be activated by a variety of agents, termed *mitogens*. The circumstances under which this may happen may be listed:

1 Interaction of antigen-specific receptor with

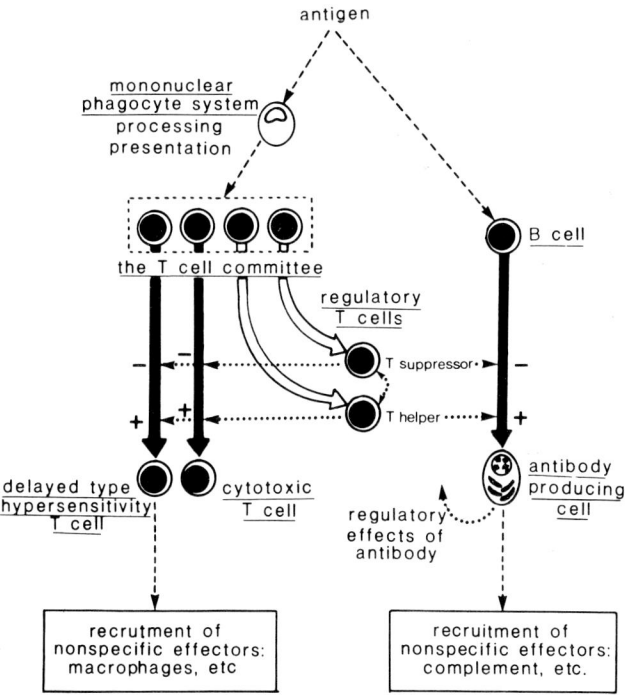

Fig. 10.1   The specific immune response, emphasizing the three principal antigen-specific effector mechanism – delayed-type hypersensitivity, cytotoxic T cells, and antibody. Regulation occurs through antigen-presenting cells, and antibody.

antigen or specific anti-receptor (anti-idiotype) antibody, leads to clonal proliferation.

2 *Lectins and other mitogens:* lectins, many of which are derived from plants, are carbohydrate-binding glycoproteins. Bacterial lipopolysaccharide is also a mitogen. The stimulation by these agents is non-specific and therefore polyclonal.

Lymphocyte activation generally requires multiple signals, especially when this activation occurs through the antigen-specific receptor. These signals may be interleukin-1 (IL-1) which macrophages release, interleukin-2, which helper T cells release, or other interleukins.

Following receipt of the appropriate signals, lymphocytes undergo a variety of changes the most obvious of which is blast transformation.

Blast transformation

Blast transformation is a dramatic change in the morphology and size of the cell. Within 12–24 h of stimulation the lymphocytes increase in size due to the production of abundant cytoplasm containing polyribosomes and a Golgi complex. There is a change in the nuclear chromatin pattern, and nucleoli make their appearance. This process of blast transformation is an indication of a greatly increased protein synthesis and preparation for cell division, following which there is differentiation. The activated B cells are rapidly dividing lymphoblasts, and the number of functioning daughter cells increases as the clone expands and with it the production of immunoglobulins. Initially IgM is produced but under conditions of optimal receipt of appropriate helper T-cell signals, immunoglobulin of another class is produced, e.g. IgG or IgA. This event is termed the *class switch*. B cells eventually become plasma cells.

Following clonal stimulation, T cells differentiate and acquire effector and regulatory functions.

Immunological memory

In addition to producing differentiated cells the lymphocyte clones generate new resting cells. These cells become memory cells once the stimulus is removed, 'Memory' meaning the capacity to mount an increased response should the same antigen be encountered again (see secondary response, below). The persistence of antibody and the ability to generate a rapid response to a second exposure to the antigen is of great importance in providing immunity to infection.

THE B-CELL RESPONSE: ANTIBODY PRODUCTION

The primary versus secondary antibody response

The *primary antibody response* tends to generate considerable IgM, low affinity antibody. The antibody production is delayed for 7–10 days after the antigen administration, and its titre is low. The *secondary response* to the same antigen will have less IgM and much more IgG, more total antibody and a higher affinity for antibody–antigen binding. The onset is more rapid often commencing as early as 2 days after antigen challenge (Fig. 10.2) These characteristics reflect the existence of memory cells Thus immunity, once induced, can be readily boosted periodically by smaller amounts of antigen. The tendency for more rapid and vigorous antibody production in the secondary response is referred to as the *recall response*.

THE STRUCTURE OF IMMUNOGLOBULINS

Immunoglobulins are composed of four polypeptide chains—a pair of light (L) chains and a pair of heavy (H) chains in the basic arrangement L_2H_2. There are two types of L chains, lambda (λ) and Kappa (κ) Each antibody molecule contains two λ chains or two κ chains, never one of each (Fig. 10.3). There are five classes of immunoglobulin dependent upon the type of heavy chain present: either gamma (γ), alpha (α), mu (μ), delta (δ) or epsilon (ε). Thus the composition of the monomeric forms of each immunoglobulin is as follows: IgG (γ_2L_2), IgA (α_2L_2); IgM (μ_2L_2); IgD (δ_2L_2) and IgE (ε_2L_2). Each B cell makes antibody of only one specificity and one type of L chain and one type of H chain at a time, but if there is a class switch the type of H chain changes. Each chain consists of a series of globular, folded areas (called *domains*), separated by unfolded regions of the chain. The foldings are held in place by disulphide bonds. Each L chain has two domains, one of which is *variable* (the V_L region), the other *constant* (the C_L region). Each H chain has four domains (five in the case of IgM and IgD), one variable (the V_H region) and three constant (the C_H1, C_H2, and C_H3 domains). Within each variable domain(V_H or V_L) there are three short regions of the chain which are much more variable than the others, known as the *hypervariable regions*. The exact amino-acid sequence in the hypervariable regions determines

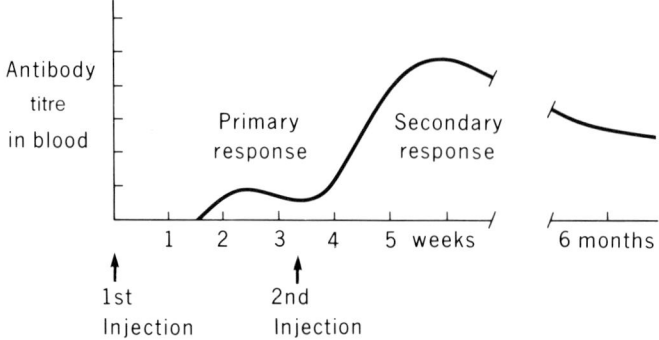

Fig. 10.2 Diagram showing the differences between a primary and a secondary response to an antigenic stimulus. (Drawn by Margot Mackay, University of Toronto.)

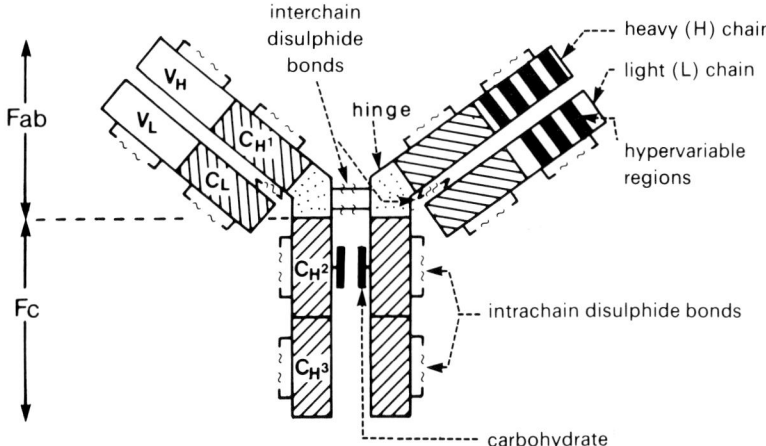

Fig. 10.3 The structure of IgG. The site of pepsin cleavage, which generates the F (ab')2 portion, is shown. Cleavage by papain occurs above the interchain disulphide bonds, leaving the F(ab) portions and one Fc portion (see text).

the antigen-binding specificity of the molecules, i.e. the hypervariable regions of the L and H chains, held in proper three-dimensional relationship by the less variable segments, and by the C regions, determine the shape of the areas in the V region of the antibody molecule which an antigen must match.

The immunoglobulin molecule (Fig. 10.3) can be digested by papain, an enzyme that cleaves the heavy chains above the interchain disulphide bonds, to create two antigen-binding fragments or Fab, and one fragment which crystalizes readily—the crystalizing fragment or Fc.

The characteristics of the various immuno-globulin classes are as follows :

IgG

This is the most abundant immunoglobulin in the blood and is the only one to cross the placenta to reach the fetus.

IgM

IgM (Fig. 10.4) which exists in two subclasses IgM1 and IgM2. Each IgM molecule is a pentamer of five monomer IgM subunits, each composed of two L and two μ chains, plus a special joining or J chain; the number of antigen-

combining sites capable of binding antigen is five, compared with two for IgG. (Indeed, in an IgM pentamer there are 10 combining sites, two per monomer, but for unknown reasons five participate in antigen binding). IgM is the first immunoglobulin (Ig) to appear in an immune respones. IgM exists in a membrane-associated monomeric form as well as in free pentameric form. This membrane-associated IgM monomer

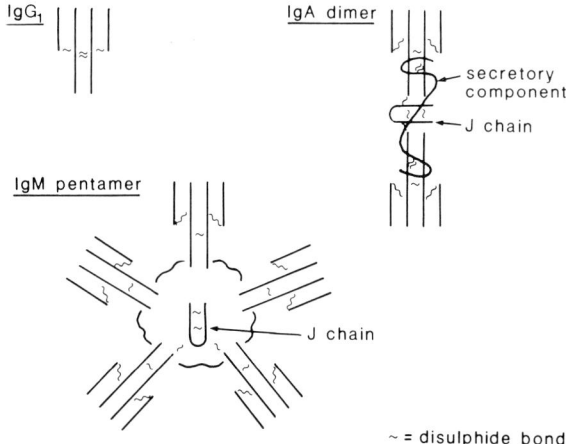

Fig. 10.4 Relative size and arrangement of the IgG, molecule, the secreted IgA dimer, and the circulating IgM pentamer. Note the J chain in the IgM pentamer molecules and the secretory component in the IgA dimer.

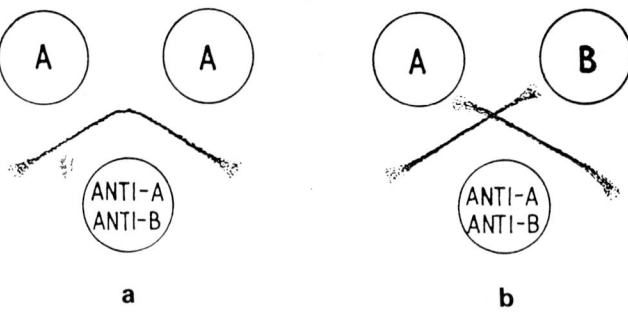

Fig. 10.5 Ouchterlony plates showing precipitin reactions In (a) the precipitin lines join together, as they are both due to the same A–anti-A reaction. In (b) the lines cross, as they are formed by different antigen–antibody reactions.

is the principal antigen-specific receptor for unstimulated B cells.

IgA

The IgA monomer is the second most abundant Ig class in serum, being about 25% as abundant as IgG. However, it is the predominant Ig in secretions such as saliva. In the production of secretory IgA, the plasma cells in the submucosa produce IgA monomers plus J chain, which are assembled to form IgA dimers. The dimers bind to *secretory component* before being transported through the epithelial cell such as those of the salivary glands. The secretory component is wound around the Fc portions of the two IgA molecules (Fig. 10.4). This appears to protect IgA from enzymatic breakdown so that it can perform its protective role on epithelial surfaces, such as in the mouth, gut or bronchi.

IgD

Relatively little is known about the role of IgD. It probably serves as antigen-specific receptor.

IgE

Although IgE exists in serum in only trivial amounts this important immunoglobulin is the mediator of typical allergy, and as such is of considerable clinical interest. The Fc portion of IgE causes it to bind avidly to Fc receptors for IgE on mast cells and basophils. Addition of antigen to these mast cells triggers the release of such mast-cell products as histamine.

DIVERSITY AND SPECIFICITY OF B CELLS

For many years a central problem in immunology has been to explain how a B cell could produce a specific antibody, the properties of which depended on a unique chemical structure. Protein synthesis is coded by specific RNA, itself modelled on nuclear DNA. If each antibody were to be modelled on one gene, a vast number of genes would be required in the genome of every cell to explain how the equally vast number of antibodies could be produced during the lifetime of the individual. The explanation is that the nuclear material of lymphocytes undergoes a type of gene rearrangement. *This is antigen-independent,* and the reader is referred to immunology texts for details.

ANTIGEN–ANTIBODY INTERACTIONS

The particular amino-acid composition of the receptor sites of the immunoglobulin creates a three-dimensional site which serves as a 'lock' into which an antigenic 'key' will fit. One antigen-combining site is composed of the hypervariable regions of the adjacent light and heavy chains. When the lock and key fit well, a variety of forces bond the antigenic determinant to the combining site. The result of this may be a direct effect or there may be involvement of other components, e.g. complement or cells.

The principle direct effects of antibody on antigen are precipitation, agglutination, and neutralization. *Precipitation* is the appearance of an insoluble precipitate when antibody interacts

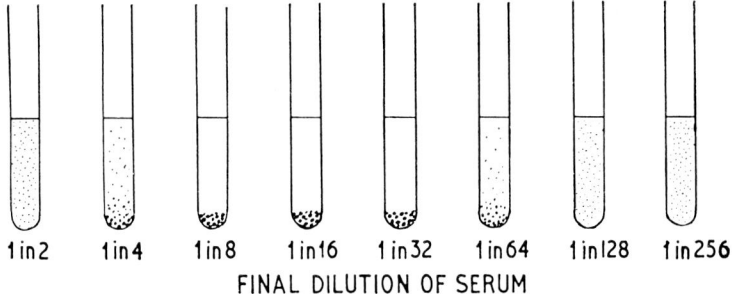

Fig. 10.6 Agglutination test. The titre of antibody is 1 in 64. The failure of the first tube (1 in 2 dilution) to show agglutination is known as the prozone phenomenon, and is not uncommonly seen in Brucella agglutination tests.

with a soluble antigen (Fig. 10.5). Agglutination is the clumping together of antigen-bearing particles, typically bacteria, erythrocytes or artificially coated latex particles (Fig. 10.6). Both precipitation and agglutination are dependent on the ability of one antibody molecule (which has at least two antigen-binding sites, depending on the class) to link two antigen molecules or antigen-bearing particles together. *Neutralization* is an important function of antibody in the host's defence against microorganisms. For example, antibody against bacterial antigens may prevent adherence, which is important to invasiveness or pathogenicity. Antibodies against toxins can neutralize toxic effects, and antiviral antibody can prevent viruses from binding to and invading cells.

Precipitin and agglutination reactions are widely used in clinical and research settings. Each test can be standardized to analyse unknown specimens for antibody titre (using a standardized antigen preparation), or for antigen estimation (using a standardized antibody preparation). Agar gel diffusion, radioimmunoassay (RIA), enzyme linked immunoabsorbent assay (ELISA), immunofluorescence and immunoperoxidase tests are other techniques.

The complement system

The complement system consists of a set of soluble serum proteins which have an important role in host defence. When activated the complement system can lyse organisms, bind them to important host cells, or can release active peptides that contribute to an inflammatory response (Fig. 10.7). As would be expected, there are a number of inhibitors that prevent excessive complement activation.

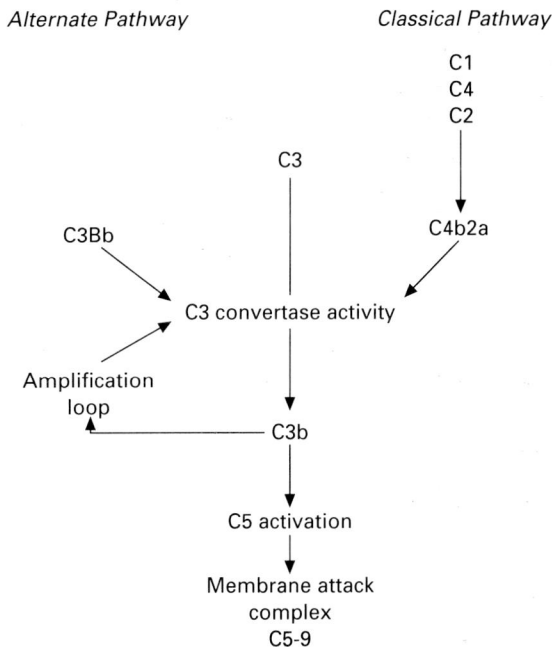

Fig.10.7 A simplified diagram to illustrate the activation of the complement system. A C3 activator is formed either via the alternate pathway (C3bBb) or the classical pathway (C4b2a). In either case there is an amplification loop whereby C3b can itself become a C3 convertase. C3b activates C5 and subsequent formation of C5-9, the membrane attack complex which when bound to a cell membrane, damages the membrane and leads to cell lysis.

Activation of complement by the classical pathway

Antigen-antibody interaction activates the component C1q which leads to activation of the other components of C1, and then in turn C4, and C2 to form C4b2a. This is the C3 convertase of the classical pathway. By its action on C3, C3b is formed. There is a natural inhibitor of C1 called C1 esterase inhibitor or C1-1NA

Activation of complement via the alternate pathway

This pathway can be activated in a variety of ways that do not involve an immunological reaction. These include the action of microbial polysaccharides and aggregated IgA or IgG. The activation results in the formation of the C3 convertase C3bBb. This substance is normally inhibited by properdin (a naturally occurring inhibitor).

The amplification loop. C3Bb can itself become a C3 convertase thus triggering more C3b formation. This causes amplification of both pathways.

Further steps in the complement cascade. C3 convertase (C4b2a in the classical pathway and C3Bb in the alternate pathway) can combine with C3b to become a C5 convertase. The sequential activation of the remaining complement components leads to the formation of the membrane attack complex C5b-9, so named because when membrane bound it leads to cell-membrane damage and lysis.

Effect of complement activation

These may be listed:

1 *Assembly of the membrane attack complex.* This leads to cell lysis.
2 *Adherence of complement components (e.g. C3b) to cells (e.g. bacteria).* This facilitates the effector function of cells such as polymorph and macrophages that have C3b receptors. Thus complement activation encourages phagocytosis, and cell mediated cytotoxicity as described below.
3 *Release of active peptides.* These include C2b kinin and the anaphylatoxins C3a and C5a which act on mast cells and cause the release of granule contents such as histamine. They also act as chemotactic mediators of inflammation.

Antibody-dependent cell mediated cytotoxicity

Antibody-coated cells and microorganisms can be killed by host cells with Fc receptors. The effector cells vary with the class of the antibody, and the characteristics of the target cell. The best known cell in antibody dependent killing cell is the K cell, a large granular lymphocyte which can kill IgG-coated nucleated cells very actively.[*] Neutrophils can also kill IgG-coated cells. Monocytes can lyse anti-Rh-coated red cells in a similar manner via their Fc receptors. Eosinophils can kill Ig-coated parasites, e.g. schistosomes. The exact killing mechanism in each case probably varies according to the cell involved.

Other effector mechanisms of humoral immunity

Platelets, polymorphs and macrophages all have Fc receptors and receptors for C3b or other complement components. This may trigger other reactions, e.g. phagocytosis and mast cell degranulation.

THE T-CELL RESPONSE

The progenitor cell of the T cell lineage is the pre-T cell. It migrates to the thymus and undergoes massive proliferation under the influence of the thymic hormones, thymosine and thymopoietin, produced by the thymic epithelium. As with B-cell maturation, genetic rearrangement occurs and results in the formation of a large number of cells, each with a specific receptor. Furthermore self-reactive cells are either eliminated or so controlled that they do not react to self antigen (see also p. 120). The mature T cells subsequently emerge from the thymus to populate the T-cell dependent areas of the peripheral lymphoid system.

The T cell antigen-specific receptor consists of

---

[*]K cells are probably the same as natural-killer (NK) cells but differ in that, in this context, they kill cells that are coated with immunoglobulin.

a dimer of two non-identical glycoprotein chains, the α chain being encoded on chromosome 14, and the β chain on chromosome 7. The T3 complex is a set of proteins distinct from the T-cell receptors but useful as a T-cell marker. Other markers are T4 (helper–DTH cells) and T8 (suppressor–cytotoxic cells). In the blood the normal T4/T8 ratio is 1.5–2.0.

Less is known about T-cell responses than B-cells reactions. T-cells are activated by antigen binding to their antigen-specific receptors in the context of the MHC class I or II products of the antigen-presenting cell. In addition, T cells can be activated by anti-receptor antibodies, and by polyclonal activators called mitogens. Other signals are usually required, e.g. interleukin-1 or interleukin-2. Then T-cell activation, clonal expansion, and differentiation begin. This leads to the emergence of *effector cells (delayed-type hypersensitivity T cells* and *T cytotoxic cells)*, and *regulator cells* (either *helper T cells* or *suppressor T cells)*.

DELAYED-TYPED HYPERSENSITIVITY (DTH)

In a delayed-typed hypersensitivity reaction, encounter with an antigen leads to an inflammatory reaction within 48–72 h. The tuberculin or Mantoux reaction is a typical example (p. 141). The pathogenesis is as follows. T cells with the specific marker, and usually with the T4 phenotype, encounter antigen on the surface of an antigen-presenting cell in the tissues in association with class-II HLA products. The presenting cell is a macrophage, or some other member of the MPS such as a dendritic cell or Langerhan's cell. The T cell responds by activation, clonal expansion and differentiation. It releases many active compounds that are collectively called *lymphokines* (see later). One such factor is *gamma interferon*, another is *lymphotoxin* which can non-specifically kill certain other cells. Of greater importance are chemotactic factors, the action of which leads to the accumulation of macrophages. These cells are immobilized by *macrophage chemotactic factor* (MCF) and *macrophage migration inhibition factor* (MIF), and then activated by *macrophage activating factors*. The macrophage in turn releases other factors, and by

its activities produces the characteristic changes of the DTH reaction, such as vascular damage, oedema and activation of the coagulation system with fibrin formation. It is the fibrin that causes much of the induration that is characteristic of the reaction. Another effect of T-cell activation is activation by IL-2 of natural killer (NK) cells which are large granular lymphocytes that can kill cells non-specifically.

Delayed-type hypersensitivity is thus initiated by a highly specific reaction involving T cells with specific markers, but much of the damage caused is non-specific and caused by macrophages and activated NK cells.

CYTOTOXIC T CELLS

In many systems in which the immune system is responding to membrane-associated antigen, it is possible to demonstrate a population of effector T cells that are able to lyse the target cells bearing that antigen. This phenomenon is demonstrable with transplantation antigens, viral antigens, and chemicals that modify self antigens such as those that cause 'allergic' contact dermatitis. Such T cells arise from committed cytotoxic cells bearing the T8 marker in man. They recognize antigen in association with class I antigens of the MHC, and respond by clonal expansion and differentiation before their cytotoxicity can be detected. This process takes several days and is dependent on the presence of IL-2. The role of cytotoxic T cells in vivo is not known. Their most likely role is to destroy virus infected cells and thereby limit an infection.

Lymphokines and interleukins

Lymphokines were originally described as soluble factors produced by lymphocytes and released after lymphocytic stimulation. Many of them were poorly categorized, and the names attached to them referred to a biological activity rather than a specific composition. The situation is changing as individual factors have been isolated. The term *cytokine* has been used to refer to any growth promoting or growth inhibiting substance. It has also been used to describe lymphokine-like substance produced by non-lymphoid cells. Thus

NO ANTIGEN   OVALBUMIN   TOXOID

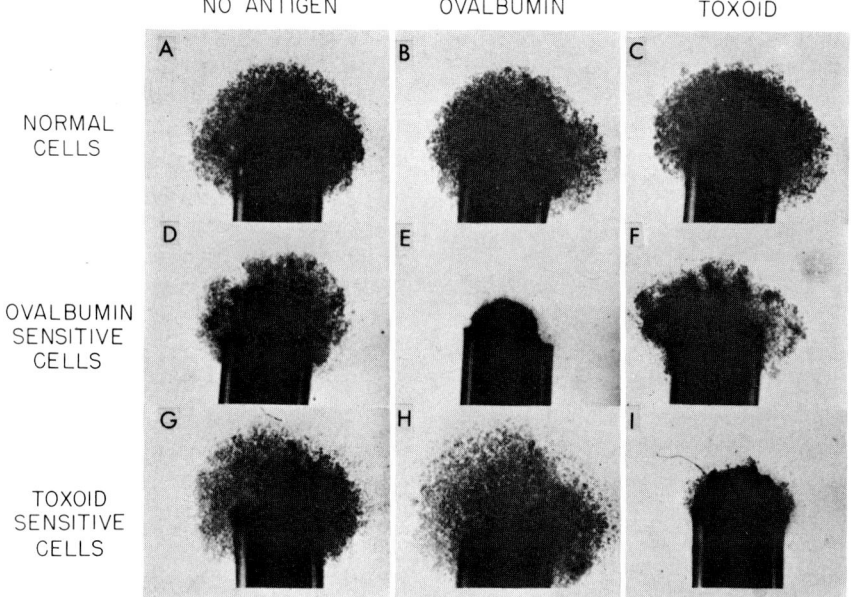

NORMAL CELLS

OVALBUMIN SENSITIVE CELLS

TOXOID SENSITIVE CELLS

Fig. 10.8   Time relation between fall of circulating antigen, formation of antigen-antibody complexes, lesions of serum sickness (glomerulonephritis), and rise of circulating antibody in rabbits injected with large doses of ^{131}I-labeled bovine serum albumin. (From Gladstone G P 1961. In Florey H W *General Pathology* 3rd edn, after Dixon J F et al in: Lawrence H S *Cellular and humoral aspects of the hypersensitivity states*. Harper and Row, New York, p345.)

a macrophage derived *tumour necrosis factor alpha* (TNFα) is identical to cachexin. The term cytokin may in fact be used as a general term that includes the lymphokines (released by lymphocytes) and monokines (released by monocytes and macrophages). The interleukins are cytokines that are made by white cells that act on other white cells. They have been numbered starting at one; the following is a very brief overview of these factors and it must be stressed that others are known and that they have many complex actions.

Interleukin-1

This was first described as being produced by monocytes but is now known to be derived from other cell types as well. It is necessary for the activation of T cells and plays a part in the proliferation and differentiation of B cells. It is chemotactic to lymphocytes, and acts as a pyrogen.[*]

Interleukin-2

Interleukin-2 is a product of helper T cells and is essential for cell division and activation of many clones of T cells after they have been stimulated by antigen. The development of IL-2 receptors by antigen stimulated cells is an essential step in this process.

Interleukin-3

This is a growth factor for haematopoietic cells and pre-B cells.

Interleukins 4 and 5

These factors are growth factors for various subsets of B and T cells.

Interleukin 6

This stimulates B cells, and induces the synthesis of acute phase proteins in the liver.

---

[*]It should be noted that interleukin-1 is not a lymphokine; it is a monokine produced by monocytes and macrophages.

γ-Interferon

This protein is produced by antigen-stimulated T cells. It induces an increased production and expression of class I and class II products of the MHC in macrophages, fibroblasts and many types of epithelial cells. It induces differentiation and inhibits proliferation of many cell types, and activates macrophages. It increases the cytotoxicity of NK cells.

Macrophage inhibition factor (MIF)

This factor inhibits the migration of macrophages, an effect that can easily be assessed in vitro and used as an assay method for specific lymphocyte responsiveness to an antigen (Fig. 10.8).

Macrophage activating factor

This substance is released by activated helper T cells. It acts on macrophages in such a way as to increase their ability to kill ingested bacteria, and to kill tumour cells. The relationship between this factor and γ-interferon is uncertain; possibly they are identical.

The most controversial lymphokine is *transfer factor*. This is said to be a low-molecular-weight dialysable factor that can transfer the ability to express an antigen-specific delayed-typed hypersensitivity response from an immune host to an non-immune recipient. There is no known mechanism whereby such a transfer could be effected by such a low-molecular-weight compound and it is doubtful whether a single entity with 'transfer factor' activity in fact exists.

HELPER T CELLS

The rate of emergence of any effector cell in the immune response—DTH T cells, cytotoxic T cells, or antibody-producing B cells—is regulated by the availability of certain interleukins produced by T cells known as helper T cells; they usually have the T4 surface marker.

In some systems the antigen is in the form of a hapten on a protein carrier: the B cell responds to the hapten, the T cell to the carrier. The T helper cell must recognize the carrier determinants in association with class II MHC molecules on an antigen-presenting cell such as a macrophage.

The T helper cells which help DTH T cells have been less well studied than those for B cells, but are probably rather similar.

The T helper cells which help cytotoxic T cells seem to act to a large extent by releasing IL-2. In a typical mixed lymphocyte culture (see p. 133) the principal IL-2 producing cells are those T4-positive cells which recognize class II antigen, while the T8-positive cytotoxic T cells, which are mostly directed against class I antigens, are highly IL-2-dependent. In many other cytotoxic T-cell responses (e.g. against virus-infected or chemically-modified cells) an IL-2-producing cell is presumably essential for the clonal proliferation of the IL-2-dependent cytotoxic T cells.

SUPPRESSOR T CELLS

Not unexpectedly, suppressor T cells have many features in common with helper T cells. Suppressor T cells (generally T8-positive) recognize antigen in association with MHC class I antigen and exert their effects by direct binding to the target cell, or by the release of soluble factors which bind to the target molecule. In addition, the specific suppressor cells may release non-specific suppressor molecules, presumably similar to the non-specific factors released by polyclonally-activated suppressor cells.

The target of the suppressor T cell varies: the macrophage, as described above, the effector cells (cytotoxic T, DTH T, and B) or their precursors, or the helper T cells.

THE T-CELL RESPONSE AND IMMUNE REGULATION

A highly sophisticated control mechanism exists to ensure a prompt, well-aimed T-cell response with minimal damage to normal structures, but which subsides promptly when the stimulus is removed. Both positive and negative regulatory signals act on each effector cell, and even the regulatory cells seem to be regulated. Cells producing positive signals are the helper cells, and those producing negative signals the suppressor cells.

A recurrent theme in the regulation field is the role of *anti-antibody reactions* or as it is often called an *idiotype anti-idiotype reaction*. The concept is that each B-cell receptor (an antibody molecule) or T-cell receptor has a unique combining site called an *idiotype*. This site exists in such tiny amounts in the unstimulated state that no tolerance for the combining site exists. An immune response rapidly expands the stimulated clones, increasing the quantity of cells (and their product) bearing these idiotypes and provoking an anti-idiotype immune response. This, in turn, rapidly expands the reciprocal clones, with anti-idiotype specificity, provoking an anti-anti-idiotype response. This sequence can theoretically continue indefinitely. Good experimental evidence for the anti-idiotype and anti-anti-idiotype response exists. Various models have been proposed whereby this mechanism might regulate the immune response.

TOLERANCE

It is obvious that some mechanism must operate to prevent clones of immune T or B lymphocytes from producing responses which could destroy the individual. Each person has unique self-markers, particularly the highly polymorphic MHC molecules, which means that one animal's definition of self is another's definition of foreign. Each person must have a mechanism for deleting self-reactivity.

The general term for the mechanism by which self-reactivity is eliminated or controlled by exposure to antigen is tolerance. Tolerance means specific suppression of certain clones of lymphocytes by exposure to antigen under special circumstances. In general the mechanisms of tolerance are :

1. *Clonal abortion:* the prevention of maturation of self-reactive clones
2. *Clonal elimination:* the destruction of self-reactive clones once they emerge
3. *Receptor paralysis:* the tying up of and cross-linking of available cell receptors by high concentrations of antigen, without permitting the receptors to signal the cell to respond
4. *Regulatory T cells,* particularly suppressor T cells, which prevent self-reactive clones from responding even though they exist

5. *Anti-receptor (anti-idiotype) antibodies* which could block or destroy cells with undesirable receptor specificities.

The role of each of these mechanisms in tolerance varies with the antigen, with the maturity of the lymphocytes and of the individual, and with the nature of antigen exposure. Certain antigens (e.g. monomeric proteins, rather than aggregated proteins), promote tolerance. The antigens present during fetal life, and to a lesser extent in neonatal life, usually promote tolerance in the organism rather than a positive response. The T cells are much more prone than the B cells to becoming tolerant, and many antigens seem to be recognizable by B cells in the adult but the necessary T cells to produce help are lacking. Immaturity favours tolerance, probably as an aid to the elimination of self-reactive clones.

The T-cell precursors that migrate to the thymus do not express antigen receptors until they have undergone genetic rearrangement. Presumably exposure to antigen in the thymus results in elimination of any clone that could react to self antigen. It is known that the rapid multiplication of cells in the thymus is accompanied by extensive cell necrosis. Those cells that do emerge do not have receptors for any antigen present in the thymus. Some cells could have receptors for self antigens not expressed in thymic cells, for example those of thyroid tissue. These lymphocytes do not normally react with thyroid cells because the latter do not express MHC class II antigen. However, under abnormal conditions (e.g. due to the effects of interferon induced by a viral infection) MHC class II antigens become expressed, helper T cells are activated and in turn stimulate B cells capable of producing specific antithyroid antibodies. This is one explanation of an autoimmune process (see also p. 143).

The prevention of autoreactivity varies in its completeness: autoantibody or cytotoxic T cells against unmodified self MHC molecules seldom occurs in vivo. On the other hand, many normal individuals develop low levels of antibody reactive with other autologous antigens e.g. rheumatoid factor (IgM specific for a determinant on autologous IgG) and anti-DNA.

An encounter with antigen in very low doses or in very high doses produces tolerance. This can be shown by the subsequent failure to immunize with a moderate dose which normally elicits a response. Both low and high-zone tolerance may exist for self antigens in vivo, since certain self antigens, such as thyroglobulin or glomerular basement membrane, would normally be at very low concentractions in lymphoid tissues, while albumin is at a high concentration.

IMMUNOSUPPRESSION

Immunologic responsiveness can be reduced by a variety of methods, some antigen-specific and others non-specific. Immunological responses are a common pathogenetic mechanism, and the control of such responses is frequently a desirable clinical end. It is noteworthy that every agent is more effective in preventing a response than in suppressing it, and more effective in a primary than in a secondary response. Many of these agents probably exert their immunosuppressive effects at least to some degree by acting in concert with suppressor T cells.

ANTIGEN-SPECIFIC IMMUNOSUPPRESSION

Antigen-specific antibody

The best example of this mechanism is passive administration of anti-Rh antibody in women who have just given birth to, or aborted, a Rh-positive infant. The antibody acts in part by promoting antigen uptake by the MPS, but may also alter the regulatory balance in favour of unresponsiveness. Such prophylaxis must be repeated after subsequent Rh-positive pregnancies. Antibody likewise has a similar effect in tissue transplantation, as outlined in the discussion of *enhancement.* The use of allergen to 'desensitize' an allergic individual is another example: this is believed to work by inducing non-IgE antibodies, the so-called *blocking antibodies.*

Antigen-induced specific immunosuppression (tolerance)

Transfusion of donor blood prior to living donor renal transplantation (see p. 134) is an example of this approach. This may be the first of many ways of inducing antigen-specific unresponsiveness by the administration of antigen, i.e. a form of tolerance induction.

NON-SPECIFIC IMMUNOSUPPRESSION

Glucocorticoids

Although extensively used the precise mode of action is unknown.

Cytotoxic drugs

These agents, which include both alkylating agents (such as cyclophosphamide) and antimetabolites (such as the purine analogue azathioprine), act on dividing cells, and thus manifest their efforts after 7–10 days, when the cycle of cell division and clonal expansion would be expected to be producing new cells.

X-Irradiation

Irradiation of the whole body, and more recently of lymphocyte-bearing areas (total lymphoid irradiation), is a potent immunosuppressive, but is obviously difficult to reverse, and is toxic to many types of cells. Since suppression T cells are much more sensitive to radiation than other types, a single dose of ionizing radiation can *augment the immune response.*

Antilymphocytic antibodies

This approach is based on the simple idea of injecting human lymphocytes into animals, and injecting the antilymphocytic serum (ALS) or separated globulin (ALG) into a patient to suppress his immune response. Because of the complexity of ALS, the precise mechanism of the action is unknown.

Cyclosporin

Cyclosporin, derived from a fungus, is a potent immunosuppressive agent, particularly for T-cell mediated reactions such as graft rejection. The drug prevents IL-2 production, and without this stimulus clonal expansion of DTH and cytotoxic T cells is impaired. The affected lymphocytes are not killed, and the withdrawal of cyclosporin can be followed by a rapid return of the undesired immune response which originally prompted the treatment.

The relationship between immunosuppression and malignancy or opportunistic infections are considered elsewhere.

GENERAL READING

Chapel H, Heaney M 1984 Essentials of clinical immunology, Blackwell Scientific, Oxford

Halloran P 1987 Chapters 12–16. In: Walter J B, Israel M S, General Pathology, 6th edn. Churchill Livingstone, Edinburgh

Klein J 1982 Immunology, the science of self-nonself discrimination. John Wiley & Son, New York

Paul, W E 1984 Fundamental immunology. Raven Press, New York

Stites, D P, et al 1984 Basic and clinical immunology. Lange Medical, Los Atos CA

11. Immunity to infection

Immunity to infection may be divided into two main classes, non-specific and specific, depending on whether it is related to previous contact with the organism or its antigens.

NON-SPECIFIC IMMUNITY

All individuals possess an inherent ability to destroy invading microorganisms that is dependent on neither an immune response nor previous contact with the organism. The subject can be considered under three headings: cellular, humoral, and genetic factors.

Cellular factors

The role of phagocytes both polymorphonuclear leucocytes and macrophages, and the ingestion and destruction of invading organisms in the inflammatory reaction has been described in Chapter 5. Natural killer (NK) cells are considered in Chapter 10.

Humoral factors

Blood and serum possess bactericidal power, and of the substances involved the components of the complement system are the best defined. This has been described in Chapter 10.

Natural opsonin. Normal serum contains a protein that can coat relatively avirulent organisms and render them more easily phagocytosed by polymorphs. A deficiency in natural opsonin for pneumococcal phagocytosis is found in patients with sickle-cell disease, and these patients are unduly susceptible to infection with this organism. The nature of the missing factor is not known.

Genetic factors

Species immunity is the most absolute immunity known. The human species has almost complete immunity to many animal diseases, e.g. distemper and foot and mouth disease, while certain typically human diseases, e.g. syphilis, AIDS, and leprosy, do not usually affect animals. This type of immunity is probably governed by genetic factors, and in some cases the resistance is due to a lack of appropriate receptors on the host cell to which the organisms can adhere. To this type of immunity the terms 'innate' or 'inborn' are applied. *Racial immunity* is illustrated by the selective breeding of disease-resistant plants and animals. In the human, the position is difficult to assess, because environmental factors are also involved. Races with a high incidence of sickle-cell anaemia are resistant to *Plasmodium falciparum* malaria because the sickle-cell trait provides protection. The existence of *individual immunity* is difficult to prove either in humans or animals. However, since the immune response is related to an individual's HLA type, this would suggest that an individual's genetic makeup is related to his immunity to infection.

SPECIFIC IMMUNITY

Specific immunity is related to a specific immune response to the organism or its products, and is always associated with the presence of antibodies or effector T cells. When the host produces its own antibodies or specific effector T cells, the immunity is called 'active'. When the immunoglobulins are donated to the host from another source, e.g. the serum of a convalescent patient or an immunized horse, the immunity is described as 'passive'. Passive transfer of effector T cells is not currently available.

Active immunity

Natural active immunity

This follows an attack of the disease, either overt or subclinical. Subclinical attacks are very common with some infections, e.g. poliomyelitis.

Artificial active immunity

This follows the injection of toxoids or vaccines.

Passive immunity

Passive immunity results from the transference of immunoglobulins.

Natural passive immunity

At birth the body is poorly equipped for making antibodies, nevertheless it has immunoglobulins in considerable quantity, which confer immunity.

These are IgG of maternal origin, and pass across to the fetus, either via the placental or the vitelline circulation, according to species.

Artificial passive immunity

This type of immunity is induced by injecting immunoglobulins for prophylactic or therapeutic purposes. The protection afforded is short-lived, because the antibodies are metabolized. Serum containing antibodies to hepatitis A virus is commonly given to those who are travelling to areas where hepatitis is prevalent and hygiene is poor. Passive immunity may be obtained by grafting cells of the immune system. Bone-marrow grafts are used in an attempt to reconstitute an immune system absent through inherited defect, or impaired by disease or its treatment (e.g. leukaemia).

IMMUNITY AGAINST INFECTION BY MICROORGANISMS

The importance of local defence mechanisms, the inflammatory reaction, complement, and the blood phagocytes are discussed elsewhere. The following section describes the mechanisms of defence that are directly related to the immune response.

DEFENCES AGAINST BACTERIA

Bacteria produce their effects in many ways. Some damage is produced by the effects of a potent exotoxin, while for the most part it is caused directly by the organisms invading the tissues.

Antitoxic immunity

Some organisms produce their major effect by secreting potent exotoxins. Since these toxins are highly antigenic, the host responds by making antitoxins that protect the individual against future disease. Diphtheria will be described as the prototype.

Diphtheria bacilli colonizing a mucous membrane elaborate an exotoxin that acts locally to cause tissue damage, evident as a sore throat; toxin absorbed into the blood stream causes damage at distant sites. If the host has a high antitoxin level in the blood and secretions, the toxin is rapidly neutralized, and the individual is immune to the infection.

Virulent organisms may sometimes persist in the nose or throat in spite of a high level of circulating antitoxin. This constitutes the *carrier state*, and the individual, although not suffering any ill-effects from this colonization, is nevertheless a source of danger to non-immune contacts. Immunity to diphtheria can be induced artificially by injecting toxoid (toxin altered by treatment with formaldehyde to render it less toxic) to produce active immunity. In patients suffering from the disease immunity can be rapidly boosted by the injection of antitoxins.

Other organisms that produce potent exotoxins include *S. pyogenes*, *C. perfringens*, *C. botulinum*, *C. tetani* and some enterotoxic strains of *E. coli*.

Antibacterial immunity

Antibacterial immunity is much more complex than antitoxic immunity because of the antigenic complexity of organisms, and the absence of well-defined toxins. The immunoglobulin antibodies formed against the invasive organisms are described as being antibacterial. Invading bacteria are destroyed in the body by one of several mechanisms. They may be killed in the cytoplasm of phagocytes (polymorphs or macrophages) or killed by the mechanism of antibody-dependent cytotoxicity. Activation of complement is another mechanism. Often these mechanisms work hand in hand. Complement activation results in the formation of potent mediators, C3a and C5a, that augment the inflammatory reaction. C3a and C5a also act as opsonins. Antibacterial antibodies play an important role in mobilizing the antibacterial activities. Sometimes, as with pneumococcal infection, the opsonic effects appear the most important. At other times complement activation is of prime importance.

One important aspect of immunity to bacterial infection of epithelial surface is the action of secretory IgA in preventing bacterial adherence. IgA-dependent killing of bacteria by macrophages or other cells could also be important in some sites.

The multiplicity of bacterial antigens leads to the formation of a large number of different antibodies when an animal is infected. Because only a few of the bacterial antigens are responsible for invasiveness or virulence, it is only the corresponding antibodies that are of protective value. Many other antibodies may also be present, but they play little if any part in providing immunity. On the other hand, their presence may be of great diagnostic help, e.g. the Widal reaction of typhoid fever. A rising titre is good evidence of an infection.

T cell-mediated immunity in bacterial disease

The cell-mediated immune response is also an important defence mechanism, particularly to intracellular organisms such as mycobacteria, and *Trep. pallidum*.

When delayed-typed hypersensitivity T cells react with antigen there is an extensive destructive inflammatory lesion in which organisms as well as host cells are destroyed. In addition there is activation of macrophages so that these cells become more phagocytic and better able to destroy the organism.

Anergy, indicating a lack of cell-mediated responses, can lead to an increased susceptibility to infection, particularly to viruses, fungi, and some bacteria. This particularly affects patients on heavy immunosuppressive therapy and those with AIDS.

ARTIFICIAL IMMUNITY

The artificial production of immunity to invasive organisms is much more difficult to accomplish than immunity to organisms in the toxic group. Suspensions of whole organisms are used (*vaccines*). Sometimes dead vaccines are effective (e.g. typhoid and pertussis, and Salk vaccine for poliomyelitis); for other diseases a vaccine containing live, attenuated organisms must be used (e.g. BCG for tuberculosis, Sabin vaccine for poliomyelitis). The techniques of gene cloning are likely to lead to the production of much better vaccines in the future; recombinant hepatitis B vaccine is already on the market.

ANTIVIRAL IMMUNITY

The role of antibody in the defence against viruses tends to be preventative. IgA antibodies in the secretions covering a mucous membrane will prevent infection, while IgG-neutralizing antibody in the plasma limits dissemination should infection occur; for example, in the presence of an adequate level of specific antibody, poliomyelitis remains an enteric infection and central nervous involvment does not occur. The T-cell response to virus infection is directed against the products of genes encoded by the virus in combination with a product of the HLA complex of the cell. Specific cytotoxic T cells destroy the virus-infected cells. Activated NK cells play a part, and other effector T cells produce a classic delayed-type hypersensitivity reaction with macrophage infiltration, endothelial-cell damage and widespread tissue injury. Release of immune interferon(γ–interferon) is another defence mechanism (see also Chapter 16).

Certain types of viral infection can directly affect the immune response. For example, in an acute measles infection there is a period of anergy which affects many other immune responses. For this reason a tuberculous focus may become activated. In AIDS, there is destruction of the T4 helper population, and the infections that ensue are devastating.

Immunological complications of viral infection

Immunological disease may directly complicate viral illnesses. Examples are legion: post-infectious or post-vaccination encephalomyelitis, and the Guillain–Barré syndrome following influenza or influenza vaccine are two examples. Autoantibody responses are not infrequent in virus infections, such as the acute haemolytic anaemia which can accompany some cases of Epstein–Barr virus infection (infectious mononucleosis). Another complication of acute or chronic virus infection is the formation of immune complexes, as occurs with hepatitis B virus, leading to glomerulonephritis, urticaria and polyarteritis.

IMMUNITY TO FUNGI

In general fungal immunity is believed to be T-cell mediated by the delayed-type hypersensitivity mechanism. However, antibody against fungi can also be produced, and then mediate disease (see Extrinsic allergic alveolitis, p. 141).

IMMUNITY AGAINST PROTOZOA AND HELMINTHS

The immune response of the body to different parasites is very variable. Some do not appear to stimulate an effective immune response (e.g. *Trypanosoma cruzii* causing Chagas' disease in South America), and the disease tends to be progressive and fatal. Most parasites, however, evoke an immune response. Antibodies can damage parasites by acting as opsonins, by activating complement, and via antibody-dependent cell-mediated cytotoxicity. Release of the eosinophil chemotactic factor of anaphylaxis is probably responsible for the heavy eosinophil accumulation around many helminths. Eosinophils appear to be able to attack and destroy some parasites, perhaps by IgE-dependent cell-mediated cytotoxicity.

A striking feature of some helminthic infections is the production of IgE antibody. This explains the asthma, urticaria and maculo-papular rashes that accompany some infection, e.g. ascariasis, particularly in children. Parasites have evolved various means of evading the potentially lethal consequences of the immune response. Some, for example the agent of African trypanosomiasis, exhibit rapid antigenic variation. With each peak of parasitaemia, organisms change their surface antigens, thereby evading the host's developing humoral response to the previous antigenic coat. The disease therefore pursues a relapsing course over many months. Some agents are ingested by macrophages and appear to be protected in these cells, while other are even more ingenious. They acquire a coating of host antigen and act like a wolf in sheep's clothing, in that the parasite is no longer recognized as foreign and is ignored by the host's immune defences.

IMMUNOLOGICAL DEFICIENCY DISEASES

The primary immunodeficiency states are uncommon and may be classified into those with predominantly antibody deficiencies and those with predominantly T-cell immunity deficiencies. The situation is, however, more complex than would at first appear, for although there are examples of diseases in which there is either a defect in immunoglobulin production or T-cell function, there are many instances where both arms of the immune response are abnormal.

As a generalization, antibody defects are associated with recurrent pyogenic infections, but occasionally they are associated with unusual viral infections or *Pneumocystis carinii* pneumonia. The T-cell defects tend to present with viral infections (such as overwhelming varicella, herpes simplex, and cytomegalovirus infections), candidiasis and other systemic fungal infections, *Pneumocystis* pneumonia, diarrhoea, and at times tuberculosis.

Immunodeficiencies with predominantly antibody defects

In *congenital sex-linked agammaglobulinaemia* the patients show a susceptibility to repeated, serious, pyogenic bacterial infections that invariably lead to death. *Selective IgA deficiency* is present in about 1 in 700 apparently normal persons. Some cases are associated with recurrent, generally mild, upper-respiratory-tract infections. There is also an increased incidence of bronchial asthma, perhaps because in the normal state the IgA in the secretions acts as a blocking antibody to prevent antigen from reaching the IgE on the mast cells. People with IgA deficiency can produce anti-IgA antibodies if given blood products. Severe hypersensitivity reactions can occur on a subsequent exposure.

Immunodeficiencies with predominantly T-cell-mediated defects

Severe combined immunodeficiency (SCID) is a group of diseases in which affected infants have severe lymphopenia, particularly affecting T cells. The principal manifestations are failure to thrive, skin eruption (due to graft-versus-host disease, as the mother's lymphocytes attack the infant's tissues), candidiasis, diarrhoea, and *Pneumocystis carinii* pneumonia.

Other types of immunodeficiency are known in which both T- and B-cell responses are abnormal.

ACQUIRED IMMUNODEFICIENCY SYNDROME (AIDS)

When previously fit young men became ill with two uncommon diseases—*Pneumocystis carenii* pneumonia and an aggressive form of Kaposi's sarcoma—it became apparent that a new disease had emerged. The disease was first noted in North America about 1978 and affected particularly male homosexuals, drug addicts, and haemophiliacs. The disease has now been recognized in all parts of the world, and the number of victims has steadily increased. The number of US cases reported to the Centers for Disease Control, Atlanta, Georgia now exceeds 100 000.

The cause of this new epidemic is infection with human immunodeficiency virus (HIV), a RNA retrovirus that was originally called lymphadenopathy associated virus (LAV), and later human T-cell lymphotropic virus, type III (HTLV III). A related strain (HIV-II) has subsequently been recovered from cases of AIDS in Africa. The origin of the virus is debated. Probably it arose in Africa as a mutation of a simian virus.

In the USA approximately 70–75% of cases of AIDS are male homosexual or bisexual males. HIV is carried in the semen, blood and other body fluids. It is thought that the virus can penetrate mucosal surface even in the absence of obvious trauma. Passive anal intercourse appears to be the major hazard. About 20% of cases are intravenous drug addicts who acquire their disease by sharing needles and intravenous equipment with other drug users. The remaining cases are female partners of infected bisexual males, customers of infected prostitutes, infants of infected mothers, and patients who have had transfusions with contaminated blood or who have received contaminated blood products such as clotting factors. Blood donors are now screened for HIV antibodies and this has almost eliminated the dangers of transfusion—absolute safety cannot be insured because some carriers of the virus may not possess antibodies. Heat treatment of factor VIII preparations has virtually eliminated the dangers of transmitting the disease to haemophiliacs, but unfortunately up to 70% of sufferers who were treated previously are already infected with the AIDS virus. Some cases of infection have followed artificial insemination. There is no evidence that the disease can be acquired by casual contact with patients, or even with close household contacts.

AIDS in relation to dentistry

In dentistry the possibility of accidental innoculation injury of contaminated blood and the likelihood of generating aerosols by low and high-speed drills, ultrosonic scalers and irrigation/air syringes emphasizes the need to wear protective eyewear, rubber gloves and a mask when working with known HIV antibody-positive patients. Indeed, in view of the fact that many infected patients remain undetected the only safe way to treat all patients must be to assume that all blood and saliva is infected until proven otherwise.

Although HIV has been identified in saliva there does not appear to any danger to health care workers.

Based on the examination of the mouths of HIV-positive patients, certain signs are most likely to be seen by the dental surgeon. Candidiasis (oral thrush) is not unusual in some patients (e.g. diabetics, those taking steroids or antibiotics, patients with cancer and other debilitating diseases), but is most unusual in the mouth of a young man. Again angular cheilitis is not unusual in some patients, but very unusual in those who are dentate. Intractable and recurrent gingivitis with ulceration and punched out dental papillae, which resembles acute necrotizing ulcerative gingivitis and does not respond to treatment, should also arouse suspicions. Rashes appearing on the face either in the form of seborrhoeic dermatitis or molluscum contagiosum must be viewed with suspicion as should intra-oral warts and severe forms of apthous ulceration.

Hairy leukoplakia has been observed with increasing frequency in homosexual men and patients with AIDS or AIDS-related complex (ARC). This occurs almost exclusively on the lateral border of the tongue as small whitish finger-like projections. Kaposi's sarcoma is relatively rare in the general population but may occur as a presenting symptom in around a third of AIDS/ARC patients.

Pathogenesis of AIDS

The virus infects helper T cells and the proviral DNA becomes incorporated into the nuclear DNA. Here it may remain dormant for an indeterminate period, but ultimately the cell dies. There is depletion of T-helper cells, and the resultant immunodeficiency state leaves the subject vulnerable to a wide array of infections and other effects including malignancy.

Following infection a number of syndromes can be recognized but they do not affect all subjects. About 7–14 days after infection a mild illness resembling influenza or infectious mononucleosis may occur. Next there may be persistent generalized lymphadenopathy (*PGL syndrome*), and the nodes show hyperplastic changes only. ARC consists of fatigue, fever, night sweats, weight loss, lymphadenopathy and diarrhoea. Pathologically there is lymphopenia with a decreased T-helper cell count, hypergamma-globulinaemia and anergy. Opportunistic infections are not a feature of this stage. Finally, AIDS develops. It is characterized by the presence of immunodeficiency in the absence of other causes, opportunistic infections as described below, and the presence of antibodies indicative of HIV infection. As the disease develops the antibody level decreases and antigenaemia increases. Weight loss is a striking feature and becomes extreme in the later stages of the disease. Indeed, in Africa 'slim disease' was recognized before its connection with HIV infection was appreciated.

Clinical features of AIDS

The severe state of immunodeficiency renders the subject liable to serious infections that can affect virtually any organ. 60% of cases present with pneumonia, the great majority being due to *P. carinii*. This is the major cause of death. Progressive fever, dyspnoea and a non-productive

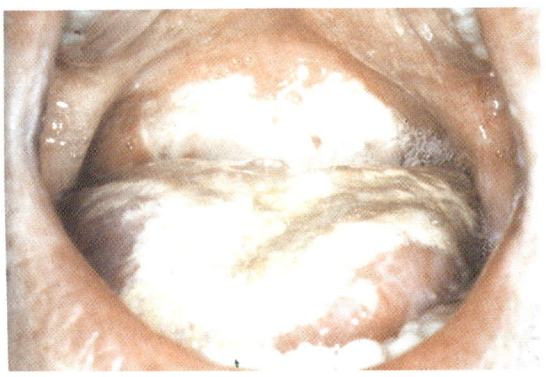

Fig. 11.1 Candida infection of the mouth in a 19-year-old haemophiliac patient who contracted AIDS as a result of receiving a transfusion of infected blood. (Photograph by courtesy of Professor A M Geddes, University of Burmingham.)

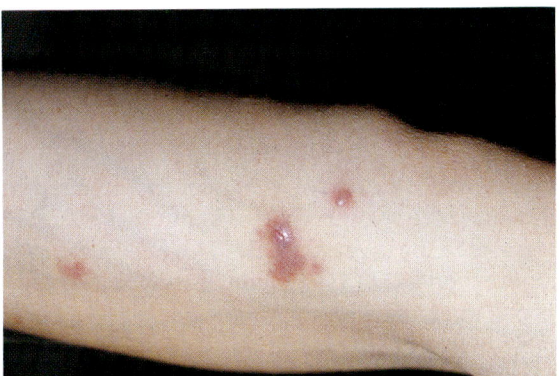

Fig. 11.2 Kaposi's sarcoma in a patient with AIDS. The patient developed scattered nodules in the skin; they varied in colour from bright red to dusky purple.

cough are the main features. *Severe persistent diarrhoea* is common and leads to the characteristic wasting. Colonic perforation requiring colectomy is a common complication. The cause of the diarrhoea is infective, and one or more of the following organisms may be found: *Isospora beli*, *Entamoeba histolytica*, *Giardia lamblia*, atypical mycobacteria, salmonella, shigella and cytomegalovirus. *Cryptosporidiosis* is another cause and is particularly resistant to treatment; the organism is an acid-fast protozoan and is detected by performing the Ziehl–Neelsen stain on faeces or tissue.

Involvement of the central nervous system is now recognized as being common; dementia with subtle loss of short-term memory is common and may be the presenting feature. It may be due to

HIV infection (AIDS encephalopathy), other infections (cryptococcosis, toxoplasmosis, etc.), progressive multifocal leucoencephalopathy or lymphoma.

Widespread infection with atypical mycobacteria, in particular *Mycobacterium avium intracellulare* is a common event and is characterized by fever, weight loss, sweating, lymphadenopathy and gastrointestinal symptoms. The organism is often present in vast numbers in the tissues. The infection is difficult to treat because the organism is highly resistant to standard antituberculous therapy.

Other infections include cytomegalovirus infection involving the gastrointestinal tract, the central nervous system, the liver and the eye. *Candida* infection of the mouth (*thrush*) (Fig. 11.1) is almost universal, and an oesophagitis (causing dysphagia) is common. It may also be due to *herpes simplex virus* an organism that also causes persistent perianal infection producing chronic ulceration and blistering.

Kaposi's sarcoma was the first *malignant disease* to be noted in patients with AIDS. Scattered erythematous or purple nodules appear in the skin of the trunk and limbs (Fig. 11.2). The hard

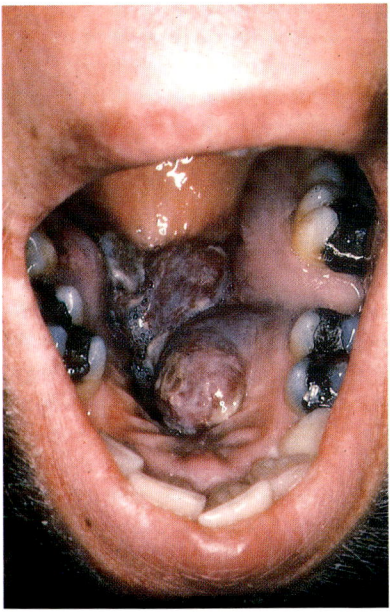

Fig. 11.3 Kaposi's tumour in a 28-year-old homosexual. (Photograph by courtesy of Professor A M Geddes, University of Birmingham.)

palate is a common site and the disease may first be noted by the dentist (Fig. 11.3). Tumours also involve internal organs, being particularly common in the gut. For reasons that are not apparent, Kaposi's sarcoma is now less common in AIDS than it was at the onset of the epidemic. Curiously enough, those patients who present with Kaposi's sarcoma have a better prognosis. Non-Hodgkin's B-cell lymphoma is also common, and as noted previously a diffuse lymphoma may be found involving the brain.

In children, AIDS has some features not commonly encountered in adults. These include lymphocytic interstitial pneumonitis due to Epstein–Barr virus infection, parotid enlargement and a terminal Gram-negative septicaemia.

Epidemiology, treatment and prognosis

The presence of antibodies to HIV is considered reliable evidence of infection and infectivity. The ELISA technique is used as a screening test and confirmed by Western blot, RIPA (radioimmunoprecipitation assay) or IFA (immunofluorescent antibody) methods. Once infected, the individual is thought to remain infective for life. Furthermore, it is probable that AIDS eventually develops in all such people but the incubation period is long; thus in one group, 34% of homosexuals with HIV-positive serum developed AIDS within 3 years.

The incidence of infection in the general population varies greatly from one part of the world to another. There are parts of Africa where 12% of the population are seropositive. Here the transmission appears to be heterosexual contact. African prostitutes have shown a seropositivity rate of 50–88% and presumably form an important source of infection. In the USA and Europe the incidence ranges from 0.005 to 0.52%.

As yet there is no curative treatment available for AIDS, but supportive and antimicrobial agents can prolong life. The antiviral drug azidothymidine (AZT) is being assessed and the results are encouraging. The drug halts DNA synthesis, especially that associated with viral RNA-dependent DNA polymerase. The overall prognosis of AIDS is about 49% survival at 1 year and 15% at 2 years. Few patients live beyond 3 years.

OTHER ACQUIRED IMMUNOLOGICAL DEFICIENCY STATES

The immune reaction is impaired in a number of other acquired diseases:

Infection

During measles, rubella and following measles immunization, there is depression of cell-mediated reactions. Likewise there is anergy in lepromatous leprosy.

Lymphoma

The immune response is frequently impaired in patients with lymphoma—a state that is often aggravated by treatment. In *Hodgkin's disease* a suppression of T-cell functions results in a liability to infection with the tubercle bacillus, viruses and fungi. In *multiple myeloma* and *Waldenström's macroglobulinaemia* there is suppression of normal immunoglobulin production that results in a tendency to bacterial infection. In *lymphocytic lymphoma* and *chronic lymphatic leukaemia* both arms of the immune response are impaired.

Iatrogenic immunological deficiency.

Heavy dosage of glucocorticosteroids and cytotoxic drugs cause a severe depression of the immune response. This often compounds the effects of the primary condition, such as a lymphoma.

GENERAL READING (see also Ch. 10)

Cohen S, Warren K S (eds) 1982 Immunology of parasitic infections. Blackwell Scientific, Oxford
Farthing C F, et al 1986 A colour atlas of AIDS. Acquired Immodeficiency Syndrome. Wolfe Medical Publications Ltd, London
Friedland G H, Klein R S 1987 Transmission of the human immundeficiency virus. New England Journal of Medicine 317: 1125

Hilgartner M W 1987 AIDS and hemophilia. New England Journal of Medicine 317: 1153
Kingsley L A 1987 Risk factors for seroconversion to human immunodeficiency virus among male homosexuals. Lancet 1: 345
Leading article 1989 Oral hairy leucoplakia. Lancet 2: 1189
Rothenberg R, et al 1987 Survival with the acquired immunodeficiency syndrome. New England Journal of Medicine 317: 1297

12. Tissue transplantation

In addition to its practical value in surgery, the transplantation of tissue has greatly extended our knowledge of the body's response to foreign tissue. The factors determining the fate of grafted tissue may be summarized:

1. Tissue transferred from a donor to a genetically identical recipient survives (i.e. *isografts survive*)
2. Tissue transferred from a donor to a genetically non-identical individual of the same species is rejected (i.e. *allografts are rejected*)
3. The genes that encode transplantation antigens are codominant, that is, both alleles can be detected in each individual, and the individual possessing a particular antigen is tolerant of that antigen and does not recognize it in a graft.

It is evident that, all other things being equal, the fate of a graft is dependent on the genetic compatibility between donor tissue and the host.

THE FATE OF ISOGRAFTS

Tissue transplantable from one part of an individual to another area in the same individual (termed an *autograft*) or to an identical twin both constitute an *isograft* and do not provoke an immune reaction. Provided local conditions are satisfactory and the graft acquires a blood supply, such grafts survive. Autographs have found extensive use in plastic surgery, either as whole-thickness flaps of skin used as pedicle grafts, or alternatively as free grafts applied to a raw surface, e.g. following a burn. Teeth have been transplanted successfully from one part of the mouth to another.

Great interest is centered on the fate of *allografts*, firstly because of the practical value of grafting tissue from one individual to another, and secondly, because of the fundamental biological properties that the allograft reaction has revealed. These have far-reaching implications in many branches of medicine.

Before proceeding to discuss the fate of allografts, some details of the major histocompatibility complex will be described.

THE MAJOR HISTOCOMPATIBILITY COMPLEX

The major histocompatibility complex (MHC) of man is a set of closely linked genes situated on the short arm of chromosome 6. These genes code for the transmembrane glycoproteins that are widely distributed in the tissues. In humans they are called the *HLA antigens* because they were first identified as *human leucocyte antigens*. The external portions of these glycoproteins act as membrane markers and can be identified by tissue typing. These are of two types:

Class I products. These are designated the A, B, and C antigens.

Class II products. These are D antigens. Subgroups are designated DP, DQ, and DR, the best known being DR.

There may be one of many possible alleles at any one locus; thus there are at least 18 alleles at A locus, 41 at B, 8 at C and 20 at D. The MHC products (HLA antigens) function as the targets of T-cell recognition of T-cell responses to antigen, and help to determine the individual's immune responses to antigenic stimulation. The MHC is important in transplantation: its name derives (originally in the mouse) from its antigenic products being the major targets for rejection of allografts.

Class III genes of the MHC are genes that code for several enzymes and components of complement.

Tissue distribution of HLA antigens

Class I antigens are found on many cells but the amount differs enormously from one cell type to another. The greatest amount is present in the lymphoid and mononuclear phagocyte systems, and on vascular endothelial cells. Class II molecules have a restricted distribution, being present on B lymphocyte, macrophages and dendritic cells, but not under normal circumstances on most other types of cell.

A vigorous systemic immune response can greatly increase the expression both of Class I and Class II products, the change in Class II being the more dramatic because in many tissues they are normally in very low concentration. One mediator of these changes is γ-interferon, produced by stimulated T lymphocytes. The significance of these changes in Class I and Class II product expression induced by immunological reactions could be to augment T-cell functions in these tissues, since the amount of MHC product on a cell is an important factor in the ability of the T cell to recognize foreign antigens.

The genetics of the major histocompatibility complex

Use of the new tools of molecular biology, using DNA probes has added much to the knowledge obtained by using classical genetic techniques to study the alleles occurring in the population.

Each MHC gene is divided into exons separated by introns. An exon frequently controls an individual domain of a protein. Thus the typical Class I gene (such as the HLA-A locus) contains three exons coding respectively for the α_1, α_2 and α_3 domains, with other exons coding for transmembrane and intracytoplasmic portions of the molecule. These individual genes are organized into one complex. In the human HLA complex the order of the genes, proceeding from the centromere, is: Class II genes, followed by Class III genes, followed by the Class I genes.

The loci of the MHC are tightly linked and tend to be inherited as a unit called a *haplotype*. Within a family, the inherited haplotypes behave as if they were single genes. If the mother's haplotypes are designated (a,b) and the father's haplotypes are designated (c,d), then their children can have the following combination of haplotypes: (a,c), (a,d), (b,c) and (b,d). The probability that any two siblings will inherit the same two haplotypes (i.e. will be HLA identical) is 25%. Each parent will always be one haplotype identical with each child, but never two haplotypes identical, unless the parents are themselves close relatives and share one or two haplotypes.

The identification of MHC alleles—tissue typing

The typing of the MHC loci is based on serological testing using specific antibodies against MHC allele products. The antibodies have been derived from several sources, typically alloimmune human sera from either multiparous women, transfused persons, or those who have received transplants. The antigens have been given consecutive numbers, and the identification and naming of each specificity is coordinated by large international, collaborative workshops that eventually define each new allele. While being studied the number is preceded by 'w', (for workshop), e.g. HLA-DRw4

The method of tissue typing depends on the phenomenon of complement dependent cytotoxicity. For type I class products a suspension of lymphocytes and monocytes is prepared from blood and a small quantity is placed in separate wells on a plate. To each is added a specific antibody, and the plate is incubated. Complement is then added. If antibody has been bound, the complement is fixed to the cell surface, the membrane attack complex is assembled, and the cell dies. This is detected by adding a dye which readily enters cells having damaged membranes. Dyed cells are dead cells! Since T lymphocytes are class II negative a preparation of monocytes is needed for class II typing. Other techniques can be used for typing certain MHC products. The *mixed lymphocyte culture* (MLC) test is the best known. It is based on the principle that if immunocompetent T cells of one individual are incubated with cells bearing the MHC products of another genetically different individual, the T cells of the first individual proliferate. Such proliferation can be detected by the incorporation of radioactive nucleic-acid precursors. The MLC test takes several days and is not suitable for routine typing purposes.

MHC AND DISEASE

The discovery in 1973 that the class I antigen HLA-B27 is frequent in patients with ankylosing spondylitis, in comparison with the general population, has lead to the discovery of many other associations of a particular disease with one or more HLA antigens. For example, type I diabetes mellitus is associated with HLA-DR3 or HLA-DR4.

HLA AND THE INTENSITY OF THE IMMUNE RESPONSE

The ability of an individual to respond to a particular antigen is related to the MHC alleles inherited by the individual. This is because the MHC products (particularly class II products) are antigen-presenting structures, and the different alleles have differing abilities to present a particular antigen to T cells.

BIOLOGICAL SIGNIFICANCE OF THE MHC

The reason for the existence of the MHC is not clear. It provides a context for T-cell recognition of foreign antigens, but the advantage of this procedure over direct recognition, as exhibited by B cells, is not evident.

The reason for the polymorphism is more apparent. Particular alleles are more adept at presenting an effective signal to the immune response in the event of a particular infection. A heterozygous individual will therefore have a greater chance of responding and overcoming an infection, and a heterogenous community will have a better chance of surviving an epidemic caused by a new infectious agent.

THE FATE OF ALLOGRAFTS

Allografts are usually rejected, and three patterns of this allograft rejection phenomenon may be recognized:

1. Acute rejection
2. Second-set phenomenon
3. Chronic rejection.

Acute rejection

Free allografts become vascularized in much the same way as isografts. The graft remains viable for a limited period and is rejected. This is T-cell mediated. The organ undergoing rejection shows oedema and an infiltration by host cells. If the recipient has previously been immunized against the donor (e.g. by the receipt of a previous graft), the rejection occurs much earlier (by day 2 or 3) and is more vigorous. This is called the *'second-set' rejection*, and is a reflection of specific immunologic memory for the antigens of the graft. In a highly sensitized animal, a 'white graft' occurs: this reaction is so early that the graft never becomes vascularized because its vessels thrombose. If the graft is connected by vascular anastomosis, as occurs with a kidney transplant, this type of reaction is termed a *hyperacute rejection* and is mediated by antibodies. Hyperacute rejection is usually a complement-mediated destruction of the vasculature of the graft.

Chronic rejection

The graft appears to be accepted, but its vessels gradually become obstructed by intimal thickening. This type of rejection has been most studied in patients with renal and heart transplants, and can occur months to years after transplantation. In many cases it is antibody-mediated.

FACTORS WHICH MAY DETERMINE LONG SURVIVAL OF ALLOGRAFTS

Allografts are usually rejected as described above, but there are exceptions. Cartilage and cornea are found to be capable of long survival. For this reason corneal transplantation is widely used. Grafts placed in special sites such as the anterior chamber of the eye seem to be protected against immune rejection. However, with these exceptions, the antigenic compatibility between the graft and the host is the single most important factor determining the fate of a graft. The antigens most concerned are major histocompatibility or HLA antigens, and careful tissue matching reduces the severity of the rejection phenomenon. Suppression of the immune response by administration of prednisone, cyclosporine or other drugs is widely employed to prolong the life of grafts.

GRAFT RECOGNITION BY THE HOST

When a graft of foreign tissue is transplanted to an allogeneic host, the host encounters the graft antigens either through host cells patrolling the donor tissues, or through antigen or cells from the graft being released and carried to the lymphoid organs. The relative importance of the two alternatives is debatable. Two other factors must be considered:

1. Passenger leukocytes in the graft
2. Changing immunogenicity of the graft.

Passenger leukocytes in the graft

Donor leucocytes are strongly positive for class II antigens of the MHC, and their presence in the graft may stimulate a strong immune response. Pretreatment of a graft by radiation or by in vitro culture can reduce its immunogenicity, an effect attributable to the destruction of its content of white cells.

Changing immunogenicity of the graft

Many cell types, including epithelial cells and endothelial cells, express little class II antigen under normal conditions. However, they become strongly positive when exposed to immunological stimuli from lymphocytes. γ-Interferon and other products of lymphocytes are important in this regard. It is evident that once initiated, the immune reaction can stimulate increased expression of HLA antigens in the graft cells, and this in turn may evoke stronger stimulation as well as make the cells better targets for the response.

Enhancement

Enhancement is the phenomenon whereby an immunized host does not reject a graft in a second-set manner, but will instead allow prolonged graft survival. Blood transfusion from a proposed donor is used in human transplantation work in an attempt to utilize this phenomenon. Enhancement is probably mediated by antibody to the class II antigens of the graft, which by destroying the most immunogenic passenger leucocytes of the graft leave the remainder of the graft much less immunogenic.

THE STATUS OF TRANSPLANTATION IN CLINICAL MEDICINE

KIDNEY

Kidney transplantation is the most widely used type of solid organ transplant. In living donor transplantation, HLA identity of one haplotype identity, as well as blood group compatibility, is usually mandatory. Furthermore donor blood can be infused on several occasions into the future recipient in the months before the transplantation, so that rejection is inhibited by the process of enhancement.

In cadaver donor transplantation tissue matching is of less importance in influencing graft survival than between related individuals. There are several possible reasons why HLA matching is of less value. The present techniques for tissue matching do not type all HLA loci, so that a 'good match' between unrelated individuals is by no means as perfect as it may seem. On the other hand, related individuals who share haplotypes are likely to be compatible at all loci—even those that are not investigated in routine techniques. A second factor is the minor histocompatibility (non-HLA) antigens which cannot be typed or matched.

BONE MARROW

The transplantation of marrow cells to cure aplastic anaemia, leukaemia, or genetic defects of the stem-cells is gaining in popularity. Often the patient's bone marrow is first destroyed by total body radiation or high doses of cyclophosphamide. The graft includes large numbers of immunocompetent cells that are capable of recognizing alloantigens in the recipient. The result of this is a *graft versus host (GVH) reaction*, characterized by skin eruptions, lung infiltrations, marrow failure, diarrhoea, and eventually death. Some individuals develops a chronic form of the disease, in which scleroderma-like changes occur in the skin and the liver develops a condition resembling biliary cirrhosis. Oral lesions resembling lichen planus and the sicca complex are common. Because of the severity of the GVH reaction only HLA-identical sibling donors have been used successfully, but perhaps newer immunosuppressive methods will change this.

LIVER

Cadaveric liver transplantation is becoming a more common procedure, and with the advent of cyclosporine the results are nearing a 75% 1-year survival.

HEART, HEART–LUNG AND LUNG

Heart transplantation and heart–lung transplantation are being performed with considerable success. Isolated lung transplants have not been so successful due to the complex problems related to anastomosis of donor bronchus to recipient bronchus. However, where only the lungs are affected as in cystic fibrosis, a heart–lung transplant may be performed and the recipient's heart then used for another patient.

CORNEA

Allografts of cornea usually remain clear for a long time and are widely used.

THE FETUS AS A GRAFT

The fetus is usually allogeneic to its mother and there is no doubt that mothers can mount an immune response to the paternal HLA antigens expressed in the fetus. Multiparous females frequently have antibodies against the HLA antigens of their husband, but successful pregnancy is clearly the rule. How this occurs has provided more questions than answers. Important factors appear to be the poor immunogenicity of the placenta—it expresses only class I antigens, a mild state of immunosuppression induced by pregnancy, and a barrier function of the placenta.

GENERAL READING (see also Ch. 10)

Bodmer W F 1987 The HLA system: structure and function. Journal of Clinical Pathology. 40:948
Demean A M 1985 Graft versus host disease: new versions of old problems. British Medical Journal 290:658
Morris P 1985 Kidney transplantation. Academic Press, London
Snell G D, Dausset J, Nathenson S 1976 Histocompatibility. Academic Press, New York

13. Diseases mediated by immunological mechanisms

Immunologically mediated tissue injury (often termed hypersensitivity) can be classified into four groups as suggested by Gell and Coombs:

Type I: IgE-mediated—'immediate hypersensitivity'

Type II: mediated by direct binding of antibody (usually IgG or IgM) to a membrane antigen, where it activates complement

Type III: mediated by deposition of immune complexes in the tissues—complement activation is involved

Type IV: mediated by delayed-type hypersensitivity—a T-cell-mediated response

This classification omits a mechanism involving the direct lysis of target cells by cytotoxic T cells.

TYPE I: IgE-MEDIATED REACTIONS

Generalized anaphylaxis and allergy, with its subset atopy, are the major types of this response.

Generalized anaphylaxis

Richet and Portier, while attempting to immunize dogs against the toxins of the sea-anemone, noted that animals that had survived a sublethal injection of toxin were unduly sensitive to a second injection—so sensitive, indeed, that quite small doses produced a severe reaction, often resulting in death. Richet called the reaction 'anaphylaxis' because it seemed to represent the antithesis of immunity (Gr. *ana*—against, *phylaxis*—protection). It was later demonstrated that anaphylaxis was mediated by 'reaginic antibody', and finally that reagin was IgE.

For anaphylaxis to occur the individual must have been exposed to the antigen previously. IgE is formed and becomes fixed to mast cells. Subsequent encounters with the antigen causes a severe reaction, due to the sudden release of mediators, especially histamine.

The principal clinical features in humans are hypotension, bronchospasm, and oedema of the larynx or skin. The treatment of such a medical emergency consists of the immediate administration of epinephrine. Antihistamine drugs, glucocorticoids, intravenous fluids, and cardiopulmonary life-support measures may also be necessary.

Anaphylactic shock is usually encountered in humans following the injection of foreign serum, the bite of a bee or wasp, or the injection of a drug, e.g. penicillin. In the latter event the drug acts as a hapten. The capacity to develop anaphylactic shock has a genetic basis but the details of the inheritance are unknown. Atopic individuals are more susceptible but not all subjects who have a history of anaphylaxis are atopic.

Cutaneous 'anaphylaxis'

If a small quantity of antigen is injected into the skin of a sensitized subject, an immediate local weal and flare develop. This test may be used clinically to detect IgE sensitivity and is used clinically in the investigation of patients suspected of having an atopic disease. The results of such skin tests cannot be used to assess possible sensitization to anaphylaxis. The safest procedure when administering foreign sera is to give a small dose subcutaneously and watch for any mild general reaction. Trained staff with adrenalin and a syringe should, of course, be at hand.

Allergy and atopy

Allergy[*] is defined as a clinical disorder caused by inappropriate IgE responses. The antigens involved in allergic states are often called *allergens*.

Although allergy is mediated by IgE, it does not follow that there has to be excess formation of IgE in order to produce allergic symptoms. Other mechanisms could involve inadequate formation of blocking IgG or IgA thereby permitting excess antigen to reach the IgE sites on mast cells.

Atopy is a subset of allergy in which there is an hereditary tendency to develop IgE-mediated illness in response to antigen exposure.

Atopy includes a variety of IgE-mediated clinical syndromes that are grouped together because of their familial incidence, although the exact mode of inheritance is not known; they include: allergic rhinitis (hay fever), bronchial asthma, urticaria, angioedema, atopic dermatitis (eczema), and some gastrointestinal allergies. The diseases may occur in different members of one family, and several diseases may affect one individual, e.g. infantile eczema may be replaced by atopic dermatitis, hay fever or asthma in later life. It should be noted that each of the clinical syndromes can also be due to non-IgE and non-immunological mechanisms.

Allergic rhinitis is a clinical picture of sneezing, nasal discharge, and nasal congestion after exposure to antigen such as ragweed pollen by inhalation. The nasal discharge contains copious eosinophils. The reaction is immediate, and the principal mediator appears to be histamine. *Extrinsic asthma* is described in Chapter 30. *Infantile eczema* and *atopic dermatitis* are described in Chapter 37.

THE IMMEDIATE HYPERSENSITIVITY RESPONSE AND ITS CHEMICAL MEDIATORS

When IgE, bound to mast cells and basophils, binds antigen, the bridging of two IgE molecules by an antigen molecule triggers the mast cell to release the contents of its granules, which cause the manifestations of immediate hypersensitivity. The principle mediators are:

1. Histamine
2. Slow-reacting substance of anaphylaxis (SRS-A) (leukotrienes C4, D4 and E4)

---

[*]The term allergy has often been used in a different way—allergic contact dermatitis, bacterial allergy to the tubercle bacillus, drug allergy, etc. In these instances IgE is not necessarily involved. In this book, allergy will be used to describe IgE-mast cell reactions, except where tradition demands differently, e.g. allergic contact dermatitis.

3. Other factors, including eosinophil-chemo-tactic factor (ECF-A), neutrophil-chemotactic factor, heparin, and many others.

The effects of these mediators vary with the organ. The lungs respond with bronchoconstriction (in response to histamine and SRS-A), mucosal oedema (due to histamine and other factors), and increased mucus production (due to histamine). Hypotensive shock can follow if the reaction is severe enough for mediators, particularly histamine and SRS-A, to enter the circulation.

Involvement of eosinophils and platelets in allergic responses

Eosinophils are characteristic of allergic reactions in tissues (perhaps in response to eosiniphil-chemotactic factor), but their precise role has been incompletely defined. They can phago-cytose basophil granules, inactivate histamine, and SRS-A, and inhibit PAF. The eosinophils are involved in the IgE-mediated attack on parasites.

Platelets can release arachidonic-acid meta-bolites (prostaglandins and thromboxane) and serotonin. Platelets have an IgE receptor, and can kill IgE-coated parasites such as schistosomes.

Mast cell degranulation by non-IgE-mediated mechanisms

Mast cells can be degranulated by mechanisms not involving IgE (e.g. the anaphylatoxins C3a and C5a). It follows that every atopic clinical syndrome can also be caused by non-IgE-mediated mechanisms: for example, angioedema may be due to a deficiency of C1-estrase inhibitor, and may have nothing to do with IgE, being mediated by anaphylatoxins generated through inappropriate complement activation; urticaria is frequently idiopathic with no clear relationship to allergens.

TYPE II HYPERSENSITIVITY

Type II reactions are mediated by antibodies that are cytotoxic to tissue cells, often by complement activation. Examples include autoimmune haemolytic anaemia, autoimmune thrombocytopenia,

and Goodpasture's syndrome. Graves' disease has been included in this group, but because the autoantibody stimulates the thyroid cells rather than destroying them, some workers prefer to classify it separately as a 'type V reaction'

TYPE III HYPERSENSITIVITY— IMMUNE-COMPLEX REACTIONS

Some types of antibodies have the property of combining with their respective antigen to form complexes that can activate complement. Chemotactic factors are liberated, and polymorphs, which are attracted to the complexes, release damaging lysosomal enzymes. Four examples in which damaging immune complexes produce disease are described below.

THE ARTHUS PHENOMENON

Subcutaneous injections of antigen given to an animal at weekly intervals lead to progressively more severe local reactions after several injections. Signs of acute inflammation with oedema and redness appear in about 1 hour and haemorrhage and necrosis develop within a few hours. The pathogenesis is as follows: The injected antigen diffuses into vessel walls and encounters the specific IgG present in the blood as a result of the previous injection of antigen. Antigen–antibody complexes form in the vessel wall, and activate complement. Released chemotactic factors cause polymorphs to accumulate, they release their damaging lysosomal enzymes and thrombosis follows (Fig. 13.1)

SERUM SICKNESS

Serum sickness is a condition characterized by *fever*, *joint pains*, and *urticarial eruptions* that occurs 10–14 days after the administration of a *large dose* of foreign serum, e.g. horse γ-globulin. The pathogenesis is explained in Fig. 13.2 The injected antigen persists in the blood until the 10th day. At this time the immune response becomes evident by the disappearance of antigen from the blood (immune catabolism) and the appearance of immunoglobulins in the plasma. At first they form complexes with antigen, but as

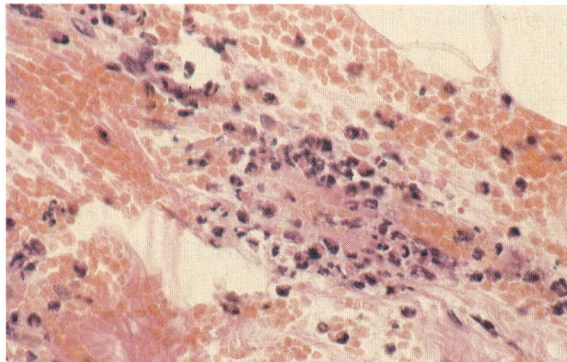

Fig. 13.1   Arthus reaction. A small vessel is surrounded and infiltrated by numerous neutrophils some of which have broken up into nuclear fragments (nuclear dust) as a result of karyorrhexis. The vessel is occluded by pink fibrinous material; surrounding it there are extravasated red cells. These changes are typical of an acute leucocytoclastic vasculitis.

these are eliminated, free antibody appears in the plasma. The lesions of serum sickness are due to the damaging effect of immune complexes deposited at certain sites—skin, etc. Complement is activated, and polymorphs accumulate and release damaging lysosomal enzymes.

Microscopically the lesions of serum sickness are similar to those of the Arthus reaction, but

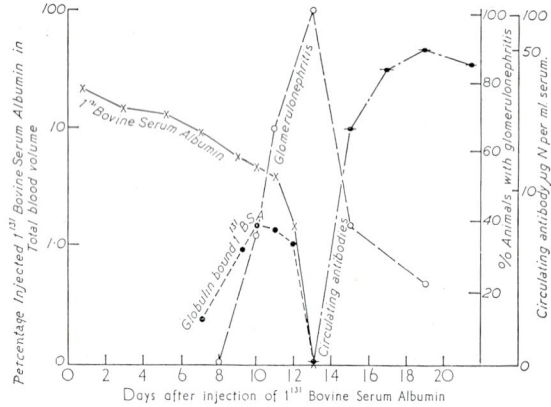

Fig. 13.2   Time relations between fall of circulating antigen, formation of antigen-antibody complexes, lesions of serum sickness (glomerulonephritis), and rise of circulating antibody in rabbits injected with large doses of ^{131}I-labelled bovine serum albumin. (From Gladstone GP 1961. In: Florey H W *General Pathology* 3rd edn, after Dixon J F et al 1959 in: Lawrence H S *Cellular and humoral aspects of the hypersensitivity states*. Harper and Row, New York, p 345.)

are less severe. There is an acute vasculitis with polymorphs infiltrating the vessel walls. In addition, a glomerulonephritis is characteristic.

Chronic immune-complex disease

If daily injections of antigen are given to an animal in doses such that antigen–antibody complexes with antigen excess are formed in the blood, a chronic glomerulonephritis develops. It is believed that some type of human glomerulonephritis have a similar pathogenesis, for example the renal lesions of systemic lupus erythematosus.

CLINICAL EXAMPLES OF HYPERSENSITIVITY MEDIATED BY IMMUNOGLOBULINS

In clinical practice it is sometimes the case that hypersensitivity reactions are mediated by several mechanisms, commonly a combination of type I and type III responses. Three examples will be described: acute leucocytoclastic vasculitis, drug hypersensitivity, and allergic lung disease.

Acute vasculitis

Many forms of acute vasculitis are believed to be examples of immune-complex disease. These include the vasculitis seen in the skin lesions of *Strep. viridans* endocarditis, meningococcal septicaemia, and gonococcal septicaemia. Histologically the lesions closely resemble those of the Arthus reaction.

Drug hypersensitivity

Hypersensitivity to drugs is a common clinical event and is due to the drug, or one of its degradation products, acting as a hapten and stimulating the formation of sensitizing antibodies. Virtually any drug can produce a reaction, but common offenders are penicillin, sulphonamides, para-aminosalicylic acid (PAS), barbiturates, and quinine. Relatively few people given a drug manifest hypersensitivity, and the tendency to do so is probably inherited. Thus atopic individuals are particularly at risk, especially for IgE-mediated effects.

Types of drug reaction

Drug reactions may be immediate and mediated by IgE; if the drug is given by injection a reaction can occur within a few minutes. Urticaria is common, and in severe cases the features are those of anaphylactic shock.

Later drug reactions begin several days after the administration of the drug and are due to the formation of IgG or IgM that cause a disease resembling serum sickness. *Late drug effects* are thrombocytopenia, haemolytic anaemia, erythema multiforme, cholestatic jaundice, and a syndrome resembling systemic lupus erythematosus. Methicillin is responsible for some cases of acute interstitial nephritis, and is accompanied by anti-renal-tubule basement-membrane antibodies. The pathogenesis of many of these effects is obscure. In some instances, e.g. haemolytic anaemia, cytotoxic antibodies are present (type II reaction).

Immunological lung disease

Lung tissue is a common site for immune-mediated disease. Several patterns of reaction can be found:

The extrinsic type of bronchial asthma. This is an IgE-mediated disorder.

Extrinsic allergic alveolitis. The best known example is Farmer's lung, a type III reaction in the alveoli caused by inhaling fungal antigen derived from mouldy hay.

Pulmonary infiltrates and eosinophilia (PIE syndrome).

Goodpasture's disease. A type II reaction.

TYPE IV REACTIONS

As the main features and pathogenesis of immunoglobulin-mediated hypersensitivity were clarified, it became evident that there also existed a separate, completely distinct type of hypersensitivity. Its recognition stemmed from the early observation of Robert Koch on the effects of tuberculosis infection in guinea-pigs. The type of hypersensitivity involved is T-cell-mediated and is also called delayed-type hypersensitivity.

The Koch phenomenon

If tubercle bacilli are injected into a normal guinea-pig, a nodule appears at the site of the injection after about 14 days; ulceration follows and persists until the death of the animal. The bacilli spread to the local lymph nodes, reach the blood stream, and finally lead to generalized milliary tuberculosis and death. The injection of tubercle bacilli into the skin of a tuberculous animal evokes a different type of response. A nodule appears in 1–2 days, ulcerates, and then heals. There is little tendency to spread to the regional lymph nodes. This second type of response was described by Koch, and differs from the primary response of a normal animal in three important respects:

1 The incubation period is greatly shortened—this may be described as hypersensitivity
2 The lesion heals quickly
3 There is no spread.

These are the features of immunity.

The heightened tissue response of the tuberculous animal can be demonstrated not only to the living tubercle bacillus but also extracts of organisms. Koch originally used 'old tuberculin', but more recently a purified protein derivative (PPD) has been introduced.

The intradermal injection of a small quantity of PPD into a normal animal results in a negligible inflammatory response. In the tuberculous animal, however, there develops a raised erythematous lesion appearing within 24 h and reaching a peak by 72 h. This is the Mantoux or tuberculin test, and a positive result indicates the existance of hypersensitivity to tuberculoprotein. The delay in the appearance of the reaction is noteworthy, and contrasts with the rapid appearance of the weal and flare effect of IgE-mediated reactions. Under natural conditions, delayed-type hypersensitivity to an organism occurs only as a result of infection. A conversion from Mantoux-negative to positive during the course of an undiagnosed illness is therefore good evidence of its tuberculous aetiology. If the infection is completely eradicated, the test may, over a period of years, revert to negative. Hence, the Mantoux test is of great importance clinically because a positive reaction indicates a past or present tuberculous infection. Indeed in communities where tuberculosis is uncommon, a strongly positive tuberculin test is highly suggestive of active tuberculosis.

Delayed-type hypersensitivity in other infections

Hypersensitivity reactions akin to the Mantoux test are of diagnostic value in other infections, and indicate the existance of sensitization. The following tests may be cited: coccidioidin, histoplasmin, blastomycin, and lepromin (Fernandez reaction). Hypersensitivity to *Candida* antigen, mumps antigen, steptokinase, streptodornase, and trichophytin is very common in normal people. A negative response to these, and to tuberculin (and coccidioidin in California), indicates an abnormal state termed anergy.

ROLE OF TYPE IV REACTIONS IN DISEASE

There can be little doubt that the tissue destruction caused by delayed-type hypersensitivity reactions is responsible for the necrosis (e.g. caseation) that occurs in some infections. Indeed the excessive and continued tissue destruction is the cause of the chronicity that characterizes mycobacterial, fungal and some other infections.

Allergic contact dermatitis

'Allergic' contact dermatitis, typified by poison ivy and nickle dermatitis, is also a type IV reaction (see Chapter 37).

OTHER DISEASES MEDIATED BY ABERRANT IMMUNE MECHANISMS

Although it is convenient to described the four types of hypersensitivity and the human diseases in which they play a dominant role, there are many instances in which the reactions are more complex. Immune complexes may form in situ rather than be formed in the circulation as in the classic type III reaction. In some diseases several types of reaction combine to produce complex lesions. Sometimes the antigen involved is a self protein and the disease is labelled autoimmune. Lupus erythematosus is a typical example.

AUTOIMMUNE DISEASE—THE CONCEPT OF 'AUTOIMMUNITY'

The idea of the host's defence system attacking and destroying the host's own tissues is attributed to Paul Ehrlich, who in 1900 described the 'horror autotoxicus', by which he implied the fear of damaging one's own tissues by a specific immune reaction against them. The description of autoimmune haemolytic anaemia and autoimmune thyroiditis in the 1950's enshrined autoimmunity firmly in the thinking of medical people—perhaps too firmly. It became convenient to use the term autoimmunity as a label for any disease of unknown aetiology in which there was any hint of an inflammatory infiltrate in the lesions or any autoantibodies in the serum.

Autoimmunity may be defined as a condition in which a major effector mechanism—humoral or cellular—reacts specifically with a self component that is not altered by foreign antigen. To some the issue of whether the foreign antigen, (e.g. a virus) does or does not alter a self antigen is a matter of semantics, because the immune response, particularly the T-cell component, is highly dependent on self antigens in the form of the HLA antigens. Autoimmunity describes the pathogenesis of some disease but does not indicate the cause. Had previous generations labelled syphilis, an autoimmune disease perhaps our knowledge of its aetiology and therapy would not have been furthered.

The role of the autoantibody in autoimmune diseases varies from being essential to the pathogenesis to being an epiphenomenon of no known significance. Some autoantibodies are organspecific, some not. It is evident that for a complete understanding of an autoimmune disease, one must not only understand the immune mechanisms that produce the lesions, but also the cause or precipitating agent.

Aetiology and precipitating factors in autoimmune disease

An autoimmune disease may develop in a

patient with a genetic susceptibility; this may be associated with a particular HLA group or a defect in a class III gene of the MHC (p. 132). The precipitating cause may be some external event such as an infection, drug administration, or trauma.

There are several suggestions as to how external agents (e.g. a virus) can trigger an autoimmune reaction. One mechanism is presented in Figure 13.3. In the normal state autoreactive B cells exist but cannot be triggered because T cells have been tolerized. A foreign protein may carry the determinant recognizable by B cells in association with a determinant that triggers helper T cells.

A second popular theory is illustrated in Figure 13.4. A virus binds to its complementary structure (receptor) on the cell membrane. We may then think of virus as the 'key' and its cell-membrane receptor as the 'lock'. Antibody is made against the virus key, but the antibody-combining site now itself must resemble the lock. Therefore, if an anti-idiotype response occurs (i.e. an antibody response against the anti-virus antibody combining site, see p. 119), the anti-anti-virus antibody will be anti-lock, i.e. able to bind to the virus receptor on the target cells of the virus. In other words, the anti-idiotype type response triggered by anti-virus antibody could lead to autoimmunity against virus receptor on cell membranes.

Another approach to the pathogenesis of antoimmunity has been described on page 120. An event such as a virus infection could encourage expression of class II HLA antigen so that reactive T cells can be stimulated and in turn lead to antibody production or the formation of effector T cells.

EXAMPLES OF IMMUNOLOGICALLY MEDIATED DISEASES

Renal disease

An autoimmune reaction is involved in several types of glomerulonephritis.

Liver disease

There is little doubt that an immune mechanism is responsible for liver cell necrosis in acute viral hepatitis, but the precise pathogenesis is not clear. Non-organ-specific autoantibodies are found in several types of chronic liver disease—chronic active hepatitis, primary biliary cirrhosis, and some cases of cirrhosis of unknown cause (cryptogenic cirrhosis). These have been grouped as 'autoimmune liver disease' but the

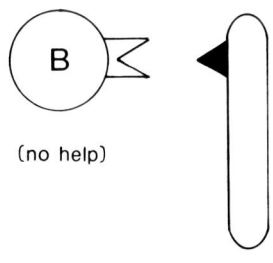

no T cell help
potential B cell response

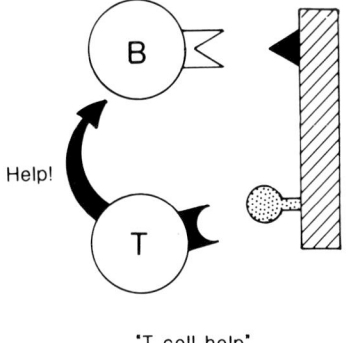

'T cell help'
autoantibody vs ◄

Fig. 13.3   A mechanism for explaining the ability of foreign antigen (e.g. infectious agent) to trigger autoantibody formation. In the normal state (left), potentially autoreactive B cells exist, but are not triggered because T cells have been tolerized. A foreign protein (right) may carry the determinant recognizable by B cells in association with a determinant which triggers helper T cells.

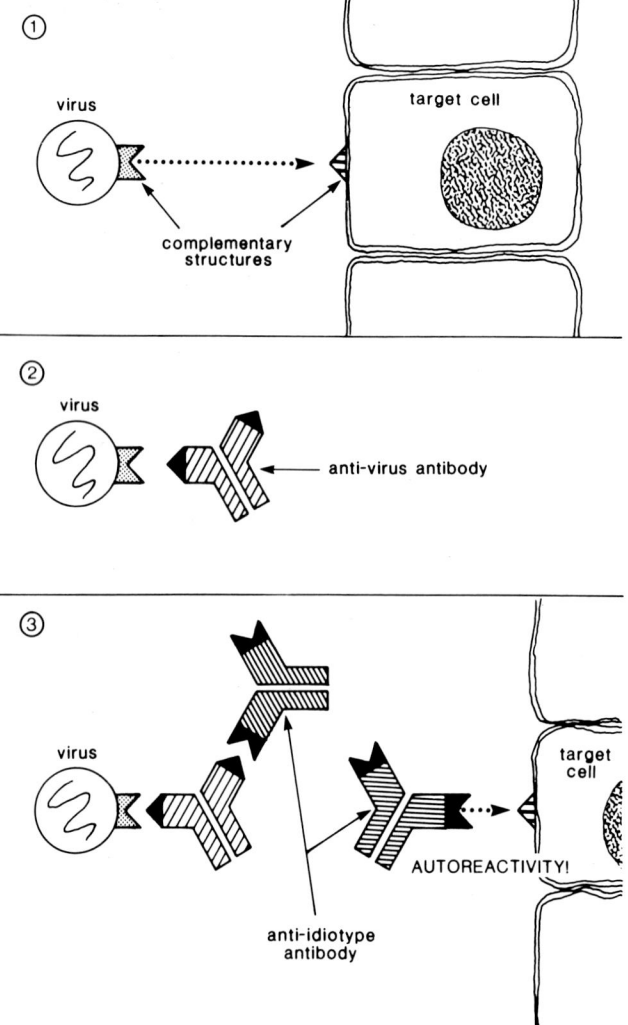

Fig. 13.4 Virus may induce autoantibody against cell-membrane structures by an idiotype-anti-idiotype mechanism. In 1, virus has a complementary structure by which it fixes to its target cell. In 2, antibody is produced against this structure. In 3, this antibody triggers an anti-idiotype response, which is capable of recognizing the virus-receptor structure on the normal cell, i.e., is an autoantibody.

relationship between the antibodies, anti-smooth muscle (in chronic active hepatitis) and anti-mitochondrial antibody (in primary biliary cirrhosis), and the pathogenesis of the disease is unknown.

Skin disease

Antibodies to skin components are found in pemphigus vulgaris, bullous pemphigoid and dermatitis herpetiformis.

Haemolytic anaemias and other autoimmune cytopenias

Autoimmune haemolytic anaemia, thrombo-cytopenia and agranulocytosis are described in Chapter 26.

Endocrine disease

Hashimoto's disease, Graves' disease, and some cases of myxoedema and Addison's disease are associated with an autoimmune process (see Chapter 36).

Diabetes mellitus. See type I diabetes mellitus, Chapter 17.

THE COLLAGEN VASCULAR DISEASES

The term diffuse collagen disease was coined by Klemperer in 1942 to describe a group of disorders in which the primary lesion appeared to be damage to collagen. *Lupus erythematosus*, *dermatomyositis*, and *progressive systemic sclerosis* will be described in this chapter. *Polyarteritis*, *acute rheumatic fever* and *rheumatoid arthritis* can also be included in this group, and they are described elsewhere.

The concept that these diseases are primary disorders of collagen is no longer held. Nevertheless they share the following features:

1 There is involvement of the connective tissues including blood vessels
2 Non-organ-specific autoantibody formation is a salient feature and is accompanied by depression of T-cell function
3 Considerable overlap occurs between the diseases so that mixed cases are not infrequent
4 The aetiology of the diseases is unknown, but there is a strong genetic predisposition to their development.

To cover this group of diseases the terms collagen vascular disease or connective tissue disease is used.

LUPUS ERYTHEMATOSUS

Lupus erythematosus may occur as localized skin lesions or as a more serious multisystem disease. The two types will be described separately, and the interrelationship between them will be discussed later.

Chronic discoid lupus erythematosus (DLE)

This type of lupus erythematosus has been recognized for many years as a skin condition that

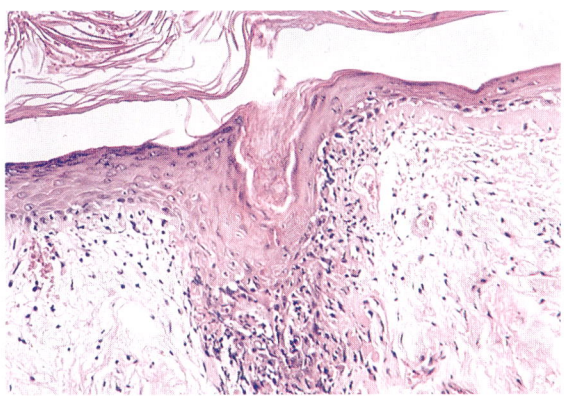

Fig. 13.5   Skin in lupus erythematosus. The epidermis is atrophic, shows hyperkeratosis and follicular plugging. The basal cell layer show vacuolar (hydropic) change; the thickened eosinophilic basement membrane zone is seen on the right side; the dermis is oedematous and infiltrated by lymphocytes particularly at the dermoepidermal interface and around the hair follicle.

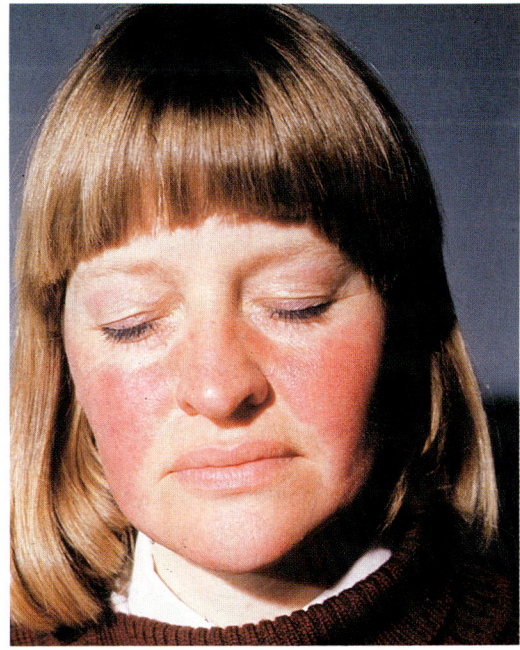

Fig. 13.6   Acute phase of systemic lupus erythematous exhibiting erythema and oedema of exposed areas of the face giving rise to the classic 'butterfly rash'. (Photograph by courtesy of Dr D G I Scott, Norfolk and Norwich Hospital.)

occurs particularly on the face and other exposed areas of the body and is made worse by exposure to sunlight. The lesions consist of well-defined erythematous, scaly papules and plaques.

The epidermis shows hyperkeratosis, atrophy, and vacuolar (hydropic) degeneration of the basal cell layer. The basement membrane zone is thickened due to a granular deposition of immunoglobulins and complement components. A periappendageal lymphocytic dermal infiltrate and dermal oedema are other features (Fig. 13.5). As the lesions heal there is dermal scarring and disturbance of pigmentation, with hypopigmentation being particularly noticeable in blacks. Telangiectasia is also often present, and the total appearance is described as poikilodermatous. Scalp involvement causes loss of hair with scarring (scarring alopecia). The oral mucosa is affected in about 15% of cases of chronic DLE, the lesions are erythematous and hyperkeratotic, so that a type of 'leucoplakia' is produced.

Systemic lupus erythematosus (SLE)

Systemic lupus erythematosus is more common in women than in men, in blacks than in whites, and the age-group 20–40 years. The lesions of the disease are widespread with involvement of skin, joints, kidney and serous sacs (commonly the pericardium). The onset of SLE may be acute with fever, malaise, weight loss, leucopoenia, elevated ESR, joint pains, lymphadenopathy, and skin rashes; severe psychotic disturbances may be the presenting symptom. On the other hand the onset of the disease may be insidious, with the development of a rash on the exposed skin, later to be followed by other organ involvement. Raynaud's phenomenon is common in SLE. The incidence of the disease appears to have increased considerably in recent years but whether this is a true increase or merely a reflection of better diagnosis and awareness of the disease is not known. The relative risk of SLE is increased by the inheritance of HLA alleles DR3 or 4.

The characteristic morphological lesions of SLE are associated with the deposition of fibrinoid material (probably immune complexes and fibrin) between connective tissue fibres (fibrinoid necrosis), in blood vessel walls (causing vasculitis) and in the kidneys (lupus nephritis) and sometimes in the skin. The areas of fibrinoid necrosis are initially associated with an acute inflammatory reaction with oedema and neutrophil infiltration. Later this may become chronic as fibrosis develops and the infiltrate changes to mononuclear cells, particularly lymphocytes.

Sites of involvement

The onset of erythema and oedema of the sun-exposed areas giving the classic 'butterfly rash' is the classical mode of presentation (Fig. 13.6). Microscopically the epidermis is atrophic and shows vacuolar degeneration of the basal cell layer (Fig. 13.5). Deposition of IgG and C3 can be demonstrated in the basement membrane zone of the affected skin; in unaffected and non-sun-exposed skin a similar band of IgG can be found—this constitutes the *lupus band test* and is not seen in patients with chronic DLE. During the course of the disease, lesions of DLE may develop.

Other features of the disease are a mild synovitis, responsible for the arthralgia that particularly affects the distal limb joints, pericarditis, pleurisy (less frequently), endocarditis, and acute vasculitis (causing palpable purpura). A glomerulonephritis is common and may cause mild haematuria, proteinuria and hypertension, and ultimately lead to renal failure. A nephrotic syndrome is not uncommon during the course of the disease.

Autoantibodies in SLE

A prominent feature of SLE is the presence of many autoantibodies in the serum. Acute haemolytic anaemia may occur, and the Coomb's test is sometimes positive. Circulating anticoagulants may be present, and there may also be thrombocytopenic purpura due to platelet antibodies. Serological tests for syphilis may be falsely positive, and the rheumatoid factor is present in about a third of the cases.

The most important antibodies from a diagnostic point of view are those that are active against nuclear components (*antinuclear anti-*

bodies). Antibodies to double-stranded DNA are virtually diagnostic of SLE.

Pathogenesis of SLE

There is good evidence that lupus glomerulonephritis is an immune-complex disorder due to the localization of soluble complexes of double-stranded DNA and antinuclear antibody in the glomeruli and elsewhere. Whether the DNA is endogenous or derived from a virus is unknown. Complement fixation is involved, and patients with active lupus nephritis often have a reduced serum level of complement. It seems probable that many of the manifestations of SLE are attributable to damaging immune complexes in the small blood vessels of the viscera, e.g. heart, joints, and serous cavities.

Genetic factors predispose an individual to develop SLE and there is an increased incidence of autoantibodies and autoimmune diseases in relatives of patients with the disease. Suggested precipitating factors include virus infection, drug administration, and exposure to sunlight. To date there is no unifying concept.

Relationship of SLE to DLE. Less than 5% of patients with chronic discoid lupus erythematosus develop the systemic variety. The diseases therefore appear to be distinct entities. Nevertheless lesions of DLE can occur in patient with SLE, and the precise relationship between the two diseases is not understood.

SCLERODERMA

As with lupus erythematosus, scleroderma was first described as a skin disease. Two types are recognized: circumscribed scleroderma, or morphoea, and systemic scleroderma, or progressive systemic sclerosis.

Morphoea

The disease is usually restricted to the skin with the formation of well-marked plaques which feel stiff and firm. The dermis first becomes thickened due initially to oedema and an infiltration of lymphocytes. This is soon followed by progres-

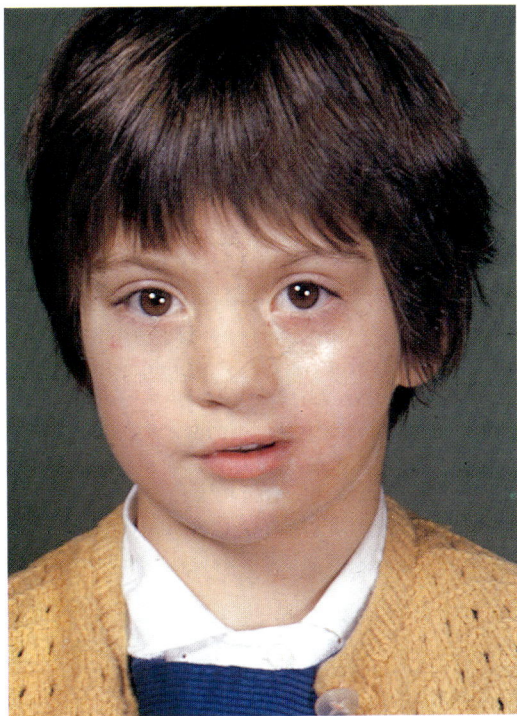

Fig. 13.7   Scleroderma affecting the soft tissues and the underlying bone on the left side of the face of this 7-year-old girl resulting in the hemifacial atrophy. (Previously published in Rock W P, Grundy M C, Shaw L Diagnostic picture tests in paediatric dentistry, Wolfe Medical Publications, London.)

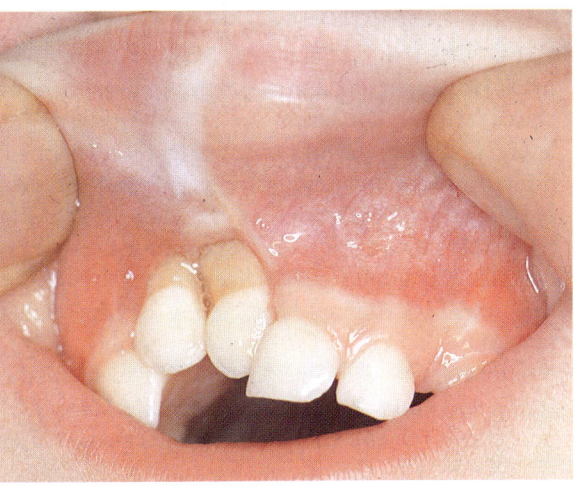

Fig. 13.8   Scleroderma affecting the upper incisor region in this 3-year-old boy which has resulted in extensive destruction of the periodontal tissues and bone supporting the maxillary right primary incisors. Note also the scar tissue in the mucosa of the lip. (Previously published in Rock W P, Grundy M C, Shaw L Diagnostic picture tests in paediatric dentistry. Wolfe Medical Publications, London.)

sive fibrosis that extends into the subcutaneous fat so that the thickened skin is firm and tethered to underlying structures. One or more plaques of affected skin are present, and they usually have a faintly purple colour, particularly at their edges. Rarely, the lesions are widespread. Sometimes they are linear, and the underlying muscle and even bone may be affected. This is particularly well marked in the fronto-parietal type (en coup de sabre, from the resemblance to a scar from a sabre cut). This lesion starts with fibrosis of the affected skin of the face. A linear, depressed groove appears on the fronto-parietal region, extending into the scalp and producing an area of alopecia. The underlying soft tissue and bone atrophy can extend to involve the facial bones, including the alveolar bone. Facial hemiatrophy and alveolar growth is affected (Figs 13.7 and 13.8).

Progressive systemic sclerosis (systemic scleroderma)

In the systemic variety there is widespread, bilateral involvement of the skin, the face and hands often being first affected. In this event the earliest feature is usually Raynaud's phenomenon. Next the skin becomes smooth, shiny, firm to touch, and bound down to underlying structures. When this affects the face, an immobile, mask-like appearance with pinching of the nose is characteristic. The hands are at first swollen, but later, as fibrosis occurs and movement becomes limited, there may be atrophy of soft tissues, particularly of the pulps of the fingers and the terminal phalanges. The appearance is then described as *sclerodactyly*. Ulceration of the finger tips and dystrophic calcification of the pulps (calcinosis cutis) is a well-recognized event. Telangiectatic vessels are commonly seen on the face, and morphologically resemble those of hereditary haemorrhagic telangiectasia. The combination of Calcinosis, Raynaud's phenomenon, Sclerodactyly, and Telangiectasia has been separated as a distinct variant called the *CRST syndrome*.

In progressive systemic sclerosis there is always involvement of internal organs. When fibrosis affects the muscle coat of the oesophagus there is oesophageal reflux leading to a foul taste in the mouth.

Radiographic motility studies are diagnostic even before the patient experiences dysphagia. A characteristic oral radiographic finding is widening of the periodontal membrane space. Fibrosis can occur in the heart, leading to heart failure, and in the lungs with diffuse fibrosis and contraction of lung substance and cyst formation. Adenocarcinoma is a well-recognized complication of scleroderma lung.

The most serious effect of systemic sclerosis is in the kidneys. The interlobular arteries show obstruction as a result of intimal thickening by mucinous collagenous material, and small vessels in the glomeruli show fibrinoid necrosis. The changes are identical to those of malignant hypertension, and the progressive vascular obstruction leads to renal failure.

Aetiology and Pathogenesis

Morphoea rarely progresses to progressive systemic sclerosis and the cause of both remains unknown. In about 50% of cases of progressive systemic sclerosis there is a polyclonal hypergammaglobulinaemia, and the rheumatoid factor and antinuclear antibodies can be demonstrated in many cases but the tendency to autoantibody formation is less marked than in SLE.

POLYMYOSITIS AND DERMATOMYOSITIS

Polymyositis is frequently included among the collagen diseases. Typically there is weakness of the proximal limb muscles and anterior neck muscles. There may also be cutaneous lesions, in which the condition is called *dermatomyositis*. The skin changes can take many forms. Erythema and oedema are common, particularly of the face. This causes the characteristic heliotrope discolouration around the eyes. Other skin lesions may resemble those of SLE or progressive systemic sclerosis. In patients over the age of 40 years there is a well-recognized association between dermatomyositis and internal malignant disease, but the precise incidence has been much debated. A tumour is probably found in about 15% of cases.

MIXED CONNECTIVE-TISSUE DISEASE

This term has been applied to a syndrome having features of SLE, progressive systemic sclerosis and dermatomyositis. Raynaud's syndrome is common, and the condition has a good prognosis since renal complications are uncommon and the response to prednisone is good.

SUMMARY

The validity of grouping these diseases under the heading of collagen vascular disease is dubious. Mixed cases occur with patients who exhibit features of several diseases. Thus some have lesions of scleroderma with vasculitis, or lupus erythematosus with rheumatoid arthritis. The occurrence of such cases suggests that there is a common mechanism, but it does not prove a common cause. The presence of autoantibodies is another feature that these diseases have in common, being the most striking in lupus erythematosus and the least evident in polyarteritis. Until the origin and pathogenesis of these diseases are discovered, it is convenient to refer to the group collectively as the 'collagen vascular diseases', since they share many features. Thus they all produce widespread lesions affecting many organs, and often they exhibit a marked constitutional effect such as fever, raised erythrocyte sedimentation rate (ESR), and hypergammaglobulinaemia. This tendency is least marked in progressive systemic sclerosis. All the diseases respond to glucocorticoid therapy as well as to other immunosuppressants such as azathioprine. Presumably, these act by suppressing autoantibody formation, thereby inhibiting the formation of new lesions. Once again progressive systemic sclerosis is the odd man out and is least responsive to therapy.

GENERAL READING (see also Ch. 10)

Cooke A, Lydyard P M, Roitt I M 1983 Mechanisms of autoimmunity a role for crossreactive idiotypes. Immunology Today 4:170

Piesetsky DS 1986 Systemic lupus erythematosus. Medical Clinics of North America 70: 337
Schatz M. Patterson R, Fink J 1979 Immunologic lung diseases. New England Journal of Medicine 300: 1310

14.   Some important bacterial infections

PYOGENIC INFECTIONS

Organisms responsible for inflammation and the formation of pus account for some of the most important lesions seen clinically. Although most of the infections respond to antibiotic therapy, surgical drainage of abscesses is still often necessary. The most important members of this group of pyogenic bacteria are:

1. **Pyogenic cocci,** e.g. *Staphylococcus aureus, Streptococcus pyogenes,* pneumococcus, meningococcus, and gonococcus

2. **Gram-negative intestinal bacilli,** viz. *Escherichia coli, Proteus* species, and *Pseudomonas aeruginosa* and organisms of the genus *Bacteroides.*

Staphylococcus aureus, Strep. pyogenes and Gram-negative bacilli are of greatest surgical moment because of their capacity to produce infections in many different sites. Furthermore,

they are of cardinal importance because they not only infect wounds and burns, but also act as secondary invaders in chronic ulcerative lesions from other causes, for instance ulcerating tumours of the skin and mucous membranes. By contrast, the pneumococcus, meningococcus, and gonococcus tend to affect the lungs, meninges, and genital tract respectively.

The pathological effects of these bacteria are all essentially similar. There is an acute inflammatory response culminating in the accumulation of an exudate crowded with neutrophil polymorphs, which attempts to destroy the organisms. If the organisms are destroyed early in the inflammatory response there is resolution; otherwise the condition proceeds to tissue destruction and suppuration. The abscess so formed may burst spontaneously on to a free surface or else be drained surgically. If the pus is successfully drained, the destroyed tissue is replaced either by the regeneration of specialized tissue or by the formation of fibrous scar tissue. If pus becomes loculated and dead tissue remains, the circumstances are ripe for the development of chronic inflammation, as explained in Chapter 9. When the pyogenic lesion becomes chronic, there is an admixture of other cells to the polymorphs already present. Lymphocytes, plasma cells, macrophages, and eosinophils are all in evidence, as well as the proliferating connective-tissue and specialized cells of the part. Indeed, these organisms are responsible for the chronic non-specific bacterial inflammation that plays such an important role in everyday clinical practice. Sometimes if the body's resistance is very poor or if the organism is extremely virulent, there may be rapid local spread and generalized dissemination of organisms. In this case a fatal septicaemia or pyaemia may ensue.

Except in very localized infections there is a general body response reflected in a polymorphonuclear leucocytosis with an increased proportion of immature neutrophils in the blood. If the infection is spreading to any extent there is a variable constitutional reaction with fever and an elevation of the ESR (p. 300).

STAPHYLOCOCCI

Staphylococci are Gram-positive, spherical organisms about 1 μm in diameter, which tend to be arranged in grape-like clusters. They are non-motile, non-sporing, and non-capsulate.

Cultural characteristics. Staphylococci are aerobes and grow easily on most media. They grow best at 37°C. On blood agar, conspicuous, shiny, convex colonies appear within 24 h, and these are white or creamy yellow in colour. *Staphyloccocus aureus* is usually creamy yellow in colour and is the most important human pathogen. It is characterized by the production of an enzyme, coagulase, that coagulates plasma. This is used as an in vitro test for the organism. Coagulase negative staphylococci, sometimes called *Staphyloccocus epidermidis*, are less virulent and cause infection only under unusual circumstances, e.g. on heart valves, or in immuno-compromized patients.

Staphylococcus aureus. This is a common skin contaminant and the anterior nares acts as the reservoir. About 15% of normal healthy adults are nasal carriers and in a hospital population the figure may rise to 70%. Organisms from such carriers can readily be transferred to patients to cause skin and other infections. Although pathogenic, not all strains of the organism are equally virulent. Three groups of staphylococci are recognized. Group II causes minor skin infections, whereas groups I and III are the important organisms causing epidemics of hospital infection. In the event of such an epidemic, it is useful to trace the source of infection by typing the organism involved.

Staphylococci are typed on the basis of serological reactions and phage typing. Bacteriophage is a virus that specifically lyses colonies of staphylococci; any one bacteriophage ('phage') can lyse only one or a few susceptible strains. Hence each

staphylococcus exhibits a distinct pattern of susceptibility to a battery of phages, and is thereby typed; thus phage type 80 has been shown to be the cause of many hospital infections.

Toxin production. The staphylococcus is an invasive organism, but the essential factors responsible for its virulence are not clearly defined. *Staphylokinase*, which lyses fibrin by activating the plasmin system, and *hyaluronidases* are produced by some strains but seldom in large amounts. Of greater importance is a number of toxins. The most important of these is the α–*toxin*, which produces local tissue necrosis, and is lethal when injected intravenously. It is also haemolytic to red cells, and destroys white cells, i.e. it is a *haemolysin* and a *leucocidin*.

In addition some strains produce exotoxins. The enterotoxin is responsible for food poisoning, while others lead to the scalded skin syndrome, scarlet fever-like syndrome, and the toxic shock syndrome.

Lesions produced by S. aureus. The typical staphylococcal lesion is a *circumscribed area of inflammation with suppuration*. Coagulase production has been suggested as an important factor in the localization of the infection by virtue of the copious fibrin formation that it induces. On the other hand, other authorities regard coagulase as a factor aiding spread of infection, because the deposition of fibrin acts as a protective covering for the organism and prevents its phagocytosis. It is evident that our ideas on the importance of coagulase in staphylococcal infection are still purely speculative. It seems likely that the local damage inflicted by the α-toxin leads to a considerable inflammatory reaction which in its turn successfully localizes and overcomes the infection.

Staphylococcal infection of the skin is common (Fig. 14.1). *Impetigo* results if the infection is superficial. Subcorneal blisters and pustules are formed. The blisters soon rupture and become covered by a honey-coloured crust. Impetigo is most common on the face and in children. Staphylococci are a common cause of suppurative *folliculitis*. If the pustules so formed are superficial the term *superficial folliculitis (Bockhart's impetigo)* is used. A deeper, more destructive folliculitis results in a *boil*, or *furuncle*. Boils are particularly common in the axillae and on the back of the neck where they are often

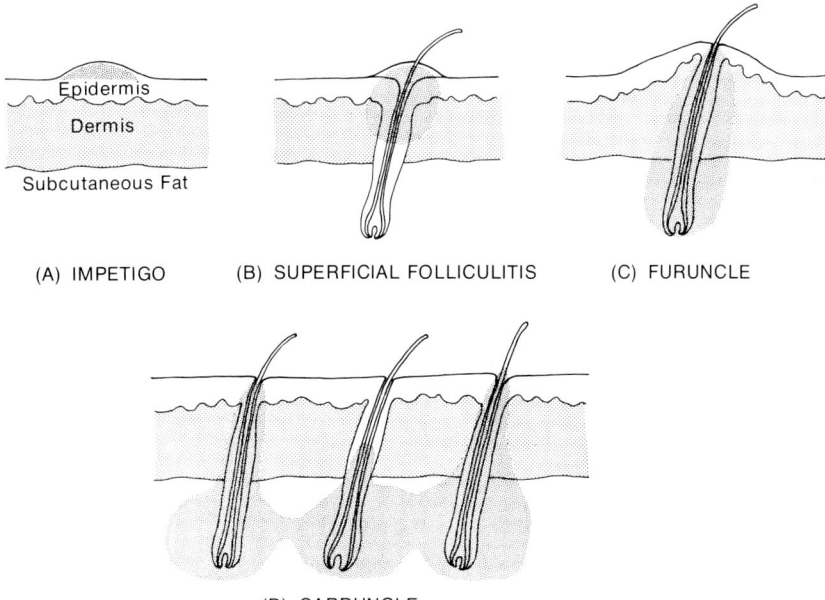

Epidermis
Dermis
Subcutaneous Fat

(A) IMPETIGO   (B) SUPERFICIAL FOLLICULITIS   (C) FURUNCLE

(D) CARBUNCLE

Fig. 14.1   Diagram illustrating some staphylococcal infections of the skin. (A) *Impetigo*. The infection is very superficial, and a pustule forms beneath the stratum corneum of the epidermis. (B) *Superficial folliculitis*. The suppurative inflammation involves the superficial part of a hair follicle. Clinically this appears as a small pustule; the condition is also called impetigo of Bockhart. (C) *Furuncle or Boil*. The infection involves an entire hair follicle, and in the inflammatory oedema produces a considerable swelling, which can be 1 cm or more in diameter. Nevertheless, a boil has one head only. (D) *Carbuncle*. The infection involves the subcutaneous tissues, and loculated pockets of pus are present. These pockets are formed between fibrous septa, which are not shown in the diagram. Note the multiple heads through which pus can be discharged. (Drawing by Margot Mackay, Department of Art as Applied to Medicine, University of Toronto. Reproduced from Walter J B (1992) Introduction to the Principles of Disease, 3rd edn. W B Saunders, Philadelphia, with permission of the publishers.)

multiple due to the large numbers of hair follicles. If the infection extends deeper to involve the subcutaneous fat, a carbuncle forms; the skin is undermined and there is a loculated abscess with multiple draining heads.

Staphylococci are a common causative organism in *wound infections* particularly as a result of infection acquired in hospital. Other important staphylococcal infections are *bronchopneumonia* and acute *osteomyelitis*.

Staphylococci may spread via the lymphatics to produce a *lymphadenitis* that may undergo suppuration. If the infection is not arrested, there will be massive blood-stream invasion to produce a fatal *septicaemia*. *Pyaemia* is not uncommon, and follows suppurative thrombophlebitis which may complicate any staphylococcal infection.

Staphylococcal food-poisoning is the only condition due entirely to the enterotoxin.

Infection associated with widespread skin manifestation

A localized staphylococcal infection may be associated with one of the three syndromes with widespread skin manifestations due to the action of one of the staphylococcal exotoxins.

Scalded skin syndrome. Following infection with *S. aureus* the patient, generally a child, develops widespread necrosis of the superficial layers of the epidermis. This gives the skin the appearance similar to a scald and must be distinguished from the effects of child abuse.

Scarlet fever. A scarlet fever-like illness due to staphylococcal infection has also been described.

Toxic shock syndrome. There is sudden onset of a severe illness that is sometimes fatal. It is characterized by high fever, generalized reddening of the skin and conjunctivae, watery diarrhoea, hypotension and renal failure. The syndrome was first described in children but more recently it has been encountered in previously healthy young women who during menstruation use tampons of a particular type with high absorbency. It is believed that the tampon acts as a site where staphylococci can grow. It can also complicate staphylococcal infection at other sites, e.g. a wound.

Lesions produced by Staphylococcus albus

Staphylococcus albus (coagulase negative) is a universal commensal of the skin and nose, and rarely produces infection. It occasionally leads to urinary-tract infections, especially in association with stones, and has recently gained prominence as a cause of opportunistic infection especially following surgery when foreign material is inserted. Thus it may cause endocarditis after open-heart surgery.

STREPTOCOCCI

Streptococci are Gram-positive, spherical organisms, slightly smaller than staphylococci. They tend to be arranged in chains which vary in length according to the method of culture. They are non-motile and non-sporing. Some strains possess very thin capsules called microcapsules.

Streptococci grow less easily than staphylococci, but are also aerobes and facultative anaerobes. A few strains are obligatory anaerobes.

They can be cultured on blood agar at 37°C, and within 24 h, tiny, transparent, dewdrop colonies develop. Around these there may be a zone of haemolysis, and according to this the organisms are classified into three main groups:

α-Haemolytic streptococci, which produce an ill-defined zone of partial haemolysis, which may be yellow or green in colour

β-Haemolytic streptococci, which produce a sharply demarcated zone of complete haemolysis

Non-haemolytic streptococci, these are also called γ-type streptococci.

β-Haemolytic streptococci are particularly important in producing serious pyogenic infec-

tions. Not all, however, are pathogenic to humans; some produce disease only in cattle and other animals. It is therefore important to distinguish between the different groups of β-haemolytic streptococci. This is done by Lancefield's method.

Lancefield grouping. β-haemolytic streptococci can be divided into 18 groups by a precipitation test, first described by Lancefield, according to the presence of a specific carbohydrate hapten, called the C antigen, in the wall of the organism. The great majority of human pathogens fall into Lancefield's group A, and a group-A organism is called *S. pyogenes*.

Streptococcus pyogenes

Streptococcus pyogenes is found in the throats of about 10% of normal people. As with *S. aureus, S. pyogenes* may give rise to epidemics and the necessity for typing the causative organisms and tracing the source of infection may then arise. Typing of the organism, by a method first devised by Griffiths, depends on the presence of M and T antigens on the surface of the organism. Over 50 serotypes are recognized. All are pathogenic and some are particularly associated with acute glomerulonephritis.

Toxin production. Like the staphylococcus, *S. pyogenes* is an invasive organism that produces powerful endotoxins; also a single exotoxin. There are two haemolysins designated *streptolysin O* and *streptolysin S*. Streptolysin O is also cardiotoxic and leucocidic, whereas streptolysin S is a pure haemolysin. As the chemical nature of endotoxins is generally so poorly understood, it is reasonable to include the *M protein* among them. This is powerfully antigenic. It acts by interfering with phagocytosis, and the antibody formed against it is an opsonin (p. 125).

The organisms produce three important enzymes; *hyaluronidase, streptokinase*, which induces fibrinolysis by activating the plasmin system, and *streptodornase* which lyses DNA. (The name streptodornase is derived from the first letters of the syllables **de**ox**y**ri**bon**ucle**ase**.)

Some strains of *S. pyogenes* produce one of three exotoxins which collectively are called *erythrogenic toxin* because they are responsible for the punctate erythema characteristic of scarlet fever.

Lesions produced. The typical streptococcal lesion is a *spreading infection of the connective tissue called a cellulitis*. The poor localizing tendency has been associated with the hyaluronidase and streptokinase produced by most strains, often in large amounts. Abscesses occur much later than in staphylococcal infections, and the pus is watery and often blood stained. It is probable that the streptodornase and streptokinase are responsible for this, because the viscosity of the pus is due to DNA and fibrin.

In recent years the virulence of *Strep. pyogenes* has declined so markedly that many of the classical streptococcal lesions which produced so much damage in years gone by are now rarely seen. By contrast, staphylococcal lesions are commoner and more severe than ever.

Streptococci are occasional causes of *wound* and *burn infections,* and are also responsible for some cases of *impetigo. Erysipelas,* a spreading infection of the dermis, is a classical streptococcal lesion. It affects the face, and is seen as a raised, bright-red plaque with a sharply defined edge that steadily advances.

Streptococci are still important causes of *tonsillitis* and *pharyngitis* (streptococcal sore throat) and these may be complicated by infection of the middle ear (*otitis media*). Streptococci have a tendency to invade the blood stream, with the development of *septicaemia.* This was a common complication of streptococcal infection of the uterus following labour (*puerperal sepsis*), which killed thousands of women before the introduction of aseptic techniques and chemotherapy.

If an infecting streptococcus produces the erythrogenic exotoxin, and the patient has no antitoxin to it, the local lesion will be complicated by the effects of this toxin. A generalized punctate erythema appears, and the condition is called *scarlet fever.*

There is an indirect relationship between streptococcal infections on the one hand and *acute rheumatic fever* and *acute glomerulonephritis* on the other. Acute nephritis occurs about 10 days after an attack of streptococcal pharyngitis; after impetigo the period is often three weeks or longer. Acute rheumatic fever follows only on streptococcal pharyngitis, almost never on skin infections; the current view is that both are manifestations of immune-complex reactions.

Other streptococci

Group-B streptococci (S. agalactiae). These organisms are not infrequently found in the female genital tract, and are recognized as a common cause of severe perinatal infection. The manifestations are those of respiratory distress with shock, septicaemia, and meningitis.

Group-C streptococci and Group-G streptococci. These organisms may also cause puerperal infection and wound infection.

α-Haemolytic streptococci. This group is often referred to a *S. viridans,* but this is not a single species but a collective name given to α-haemolytic streptococci. These organisms are invariable commensals of the mouth and throat, and a number of strains, e.g. *S. mitis, S. mutans,* and *S. sanguis,* have been incriminated in dental caries and periodontal disease. Of greater importance, however, is the association of *S. viridans* with subacute infective endocarditis, described on page 358.

Group D streptococci. This group is usually non-haemolytic and includes *S. faecalis* which forms part of the normal flora of the large intestine. If it leaves its normal habitat this organism can cause suppurative lesions of a type and distribution similar to *E. coli.* It is a common cause of urinary-tract infection.

Anaerobic streptococcal infections. Anaerobic streptococci are normal inhabitants of the bowel, vagina, and mouth (particularly the gingival sulci). These were important causes of puerperal sepsis in the past, and occasionally are associated with *wound infection.* They may also be found in gangrenous lesions (p. 48).

STREPTOCOCCUS PNEUMONIAE

Streptococcus pneumoniae, also called the pneumococcus, is an oval or lance-shaped coccus. The organisms are arranged in pairs with the long axes in line with each other. It is the same size as the streptococcus, and similarly is Gram-positive, non-motile, and non-sporing. An important feature is the presence of a prominent capsule.

It resembles the α-haemolytic streptococcus very closely, and both produce a diffuse greenish haemolysis of the surrounding blood agar.

An important feature of the organism is the presence of a prominent capsule which contains a polysaccharide polymer related to the type and therefore the virulence of the organism. Over 80 types have been recognized and type 3 is the most virulent. Together with some other types it is responsible for most cases of lobar pneumonia. The other types of pneumococci, commensals of the nose and throat, cause infection in debilitated subjects but little harm to healthy individuals.

Lesions produced. The most important pneumococcal lesion is *lobar pneumonia,* which is caused by one of the virulent strains, usually type 1, 2, or 3. Other types of pneumococci are sometimes implicated in bronchopneumonia (p. 368). Other primary pneumococcal conditions are *otitis media* and *suppurative sinusitis,* both of which may lead to *meningitis.*

NEISSERIAL INFECTIONS

Organisms of the genus *Neisseria* are Gram-negative kidney-shaped diplococci. Included are the common oral commensals, *N. sicca, N. sub-flavum,* etc., and the related *Branhamella catar-rhalis,* in addition to the two pathogens *N. meningitidis* (the meningococcus) and *N. gonor-rhoeae* (the gonococcus). Both these latter organisms cause an acute inflammatory reaction with the formation of pus but, unlike staphylococci and streptococci, infection is generally limited to the meninges or genital tract respectively.

Meningococcal infections

From 5 to 30% of healthy individuals carry meningococci in the nasopharynx. Epidemics of meningococcal infection occur periodically and are preceded by an increase in the carrier rate. The portal of entry appears to be the nasopharynx but the first clinical manifestation is that of septicaemia with fever, severe constitutional symptoms, a widespread petechial rash due to acute vasculitis of the skin, and purulent meningitis. The reason for this specific localization is unknown.

Gonococcal infections

The gonococcus is generally transmitted by sexual intercourse and causes the important venereal disease gonorrhea. It usually invades the mucosal surfaces of the genitourinary tract and its appendages. In the male, an acute urethritis with a purulent penile discharge appears 2–8 days after infection. If untreated, the infection can become chronic and cause urethral stricture.

Gonorrhea is manifest as acute urethritis and cervicitis in the female but the symptoms may be mild and go unnoticed. Infection persists, however, and asymptomatic females are the main reservoir of infection. Spread to involve the fallopian tubes leads to *acute salpingitis.* Infection of the throat causing *gonococcal pharyngitis* may occur in members of either sex who practise orogenital sex. *Proctitis* may follow sodomy. Infection of the baby's conjunctiva during delivery results in an acute purulent conjunctivitis.

The gonococcus may occasionally spread beyond the genital tact; bacteraemia, septicaemia, vasculitis and arthritis are all recognized complications.

THE GRAM-NEGATIVE INTESTINAL BACILLI

The members of this group which are important causes of pyogenic infections, are *Escherichia coli, Proteus* species, and *Pseudomonas aeruginosa.* Most of these organisms belong to the family *Enterobacteriaceae* which includes the numerous genera conveniently grouped together as the 'coliform organisms'. Of these the most important pyogenic member is the genus *Escherichia.*

Proteus is included, but *Pseudomonas* is excluded from it, because *P. aeruginosa* is only occasionally found as a commensal of the bowel, whereas the true *Enterobacteriaceae* are all native to the intestinal tract.

The group also includes the genus *Salmonella,* responsible for typhoid fever and food-poisoning, and the genus *Shigella,* responsible for bacillary dysentery. These two groups of organisms are not distinguished by suppuration, and are not described further.

The *Enterobacteriaceae* are all Gram-negative

rods 1–4 μm long. Most of them are vigorously motile, but there are some exceptions, e.g. *Klebsiella* species which are non-motile, as are the *Shigella* species.

The organisms grow easily at 37°C, being aerobic and facultatively anaerobic. On blood agar, large greyish-white, irregular, shiny colonies are produced within 24 h.

The most important biochemical property of these organisms is their ability to ferment various sugars. This is used in their laboratory identification. Thus *E. coli* ferments lactose, whereas *Proteus, Pseudomonas, Salmonella,* and *Shigella,* are unable to do so.

Pathogenicity. The pathogenic action of these organisms is believed to be due to an endotoxin, which as yet has been poorly defined. When they escape from the lumen of the bowel and invade the tissues, suppurative lesions ensue. Endotoxin is probably responsible for shock when large numbers of Gram-negative organisms enter the circulation (p. 298).

Lesions produced. *Escherichia coli* and the other coliform organisms are always predominant in infective lesions derived from the bowel contents, e.g. *appendix abscess* and *generalized peritonitis following perforation of a hollow viscus.* Furthermore, the organism is the commonest agent in *urinary-tract infections.*

Escherichia coli is not infrequently present in sputum, and it may be an agent in producing *pneumonia.*

It should be noted that although *Esch. coli* is an inevitable and harmless inhabitant of the bowel, in recent years certain enteropathogenic strains have been isolated. These are of no special importance as causes of suppuration but they may produce epidemics of *infantile gastroenteritis* and traveller's diarrhoea.

Proteus organisms and *Ps. aeruginosa* have a similar range of pathogenicity, but as they are less frequently commensals of the bowel, they are much more frequently transmitted by cross-infection. Both are important causes of urinary-tract, respiratory, ear, and wound infections.

Salmonella typhi infection is described in Chapter 7. Intestinal infections due to *Salmonella* and *Shigella* organisms are considered in Chapter 31.

ANAEROBIC WOUND INFECTIONS

These infections are of great importance in clinical practice, not because they are common but because when they do occur they are serious. With the exception of infections with the anaerobic streptococci, bacteroides, and actinomyces, all are due to the clostridial group of anaerobic spore-bearers. The clostridial organisms are responsible for two extremely serious conditions, *gas-gangrene* and *tetanus*. Gas-gangrene is produced by the combined action of a number of clostridia, the most important of which are *C. perfringens, C. novyi* and *C. septicum*, whereas tetanus is caused by a single organism, *C. tetani*. The rare, lethal form of food-poisoning, botulism, is produced by another clostridium, *C. botulinum*. This is not a wound infection but an intoxication which usually follows the ingestion of a heat-stable, potent exotoxin produced by the organism in poorly prepared food during its period of storage.

CLOSTRIDIAL INFECTIONS

The clostridia are large, Gram-positive bacilli approximately 5 μm long. The most characteristic feature is the spore, which is produced whenever the organism finds itself in adverse conditions. It is usually central or subterminal, but in the case of *C. tetani* it is situated terminally. These organisms are all motile and non-capsulate, with the exception of *C. perfringens*, which is non-motile and possesses a capsule.

They all grow quite easily but most of them demand anaerobiosis, i.e. they are obligatory anaerobes.

Fermentation reactions are of considerable importance. Clostridia are divided into two categories saccharolytic and proteolytic.

Saccharolytic clostridia ferment many sugars, e.g. lactose and glucose. They do not break down proteins. The main pathogens of gas-gangrene, viz. *C. perfringens, C. septicum* and *C. novyi*, come into this category.

Proteolytic clostridia break down protein, and produce foul-smelling gases like hydrogen sulphide and ammonia. These organisms are also able to ferment sugars, but they are less active than the first group. The secondary putrefactive saprophytes of gas-gangrene, e.g. *C. sporogenes* and *C. histolyticum*, come into this category.

Saccharolytic clostridia are the important pathogens in gas-gangrene and the proteolytic clostridia mostly saprophytes. However, the demarcation is not clear, since the proteolytic clostridia have some saccharolytic capacity, and, in addition, *C. histolyticum* is also pathogenic despite its predominantly proteolytic activity.

Toxin production. The clostridia are excellent examples of toxic organisms, the lesions they produce being due entirely to exotoxins. The infection is localized, but the systemic effects are far-reaching.

In the gas-gangrene groups most work has been done on *C. perfringens*. Five types have been described, type A being the human pathogen and causing gas-gangrene and food-poisoning. The important toxin of type A is called α-toxin. It is a lecithinase. In animals a local injection causes tissue necrosis, and larger doses are lethal. By virtue of its lecithinase activity it destroys the phospholipid components of red-cell envelopes, and is thus a powerful haemolysin.

The other toxins of *C. perfringens* include *hyaluronidase*, a *deoxyribonuclease* and a *collagenase*. These enzymes play an important part in breaking down the intercellular ground substance and collagen fibres of tissues which are infected with *C. perfringens*, and so aid the local spread of the organism.*

Clostridium septicum and *C. novyi* produce powerful haemolytic and necrotizing exotoxins. *C. novyi* also yields small amounts of a lecithinase.

By contrast, *C. tetani* produces only two exotoxins. The important one is a neurotoxin called *tetanospasmin*, which is, of course, responsible for the convulsions of tetanus. It is an immensely potent poison, being second only to the exotoxin of *C. botulinum* in this respect. The other exotoxin is haemolytic, and is known as *tetanolysin*.

The spores of these organisms are widely dispersed in nature, and are especially plentiful in

soil. The clostridia are commensals of the human and animal intestine, and their spores are excreted in the faeces and returned to the soil in the form of manure. These spores must be expected in all environments. They are resistant to heat and desiccation. Only well-devised sterilizing methods can destroy them.

Apart from the role played by *C. perfringens* in gas-gangrene, certain specific strains are an important cause of *food-poisoning* when they contaminate meat in heavy culture. The symptoms, which may be quite severe and occasionally fatal, are dysenteric in type.

GAS-GANGRENE

Gas-gangrene may follow the contamination of a wound with the spores of the pathogenic clostridia. Considering the ubiquitous presence of these spores and the rarity of gas-gangrene in civilian practice, it is evident that healthy incised wounds so contaminated do not develop infection. The essential factor necessary for spore germination is a reduced oxygen tension. This is present in irregularly contused or lacerated wounds containing much dead tissue, which has been devitalized as a result of compression or impaired blood supply. Foreign bodies like shrapnel or pieces of clothing will exert local pressure, and also favour pyogenic infection. Soil is particularly dangerous, in that the ionizable calcium salts in it lead to considerable tissue necrosis. Finally, any coincidental infection by aerobic pyogenic organisms serves to augment the anaerobiosis. The local injection of adrenaline has a similar effect by causing vasoconstriction.

It therefore follows that most gas gangrene is exogenous in origin, and is due to the gross contamination of severely lacerated wounds. It is usually seen in battle casualties or in agricultural accidents. Occasionally gas-gangrene is endogenous, and occurs when a wound is contaminated with the patient's faeces.

Pathogenesis and Lesions. Gas-gangrene is never due to infection by a single type of clostridia organisms; it is the result of a combined assault by numerous saccharolytic and proteolytic species working together. The main pathogens—*C. perfringens*, *C. septicum* and *C. novyi*—

---

*The description of proteolytic enzymes in saccharolytic organisms seems to be a contradiction in terms. But 'proteolytic' refers to the putrefaction of complex protein, and this is not done by the saccharolytic group.

germinate, and the powerful exotoxins which they liberate produce local tissue necrosis. At this stage the proteolytic *C. sporogenes* and *C. histolyticum* flourish in the dead material, and break it down into putrid products.

If the wound is superficial, it will discharge foul-smelling fluid in which there are bubbles of gas. If it is extensive enough to implicate the underlying muscles, the florid anaerobic myositis typical of gas-gangrene develops.

When muscle is infected the organisms spread rapidly due to the destruction of local tissue barriers by the hyaluronidase and collagenase present as components of the exotoxins. A whole muscle bundle may be affected with great rapidity. Indeed, gas-gangrene resembles an invasive infection in the extent of its local spread, but the organisms remain localized to one area. The muscle carbohydrate is fermented by the clostridia. Lactic acid and gas (mostly hydrogen and carbon dioxide) are formed. This is the origin of the 'gas' in gas-gangrene. At this stage it is odourless. The local pathological effect of the clostridial infection are those of acute inflammation with marked oedema. Polymorph infiltration is not conspicuous, at least not while the process is advancing. The absence of polymorphs is strange; perhaps the powerful exotoxins exert a negative chemotactic influence. As the infection spreads, so the necrosis increases, due not only to the liberated exotoxins but also to the effect of ischaemia engendered by the pressure of the gas and exudate on blood vessels. The area is tense, oedematous, and crepitant; the muscle is odourless and brick-red in colour.

Following in the wake of the extensive necrosis there is progressive putrefaction, brought about by the proteolytic clostridia. These decompose the dead muscle and cause it to become greenish-black in colour. Necrosis with superadded putrefaction is called gangrene and in this way these saprophytes complete the evolution of gas-gangrene. It is at this stage that the characteristically foul odour appears.

The clostridia show no tendency to invade the blood stream except terminally; however, the powerful toxins released by the organisms cause a profound general toxaemia manifested by shock and rapidly developing haemolytic anaemia, which is secondary to the effect of the lecithinase on the red-cell envelopes. It is this toxaemia which brings about the death of the patient.

Treatment. The treatment of gas-gangrene entails giving an antiserum against the exotoxin of the three main pathogens, as well as the administration of suitable antibiotics. For prophylaxis in cases of grossly contaminated wounds, debridement with removal of all necrotic and foreign tissue combined with antibiotic therapy has replaced antiserum therapy. An additional aid is the use of hyperbaric oxygen.

TETANUS

The spores of *C. tetani* not infrequently contaminate wounds, but as with the gas-gangrene organisms a reduced oxygen tension is essential for germination. Local conditions must be favourable for growth of the anaerobic *C. tetani*, but quite often the degree of trauma appears to be very mild, because an insignificant punctured wound, like the prick of a contaminated thorn, has quite commonly been the site of origin of a fatal tetanus infection.

Exogenous infection has also resulted in *surgical tetanus*, i.e. the introduction of spores into a wound during the course of a surgical operation. For such spores to germinate they must be presented with a nidus where conditions are relatively anaerobic. Foreign materials embedded in the tissues, e.g. contaminated catgut, talc, or cotton-wool, provide the necessary nidus, and these are the causes of surgical tetanus, which nowadays is fortunately very rare indeed owing to modern methods of sterilization.

Although tetanus is now uncommon in the Western world, the situation in the poorer countries is quite different; in them it is a leading cause of death among hospital admissions. Among the ways by which spores may be introduced into the tissues of the unprotected population are injecting quinine (for malaria), ear piercing, and applying soil (or even dung) to the umbilicus of the newborn.

Clinical features. The incubation period varies from a few days to several weeks, and the shorter it is, the worse is the prognosis. Tetanus developing from wounds of the upper extremities, neck, and face is said to be more frequently lethal than that arising after injuries to the lower parts of the body.

Tetanus is clinically a disease of the central nervous system. The local lesion may be so mild that only very careful search will reveal it, yet the exotoxin produced may be sufficient to cause death. The toxin reaches the central nervous system probably by passing along the motor trunks; it acts by interfering with the inhibitory impulses reaching the motor neurons. This accounts for the generalized increase in tone. This is the early tendency to spasms of those muscles controlled by the same spinal segment as that supplying the area infected. At first there is stiffness, but this is soon followed by increase in muscular tone and spasms. This is termed local tetanus. Subsequently the spasms involve other muscles. Spasm of the masseter muscles results in trismus (inability to open the mouth, or 'lockjaw') while spasm of the facial muscles produces the characteristic *risus sardonicus*. Finally generalized tetanic convulsions occur. Death is due to asphyxia following involvement of the respiratory muscles.

Prophylaxis. Tetanus may occur following quite trivial wounds and by far the best method of prophylaxis is active immunization by giving a course of three injections of tetanus toxoid, a formalized preparation of the exotoxin adsorbed on to aluminium hydroxide or phosphate. The second injection is given about 8 weeks after the first, and the third from 6 to 12 months after the second. This regime should be carried out on all infants, and is mandatory for people whose occupation carries a hazard of injury. Booster doses are recommended at 10-year intervals.

In cases of deep wounds, particularly those with much ragged laceration of tissue or of a punctured type, prophylaxis is essential, and the procedure to be adopted depends on whether there has been previous active immunization or not.

If the patient has had a complete basic course of toxoid injections or a booster within the past 5 years, immunity is adequate and nothing further should be done apart from local treatment of the wound. If the period since the last dose of toxoid exceeds 5 years, but is less than 10 years, a booster dose should be given. If, however, the

period exceeds 10 years, immediate passive immunization must be performed, since any residual immunity may not be adequate to protect the patient even under the stimulus of a booster dose. If there is no history of active immunization, the need for passive immunization is even stronger. This is carried out by giving *human tetanus immunoglobulin,* also called *tetanus immune globulin (human),* 250 units intramuscularly. In addition, a dose of toxoid is also administered, but into a different limb. In the case of a patient who has never been immunized actively before, this constitutes the first of the three immunizing doses; in one who has allowed the respective immunity to lapse for more than 5 years, this is a booster dose. Since the toxoid is of the adsorbed type and is administered at a distance from the immunoglobulin, its action is not interfered with by the initially high level of passive immunity.

Immunization against tetanus is always advisable before surgery is performed on old war and agricultural wounds because spores have been known to remain dormant for many years in healed wounds, and to have germinated following surgical intervention.

GRAM-NEGATIVE ANAEROBIC INTESTINAL BACILLI

The Gram-negative intestinal organisms of the genus *Bacteroides* form the bulk of organisms in the faeces, and are present also as part of the normal flora of the mouth and vagina. They are non-spore-bearing, strict anaerobes. They cause wound infection, pelvic abscesses, otitis media, puerperal sepsis, and oral infections (p. 48), but in these instances their role is probably secondary to infection with more pathogenic organisms. Their presence should be suspected in any infection associated with a foul odour. The organisms may invade the blood stream and cause septicaemia and Gram-negative shock.

OTHER CLOSTRIDIAL INFECTIONS

BOTULISM

Botulism is a disease caused by the action of the neurotoxin of *Clostridium botulinum*. Three types are known. In the well-recognized *food-borne botulism* there is an intoxication caused by the ingestion of preformed toxin in improperly preserved food. Occasionally *C. botulinum* colonizes traumatized tissue and leads to *wound botulism*. *Botulism* is occasionally due to the absorption of toxin formed by organisms that colonize and multiply in the intestinal tract. Children are usually affected but it has been reported in adults.

CLOSTRIDIUM DIFFICILE PSEUDOMEMBRANOUS COLITIS

C. difficile is a normal inhabitant of the large intestine, and under some circumstances can proliferate to produce a toxin which causes necrosis of the colonic mucosa. The result is *acute pseudomembranous colitis*. This is a serious disease characterized by the sudden onset of severe diarrhoea and having an appreciable mortality. The disease usually occurs as a complication of the administration of an antibiotic, particularly clindamycin or lincomycinin. It can also occur postoperatively or in debilitated subjects.

ACTINOMYCOSIS

Actinomycosis is characterized by chronic, loculated foci of suppuration occurring particularly in the region of the jaw. It is caused by infection by *Actinomyces israeli,* an anaerobic organism that is now classified as a bacterium of the family Actinomycetaceae, which also includes the genus *Nocardia*. The organism is Gram-positive and grows as a filament that has a tendency to branch. In animal tissue the filaments form a felted, radially arranged mass that becomes encrusted by lipid of host origin forming a projecting fringe of club-shaped excrescences or clubs. These are visible to the naked eye and having a greyish-yellow colour are called *sulphur granules*. Diagnosis of the disease depends on finding these granules in pus and identifying them by microscopy and culture.

The organism is a normal commensal of the mouth and colonies of them are frequently found in the tonsillar crypts. The disease can follow dental extraction, though considering the widespread distribution of the organism, the disease is surprisingly infrequent. It is not understood what local conditions must be fulfilled before the organism can invade the tissues and set up a progressive inflammatory reaction. It has been known to produce infection in a hand wound caused by hitting an assailant in the teeth ('punch actinomycosis').

The lesions. Actinomycosis commonly occurs in the *cervico-facial* region. Primary *ileo-caecal* infection is uncommon, and *pulmonary* lesions are rare.

The actinomycotic lesion starts as an acute suppurative inflammation, which then persists and progresses to intractable chronicity. As the organisms spread by direct continuity, large numbers of abscesses are produced. Some of these fuse together, but there is a tendency for individual foci of suppuration to remain discrete owing to the persistence of fibrous septa. This produces a characteristically loculated appearance, which is seen most typically in actinomycotic lesions of the liver (*honeycomb liver*).

Histologically the abscess cavities are crowded with pus cells which surround actinomycotic colonies (Fig. 14.2). The narrow septa between the abscesses are composed of fibrous tissue which is heavily infiltrated by polymorphs, lymphocytes, macrophages, and plasma cells. These fibrous septa are not merely the remains of destroyed parenchyma; they are produced by attempts at healing by repair, and the entire lesion is surrounded by a similar dense zone of fibrous tissue.

Spread of infection. The main mode of spread of the disease is by direct contact. Whereas other organisms move in the tissue spaces along preformed planes, the actinomyces extends slowly and inexorably onwards through the tissues. In cervico-facial actinomycosis there is direct spread to the adjacent muscles and bones. The mandible is the bone usually involved, but sometimes there is extension to the maxilla, and eventually the meninges and brain become infected. There is also progressive cutaneous involvement and the abscesses discharge with the production of many sinuses. The appearance of a diffuse, indurated, painless

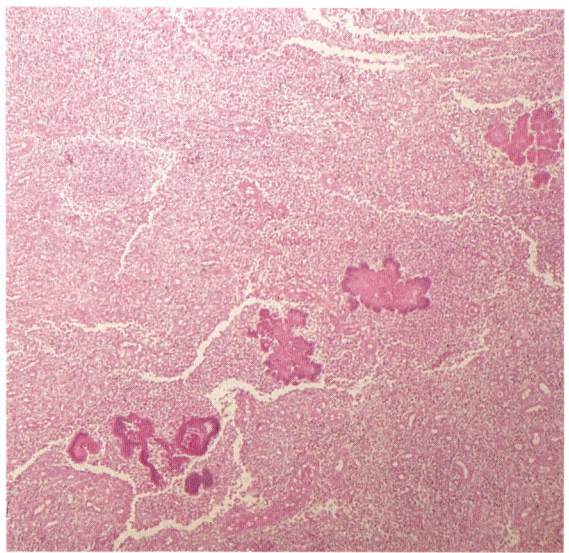

Fig. 14.2 Actinomycosis. The section is of an abscess containing sulphur granules which appear as deeply staining masses composed of colonies of actinomyces organisms. The individual neutrophils in the abscess cannot be resolved at this magnification.

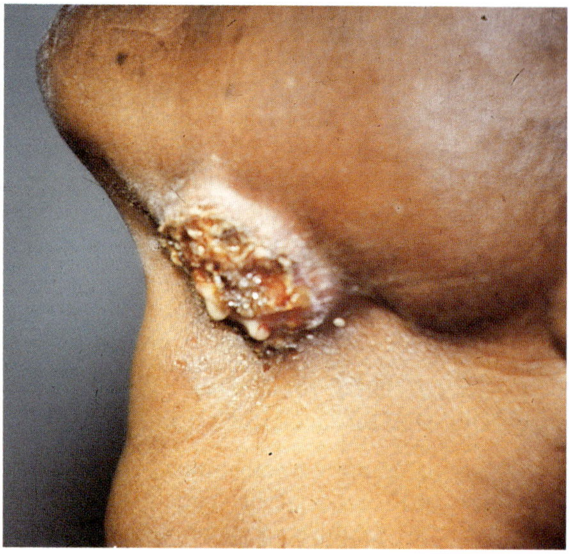

Fig. 14.3 This 40-year-old Nepalese woman had a fluctuant purplish swelling with multiple sinuses on the lower border of the mandible. The thick pus which was expressed contained 'sulphur granules', colonies of actinomyces organisms. (Photograph by courtesy of Miss C E R Spinks.)

area of suppuration in the area of the mandible discharging to the exterior through multiple sinuses is very characteristic of actinomycosis (Fig. 14.3).

Similarly, ileo-caecal actinomycosis spreads through the anterior abdominal wall with the development of discharging sinuses, and pulmonary actinomycosis erupts through the wall of the chest.

Lymphatic spread does not occur in actinomycosis; perhaps the filaments are too large to be accommodated in the lymphatic channels. Any regional lymphadenitis that may occur is attributable to secondary bacterial infection by staphylococci and coliform organisms.

Blood-borne spread, on the other hand, is important, and is typified by the spread of ileo-caecal disease by the portal vein to the liver, where the loculated actinomycotic abscesses of honeycomb liver are produced.

Treatment. Actinomyces organisms are very sensitive to the commonly-used antibiotics, and in practice penicillin and lincomycin are the most useful.

GENERAL READING

Braude A I 1981 Medical microbiology and infectious diseases. Saunders, Philadelphia

Lennette A, et al (eds) 1985 Manual of clinical microbiology, 4th edn. American Society for Microbiology, Washington DC

Youmans G P, Paterson P Y, Sommers H M 1987 The biologic and clinical basis of infectious diseases, 2nd edn. Saunders, Philadelphia

15. Tuberculosis, leprosy, syphilis and some fungal diseases

Whereas the pyogenic infections produce an overt acute inflammatory reaction which may or may not terminate in resolution, there are a great number of other organisms which tend to set up the condition of chronic inflammation. In these there is usually great tissue destruction so that resolution is impossible and a chronic course invariable. During the progress of these infections acute exacerbations of an exudative type are not infrequent, and these are immunologically mediated. Tuberculosis, syphilis, actinomycosis, and the fungal, protozoal, and helminthic infections all come into this category.

There are no histological features common to all these infections; in tuberculosis and histoplasmosis the macrophage is the prominent cell type, in actinomycosis there is chronic suppuration with a polymorph infiltration, while in syphilis there is a non-specific infiltration of lymphocytes and plasma cells. The helminthic diseases are often associated with heavy eosinophil accumulations.

In the acute bacterial infections the causal organisms appear to produce damage by some direct action often by producing powerful toxins. From many of the organisms responsible for chronic infection no satisfactory toxin has been isolated. Their destructive effect is the result of the development of delayed-type hypersensitivity.

In the acute bacterial infections a long-lasting immunity often ensues, and this is usually due to the presence of immunoglobulins in the circulation. In chronic infections immunoglobulins may also be present, but though they may be valuable in the diagnosis of the disease, e.g. in the serological diagnosis of syphilis, they do not produce immunity against the disease. There is evidence in some of these infections, notably tuberculosis, that a degree of immunity is acquired after an infection, but this is cell-mediated rather than being due to the development of specific immunoglobulins.

The body's general reaction to these infections depends on whether they are localized or generalized. In the latter case, there is fever, and severe constitutional disturbances are common. The ESR is considerably elevated and there is hyper-gammaglobulinaemia of the polyclonal type (p. 259).

MYCOBACTERIAL DISEASES

The two important mycobacterial diseases are tuberculosis and Hansen's disease (leprosy). In addition there are a number of atypical myo-bacteria that cause less serious infections, parti-cularly of the skin.

TUBERCULOSIS

Tuberculosis ('consumption') is caused by an infection with *Mycobacterium tuberculosis* of which there are two strains of importance in human disease. The *human strain* infects humans exclu-sively, and the mode of infection is by inhalation of organisms present in fresh droplets or the dust of dried sputum expectorated from the lungs of an open case of pulmonary tuberculosis. The *bovine strain* affects cows and is excreted in the milk to cause tonsillar or intestinal infection in humans.

In the past, tuberculosis has been a common and serious disease. It was a disease of poverty and overcrowding, and its declining incidence has largely been due to improvement in social con-ditions, and the eradication of tuberculous herds of cattle. The availability of effective chemo-therapy has also contributed to its decline. Nevertheless the disease is still encountered in underprivileged areas and in those whose immu-nity is impaired. During the first 5 years of life the body's resistance to infection is poor and the mortality rate is high. From 5–15 years resis-tance is at its peak, but it breaks down during the early adult period of 15–30 years, particularly in women. After the age of 30 years resistance is quite high, but it breaks down again in old age, particularly in men. The presence of silicosis predisposes to infection. The general health of the individual is important. Malnourishment and overcrowding, as in prison camps or slums, pre-disposes to the rapid spread of disease throughout the community. Alcoholism, diabetes mellitus and other chronic debilitating diseases predispose to a rapidly spreading type of infection. Likewise, impaired immunity, particularly with respect to T-cell function, renders an individual susceptible to infection. This situation is encountered with lymphoma, AIDS, and following the admini-stration of immunosuppressive drugs, particularly glucocorticosteroids. These drugs should be used with great caution in patients known to have, or to have had, tuberculosis.

Bacteriology. *Mycobacterium tuberculosis* is a slender bacillus about 3 μm long, non-motile and non-sporing. Its most conspicuous feature is its waxy content which makes it impermeable to the usual stains. It slowly takes up heated stains, e.g. carbol fuchsin in the Ziehl–Neelsen method, and then resists decolorization even by strong acids and alcohols, i.e. it is *acid-fast* and *alcohol-fast*. It is Gram-positive, but Gram-staining is not per-formed because the methyl violet penetrates only with great difficulty. It grows very slowly on standard media such as Lowenstein-Jensen me-dium, but recently the organism can be more rapidly identified by using a medium containing a substrate labelled with ^{14}C and detecting the liberation of free $^{14}CO_2$.

Atypical, or *anonymous*, mycobacteria are des-cribed later in this section.

Mycobacterium tuberculosis is very resistant to drying, and it can survive in dust for several months. It is, however, very sensitive to the effect of ultraviolet radiation, and is rapidly killed in sunlight.

Evolution of the tuberculous lesion. The immediate tissue response to the tubercle bacillus is a mild acute inflammation. The neutrophil infiltration is soon replaced by macrophages derived from blood monocytes. In a short time these cells enlarge, lose their phagocytic powers and become converted into epithelioid cells. Some fuse to form giant cells, mostly of the Langhans' type (Fig. 15.1). The tubercles so formed have a surrounding mantle of lympho-cytes and later fibroblasts. Within 10–14 days necrosis, called caseation, occurs in the centre of the follicle, which consists of epithelioid cells and cells peculiar to the tissue of the part. The *caseation* of tuberculosis is a very firm, cheesy type of coagulative necrosis, and it differs from other types of necrosis in that it has a very high content of lipid material, and shows little ten-dency towards autolysis. Histologically, caseation is associated with such great tissue disintegration that scarcely any structure is recognizable. Every-thing is merged into a brightly eosinophilic mass of amorphous debris. Caseation is produced by a delayed-type hypersensitivity reaction to tubercu-loprotein; it is not the effect of a bacterial toxin.

The fully formed *tubercle follicle* consists of a

central mass of caseation surrounded by epithelioid cells and giant cells, which in turn are surrounded by a wide zone of small round cells (Fig 15.2). The appearance is characteristic of tuberculosis, though it is sometimes also seen in fungal infections.

Variations in the reaction to the tubercle bacillus. The common type of lesion described above is called *productive*, or *proliferative*, because its main components are cells rather than a fluid exudate. The acute caseous, and the chronic caseous, fibrocaseous, and fibroid types of tuberculosis are described in connexion with the lung (p. 167).

Another well-known type of lesion is the *exudative* form of tuberculosis. It is characterized by the outpouring of an inflammatory exudate rich in fibrin. There is a considerable infiltration of lymphocytes, and often many polymorphs are present, but epithelioid and giant cells are scanty. Exudative lesions are typical of tuberculosis of serous cavities. They are not necessarily more serious than productive ones.

The most serious type of lesion is *non-reactive tuberculosis*, in which there are extensive foci of caseation teeming with bacilli but showing virtually no cellular reaction around them. This type of disease is seen in patients with immunological deficiency and subjected to overwhelming infection: thus it may occur as a complication of leukaemia. The tuberculin test is usually negative in this type of tuberculosis.

The fate of the tuberculous lesion. The caseous focus may either cease to progress and heal by fibrosis, or it may soften and spread.

The hallmark of healing is fibrous tissue, and this is produced by the proliferating fibroblasts at the periphery of the lesion. In due course the area of caseation may be replaced by a solid fibrous nodule. Sometimes only a ring of fibrous tissue forms around the periphery, while the central mass of caseation undergoes slow *dystrophic calcification*. In this calcareous nodule organisms may still survive, and years later, when the resistance of the host breaks down, they may become active again.

The hallmark of activity is caseation and softening. If the lesion is spreading, bacilli are carried by macrophages into the surrounding lymphatics and tissue spaces. There they settle and set up satellite follicles, which by fusing with the primary enlarging lesion, produce a *conglomerate tubercle follicle*. Caseous material does not soften rapidly, due possibly to the presence of phosphatides that inhibit autolytic enzymes. Sometimes, however, *liquefaction* does occur, and this is attended by serious consequences.

There is no really satisfactory explanation for this softening. There is no doubt that it is associated with spread, and that the liquefied debris contains many bacilli, but it is not known whether this multiplication of organisms is the cause or the result of the softening. It has been suggested that the liquefaction is due to secondary infection, but this is untrue. Pyogenic infection may certainly complicate a tuberculous lesion, but liquefaction often occurs in the absence of such infection. The element of hypersensitivity is probably of considerable importance.

Once liquefaction has occurred, the debris contains large numbers of tubercle bacilli, and the whole is often called a *cold abscess*. Unlike a pyogenic abscess there are comparatively few cells present, and most of these are disintegrating. The term 'pus' is therefore inapplicable, as there are no pus cells. The term 'cold abscess' is equally inapplicable. In practice it is reserved exclusively for tuberculous lesions, even though in fact the suppurative lesions of actinomycosis may also be 'cold', as neither the heat, pain, nor redness seen in acute pyogenic infection is a marked feature of them. The liquefied debris ('pus') tracks towards a free surface and discharges there. In a lesion of the lung rupture soon occurs into a bronchus, and the disease spreads to other parts of the lung; much infectious material is also coughed up. A tuberculous abscess is lined by tuberculous granulation tissue. This consists of systems of tubercle follicles irregularly disposed in a mass of newly-formed fibrous tissue which is heavily infiltrated with lymphocytes and macrophages.

Whenever a tuberculous abscess opens to the exterior, the disease becomes more serious, firstly because of its *open*, infectious character, and secondly because the tubercle bacillus is an aerobic organism and proliferates much more profusely in an atmosphere of air. These features are well

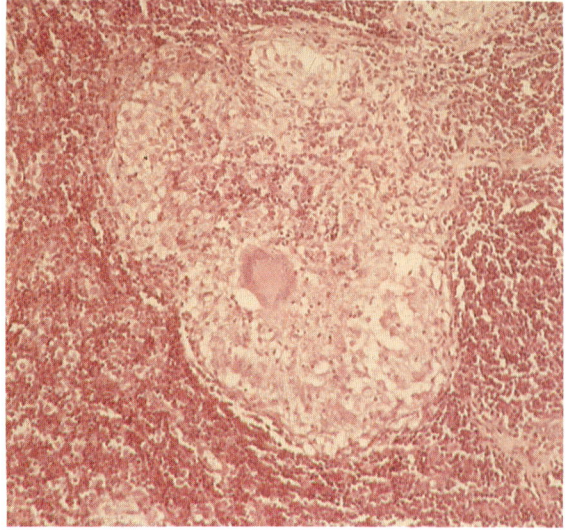

Fig. 15.1 Early lesion of tuberculosis in lymph node. The tubercle consists of a mass of epithelioid cells and one Langhans' giant cell, but no caseation.

illustrated in the open, cavitating type of pulmonary tuberculosis.

Spread of tuberculosis in the body

The principles differ in no significant way from those of most other infections.

Local spread. The spread by macrophages has already been described.

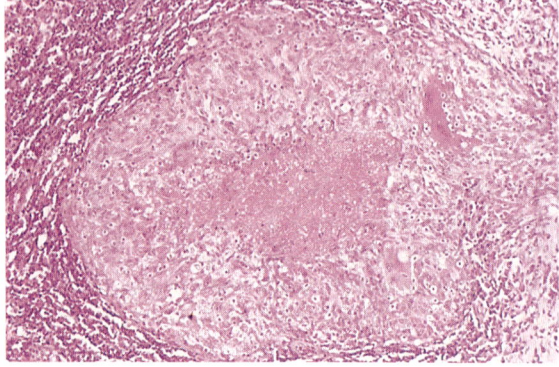

Fig. 15.2 Caseating tuberculous lesion. The tubercle is composed of epithelioid cells with occasional giant cells; the central area consists of structureless eosinophilic caseous material.

Spread in serous cavities is seen in the diffuse pleurisy that may complicate lung lesions, the localized peritonitis found in cases of tuberculous salpingitis, and in tuberculous meningitis.

Spread along epithelial-lined surfaces is typified by the intrabronchial spread of tuberculosis that occurs when sputum is inhaled into adjacent lung segments. If the sputum is coughed up, it can produce *tuberculous laryngitis*. Tuberculous infection occasionally occurs on the tongue, lips, or gingivae. The ulcer so formed has an irregular outline with undermined edges. The most frequent lesion is an ulceration of the tongue, and the adjacent skin (*tuberculosis cutis orificialis*). The laryngeal and oral lesions are extremely painful, and fortunately are now rare.

If sputum is swallowed, the bacilli may infect the ileo-caecal area of the bowel and lead to tuberculous enteritis.

Lymphatic spread. This is a continuation of local spread. The result is a regional tuberculous lymphadenitis.

Blood spread. Organisms may reach the blood stream in one of two ways:

As an extension of lymphatic involvement. In an overwhelming infection the organisms enter the blood stream to produce *miliary tuberculosis*. The lungs, spleen, liver, kidney, and to a lesser extent other organs, are seeded with tubercle bacilli which produce numerous follicles about 1 mm in diameter. Clinically the patient is seriously ill and has a high fever. Sometimes only a few organisms enter the blood stream, and become lodged in various organs to produce metastatic lesions (see below).

Direct involvement of a vein. Blood spread also occurs when caseous hilar nodes directly implicate the adjacent pulmonary vein. If there is a discharge of large numbers of organisms into the blood stream, miliary tuberculosis occurs, but the lungs are often spared.

Tuberculous meningitis is almost invariably present in miliary tuberculosis, and is due either to involvement of the choroid plexus, or else to a small subcortical lesion (*Rich's focus*) rupturing into the subarachnoid space. Miliary tuberculosis is much more common in young children than in adults.

Metastatic lesions. In older children and adults it sometimes happens that only a few bacilli invade the systemic circulation. These may be destroyed by the MP system, or else become lodged in various sites to give rise to metastatic disease. Such a lesion may progress immediately to produce clinical effects, or else remain quiescent, only to undergo reactivation years later. This type of lesion is called *local metastatic tuberculosis*, and it accounts for most of the disease seen in surgical practice. Organs sometimes involved in this way are the *kidneys, adrenals, uterine tubes, epididymes,* and the *bones, joints,* and *tendon sheaths.*

Morphology of tuberculous infections

It has been recognized for a long time that the behaviour of tuberculous infection is quite different in children as compared to adults. At all ages the lung is the organ principally affected.

Childhood. In childhood the primary focus (*Ghon focus*) is a small wedge-shaped area situated at the periphery of the lung field. This subpleural focus may heal and produce no clinical illness, or else the infection spreads to the hilar lymph nodes, which become greatly enlarged and caseous. A conspicuous *primary complex* is the result. It either heals and calcifies, or else it spreads and the child dies of *miliary tuberculosis with meningitis.*

In days gone by the primary lesion was frequently in the pharynx, tonsil, gingiva, or palate. It appeared as a painless ulcer and was acquired by the ingestion of contaminated milk. Sometimes the primary lesion was in the oesophagus or small intestine and usually escaped clinical attention. In most cases the primary lesion was small and the major feature was the enormous enlargement of the regional lymph nodes— *mesenteric* or *cervical.* In all childhood lesions the feature in common is the small size of the primary focus and the tendency to extensive lymph-node involvement with the danger of spread to the blood stream and fatal termination.

Adult life. In adult life the pulmonary focus is almost always apical or subapical (*Assmann focus*). The lesion either heals, or else it progresses, softens, and produces a cavity. Haemoptysis

(the coughing up of blood), chronic cough, weight loss, low-grade fever, and a raised ESR are the main clinical features. Depending on the resistance of the patient there is a tendency for either fibrosis or extensive cavitation to occur. In severe cases great destruction of lung tissue eventually results (Fig. 15.3) and a large cavity may be formed. At any time caseous debris may be inhaled into other bronchi to produce tuberculous bronchopneumonia. This may occur on a small scale and result in extension of the disease, but if widespread it causes rapid caseation of a

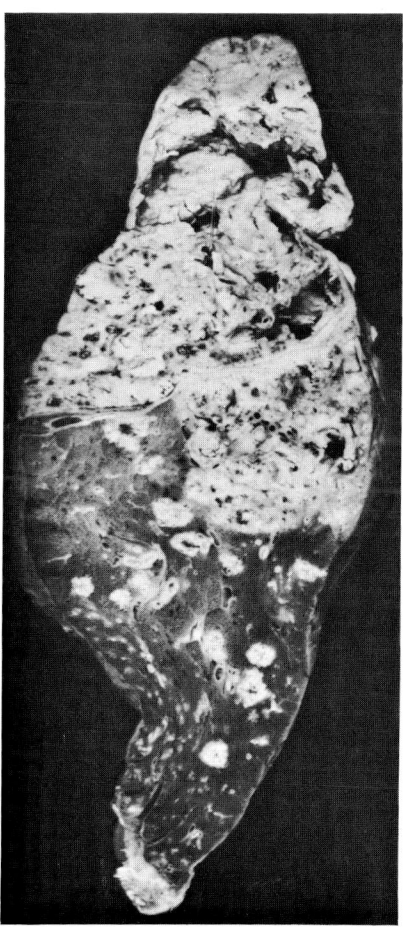

Fig. 15.3 Caseous tuberculosis of lung. The entire upper lobe and part of the apex of the lower lobe have been destroyed by caseous tuberculosis with extensive cavitation. Discrete areas of infection are present in the remainder of the lower lobe. (R37.1, Reproduced by permission of the President and Council of the Royal College of Surgeons of England.)

great area of lung tissue. The latter is associate with intense hypersensitivity, and the disease remains localized to the lungs. Lymph-node involvement is inconspicuous, and blood-spread dissemination is unusual. Death is the result of the local lung lesion which is called *acute caseous bronchopneumonia*. There are severe constitutional symptoms due probably to the effects of hyper-sensitivity—these are described clinically as tox-aemia, but no definite toxins have been isolated.

Chronic tuberculosis. Here the immunity of the host is adequate to cause some destruction of the bacilli, and healing by fibrosis occurs side by side with caseous destruction. Three types of chronic pulmonary tuberculosis are recognized: caseous, fibro-caseous, and fibroid, depending on the rela-tive degrees of caseation and fibrosis. In long-standing fibroid tuberculosis the lung may be converted into a contracted mass of dense fibrous tissue, in which there may be little recognizable evidence of active tuberculous infection. Bronchi-ectasis is a frequent complication of this type of disease, which is characterized clinically by dysp-noea, respiratory failure, and right-sided heart failure.

Another type of cutaneous tuberculosis, apart from tuberculosis cutis orificialis is *lupus vulgaris*. It nearly always involves the face with the ears and nose being commonly affected. The dermis shows a typical non-caseating tuberculoid re-action and the disease spreads by continuity. The course of lupus vulgaris is prolonged, and ultimately great tissue destruction and scarring result. Nevertheless, few organisms can be found in the lesions and the disease appears to be an infection in a person with considerable immunity. The source of the infection may be from a pre-vious pulmonary lesion, but often no other active tuberculosis can be detected.

Skeletal tuberculosis usually starts in the meta-physeal area of a bone, and it causes great local destruction. Unlike pyogenic osteomyelitis it destroys the epiphyseal cartilage with ease, and soon the neighbouring joint is affected. When softening occurs a 'cold abscess' is produced. Tuberculosis of the spine used to be quite com-mon (Pott's disease), and was responsible for col-lapse of the affected vertebrae and great defor-mity. Tuberculous 'pus' sometimes entered the

posas muscle sheath and tracked down, dis-charging on to the skin of the groin below the inguinal ligament.

The feature that all these adult lesions have in common is the tendency to extensive local destruction without much lymphatic involve-ment.

It is traditionally believed that the adult lesion is always secondary to a 'primary' lesion acquired during childhood, and that the difference in course of the two infections can be explained on the basis of hypersensitivity and immunity acquired during the 'primary' infection. Just as in the Koch phenomenon (p. 141), where the second dose of organisms remained localized and did not spread to the regional nodes so it is that the 'secondary' adult lesion remains localized to the lungs and does not spread further afield.

It is becoming increasingly apparent that more and more young adults are Mantoux negative, a proof that they have not had tuberculosis in childhood, yet the incidence of the 'primary' Ghon type of lesion with massive hilar lymph-adenopathy is not increasing in the adult popul-ation. It seems that even primary infections in adults start at the apex of the lung and do not produce much lymphatic involvement. Further-more, there are very definite differences between the adult lesion and the Koch phenomenon. There is lymph-node involvement in the adult, though it is of microscopic extent only, and the lesion shows no particular tendency to heal as in the second infection of the tuberculous guinea-pig. The essential difference in behaviour between childhood and adult lesions appears to be due to tissue maturation; the older the patient, the less is the tendency towards gross lymph-node involvement. The effect of a previous infection as an additional modifying factor cannot be excluded, but it is unjustifiable to label all adult lesions as secondary. The terms childhood and adult tuberculosis are much more accurate than 'primary' and 'secondary' tuber-culosis.

The source of the organisms causing adult-type tuberculosis has been the centre of much discus-sion in the past. The pulmonary lesions were regarded as due either to *reactivation* of a quiesc-ent primary lesion or to the development of a new lesion produced by a *reinfection* from some external source. In the past reinfection was probably of great importance, but nowadays it seems that adult-type lesions are themselves primary infections. In the case of other organs, e.g. kidney and bone, it is almost certain that tuberculosis is due to the reactivation of small lesions which were produced during a bacteraemic phase of a previous pulmonary infection.

Immunity and hypersensitivity in tuberculosis

A primary infection with the tubercle bacillus induces a state of immunity as was first described by Koch using guinea-pigs. The immunity is related to the development of delayed-type hypersensitivity to tuberculoprotein. This hypersensitivity is evident by a positive tuberculin (Mantoux) reaction. The interaction of bacillary antigen and specifically reacting T cells leads to tissue necrosis, and also leads to the recruitment of inflammatory cells, particularly macrophages, which are also activated and more able to phagocytose and destroy the bacilli.

The immunity to tuberculosis induced by a primary infection is not as effective as is seen in some other disease, e.g. diphtheria. Nevertheless it induces a useful degree of immunity and, on this supposition, depends the use of a vaccine for active immunization. The strain commonly used is BCG (Bacille Calmette–Guérin), an attenuated bovine strain. It is injected intradermally and produces a mild localized infection, following which the tuberculin reaction becomes positive. The value of BCG vaccination is debatable. In Britain it is given to individuals who are tuberculin negative and are exposed to infection (e.g. medical personnel). Unfortunately it appears to be of little use in the Third World, probably because any immunity provided is more than offset by the malnutrition and chronic intercurrent infections that are rampant.

In North America the great majority of the population have never been exposed to the tubercle bacillus and are tuberculin-negative. A positive test suggests active disease. If the subject has had a BCG vaccination and is tuberculin positive, the diagnostic value of the tuberculin test is lost. Hence chemoprophylaxis is preferred as an alternative for subjects exposed to infection.

Atypical mycobacteria (MOTTS)

Mycobacteria resembling *M. tuberculosis* but differing from the classical organism in cultural characteristics, antibiotic sensitivity and animal pathogenicity are sometimes isolated from cases of human tuberculosis. The disease is generally milder than classical disease. These atypical bacteria or 'mycobacteria other than tubercle bacilli' (MOTTS) include *M. intracellular avium* and *M. kansassi*.

Mycobacterium avium intracellulare is now recognized as an important opportunistic pathogen in patients with AIDS. It causes a disseminated infection and vast numbers of organisms are found in the lungs, spleen and lymph nodes.

Skin infections, other than lupus vulgaris, due to mycobacteria have also been recognized. The best known is due to *M. marinum* acquired in swimming pools or sometimes from tropical fish tanks. Other e.g. *M. fortuitum* and *M. cheloni* occasionally cause wound infection, particularly following heart surgery.

SARCOIDOSIS

Although of unknown aetiology it is convenient to consider sarcoidosis at this point, since its histological features closely resemble those of tuberculosis. The unit of sarcoidosis is a discrete follicle composed of plump epithelioid cells, in the midst of which a few giant cells may be found. The follicle is surrounded by a rim of lymphocytes and is therefore very like a tubercle follicle, but differs in that there is rarely any central caseation (Fig. 15.4).

Sarcoidosis is a generalized disease and affects the lungs (producing miliary lesions), the bones (especially those of the hands), the skin, eye, spleen, liver, lymph nodes, salivary glands, heart, and nervous system.

The lesions tend to heal with fibrosis, and in certain situations, e.g. the eye, brain, and lung, they can produce serious effects. The disease is not uncommon in Northern European countries.

LEPROSY (HANSEN'S DISEASE)

Leprosy is caused by *Mycobacterium leprae*, which although one of the first bacteria to be incrim-

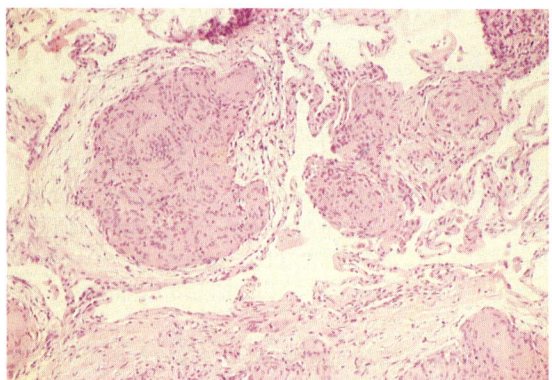

Fig. 15.4   Sarcoidosis of lung. The tubercles are composed of epithelioid cells and occasional giant cells. There is no surrounding lymphocytic reaction and the tubercles are described as 'naked'.

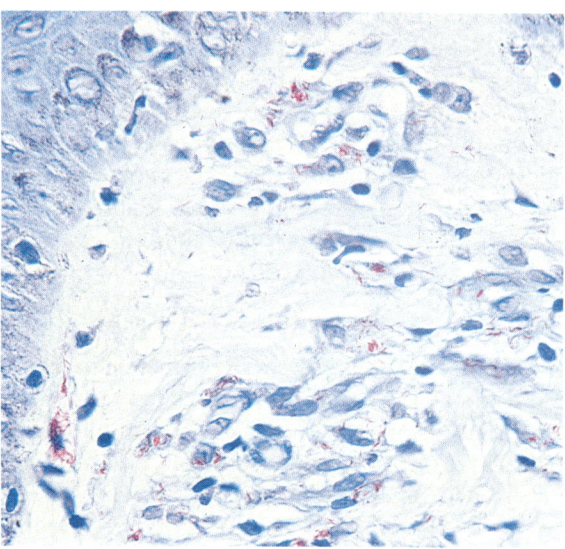

Fig. 15.5   Leprosy of skin. The section has been stained by the Fite method and shows numerous red staining organisms situated within the cytoplasm of macrophages.

inated as a cause of human disease has never been cultured in an artificial medium. Investigation of the disease, in particular the sensitivity of the organism to antibiotics, has been greatly hindered by our inability to grow the organism and the great difficulty encountered in infecting laboratory animals. So far, the organism has only been grown in the foot pads of mice and in the armadillo. In practice, pathological diagnosis depends on demonstrating the organism in smears or sections by the Fite stain (Fig. 15.5), a modification of the Ziehl–Neelsen stain.

Although the disease is of great antiquity its precise origin is unknown. It is believed to have been present in India during the sixth century BC and to have been introduced into Europe by the armies of Alexander the Great returning from the Indian campaign in 327–326 BC. Later the armies of Rome and the Crusaders returning from the Middle East are credited with further disseminating the disease. Leprosy was common in Europe during the Middle Ages but, for reasons that are unclear, rapidly declined. Decimation of the population by plagues, and later improved living conditions have been held responsible. Leprosy is still endemic in areas of poverty in the Far East, India, the Middle East, Africa, and Central and South America. The disease was probably introduced into the United States by the Negro slaves, and is still endemic in some southern states and Hawaii.

The mode of infection is not known for certain but the disease is probably acquired by inhala-

tion, being spread by contaminated nasal secretions from a patient with lepromatous leprosy. The disease is generally acquired in childhood, and the first lesion is an insignificant scaly skin patch. This *indeterminate lesion* may heal spontaneously or progress to one of the two major forms of the disease.

Types of leprosy

Tuberculoid leprosy. This type of leprosy occurs in individuals with a high state of immunity. The skin lesions consist of one or several *well-demarcated* papules or plaques, which are associated with local nerves, causing the skin of the area to become anaesthetic (Fig. 15.6). Microscopically the skin and involved nerves show a non-caseating tuberculoid reaction similar to that seen in early tuberculosis. Lepra bacilli are extremely sparse.

Lepromatous leprosy. In lepromatous leprosy the lesions consist of multiple macules, papules, and plaques, which are of *widespread distribution* and tend to be *symmetrical*. The lesions are *poorly delineated*, and often there is a diffuse infiltration of the skin (Fig. 15.7). Microscopically the dermis is diffusely packed with macrophages, which are themselves stuffed with lepra bacilli. Since the

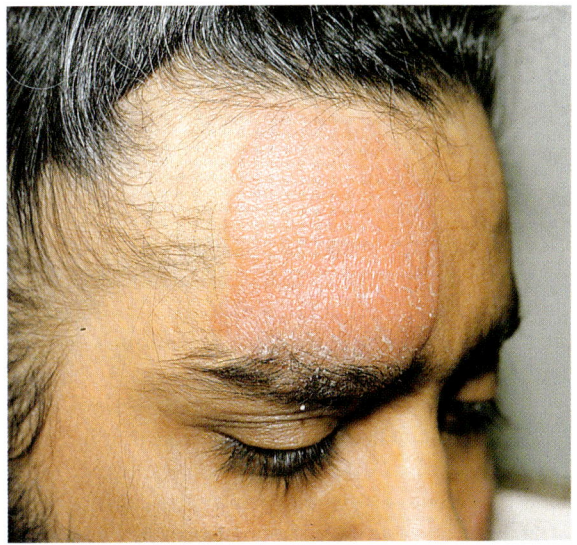

Fig. 15.6 Well-demarcated plaque associated with the opthalmic division of the trigeminal nerve in a patient with tuberculoid leprosy.

lesions tend to occur in the cold parts of the body, the hands and face are particularly affected. The diffuse thickening of the skin of the face leads to a lion-like appearance (leonine facies). There is diffuse involvement of nerves, so that symmetrical peripheral neuritis is characteristic.

In lepromatous leprosy, the nasal mucosa is also infiltrated by bacteria-laden macrophages, and the destruction of the nasal bones leads to

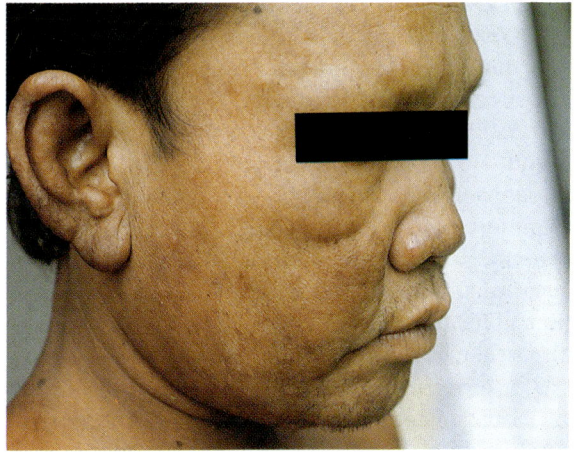

Fig. 15.7 Lepromatous leprosy. The skin of the face, including the earlobes, is thickened and nodular.

the characteristic appearance. The nasal secretions contain a large number of bacilli.

In lepromatous leprosy there is defective T-cell immunity, causing the lepromin reaction to be negative. As if to compensate for this there is an overproduction of immunoglobulins, and the hypergammaglobulinaemia is associated with *acute reactional phases* that are a great hazard in leprosy. Exacerbation of the skin lesions, iridocyclitis, orchitis, nerve damage, fever, prostration, and death can occur during these acute phases, which may either develop spontaneously or be precipitated by ill-advised vigorous treatment. The damage is probably mediated by the deposition of immune complexes with antigen excess (see Ch. 13). The large number of bacilli present in the lesions provide the antigen for the formation of these complexes.

Leprosy provides a fascinating example of the effects that an immune response has on the pattern of an infection. In the tuberculoid type, T-cell immunity is well developed, few bacilli are present in the lesions, and the inflammatory response is characterized by a tuberculoid reaction with plentiful Langhans' giant cells. The pattern of reaction is similar to that encountered in the common type of tuberculous infection. In lepromatous leprosy, on the other hand, T-cell function is in abeyance and vast numbers of bacilli are present in the lesions, which are characterized by a diffuse infiltration by macrophages ('lepra cells'). Occasionally an analogous situation is encountered in tuberculosis. In the terminal stages in miliary tuberculosis, the tuberculin test becomes negative, and the lesions teem with bacilli.

Borderline or dimorphous leprosy. Cases occur in which the clinical and pathological features are between the two polar types of tuberculoid and lepromatous leprosy. In these borderline cases, acute reactional states are particularly common, and the disease tends to terminate in one of the two major forms, often the lepromatous type.

Leprosy is a chronic disease that is now amenable to treatment with a number of chemotherapeutic drugs. The sulphones are the mainstay of these drugs, because they are not only effective but also readily available and cheap.

SPIROCHAETAL INFECTIONS

Spirochaetes are long, slender, spiral organisms belonging to three genera—*Borrelia*, *Leptospira* and *Treponema*.

BORRELLIOSIS

Various borrelia species cause *relapsing fever*. The organisms are remarkable for being able to undergo rapid antigenic variation, so that when the infected subject makes antibodies capable of clearing the body of organisms, a new variant appears and with it a new wave of infection. Repetition of this process causes the characteristic relapsing fever.

Borrelia vincentii is a large spirochaete that forms part of the normal flora of the mouth. Associated with anaerobic fusiform bacilli it causes ulcerative oral lesions when local resistance is impaired, e.g. in agranulocytosis. *Acute ulcerative gingivitis* is associated with poor nutrition and poor oral hygiene.

Borrelia burgdorferi is a spirochaete transmitted by the bite of a tick. It causes *Lyme disease* so named after Lyme in Connecticut where a major outbreak led to the identification of the causative organism. Around the site of the bite an expanding patch of erythema develops (erythema chronicum migrans); the disease is of importance because, later, more serious manifestations develop, including involvement of the meninges, heart and joints. Arthritis can be severe.

LEPTOSPIROSIS

Leptospirosis is a disease of many animal species including dogs and rodents, and the organism is excreted in their urine; humans are infected by contact with contaminated water. The severity of the disease varies greatly but fever, meningitis, and liver and renal damage are the main features of a severe infection.

TREPONEMAL DISEASES

The most severe treponemal disease is *syphilis* or, more exactly, *venereal syphilis* which will be described first. Less well known but more common are a variety of non-venereal treponemal diseases that resemble venereal syphilis, but are less severe and are transmitted by non-sexual physical contact, usually during childhood.

Syphilis

Bacteriology and Serology. The causative organism *Treponema pallidum* is a delicate spiral filament, or spirochaete, about 10 μm long. It cannot be stained by the usual techniques, and is demonstrable in exudates by means of dark-ground illumination. In histological sections it is stained by special silver impregnation methods.

The organism has never been cultured artificially even in fertile eggs or tissue-culture systems, nor does animal inoculation play any part in the diagnosis of the disease. In fact, rabbits develop acute orchitis after the intratesticular inoculation of the organisms. This method is used to obtain a supply of spirochaetes for such procedures as the *T. pallidum* immobilization (TPI) test.

During the course of infection a patient develops immunoglobulins of great importance. Two groups are recognized:

The Wassermann antibody. This antibody fixes complement in the presence of a phosphatide extract of heart muscle (cardiolipin). This antigen is used in the *standard tests for syphilis*, namely the *Wassermann complement-fixation test* and the *flocculation tests*, of which the *Kahn* and the *Venereal Disease Research Laboratory (VDRL) tests* are the most widely used. They are more sensitive than the complement fixation test but not more specific. Since the antigen is not specific for the organism of syphilis, it is not surprising that a positive reaction is sometimes found in non-treponemal diseases, notably trypanosomiasis, leprosy, malaria, infectious mononucleosis, mycoplasmal pneumonia, and systemic lupus erythematosus. Pregnancy too, is occasionally associated with a false-positive reaction. The tests are positive in other treponemal diseases, e.g. yaws.

Treponemal antibody. The second group of antibodies which is formed reacts with treponemal protein. Some antibody activity is directed against protein common to several treponemes (group protein), whereas other antibodies are more specific. The following tests are employed.

Reiter protein complement-fixation (RPCF) test. This test is more specific than the standard test for syphilis and therefore gives fewer false positive results.

Treponema pallidum immobilization (TPI) test. When positive serum in incubated with a concentrated suspension of *T. pallidum* in the presence of complement, it leads to the immobilization of the spirochaetes as viewed under dark-ground illumination. The TPI test becomes positive a little later in the disease than do the standard tests, but it remains positive for the remainder of the patient's life with the exception of some cases in which the disease has been successfully treated early in its course. Being more specific, it is useful when there is a suspected false serology. Unfortunately the test is technically difficult to perform and needs a supply of pathogenic organisms.

Fluorescent treponemal antibody (FTA) test. Specific antibody adheres to *T. pallidum* and can be detected by applying fluorescein-labelled anti-human γ-globulin. Two antibodies are involved; one is group specific, reacting with *T. pallidum* and other treponemes, but the other is specific for *T. pallidum*. Both are formed in syphilis. The group specific antibody can be absorbed by a non-pathogenic strain of treponomes (the Reiter strain that can be cultured in vitro). The test (FTA-ABS) is as sensitive and specific as the TPI test. These two specific tests are performed only when the standard tests are equivocal, or when the results do not correlate with the clinical features of the case. No test is absolutely reliable, and none can distinguish between syphilis and yaws (page 175).

Treponemal passive haemagglutination (TPHA) test. Formalized, tanned sheep red cells sensitized with material from disrupted *T. pallidum* are used as the antigen. The test is an alternative to the TPI and FTA-ABS tests.

Acquired syphilis

Apart from congenital syphilis, the infection is almost always acquired venereally, although on rare occasions it is transmitted by a blood trans-fusion, and a primary lesion can occur on the finger of an unfortunate dentist or physician who examines an infected patient. Nevertheless, considering how frequent it must be for the hands to come in contact with the treponema, the rarity of cutaneous chancres is curious. Evidentally the organism cannot easily infect the skin. Unlike the tubercle bacillus, *T. pallidum* is very rapidly destroyed both in water and by drying. Intimate direct contact is therefore necessary for infection to occur. The spirochaete is one of the most invasive organisms known. Once it penetrates the surface integument, it spreads along the lymphatics to the regional lymph nodes, and finally reaches the blood stream within a matter of hours. There is therefore systemic dissemination long before any local manifestation appears.

The disease is divisible into three active stages.

Primary syphilis. The typical lesion of primary syphilis is the chancre, which usually appears on the genital region 2–4 weeks after infection. It is an indurated papule which breaks down to form an ulcer. It is characteristically painless, and is accompanied by a considerable *regional lymphadenitis*, which is also painless. Extragenital chancres are not uncommon, e.g. around the anus in homosexuals, and on the lips, tip of tongue, tonsils, gingiva, or other part of the oral cavity.

The histological appearance is quite non-specific, consisting merely of a dense infiltration of lymphocytes, plasma cells, and a few macrophages in the dermis.

Even without treatment the chancre gradually heals, usually with little scarring.

The fact that the spirochaetes become disseminated in the blood stream long before there is any local lesion suggests that hypersensitivity plays an important part in the process. The chancre is not comparable with a boil, for it is not a local inflammatory reaction tending to limit the infection. A possible explanation is that sensitizing antibodies are first formed in the cells at the site of entry and in the regional lymph nodes. During the incubation period the spirochaetes multiply in the MP system, and when liberated react with the sensitized tissue. This would explain the chancre and the lymphadenopathy quite well.

At a later stage the other tissues of the body

become sensitized, and then the generalized lesions of secondary syphilis become manifest.

Diagnosis. The laboratory diagnosis depends on demonstrating spirochaetes in the exudate from the chancre by dark-ground illumination.

About 2 weeks after the appearance of the chancre, antibodies first appear in the blood. The VDRL becomes positive before the TPI.

Secondary syphilis. Within 2 weeks to 6 months after exposure the disease becomes clinically generalized. When syphilis was first introduced into Europe, this stage was severe enough to warrant the name, 'the great pox'. Nowadays it is much milder, and is characterized by the development of a skin eruption. This is widespread, symmetrical, usually not pruritic, and in addition to being present on the trunk is also seen on the face, palms, and soles. The lesions are generally erythematous papules, but may be of any type except vesicular or bullous. Other lesions are less common. In moist areas, e.g. the vulva, anal region, and axillae, plateau-like excrescences are formed (*condylomata lata*). In the buccal mucosa the flat lesions are called *mucous patches*, and shallow, serpiginous areas of ulceration also occur (*snail-track ulcers*). The muco-cutaneous lesions may be accompanied by constitutional symptoms which include low-grade fever, myalgia, moderate anaemia, iridocyclitis, and a generalized painless lymphadenopathy. Histologically the secondary lesions show a non-specific inflammatory infiltrate by lymphocytes, plasma cells, and macrophages. The secondary lesions resolve spontaneously and do not form scars. This is the phase of maximum infectivity; spirochaetes ooze out of the condylomata and mucous patches.

Diagnosis. The standard serological tests are always positive in overt secondary syphilis unless the patient is severely immunodepressed as in AIDS. If a negative result is reported in the face of strong clinical indications of syphilis, the *prozone phenomenon* should be suspected (p. 115), and the test repeated with suitable dilutions so that the titre of antibody can be measured. Organisms can be demonstrated in the exudates from mucous and cutaneous lesions.

The occurrence of the *Jarish–Herxheimer* reaction confirms the diagnosis of syphilis. It consists of a transient episode of fever and malaise with an accentuation of the skin eruption within 12 h of beginning treatment—generally an injection of penicillin. The reaction is presumably due to the massive release of bacterial antigens as the organisms are killed.

Tertiary syphilis. Local destructive lesions of a truly chronic inflammatory nature may appear 2–3 years after infection and continue to erupt sporadically for at least 20 years. Such lesions are rarely encountered nowadays: this is a tribute to the efficacy of penicillin, for syphilis is as common today as ever and indeed in some parts of the world is on the increase. The lesions of tertiary syphilis are presumably due to marked hypersensitivity, since spirochaetes are few and the reaction to them is excessive. Two forms of lesions occur: *localized gummata* and *diffuse inflammatory lesions* characterized by parenchymatous destruction.

A *gumma* is a tumour-like mass with a central area of gummy, coagulated necrotic material surrounded by a zone of epithelioid cells, giant cells, lymphocytes, plasma cells and fibroblasts. The tissue reaction resembles that of tuberculosis but giant cells are less numerous and the arteries in the vicinity tend to show endarteritis obliterans. Gummata are particularly liable to occur in the liver, testes, subcutaneous tissues, and in bones, notably the tibia, ulna, clavicle, calvaria of skull, and the nasal and palatal bones. The destruction produced by gummata is exemplified by the perforated palate and the saddle-shaped nasal deformity seen in tertiary syphilis.

In the past the serious effects of tertiary syphilis fell on the cardiovascular and nervous systems. In *syphilitic aortitis* the infection causes inflammation of the vessel wall and destruction of its elastic component such that the vessel dilates and aneurysms form. The thoracic aorta is generally most severely affected and dilatation of the aortic valve ring causes aortic regurgitation.

Cerebral syphilis may be *meningo-vascular* or *parenchymatous*. In the former type there is focal meningitis and vascular occlusion due to endarteritis obliterans of the small vessels. Isolated cranial nerve palsies are quite common.

Parenchymatous neurosyphilis includes the two well-known conditions, general paralysis of the insane and tabes dorsalis. *General paralysis of the insane* is a chronic syphilitic meningoencephalitis in which the frontal lobes are particularly severely affected. This results in progressive dementia and often paralysis. *Tabes dorsalis* is a degenerative condition of the posterior columns of the spinal cord and the posterior roots of the spinal nerves. There is severe demyelination of the sensory tracts. This results in loss of sensation leading to trophic disturbances, and loss of postural sense, which produces the typical staggering gait.

The bones are sometimes affected by a diffuse type of syphilitic inflammation. There may be widespread periostitis, involving especially the tibia and the bones of the calvaria of the skull. The irregular thickening that is very apparent clinically is due to the laying down of new bone. This gives rise to the classical sabre tibia, and in the skull a rather typical worm-eaten appearance.

Diagnosis. The diagnosis of tertiary syphilis is primarily clinical, but it may often be substantiated by serological examination of the blood and cerebrospinal fluid. In most cases of overt syphilis this examination is strongly positive, and in neuro-syphilis the cerebrospinal fluid is generally more helpful than the blood.

Congenital syphilis

During the first 2 years of infection an untreated syphilitic mother is very liable to transmit the disease to her fetus, particularly after the fourth month of pregnancy, when the Langerhans' layer of the placenta becomes attenuated. Abortion may result, or else a severely affected infant may die soon after birth.

More frequently the child survives, and it may then exhibit early stigmata of infection like skin eruptions, snuffles, epiphysitis of the elbows, and wasting. Sometimes stigmata appear only in later childhood. The notched, peg-shaped Hutchinson's incisor teeth and mulberry molars (Moon's molars) due to syphilitic infection of the tooth germs during fetal life are well-known examples of this type of lesion, as are also interstitial keratitis (inflammation of the cornea), tibial periostitis (sabre tibia), and nerve deafness.

The histological appearances of these various lesions are all very similar, being combinations of the heavy cellular infiltration of secondary syphilis together with the gummatous destruction typical of the tertiary phase. In fact, congenital syphilis may be regarded as a combined secondary and tertiary syphilis occurring in a child whose primary lesion was placental.

Non-venereal treponemal diseases

The best known example of this group is *yaws*, a disease quite common in some tropical countries and caused by *T. pertenue*. The primary lesion is extragenital, and this is followed by a secondary and tertiary stage. In the latter there are destructive skin and bone lesions, and these may affect the face and nose. Significant cardiovascular and central nervous system involvement is rare as compared with syphilis. Possibly *T. pallidum* evolved as a mutant of *T. pertenue*.

FUNGAL INFECTIONS

For practical purposes four varieties can be recognized:

Moulds, which grow as long filaments (*hyphae*),

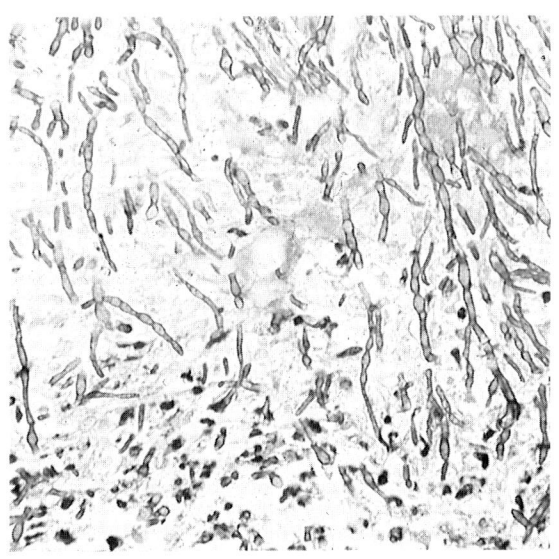

Fig. 15.8 *Candida* organisms in the base of an oral ulcer. The section has been stained by the periodic acid–Schiff (PAS) method and shows the organisms stained red. Occasional budding yeasts are present but the majority of the fungi are in the form of elongated pseudohyphae.

and which branch and interlace to form a meshwork, or *mycelium*.

Yeasts, which grow by budding only.

Yeast-like fungi, which grow partly as yeasts and partly as long filamentous forms called pseudohyphae.

Dimorphic fungi, which can grow either as hyphae or as yeast depending on the cultural conditions.

The line of distinction between some higher bacteria (e.g. the *Actinomycetales* which includes the *Mycobacteriaceae*, *Actinomycetaceae*, and *Streptomycetaceae*) and true fungi is by no means clear-cut.

SUPERFICIAL INFECTIONS BY FUNGI

A number of fungi are able to grow in the hair and the superficial layers of the epidermis, where they produce skin diseases typified by *ringworm*.

Ringworm, or tinea

Ringworm is caused by a group of fungi which are termed *dermatophytes*, and have the property of digesting the keratin of skin or hair. The dermatophytes are moulds that grow as a mycelium and reproduce by the formation of various types of spores. Ringworm is due to invasion of keratin by one of the dermatophytes and can affect any part of the skin; in general the lesions are erythematous, scaly, and sometimes vesicular, and tend to have a sharp, red, spreading border that gives the lesions a ring-like shape from which the disease acquired its name.

Scrapings of nail or keratin can be examined by direct microscopy for hyphae; and from a culture one can readily identify the particular strain of mould responsible.

Candidiasis

Infection with *Candida* species is one of the most frequent fungal infections in the human subject. The organism most commonly involved is the yeast-like fungus *Candida albicans*. The common yeast form is seen in thrush, and is 1.5–5.0 μm in diameter and intensely Gram-positive. It reproduces by budding, but sometimes the bud elongates to form a pseudohypha. (Fig. 15.8). This form can occur in cultures and is also characteristic of invasive candida infections, especially the lesions of systemic candidiasis (see Fig. 1.1). The organism is a common commensal in the oral cavity, alimentary tract, and vagina. Infections occur when local or general conditions become suitable, but it must be accepted that the factors which govern the delicate balance between host and organism are poorly understood. The superficial infections of the mucous membranes appear as white patches called *thrush*. In the mouth this is very common in infants, especially premature ones, and may be acompanied by perianal lesions. Oral candidiasis can occur at any age during the course of any debilitating disease. It may also occur under dentures and orthodontic appliances, and can complicate other erosive disease, e.g. pemphigus vulgaris. Vaginal thrush is common during pregnancy, in those on the contraceptive pill or taking tetracycline for acne vulgaris, and in diabetes mellitus. Cutaneous candidiasis occurs around the corners of the mouth (*angular cheilitis*, or *perléche*), in other moist intertriginous areas, and in the nail folds (*chronic paronychia*).

The important feature of candidiasis is that it is sometimes a serious opportunistic infection. The organism may invade the blood stream and lead to generalized systemic candidiasis in which lesions occur in many organs. Renal abscesses are usually prominent, but almost any organ may be affected and endocarditis is sometimes seen. Severe candidiasis is often encountered in patients with immunodeficiency, particularly with T-cell involvement, as in AIDS.

Less extensive candida infections are seen in particular circumstances. Endocarditis can occur as a primary event, particularly in addicts who inject themselves intravenously with narcotics. Oral lesions can spread to produce extensive gastrointestinal infection following the prolonged administration of oral broad-spectrum antibiotics. Finally the are some types of primary immunological deficiency disease affecting the T lymphocytes in which there is *chronic widespread mucocutaneous candidiasis*. These may be familial, and endocrine abnormalities particularly hypoparathyroidism, may coexist. These conditions persist for many years and do not tend to terminate in generalized spread nor is there usually a tendency for other infections to occur.

The tissue reaction to *Candida* varies. In minor and superficial infections there is some tissue necrosis accompanied by a pyogenic response. Intra-epidermal pustules are seen in the cutaneous lesions. When the infection is overwhelming, as in generalized candidiasis, there is much necrosis and very little inflammatory reaction. Indeed, the lesions show massive accumulations of fungus and few host cells.

SYSTEMIC FUNGAL INFECTIONS

In certain parts of the world fungal infections are of considerable importance. In general the organisms are found in the soil, and infection is acquired by inhalation. A primary lesion occurs in the lung and in the majority of people healing follows. Occasionally, however, the organims produce more severe damage and spread to involve other organs. These diseases therefore resemble tuberculosis in their pathogenesis. Furthermore, the tissue reaction to these organisms sometimes also closely resembles that seen in tuberculosis.

Cryptococcosis

The causative organism *Cryptococcus neoformans* is a true yeast, and of world-wide distribution. The primary lung lesion is usually small and heals by fibrosis. Occasionally the organism becomes widely disseminated and in particular causes *meningitis*. This widespread dissemination is particularly common in immunosuppressed patients.

Histoplasmosis

The causative organism *Histoplama capsulatum* is a dimorphic fungus which has a world-wide distribution, and is endemic in the Mississippi Valley of the USA. The histoplasmin test, analagous to the tuberculin test, is positive in affected individuals.

The primary lung lesion resembles tuberculosis and usually heals with calcification; rarely there is blood-borne dissemination. This occurs most commonly in infants, and many of the internal organs are involved. Large numbers of organisms are then found parasitizing macrophages. Disseminated histoplasmosis may also occur in elderly dibilitated subjects, usually men, and the infection is less widespread than in the infantile type. In some cases infection of the lips, mouth, nose or larnyx is the initial manifestation.

Coccidioidomycosis

This disease, caused by the dimorphic fungus *Coccidioides immitis*, is common in the desert regions of California and Arizona and also in the Chaco district of Argentina. Many of the inhabitants acquire a pulmonary infection, but this is either asymptomatic or accompanied by a self-limiting influenza-like illness called locally 'desert fever'. Occasionally the disease is progressive, and the destructive lung lesions closely resemble tuberculosis. Systemic spread to many organs may occur. Histologically the lesions show a suppurative tuberculoid reaction.

Blastomycosis

This disease, formerly called North American blastomycosis, is caused by infection with *Blastomyces dermatitidis*, a yeast with a thick double-contoured capsule. The primary lesion is usually pulmonary but may be cutaneous. It generally subsides spontaneously, but occasionally it progresses and widespread dissemination can then follow. Suppurative lesions occur in many sites, particularly the skin, bones, and lungs.

Paracoccidioidomycosis

This disease, formerly called South American blastomycosis, is caused by the diamorphic yeast *Paracoccidioides braziliensis* that multiplies by producing multiple peripheral buds so that the organism becomes surrounded by a 'row of beads'. The common primary site of infection is the nasopharynx, and ulcerative destructive lesions are produced. The lymph nodes are soon involved, and sometimes cervical lymphadenopathy is the presenting symptom. The disease tends to become disseminated and affect the lungs, skin, and other organs. It is commonly fatal unless treated.

GENERAL READING

Braude A I 1981 Medical microbiology and infectious diseases. Saunders, Philadelphia.

Davidson P T 1985 Tuberculosis. New views of an old disease. New England Journal of Medicine 312:1514

Drusin L M 1984 Syphilis: clinical manifestations, diagnosis and treatment.Urologic Clinics of North America 11:121

Drutz D J, Catanzano A 1978 Coccidioidomycosis. American Review of Respiratory Disease 117: 559 Essentials of medical mycology. Churchill Livingstone, Edinburgh

Hart G 1986 Syphilis tests in diagnostic and therapeutic decision making. Annals of Internal Medicine 104:368.

Holmes K K, et al (eds) 1984 Sexually transmitted diseases. McGraw Hill, New York.

Jopling W H, Harman R R M 1986 Leprosy. In: Rook A, et al (eds) Textbook of dermatology, 4th edn. Blackwell Scientific, Oxford, p. 862.

Kerdel F A, Moschella S L 1984 Sarcoidosis. An updated review. Journal of the American Academy of Dermatology 11:1.

Leading Article 1984 Tick-borne Borrelia. Lancet 2:1134

Lever W F, Schaumburg-Lever G 1990 Histopathology of the skin. See fungal diseases and leprosy, 7th edn. Lippincott, Philadelphia

Macher A 1980 Histoplasmosis and blastomycosis. Medical Clinics of North America 64:447

Metzer M 1979 Role of humoral versus cellular mechanisms of resistance in the pathogenesis of syphilis. British Journal of Venereal Diseases 55:94

Musher D M, Schell R F, Knox J M 1976 The immunology of syphilis. International Journal of Dermatology 15:566.

Steere A C et al 1983 The early clinical manifestations of Lyme disease. Annals of Internal Medicine 99: 76

16. Rickettsial, chlamydial, mycoplasmal and viral diseases

It is useful at the outset, before considering the properties of viruses, first to define those of other small organisms with which they might be confused.

Bacteria are generally unicellular, but even the smallest is within the range of the light microscope (which resolves up to about 0.2 μm in diameter). They grow with variable ease on artificial cell-free media, though in this respect *M. leprae* and *T pallidum* are exceptions, for neither has been cultured artificially as yet. The bacterial cell is complete, and contains DNA in its nuclear body and RNA in its cytoplasm.

RICKETTSIAE

Rickettsiae are unicellular organisms about 0.4 μm (400 nm) in size, and are visible under the light microscope. They resemble bacteria in reproducing by asexual binary fission, possessing both DNA and RNA, and having a *cell wall* containing muramic acid. They differ from bacteria in that they require living cells for growth, i.e. they are *obligatory intracellular parasites*. The rickettsiae produce the typhus group of fevers which have a world-wide distribution, and are transmitted by arthropods like lice, fleas, ticks, and mites, e.g. epidemic typhus is caused by *R. prowazeki* transmitted by lice. Another condition caused by a rickettsia is Q (query) fever, a febrile disease with chest symptoms. The causal organism *Coxiella burnetii* is somewhat smaller than those of typhus.

CHLAMYDIAE

These organisms have much in common with the rickettsiae but are smaller and more rudimentary. They also are obligatory intracellular parasites. Parasitized cells contain characteristic inclusion bodies, which are microcolonies of the organism.

Two species are recognized—*Chlamydia trachomatis* and *Chlamydia psittaci*.

Chlamydia trachomatis

Chlamydia trachomatis consists of a number of different serotypes which are responsible for various conjunctival and genital infections.

Hyperendemic trachoma. This is the most severe ocular disease caused by a group of serotypes and is responsible for blinding millions of people especially in Africa and Asia. It starts as a chronic conjunctivitis characterized by proliferation of the conjunctival epithelium and a heavy infiltration of the subepithelial tissues with lymphocytes and macrophages. The epithelium undergoes necrosis, and the subsequent ulceration and scarring cause the lids to become distorted by contractures. Furthermore, the inflammatory process involves the cornea and leads to ulceration. The deeper layers of the cornea are infiltrated by inflammatory cells, and there is progressive vascularization, thereby forming a *pannus*, which is subsequently replaced by scar tissue. Thus the cornea becomes opaque. The disease is transmitted from eye to eye.

Chlamydial urethritis and cervicitis. Another group of serotypes is an important cause of sexually transmitted genital infection. Chlamydial urethritis causes about half the cases of nongonococcal urethritis in males. In females the infection is often not evident clinically but it accounts for some cases of salpingitis and pelvic inflammatory disease. An acute conjunctivitis (*chlamydial ophthalmia neonatorum*) can occur as a result of infection of a baby during birth.

Paratrachoma. A variety of clinical types of conjunctivitis are caused by chlamydia; the most severe is endemic trachoma which clinically resembles hyperendemic trachoma.

Lymphogranuloma venereum. This sexually transmitted disease is caused by the L1, L2 and L3 serotypes. It is predominantly a disease of tropical countries. It starts as a small genital papule which ulcerates and is followed in about 2 weeks by regional lymphadenitis, usually of a suppurative nature. During the healing stage there may be much scarring with lymphatic obstruction. This has serious effects in the female and can cause vaginal or rectal stenosis.

Chlamydia psittaci

Chlamydia psittaci causes *psittacosis* in the human subject, and similar diseases in birds (ornithosis), particularly those of the parrot family (psittacine birds) but also in other related species. The diseases are acquired by inhaling the infected aerosol or dust from birds which may have been handled as pets or killed for eating.

The disease is an acute interstitial pneumonia and clinically may resemble influenza with rapid recovery, or else there may be progression to a severe pneumonia and death.

MYCOPLASMAS

Mycoplasmas comprise a group of minute organisms about 200–250 nm in size that are able to grow in artificial cell-free media. They possess no cell wall but only a limiting membrane. The result is *extreme fragility* and *pleomorphism*: granules, rings, coccoid forms, and fine filaments are all described. Because of their small size they pass through very fine filters, yet they resemble bacteria in being able to grow on artificial cell-free media.

The only definite human pathogen is *Mycoplasma pneumoniae* which causes a mild, but sometimes protracted form of pneumonia. It responds well to tetracyclines. Mycoplasmas are also found in the mouth and genito-urinary tract, but it is doubtful whether they are pathogenic.

L-forms. These were first described by Klieneberger-Nobel working at the Lister Institute, London (L stands for Lister). When certain bacteria are faced with adverse circumstances, they swell up (and possibly fuse) into a large mass which then disintegrates into irregularly spherical granules which are plastic, refractile, and very fragile. They are minute, measuring 100–500 nm in diameter. They are penicillin-resistant irrespective of the general sensitivity of the strain from which they are derived. L-forms have been described in *Strep. viridans*, *Esch. coli*, and many other species. They bear a close resemblance to *Mycoplasma* organisms. An L-form returns to type when conditions are normal and their role in human disease is uncertain.

VIRUSES

Viruses are small obligatory intracellular parasites that are distinct from all other organisms in that during the process of multiplication they enter a non-infective 'eclipse' phase. Viruses do not possess all the enzyme systems capable of synthetizing viral material; they are therefore dependent on the parasitized cell for survival and multiplication. Indeed, the essential difference between viruses and other organisms is that the synthetic processes that attend multiplication take place within the protoplasm of the infected cells in the case of viruses, but in the body of the organism itself in other infective agents.

GENERAL PROPERTIES OF VIRUSES

Size. Among the largest of the true viruses is the pox group responsible for smallpox, vaccinia, and similar diseases in other species of animals. These are about 250 nm in size, and a single virus particle when suitably stained is just visible under the light microscope.

Most viruses are less than 200 nm in size— varicella virus is 150–120 nm, and one of the smallest, that of foot-and-mouth disease, is only 20 nm.

Many viruses are spherical in shape, e.g. polio- virus, herpes-simplex virus, and adenovirus, some are filamentous, e.g. tobacco-mosaic virus and influenza virus, while bacteriophage has a characteristic tadpole shape. (Fig. 16.3)

Chemical constituents. The basic composi- tion of a virus particle, or *virion* (also called an

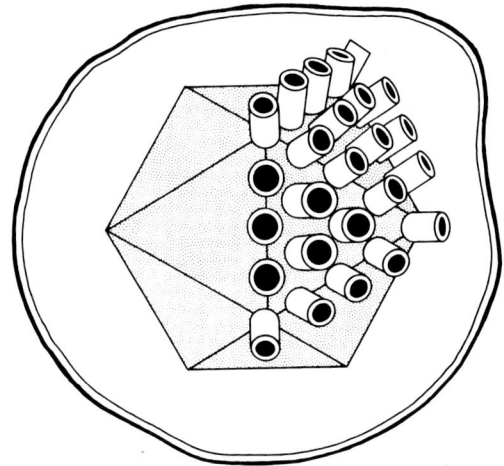

Fig. 16.2 Diagrammatic representation of a typical virus showing cubical symmetry. The core of the virus has the form of an icosahedron having 20 facets. It is covered by symmetrically arranged capsomeres, each consisting of a hollow tube. The covering of capsomeres constitutes the viral capsid. The virion (consisting of the genetic material and the capsid) has an outer membrane that is derived from the altered host plasma membrane or nuclear membrane. Not all such viruses possess an outer membrane. (Drawing by Frederick Lammerich, University of Toronto.)

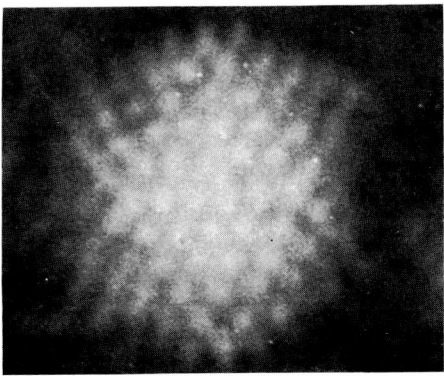

Fig. 16.1 A single particle (elementary body) of adenovirus embedded in electron-opaque phosphotungstate. The negatively-stained particle viewed under the electron microscope is seen to be composed of morphological units (capsomeres) of spherical shape packed in a symmetrical arrangement. It has been calculated that the total number of capsomeres around the central core of an adenovirus is 252. × 480 000. (From Horne R W, Brenner S, Waterson A P, Wildy P 1959 *Journal of Molecular Biology 1:84*.)

elementary body), is a nucleic-acid core surround- ed by a protein envelope called a *capsid*. In some viruses, e.g. herpesviruses and adenoviruses, the nucleic acid is DNA, whereas in others, e.g. the enteroviruses and myxoviruses, it is RNA. The heart of a virus is its nucleic-acid portion, for this controls the synthesis of new viral material when it infects a host cell.

The protein envelope is composed of sub-units built in a compact, regular manner around the nucleic-acid core. These protein sub-units are called *capsomeres*, and their arrangement is related to the shape of the virus. In spherical viruses they show a cubical or icosahedral symmetry, i.e. they are disposed around the core in the form of a regular icosahedron (a solid bounded by 20 plane surfaces each of which is an equilateral triangle). This is demonstrated in Figs 16.1 and 16.2. Filamentous (or rod-shaped) viruses are sur- rounded by a helix of protein sub-units, i.e. they are arranged in a spiral around the central rod.

The tadpole-shaped bacteriophage has a binal symmetry in its capsid, meaning that it is arranged differently around the head as compared with the tail.

Some viruses are also ensheathed in one or more outer, lipid-containing membranes, or envelopes, composed predominantly of lipid, derived from the modified host cell or nuclear membrane prior to the release of the virus. Enveloped viruses, e.g. herpesviruses, myxoviruses, and togaviruses, are vulnerable to fat solvents such as ether and bile salts. The larger viruses, especially poxviruses, also contain carbohydrates, co-enzymes, and even some enzymes, e.g. lipase, catalase, and phosphatase, but none contains all the enzymes necessary for the metabolism of its own substance. It is for this reason that viruses are obligatory intracellular parasites.

Life-cycle and reproduction. The life-cycle of a virus is intracellular, and the details vary according to the virus, but the basic steps are similar for all viruses.

The first stage is the attachment of the virus to a specific *cell receptor*, or *receptor site*, on the cell membrane. This *attachment phase* is followed by *penetration* of the virus into the cell.

With bacteriophage the naked DNA is injected into the interior of the bacterium, while the protein coat, which acts as a microsyringe, remains exterior attached to the bacterial wall (Fig.16.3). The mode of penetration of animal viruses is different, and both pinocytosis and phagocytosis

are involved. The next step is removal of the protein coat and release of the viral nucleic acid into the cytoplasm of the cell. The virus now ceases to exist as a particle. This is the all-important eclipse phase and the virus may not even be infectious; it can only be detected by a suitable probe.

The next step is viral multiplication which entails utilization of the cell's own metabolic systems and terminates with the production of new virions. The precise mechanism is complex and varies from one virus to another.

With *DNA viruses*, the DNA encodes for mRNA (by convention termed +RNA) which passes to host ribosomes and leads to the formation of enzymes that ultimately are responsible for the formation of new viral DNA and viral type proteins. When the nucleic acid and nuclear proteins are assembled a new virion is produced.

With *RNA viruses* the mode of replication is more varied. With *plus-stranded RNA viruses* the viral RNA acts as messenger RNA, and also leads to the formation of a complementary RNA molecule from which new viral RNA can be made. With *minus-stranded RNA viruses*, a complementary RNA is formed and this acts as mRNA. *Retroviruses*, some of which cause tumours, have a unique mode of reproduction. They contain a DNA polymerase that leads to the formation of complementary DNA provirus.

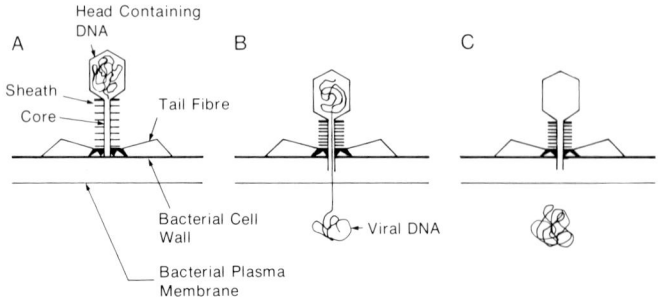

Fig. 16.3 Diagrammatic representation of the entry of bacteriophage into a bacterial cell. The bacteriophage consists of a head containing DNA, a rigid core surrounded by a sheath to which is attached a tail piece, and tail fibres. *A*. The first event in the entry of the phage is the attachment of the tail fibres to the receptors of the bacterial cell wall. *B*. Contraction of the sheath results in the injection of viral DNA into the bacterial cell substance. *C*. The protein component of the phage shown attached to the cell wall is subsequently lost, leaving the viral DNA within the substance of the bacterium. Here it can replicate and lead to lysis of the bacterial cell, or it can remain latent as prophage. (Drawn by Sue Reynolds.)

This may become incorporated into the cell's genome.

The last stage in the formation of mature virions is release from the infected cell. If the cell has been so damaged that it disintegrates the mature virus particles are released in a burst-like fashion. In other instances the viruses are released slowly and in the process may become covered by a layer of nuclear or cell membrane which forms a capsule for the virus. The membrane is not completely normal membrane but one that has been modified during the period of release, which takes about an hour. After release the virus enters other cells either by direct contact or after carriage by body fluids.

Virus-infected cells may sometimes produce a mass of homogeneous material termed an inclusion body (Fig. 16.4) either in the nucleus or the cytoplasm. The inclusion body often consists of a mass of maturing virus particles and its morphology may be of diagnostic importance, for instance the cytoplasmic eosinophilic Negri body found in the neurons in rabies. Characteristic intranuclear inclusions are found in epidermal cells in varicella-zoster and herpes simplex.

Reaction to environment. Unlike bacteria, most viruses are easily inactivated even at room temperature, and care must be taken to keep specimens frozen, if possible at $-70°C$. A few viruses are much more stable than this, however, and the viruses of poliomyelitis and vaccinia can survive at ordinary atmospheric temperatures for some weeks. The hepatitis viruses appear to be particularly resistant, but the most durable agent is that of scrapie, which withstands boiling for 3 h.

Reaction to chemicals. Viruses are destroyed without difficulty by the chemical disinfectants, such as chlorine in the form of bleach, used against bacteria; the scrapie virus is an exception, being able to survive in strong formalin solutions. One important property of viruses is their great resistance to a 50% solution of glycerol, which kills non-sporing bacteria quite rapidly. Vaccinia virus is actually preserved in glycerol. No virus is susceptible to any antibiotic therapy in current use, but a few specific chemotherapeutic agents are now known.

Cultivation of viruses. Viruses multiply only in living cells, and at first the only systems that could be used were experimental animals and chick embryos. *Animal inoculation* is reserved for those viruses which do not grow satisfactorily in *tissue culture*, e.g. some Coxsackie viruses. Nowadays the vast majority of viruses are cultivated in tissue culture, a method which is cheap, simple, and efficacious. The basis of this technique is that living cells are grown on the sides of test-tubes. Many viruses are able to multiply in these cells, in which they produce destructive changes. This is called a *cytopathic effect*, and is illustrated in Figs 16.5 to 16.7. The changes are sometimes characteristic of a specific virus, but in any case the virus can be identified by *neutralization tests* and *complement fixation* using specific rabbit antisera. If, for instance, a specific antiserum prevents a cytopathic effect in a cell system (or for that matter, if it prevents a lesion in an egg or a test animal), the virus is typed accordingly. The fluid in the tissue-culture system provides the virus antigen for performing complement fixation tests. The cell systems commonly employed in this way are monkey kidney cells, human amnion cells, and strains of cancer cells, e.g. the 'HeLa cell' derived from a carcinoma of the cervix of a woman named Helen Lane.

CLASSIFICATION OF VIRUSES.

It was once popular to classify viruses on the basis of the organ or tissue that they affected. This proved to be quite unsatisfactory because one virus can infect several different tissues and produce a wide array of clinical pictures. For example, herpes simplex virus can cause localized cold sores, a severe pneumonitis or a fulminating encephalitis. At present viruses are classified on the basis of their morphology, nucleic acid content, mode of reproduction and the disease that they cause. The classification is complex, and the reader is referred to virology texts for details.

TISSUE REACTIONS TO VIRUSES

All considerations of the effects of viruses on the tissues of the body must start at a cellular level; viruses are intracellular parasites, and the damage they produce is directed primarily at the cell. This

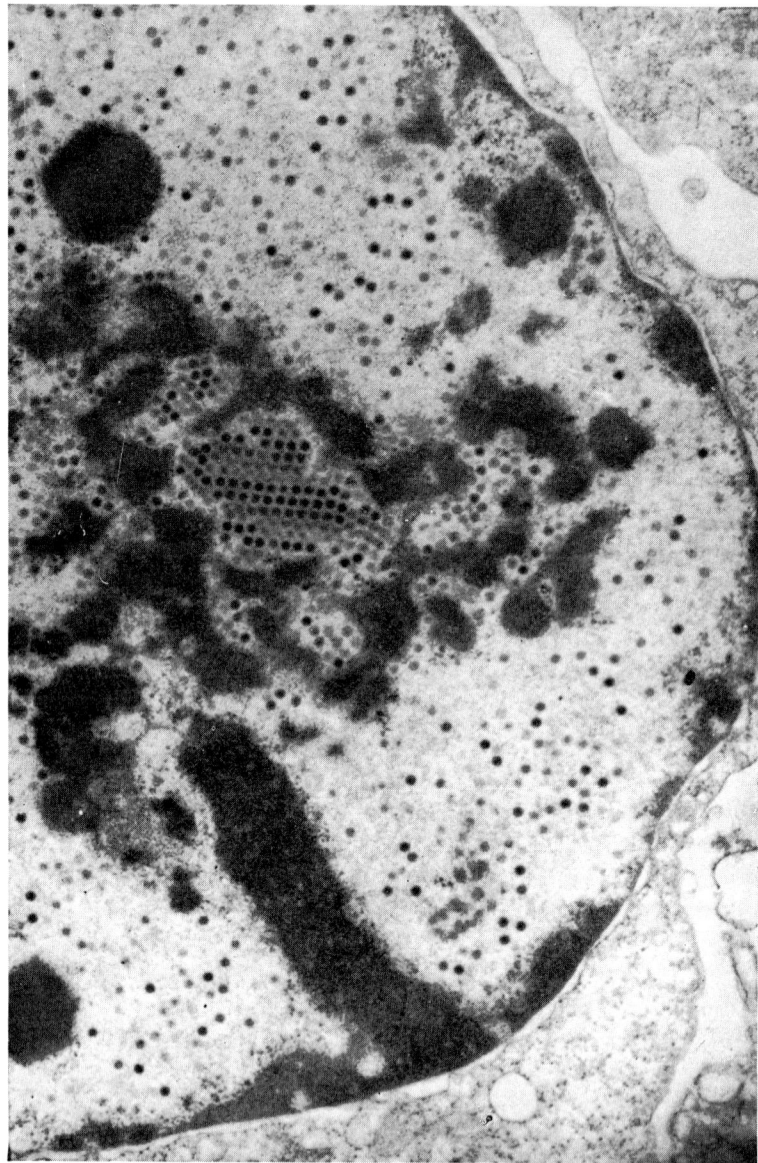

Fig. 16.4   Nuclear inclusion induced by adenovirus 12. The virus crystals in the centre are surrounded by very dense material with irregular contours. Many virus particles are dispersed in the nucleoplasm. × 24 000. (From Bernhard W 1964 In: de Reuck A V S, Knight J (eds) *Cellular injury, a Ciba Foundation Symposium.* Churchill, London, p. 215.)

is followed secondarily by a local inflammatory reaction.

Cellular reaction

A cell infected with a virus may degenerate at once, or it may undergo proliferation which may or may not be followed by later necrosis, or it may show no change whatsoever. This last effect is typical of what is called 'latent virus' infection. It is well known, for example, that many people harbour herpes simplex virus without showing any lesion. Similarly, many children are infected with certain types of adenoviruses early in life,

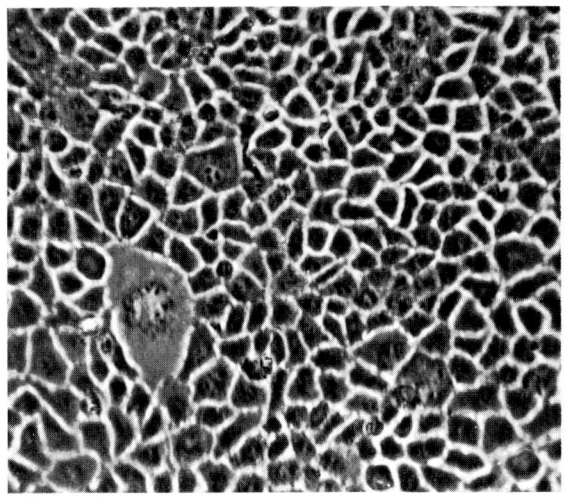

Fig. 16.5 Normal HeLa cells. Note the confluent sheet of plump polygonal cells with a conspicuous giant form. They are derived from a malignant epithelial cell line. (McCarthy phase contrast × 200.)

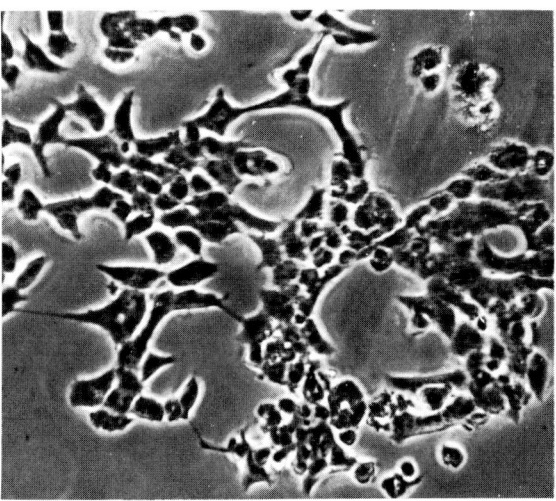

Fig. 16.6 HeLa cells infected with adenovirus. The sheet has been broken up, and the swollen, refractile cells form irregular masses. (McCarthy phase contrast × 200.)

and these remain in their tonsils and adenoids without producing conspicuous damage.

Whether a cell degenerates or proliferates depends on the type of cell involved and on the nature of the infecting virus. Labile cells, like those of surface epithelia, undergo continuous division throughout life, and so it is not surpri-

sing that some viral conditions of the skin have a proliferative tendency, e.g. verruca vulgaris.

Other cells described as permanent, e.g. neurons, cannot divide after birth, and viral infection of these is necessarily always destructive in tendency.

In most human viral diseases cellular destruction is the predominant lesion. The respiratory viruses destroy the surface epithelium, a tendency well marked in influenza, the viruses of hepatitis and yellow fever produce a characteristic necrosis of the liver, mumps produces destructive lesions of the acinar cells of the salivary glands and sometimes the pancreas, while the central nervous system may sustain permanent neuronal loss a result of poliomyelitis and viral encephalitis.

Once the infection is overcome, there is rapid healing due to proliferation of neighbouring cells. The focal necrosis of hepatitis A virus heals so rapidly that needle biopsy of the liver performed after a few months may reveal no abnormality whatsoever. Neuronal destruction can be healed only by repair, i.e. gliosis, and hence permanent damage must sometimes be expected. It should be noted, however, that not every neuron infected with poliovirus is necessarily doomed. Many recover completely.

Inflammatory reaction

Secondary to the cellular damage there is a nondescript acute inflammatory reaction in the vicinity. This takes the form of vascular dilatation and an exudate containing lymphocytes and macrophages. Polymorphs are usually few in number. Most viral diseases are acute and of short duration, terminating in either rapid death or recovery. Exceptions to this are the tumour-producing viruses and certain slow viruses.

Viral infections of epithelial surfaces are often complicated by secondary bacterial invasion: influenza is commonly followed by bacterial pneumonia.

It is noteworthy that viral infections, even the chronic ones, do not bring forth a predominantly macrophage response. Epithelioid-cell formation is never seen, nor indeed is any viral infection characterized by a granulomatous reaction.

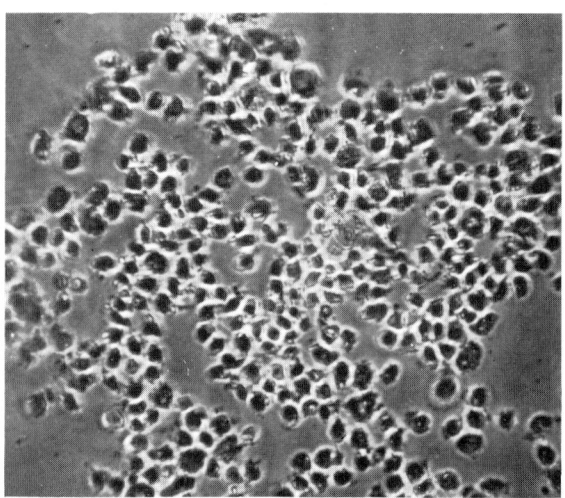

Fig. 16.7 HeLa cells infected with poliovirus. Note the severe disintegration of the cells. Poliovirus has a more destructive effect on cell cultures than does adenovirus. (McCarthy phase contrast × 200.)

THE GENERAL BODY REACTION TO VIRAL INFECTION

Localization. Like other organisms, viruses first contaminate and infect a surface integument, either by inhalation (e.g. influenza), ingestion (e.g. poliomyelitis), or by the bite of an arthropod vector (e.g. yellow fever). Some viruses remain localized to their tissues of entry, e.g. verruca vulgaris virus and the rhinoviruses, while others become disseminated throughout the blood stream, and produce lesions in an organ remote from the sites of primary infection, e.g. poliomyelitis and yellow fever, or else lead to a generalized viral infection involving many organs, e.g. measles. The systemic type of infection is associated with much more pronounced constitutional symptoms than the localized one, and a characteristic feature is the presence of high fever during the early viraemic phase. This is often followed by a remission, which is in turn succeeded by another spurt of pyrexia when the virus becomes clinically localized at its organ of destination. Localized diseases like the common cold and verruca vulgaris are accompanied by little, if any, constitutional upset.

Dissemination. The mode of dissemination of a virus in the body has been investigated with respect to mouse-pox. The virus enters the mouse's body through an abrasion in its skin, and multiplies there. Within 8 h the virus reaches the local lymph nodes, and after further multiplication it invades the blood stream and is taken up by the MP cells of the liver and spleen. There it multiplies once more, and after 6 days it invades the blood stream in large amounts, and settles selectively in the epidermal cells of the skin. This phase of viraemia is accompanied by severe constitutional effects; still another 4 days elapse before a rash appears.

The initial 6 days of infection constitute the *incubation period*; the 4 days of severe illness, which may prove fatal in overwhelming infections, are the *prodromal period*. During this time virus material may still be cultured from the blood, but once the rash appears (10th day) there is a rapidly rising level of neutralizing antibody in the circulation. Human diseases like smallpox and measles have a somewhat similar pattern of dissemination, but the route of entry is through the respiratory tract.

Transplacental infection of the fetus is important in rubella infections and may lead to congenital abnormalities. Other viral diseases transmitted across the placenta are herpes-simplex infection and Coxsackie-virus myocarditis.

Antibody response. Viral infections are accompanied by a high titre of immunoglobulins during the period of convalescence. The highest antibody response is encountered in those viruses which are widely disseminated in the circulation, and a life-long *immunity* may be expected after diseases like smallpox, measles, and mumps. Localized infections, like the common cold, also induce antibodies, but the degree of immunity is small, and recurrence is common. It must also be remembered that many viruses are of more than one type, e.g. there are three types of poliovirus and many types of human adenovirus. This is an additional reason for recurrent attacks of certain infections.

The element of *hypersensitivity* is also noteworthy in viral infections. The accelerated reaction following a second vaccination is a good example of allergy to vaccinia virus. The lesion appears within a day or two and resolves after about 1 week, whereas a primary vaccination reaction appears on the fourth or fifth day and reaches its zenith on about the 10th day. It takes about 3 weeks to heal and is occasionally complicated by systemic lesions. The close resemblance of this to the Koch phenomenon is obvious, except that here the element of immunity is much greater than in tuberculosis.

There is a strong element of hypersensitivity in the skin eruption that occurs in the course of generalized infections like smallpox and measles. In such conditions there is an incubation period of about 2 weeks, and the skin is sensitized to viral products before the virus reaches it in full force. The analogy to the later intestinal ulceration of typhoid fever is very close.

Mechanism of the pathogenic effects of viruses

Viruses produce their harmful effects by virtue of the cell destruction they cause; no factors comparable with bacterial toxins have been demonstrated. It is believed that the cytotoxic effect of viruses is due to complex biochemical disturbances that accompany virus replication. In addition, there is also a delayed type of hypersensitivity.

The cause of death in viral disease is obvious when a vital organ in damaged directly, e.g. the liver in hepatitis. In the pox diseases the mode of death is less easily explained. Clinically there is a state of 'shock' reminiscent of the toxaemia of invasive bacterial infections, and it is suggested that this is due to virus invasion and damage of vascular endothelial cells.

Immunity to viral infections

The mechanism of immunity to viral infection is complex and has several components.

Immunoglobulins. Immunoglobulins play an important part, especially in the disseminated infections. Viruses have a number of antigens, some associated with the nucleoprotein and others with the capsid and outer envelope. It is against these last two antigens that immunoglobulins act; by neutralizing them they prevent the virus attaching itself to a cell receptor. The extracellular complex is phagocytosed and destroyed. Intracellular virus is invulnerable to

antibody. These plasma, virus-neutralizing immunoglobulins belong to the 1gG class.

It is also to be noted that after recovery from an attack of poliomyelitis or following immunization with living attenuated virus administered orally, a subsequent dose of poliovirus does not flourish in the cells of the small bowel. This is due to the action of IgA antibodies produced locally in the intestine and present in the secretions. People who have been immunized with a killed suspension of poliovirus administered parenterally usually exhibit unhindered virus multiplication in the small bowel despite a considerable antibody response.

Cell-mediated immunity. This plays an even more important role in viral infections than do the immunoglobulins. Thus in states of pure immunoglobulin deficiency (hypogammaglobulinaemia) there is usually an effective host response to systemic viral infections, whereas in states of T-lymphocyte deficiency chronic, progressive, fatal viral infections, e.g. chickenpox, herpes simplex, and cytomegalic inclusion disease, are extremely common. The part the lymphocyte plays in viral infection is still obscure. It is known that a sensitized lymphocyte secretes interferon among the lymphokines; in addition, it is possible that cytotoxic lymphocytes destroy the virus-infected cell directly, thereby killing intracellular virus.

Interferons. The name interferon was coined in the late 1950s by Isaacs and Lindermann to describe a substance produced by a cell in response to viral exposure that enabled neighbouring cells to resist viral infection. It is now known that the interferons are a group of glycoproteins produced by cells in response to a variety of stimuli, including exposure to viruses, mitogens and a variety of compounds that stimulate the immune response. There are three groups depending on the cell that produces them. Interferon-α (INF-α) is produced by leucocytes, INF-β by fibroblasts and INF-γ by T lymphocytes. The secreted interferon molecules bind to surface receptors on other cells and lead to derepression of target cell genes and the production of a spectrum of proteins, of which only a few have been characterized. These proteins induce an antiviral state within the cells through interference with viral replication at many points. In addition, interferons act as immunomodulatory lymphokines which augment the antiviral effect. They also have an anti-tumour effect by inhibiting cell proliferation.

Interferons are species-specific and their investigation and use has been impeded by the limited quantities available. Recombinant DNA techniques have now yielded the larger quantities needed for therapeutic testing. Clinical trials have demonstrated activity against a variety of viruses including certain herpesviruses, papilloma viruses and hepatitis B virus. Interferons have also been used in the treatment of tumours, but unfortunately many trials have yielded somewhat inconclusive results. They are most effective against certain skin tumours, lymphomas and leukaemias. Toxic side-effects have limited their use, and clinical applications are still largely investigational.

Chemotherapy of viral diseases

The highly specific series of events that take place from initial attachment of a virus to a cell to the final release of mature virions has been closely studied, and many chemicals have been found that will block this sequence, although unfortunately many of them are toxic.

Most currently available antiviral agents are analogues of nucleosides and inhibit DNA and RNA synthesis. The original nucleoside analogues, 5-iodo-2-deoxyuridine (5-IDU) and cytosine arabinoside developed as anti-tumour drugs in the 1950s and 1960s have been largely replaced by more selective, less toxic agents. Acyclovir, a guanosine analogue, was found to have remarkable antiviral specificity. The drug is phosphorylated by virus-specified thymidine kinase. Within the infected cell it is further phosphorylated and in this active form inhibits virus-specific DNA polymerase and therefore prevents viral replication when incorporated into viral DNA polymerase. Acyclovir is therefore useful in the treatment of certain infections caused by herpes simplex types I and II, and varicella zoster. Resistance to acyclovir has been demonstrated by viral mutants with altered expression of the thymidine kinase gene. For-

tunately, drug resistance during therapy is unusual.

Ganciclovir is a closely related drug useful in the treatment of cytomegalovirus infection. Ribavin, another guanosine analogue shows activity against certain RNA viruses (e.g. influenza, parainfluenza and respiratory syncytial viruses), human immunodeficiency virus and Lassa fever virus.

Amantadine has been useful as a prophylactic agent during outbreaks of influenza. It seem to act by preventing uncoating viral particles.

Much attention has been focused recently in the use of azidothymidine (AZT) for the treatment of AIDS (HIV infection). AZT is a thymine analogue which when phosphorylated inhibits the activity of reverse transcriptase, an enzyme critical in the replication of this RNA retrovirus.

Interferons as antiviral agents have already been mentioned. The challenge for the future rests on the development of more specific, non-toxic agents, through greater understanding of viral replication cycles. It may also be important to explore new synergistic combinations of drugs to reduce toxic side-effects and prevent the emergence of resistant strains of virus.

THE DIAGNOSIS OF VIRAL DISEASE

In a few instances diagnostic *inclusion bodies* may be found (e.g. Negri bodies in rabies), or characteristic *elementary bodies* may be seen by light microscopy (e.g. Paschen bodies in the vesicles of vaccinia).

An important diagnostic procedure is the isolation of the virus from the patient's secretions using the living-cell systems already described. The virus may then be typed by means of complement fixation and neutralization tests using specific rabbit antisera. Some viruses with a characteristic shape can be identified by electron microscopy. With negative-contrast techniques virus may be detected within a few minutes of collecting the specimen, provided it is present at concentrations greater than about 10^6 per ml. For practical purposes this limits its use to examining specimens obtained from readily accessible sites which contain high concentrations of virus, e.g. poxviruses and herpesviruses from skin lesions and rotaviruses, adenoviruses, and hepatitis A virus from the faeces. The technique of immune electron microscopy can distinguish between antigenically distinct but morphologically identical viruses; it consists of the detection of immune complexes after the specimen has been pre-incubated with a virus-specific antiserum.

Immunoflourescence techniques are also valuable in the rapid diagnosis of viral disease, and they are more sensitive than electron microscopy especially now that the quality of the reagents is satisfactory enough to minimize the amount of non-specific fluorescence. They are particularly useful in examining brain material for herpes-simplex virus and rabies virus and nasopharyngeal secretions for respiratory viruses.

Various *transport media* are available for conveying unfrozen specimens to the laboratory. The media consist of neutral balanced salt solutions containing a protein (e.g. bovine serum albumin) and antibiotics. Viruses survive in transport medium for a number of hours or days according to the organism. In practice, a specimen should be sent to the laboratory as soon as possible and preferably the same day that it has been collected.

ANTIGEN DETECTION IN DIAGNOSIS

The detection of viral antigen in blood or tissue fluids is a rapid and valuable aid to diagnosis in certain viral infections. It has found particular application in the investigation of patients and carriers of hepatitis B virus. The antigens are estimated by a variety of immunological techniques. Radioimmunoassay (RIA) is the most sensitive, commonly used method, but more recently the enzyme-linked immunosorbent assay (ELISA) and countercurrent immuno-electro-osmophoresis (CIEOP) have been introduced.[*]

Examination of convalescent serum. In convalescent patients there is invariably a rise in titre of antibodies against the agent. It is therefore important to obtain a sample of serum as early in the disease as possible (this furnishes a baseline against which to judge the subsequent rise), as well as a second specimen 10–14 days later. Antibodies may be estimated by a variety of tests including complement fixation, neutralization, RIA,[*] ELISA,[*] and indirect immunofluorescent techniques.

In practice retrospective diagnosis made on serological grounds is the most important method of diagnosing viral disease.

SOME COMMON VIRAL INFECTIONS

Enteroviruses

The enteroviruses are a group of small, spherical, RNA-containing viruses found particularly in the cells of the intestine. They are members of a larger group called the *picornaviruses* (pico = small + RNA), to which the rhinoviruses that cause the common cold also belong. The enteroviruses are especially associated with neurological diseases. There are three subgroups:

Coxsackie viruses

These were first isolated in the town of Coxsackie in New York State in 1948, and are found quite frequently in the faeces of healthy children. Many types have been isolated and they are responsible for a variety of clinical pictures including an upper respiratory, cold-like condition, and an illness which resembles paralytic poliomyelitis. They also cause *herpangina*, a febrile disease of children in which there are shallow greyish ulcers in the mouth and fauces, and *Bornholm disease*, in which there is agonizing chest pain.

ECHO (enteric, cytopathic, human, orphan) viruses

There are at least 34 types. They are found quite commonly in children's faeces, and for a long

---

[*]Radioimmunoassay methods are used to estimate a wide range of substances, eg. viral antigens, antibodies, and hormones. Thus to estimate HBsAg, a quantity of antibody is attached to a suitable surface (the solid phase). This is allowed to react with patient's serum, and subsequently radioactive-labelled antibody is applied. By estimating the amount of radioactivity attached to the surface, the titre of antigen may be calculated. The enzyme-linked immunosorbent assay (ELISA) utilizes an enzyme as a marker instead of radioactive iodine. It is therefore a safer method for laboratory workers. In countercurrent immuno-electro-osmophoresis (CIEOP) the two reacting components are driven together under the influence of an electric field. This is less wasteful of reagents (and therefore a more sensitive method) than if the components simply diffused passively towards each other as in the original Ouchterlony precipitin method.

time could not be associated with any disease—hence the name 'orphan'. It is now known that they produce a variety of febrile illnesses including some which mimic poliomyelitis and the common cold.

Polioviruses

Poliomyelitis is caused by the three types of poliovirus, of which type 1 produces the most severe disease. The disease is contracted by the ingestion of material which has been contaminated by virus-containing faeces. Faecal pollution of drinking water or swimming baths is a possible danger, as is also fly-borne contamination of food. Indirect contact with excretors, whose dirty hands contaminate fomites, is another source of infection.

Spread of virus in the body. It is believed that the virus proliferates first in the cells of the pharynx and the lower part of the small bowel. If it is not arrested at this stage, it enters the general circulation via the lymphatics, and it then multiplies in various extraneural sites like the spleen and kidneys. This marks the end of the incubation period, which usually lasts 7–14 days, but may extend up to 30 days. The next viraemic phase is ushered in by a febrile reaction, but even then the infection may be overcome. If the condition proceeds, the virus settles finally in the central nervous system which it reaches by the blood stream. It localizes itself specifically in the anterior horn cells and their brain stem counterparts. Some of the infected cells die and paralysis ensues.

A second mode of spread is directly up the peripheral nerve endings of the bowel and especially the pharynx. Opinions vary about the importance of this method of spread; it probably accounts for the bulbar type of disease that sometimes follows tonsillectomy and other operative procedures in the mouth.

It is evident that much has still to be learned about the pathogenesis of the disease. Poliomyelitis is an excellent example of an infection that tends to be subclinical. Many people are infected with poliomyelitis, and either show no illness at all or else have a mild febrile reaction. Only a small unlucky minority develop paralysis.

Factors aggravating the disease. The incubation period is shortened, and the liability to nervous-system involvement increased by the following factors: heavy exercise and fatigue, pregnancy, operative procedures, and active immunization with any antigen. When the disease follows immunization, it is called *provocation poliomyelitis*; it is believed that alum and other adjuvants in the vaccines and toxoids are the important factors. The mode of action is unknown, but it has been suggested that the focus of imflammation acts as a nidus for proliferation of the virus during the period of viraemia. It might then travel up the local nerve to the spinal cord. Active immunization procedures should be postponed during a poliomyelitis epidemic. So also should minor surgery, e.g. dental extraction.

Immunization. A consideration of poliomyelitis immunization is valuable as a general exercise in comparing the relative merits of dead suspensions to those of live attenuated viruses.

The first effective vaccine was devised by Salk, who used polioviruses grown in monkey kidney cells and subsequently inactivated by formolization. It is issued in trivalent form, containing types 1, 2, and 3, and requires at least three intramuscular inoculations, the second a month after the first, and the third about 6 months after the second. A high titre of circulating immunoglobulin should be produced, though often there is a disappointing response to type-1 virus, the most dangerous of the three. Immunity depends on the presence of IgG antibody. The resistance of the cells of the small bowel to subsequent infection by poliovirus is not altered.

The live attenuated vaccine developed by Sabin is given by mouth. It causes intestinal infection that simulates the natural disease except that spread to the central nervous system does not occur. IgG antibodies are produced as with Salk vaccine, but in addition IgA is produced in the intestine. The immunized subject is therefore immune to future infection by the poliovirus. Live virus is passed in the faeces and almost inevitably infects other people. In this way large populations have been infected and the Sabin strain of virus has largely replaced the wild, more virulent strains. Indeed the few cases of poliomyelitis that do occur are usually due to

Sabin-derived strains. Thus the Sabin vaccine produces good immunity; it is easy to administer and is the more popular of the two methods.

The oral vaccine has supplanted the inactivated one because it gives a better, long-lasting immunity and it acts more rapidly in a threatened epidemic. Despite its general safety it should not be given within 3 weeks of tonsillectomy or any immunization procedure.

Poxviruses

The poxviruses are a group of large DNA-containing viruses which produce vesicular and pustular skin lesions. Many animals have their own variety of pox disease, e.g. cow-pox, mouse-pox, etc. The human disease is smallpox, a disease that has now become extinct. The last case reported was in 1978, in Birmingham, England. No known carrier state exists, and apart from strains possibly kept at reference laboratories the virus has died out.

Molluscum contagiosum is a localized skin infection caused by a pox virus.

Viruses affecting the respiratory tract

The number of viruses incriminated in respiratory infections is legion.

Orthomyxoviruses

The orthomyxoviruses are a group of medium-sized RNA-containing viruses. They are so named because they have a strong affinity for mucins. Thus, in vitro they can attach themselves to the mucoprotein receptors of red cells, and by forming bridges, cause the cells to agglutinate. The important human orthomyxoviruses are the *influenza viruses* of which there are three types. The *parainfluenza viruses* and the virus of *mumps* belong to a closely related group, the *paramyxoviruses*, which are slightly larger than the orthomyxoviruses.

Adenoviruses

The adenoviruses are small DNA-containing viruses which have proclivity for the mucosa of the upper respiratory tract and the conjunctiva.

Coronaviruses

These are a group of medium-sized, pleomorphic, RNA-containing viruses with a prominent envelope arranged into spikes, or peplomeres, which form a fringe of projections resembling petals. Their resemblance to a crown is the basis of the name coronavirus.

Many coronaviruses cause disease in animals, e.g. mouse hepatitis and avian infectious bronchitis. In the human being they are an important cause of respiratory tract infections of a cold-like type.

Rhinoviruses

The rhinoviruses cause the common cold, and are of interest in requiring a temperature of 33°C instead of 37°C for successful culture. Their habitat in the nose is probably related to this temperature requirement. More than 100 serotypes of this virus are known.

The arthropod-borne viruses

Arthropod-borne viruses cause yellow fever, dengue, sandfly fever, and a number of types of encephalitis of regional geographical distribution. Members of this group have been called *arboviruses*, but the group is in fact made up of several different families, e.g. *togaviruses* and *orbiviruses*. In addition to the diseases mentioned above, some arthropod-borne viruses cause *viral haemorrhagic fevers*. These are severe diseases which can also be caused by other viruses, e.g. the Marburg virus which was inadvertently imported from Germany in 1967.

Viral hepatitis

Although many viruses can cause hepatitis (e.g. Epstein–Barr virus and yellow fever virus), the term viral hepatitis is generally confined to a disease caused by one of at least three viruses: hepatitis A virus (HAV), hepatitis B virus (HBV), and the virus or viruses of non-A, non-B hepatitis. Clinically the three diseases cannot be distinguished.

Virus A hepatitis

This disease occurs endemically in institutions such as schools and army camps. Its main incidence is among children and young adults. Subclinical infection is common and many adults have protective antibodies.

Hepatitis A virus is a small RNA picornavirus with cubical symmetry that can be grown in special cell-culture systems. It is present in the faeces for 5 days, while the patient is incubating the disease, but soon disappears as clinical jaundice becomes evident. No carrier state exists and infection is via the faecal–oral route. The incubation period is 2–6 weeks and disease is generally mild: death or chronic hepatitis are almost unknown.

Virus B hepatitis

This type of viral hepatitis is transmitted by blood and before testing was possible was a common cause of post-transfusion jaundice. Very little contaminated blood is needed for transmission of the virus and the prick of a contaminated needle is adequate. It is a major hazard among drug addicts who share needles (mainliners). People who handle blood, such a laboratory technicians and workers in haemodialysis units, are also at risk. The virus is present in secretions and transmission by kissing and intercourse is possible. The infection is common in male homosexuals. Infected mothers can infect their baby during birth. The incubation period is 6 weeks to 6 months.

Hepatitis B virus is a double-shelled, 42 nm DNA-containing virus. It consists of core called the Dane particle and a shell. Each contains antigens. The core contains core antigen (HBcAg) as well as an e antigen, the presence of which in the blood indicates infectivity because it corresponds with the presence of intact infective particles. The surface antigen (HBsAg) was first called Australia antigen because it was originally found in an Australian aborigine. In the blood of carriers, excess HBsAg is present and forms 22nm spherical particles and long tubular structures (Fig.16.8). The delta virus is a defective

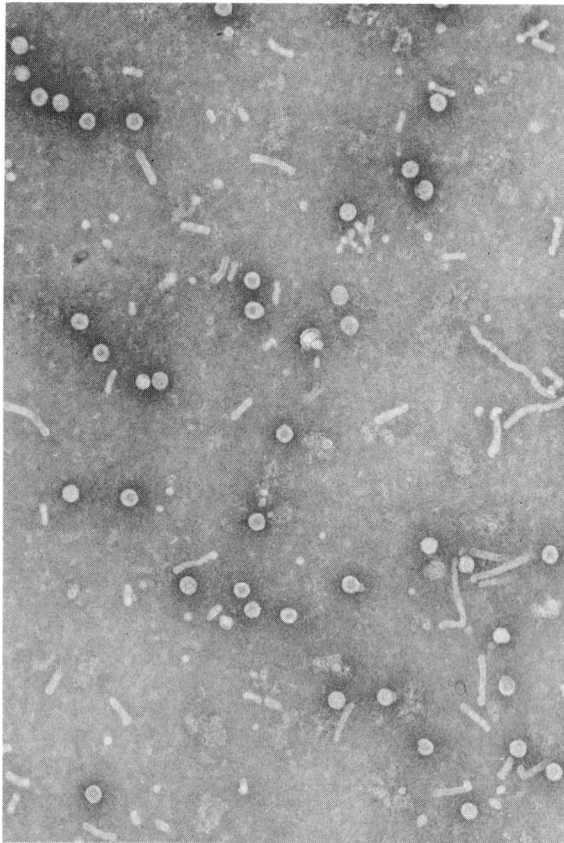

Fig. 16.8 Hepatitis B virus. This is a negative-stained preparation of hepatitis B positive serum. Three types of particles can be seen: spherical particles 20 nm in diameter; elongated, tubular filaments up to 230 nm in length; and Dane particles 42 nm in diameter and having a double shell. × 199 700. (Photograph by courtesy of Micheline Fauvel, Laboratoire de Santé Publique du Quebec, Sainte-Anne-de-Bellevue, Quebec, Canada.)

RNA virus that can only survive in the blood of carriers of HBV. Its presence contributes to the severity of HBV hepatitis.

Non-A, non-B hepatitis

The detection of HBV antigens in the serum of blood donors was an important advance and it was hoped that hepatitis would cease to be a hazard. Unfortunately, post-transfusional hepatitis continues to occur and the agent or agents have been termed non-A, non-B virus. One virus termed hepatitis C virus has been identified.

Virus A and virus B hepatitis

The diseases these two viruses produce are

pathologically very similar: a widespread focal necrosis which usually recovers by complete regeneration. Nevertheless, there are distinct clinical differences. Virus A hepatitis has a much shorter incubation period than virus B hepatitis (15–40 days as compared with 60–160 days). Although the clinical features of the two conditions are very similar, the mortality rate is 0.1% with virus A hepatitis and up to 10%, or even higher, with virus B hepatitis. Both can kill with a fulminating infection that leads to massive necrosis, but as yet there is no evidence that HAV infection leads to chronic liver disease. On the other hand, about 10% of cases of HBV infection progress to a chronic type of hepatitis, e.g. subacute or chronic active hepatitis, which may proceed to macronodular cirrhosis. Adults are more vulnerable than are children, and pregnant and older women are especially endangered. The most dangerous type of virus B infection is post-transfusion hepatitis, which has a mortality rate of from 10 to 20%. This is attributable to the large dose of virus received and the poor state of health of the patient which necessitated transfusion. The overall mortality rate is much less than this (about 1%).

Prophylactic passive immunization with γ-globulin is useful against HAV, but is of much less value in HBV infection because of the low antibody titre against HBV. Special high-titre HBV immunoglobulin is now available, and promises to be of value.

Virus B hepatitis is a good example of a condition in which antibodies can play a dangerous role in the progress of the disease. Immune-complex hypersensitivity effects, e.g. serum-sickness phenomena (urticaria and arthralgia) occur in 10–20% of cases some days or weeks before the symptoms of liver disease occur. Occasionally there may be glomerulonephritis or polyarteritis nodosa.

Furthermore, immunologically deficient people, e.g. lepromatous lepers, those on immuno-suppressants, and especially those with chronic renal failure, carry the antigen for long periods. Such people do not appear to suffer from liver damage, but they are potent transmitters of the agent. Many cases of hepatitis have occurred in doctors and nurses working in renal dialysis units, and a disturbingly high mortality rate has occurred in some centres.

In the general population the carrier rate varies from about 0.1% in the USA to over 10% in some of the Pacific Islands. Perhaps primitive conditions, including tattooing, play a part in carrying infection around the community. Transmission by mosquito bite is another possibility, as these insects have been shown to harbour HBsAg, but it has not been shown that they transmit the disease. Spread by bed bugs is a possibility.

It has been shown that HBV can spread naturally from person to person and that serum containing antigen is infectious when given by mouth. Thus the traditional teaching that HBV can be transmitted only by injection is not absolutely true; nevertheless, the great majority of infections are acquired parenterally. We know little about the excretion of the virus in the faeces and urine. The virus may also be present in the saliva, and be transmitted by kissing.

The presence of HBV in saliva presents a potential hazard to dentists. The following categories of patients have been suggested as presenting a particular hazard that requires special precautions for dental treatment.[*]

1. Patients with chronic renal failure who are receiving, or are likely to receive, regular dialysis treatment and patients who have had a renal or other organ transplant.
2. Patients receiving long-term immunosuppressive therapy.
3. Patients with haemophilia and others with haematological disorders who receive multiple transfusions of blood or blood products.
4. Patients from institutions for the mentally handicapped. (Mentally handicapped patients living at home do not constitute a special risk).
5. Known drug addicts.
6. Patients suffering from jaundice which is thought to be infective in nature and those who have suffered from such jaundice within the previous 6 months.

---

[*]This recommendation is taken from a report by the Expert Group on Hepatitis in Dentistry published by Her Majesty's Stationery Office, London, 1979.

7. Patients who either live in, or have come from, areas where the carrier rate is high, e.g. Asia.

Herpesviruses

The herpesviruses are a group of spherical DNA-containing viruses that tend to lie latent in tissues for long periods. Infected cells may fuse together to form multinucleate giant cells and intranuclear inclusion bodies are often formed. Four herpesviruses are of importance in causing human disease.

Varicella and zoster

Though the well-known clinical features of varicella (chickenpox) and zoster are poles apart, there is good evidence that they are both caused by the same virus.

Chickenpox. The pathogenesis is similar to that of mouse-pox but the site of entry is probably the upper respiratory tract. There is an enanthem involving the oral mucosa and an exanthem consisting of a vesicular skin rash. The lesions subsequently become pustular and may leave scars.

Zoster. Following an attack of chickenpox the virus may lie latent in the tissues, and in later life be reactivated by some physical or mental shock. It produces lesions specifically in the posterior root ganglia of the spinal, trigeminal, or facial nerves, and from there infection spreads down the nerve fibres to the skin. Pain followed by the development of a vesicular rash restricted to an area supplied by the nerve are characteristic (Fig. 16.9). Children exposed to a patient with zoster often develop chickenpox.

Herpes simplex

Two strains of herpes simplex virus (HSV) are known. HSV-1 is the most common and tends to infect the skin and oropharyngeal mucosa, while HSV-2 commonly affects the genital area and is sexually transmitted. Nevertheless both types of virus can cause lesions anywhere. Serological studies indicate that herpes simplex (Figs 16.10 to 16.12) is one of the most widely distributed viruses in human beings. It is estimated that

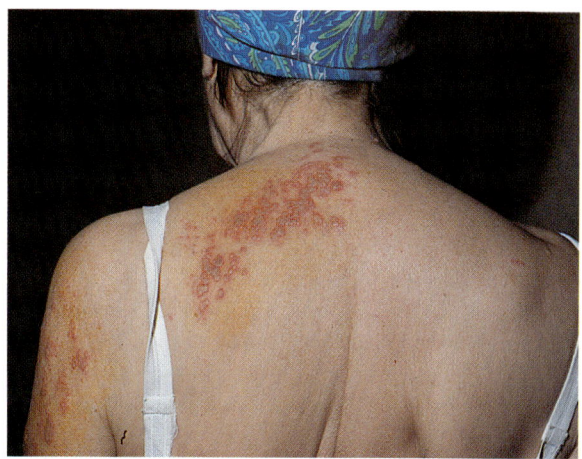

Fig. 16.9 Infection of the posterior root ganglion by herpesvirus. There are clusters of vesicles with erythematous bases, which have coalesced.

about 60% of the population are affected. Of these only 10% exhibit primary childhood lesions, such as *gingivostomatitis* (Fig. 16.11), *keratoconjunctivitis*, and *vulvovaginitis*. Rarely the infection is more widespread.

Abrasions of the skin predispose to primary herpetic infection (*traumatic*, or *inoculation*, *herpes simplex*). A good example of this is the painful *herpetic whitlow*, which is seen in nursing attendants working in neurosurgical wards. These people acquire their infection while inserting endotracheal tubes into the mouths of unconscious patients. It is also seen in dentists.

Usually, however, the primary infection remains subclinical, and the virus remains latent in the cells of the host. This symbiosis tends to be disturbed by intercurrent infections, e.g. the common cold, pneumonia, and malaria, and even, in very susceptible victims, by menstruation, emotional strain, and exposure to sunlight. There then develop typical *herpetic blisters* (cold sores). These are most common on the *lips* near the mucocutaneous junction; the oral mucosa is rarely affected, and it should be noted that the common recurrent aphthous ulcers of the mouth are not due to herpes simplex. Occasionally the *conjunctiva* or *cornea* (dendritic ulcers) are affected. *Skin* lesions are common, and may be found on any part of the body. The lesions of herpes tend to recur in the

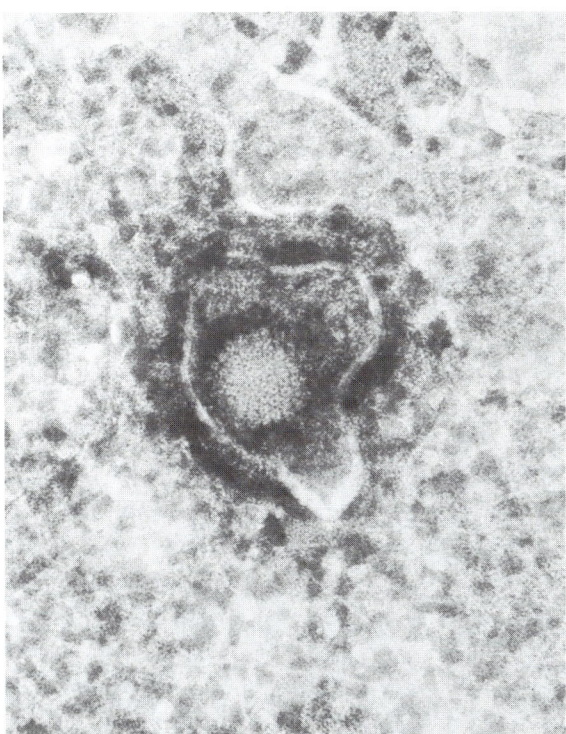

Fig. 16.10 Herpes simplex virus. The envelope, which is clearly delineated, is derived from the modified nuclear membrane of an infected cell. The hollow capsomeres of the virion are clearly visible. × 139 800. (Photograph courtesy of Micheline Fauvel, Laboratoire de Santé Publique du Quebec, Sainte-Anne-de-Bellevue, Quebec, Canada.)

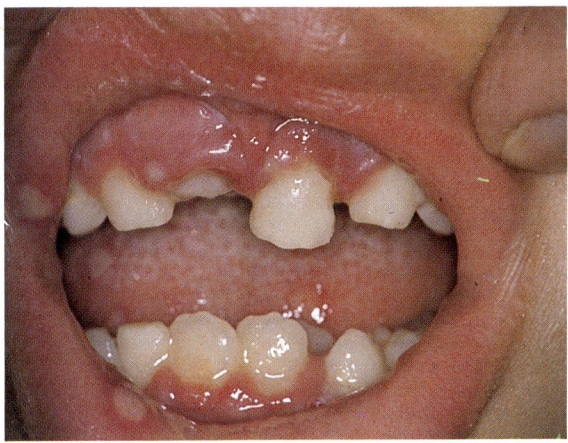

Fig. 16.11 Acute herpetic gingivostomatitis in an 8-year-old child. The gingivae are red and inflamed and there are multiple small ulcers affecting the oral mucosa.(Previously published in Rock W P, Grundy M C, Shaw L Diagnostic picture tests in paediatric dentistry, Wolfe Medical Publications, London.)

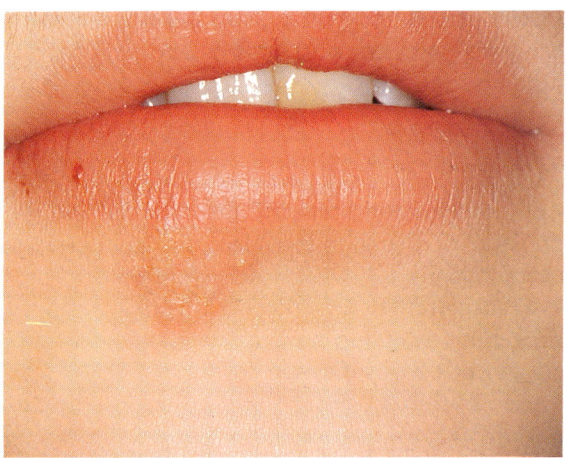

Fig. 16.12 Recurrent herpes labialis occurring on the skin at the mucocutaneous junction. (Previously published in Rock W P, Grundy M C, Shaw L Diagnostic picture tests in paediatric dentistry, Wolfe Medical Publications, London.)

same general area of skin, and this is presumably because between attacks the virus lies latent in the posterior root ganglia of the sensory nerve supplying the part.

Genital herpes affects the vulva or penis and presents as recurrent blisters which rapidly break down to form painful shallow ulcers. Involvement of the cervix is now recognized as being common, and is associated with the development of carcinoma, although the nature of the relationship is not clear. Genital herpes is now one of the major sexually transmitted diseases and as yet there is no effective cure. Babies born of mothers with active genital herpes may develop the dangerous *generalized herpes of the newborn*.

The precise localization of the virus during the latent periods has been a matter for speculation. It cannot be identified in the skin between attacks, but it has been isolated from sensory nerve-root ganglia—trigeminal or sacral—examined at necropsy. It appears that the virus remains latent in nerve cells, but when conditions are favourable it is able to infect the skin and produce typical herpetic vesicles. The mechanism is therefore analogous to that encountered in zoster.

Epstein–Barr virus

This herpesvirus causes classical *infectious mononucleosis* (glandular fever) with a positive

Paul–Bunnell test. It is also associated with Burkitt's tumour and nasopharyngeal carcinoma (see p. 259).

Cytomegalovirus (CMV)

Cells infected with this virus are enlarged and the presence of a large intranuclear inclusion body is characteristic.

Transplacental infection can cause a severe congenital infection that often leaves the survivors with brain damage. In adults, CMV can cause a disease resembling infectious mononucleosis, but in immunosuppressed patients, e.g. those with AIDS, the effects may be severe and contribute to death.

Rabies

Rabies is caused by an infection with a bullet-shaped virus, a rhabdovirus. Infection is endemic in wild animals in many parts of the world, the particular species depending on the area. The wolf, fox and raccoon are important in Europe, while in North America, in addition to these animals, the skunk is important. In parts of Central and South America and in the Caribbean the vampire bat is infected. The virus is excreted in saliva, and human infection is generally acquired from the bite of an infected dog. The virus spreads to the brain and causes a meningencephalitis. The incubation period is long and can be several months. Initial symptoms are agitation, painful muscular contractions and seizures. Painful pharyngeal contractions on attempting to swallow water have given the disease its common name 'hydrophobia'. Paralysis follows and the patient dies within a few days. The disease may be paralytic from the beginning. A particularly distressing feature of the disease is that the mind remains clear until near the end.

If a person is bitten by an animal suspected of being rabid, the animal should be captured and examined for infection. If this is positive or if the animal escapes, the victim must be immunized. The Semple vaccine prepared from infected rabbit cord as devised by Pasteur can be given, but injections are painful and occasionally complicated by the development of an autoimmune

encephalomyelitis due to the injection of foreign nervous tissue. A vaccine prepared from human diploid cells is currently recommended to avoid this danger. Antirabies serum can be given intramuscularly and into the area of the wound.

Papovaviruses*

This group includes the human papillomaviruses (HPV) of which many strains have been identified (Fig. 16.3). They have yet to be cultured in

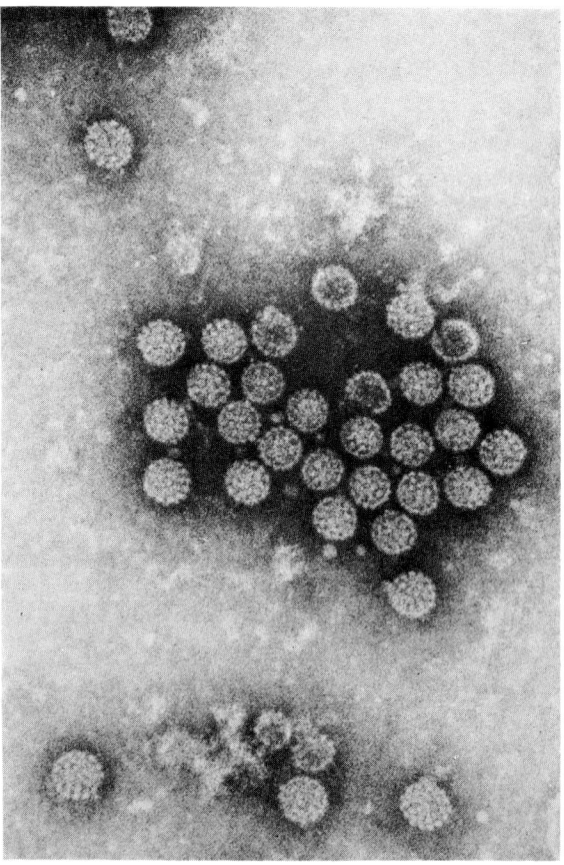

Fig. 16.13 A papovavirus (SV 40). This organism was found as a contaminant in a culture of African Green Monkey kidney cells. × 136 000. (Photograph by courtesy of Micheline Fauvel, Laboratoire de Santé Publique du Quebec, Sainte-Anne-de-Bellevue, Quebec, Canada.)

*The name papova is derived from the first two letters of the words PApilloma, POlyoma and VAcuolating agent.

vitro. They cause human warts of varying types. Those that infect the genital area to cause condyloma accuminata have been implicated in the development of carcinoma of the cervix.

The *polyoma virus*, which causes a variety of animal tumours, belongs to the group of papovaviruses as does the *JC virus*, which causes a trivial upper respiratory infection in childhood but a severe encephalitis in certain immunodeficiency disease such as AIDS.

Slow viruses

Scrapie is a lethal neurological disease of sheep which appears to be caused by an agent which is very resistant to heat and chemical disinfectants. The incubation period is several *years*. The precise nature of the agent is unclear but it appears to contain neither DNA nor RNA; it has been called a prion. Certain rare human diseases have a similar cause. The best known is Creutzfeldt--Jakob disease, which has inadvertently been transmitted to humans from corneal grafts. It is of interest that certain common viruses can remain latent, only to cause disease at a later time. As an example, the measles virus can cause a rare type of encephalitis.

CONCLUSION

The range of diseases caused by viruses is very large, and in many of them there are oral lesions; although these are often of little significance, some are useful in diagnosis. The enanthem often appears before the typical exanthem—Koplik's spots in measles are a good example of this. These resemble white grains of salt on a red background, and may be present on the buccal mucosa a day or two before the typical skin rash appears.

The increasing complexity of viral structure and reproduction which recent research has revealed is necessitating a reappraisal of the aetiology of many diseases. The phenomena of viral latency and the eclipse phase indicate that a failure to isolate a virus does not necessarily signify its absence. Similarly slow viruses, mycoplasmas, and the delicate and elusive L-forms of bacteria have not yet been sufficiently investigated for their role in disease to be assessed.

GENERAL READING

Balkwill F R 1989 Interferons. Lancet 1:1060
Belshe R B (ed.) 1984 Textbook of human virology. PSG Publishing. Littleton MA.
Bockman J M, et al 1985 Creutzfeld–Jacob disease prion proteins in human brains. New England Journal of Medicine 312:73
Brunham R C, et al 1984 Mucopurulent cervicitis—the ignored counterpart in women of urethritis in men. New England Journal of Medicine 311:1
Cassell G H, Cole B C 1981 Mycoplasmas agents of human disease. New England Journal of Medicine 304:80
Corey L, Spear PG 1986 Infections with herpes simplex viruses. New England Journal of Medicine 314:686

Haywood A.M 1986 Patterns of persistant viral infections. New England Journal of Medicine 315:939
Schachter J 1978 Chlamydial infections. New England Journal of Medicine 298:428,490 & 540
Sharpe A H, Fields B N 1985 Pathogenesis of viral infections: basic concepts derived from the reovirus model. New England Journal of Medicine 312:486
Taylor-Robertson D, McCormack W M 1980 The genital mycoplasmas. New England Journal of Medicine 302: 1003, 1063
Timbury M C 1983 Notes on Medical Virology, 7th edn. Churchill Livingstone, Edinburgh

17.   Some disorders of metabolism

Disorders of metabolism form a heterogeneous group of diseases. Some are inherited and the metabolic defect involved is known with precision. Phenylketonuria and some other inborn errors of metabolism are considered in Chapter 3. The haemoglobinopathies and some haemolytic anaemias are considered in Chapter 26. There are, in addition, other metabolic diseases in which the chemical defect and mode of inheritance are less precisely known. A good example of this type of metabolic disorder is diabetes mellitus, a disease that affects about 3% of the population. Together with gout it is considered in this chapter.

Before attempting to describe diabetes mellitus it is necessary to understand the mechanism of glucose homeostasis.

GLUCOSE HOMEOSTASIS

Glucose is the only fuel used by the central nervous system under normal circumstances and is also used by many other tissues. Its blood level is maintained between narrow limits (3.0–5.0 mmol/L) by a complex mechanism involving a number of hormones, of which insulin is the most important. The liver acts as a storehouse whereby glucose is either stored (as glycogen) or released into the blood.

Following the absorption of glucose from digested food in the intestine, the rise in blood glucose level directly stimulates the secretion of insulin from the pancreatic islets. This aids the entry of glucose into resting muscle and fat cells, which are the insulin-dependent tissues. About 15% of the absorbed glucose enters these tissues along insulin-dependent pathways. An additional 25% escapes from the splanchnic bed and is utilized to meet the ongoing glucose needs of insulin-independent tissues, especially the brain. From 55 to 60% is retained in the liver, for there is no barrier to the entry to glucose into liver cells, and this organ is well situated anatomically to intercept glucose from the portal vein and prevent it entering the systemic circulation. In the liver the glucose is utilized in the synthesis of glycogen and triglycerides.

It follows that in the normal person, even after a carbohydrate meal, the blood glucose does not rise above 9 mmol/L; this forms the basis of the glucose-tolerance test.

In this test a fasting subject, previously on an adequate carbohydrate diet, is given 100 g of glucose by mouth. The blood glucose should not exceed 5 mmol/L at the start of the test nor 9 mmol/L (160 mg/dl) an hour later; it should have returned to 5 mmol/L after 2 h. At a blood-glucose level of 10 mmol/L (80 mg/dl) glycosuria may be expected.

If an individual fasts overnight, the liver and the insulin-dependent tissues (resting muscle and fat) show little glucose uptake. The insulin-independent tissues (brain, blood cells, and renal medulla) show a continued glucose uptake at a rate of 150 to 200 g per day; the blood-glucose level is maintained by the release of glucose from

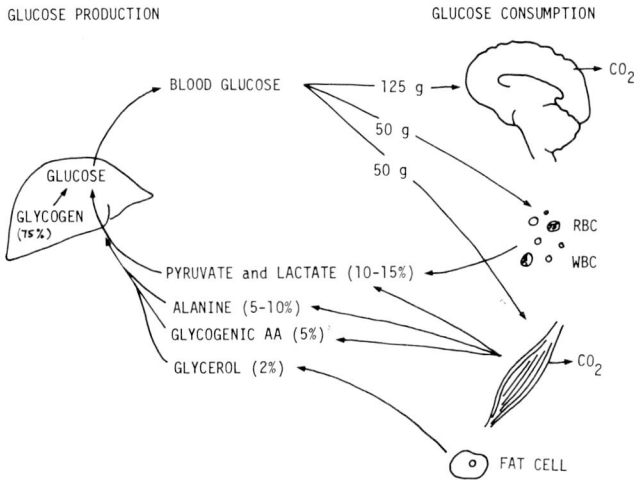

Fig. 17.1   Glucose balance in normal man in the postabsorbtive, overnight-fasted state. Alanine forms the principal amino acid released from muscle, and is utilized by the liver to form glucose. The muscle can utilize glucose to form alanine, and this constitutes the glucose-alanine cycle analogous to the Cori cycle. In the latter, lactate and pyruvate formed from glucose in the muscle are released into the blood, taken up by the liver, and there converted into glucose. (From Felig P 1975 The liver in glucose homeostasis in normal man and diabetes. In: Valance-Owen J (ed.) *Diabetes*, University Park Press, Baltimore.)

the liver (Fig. 17.1). However, the liver contains about 70 g of glycogen which provides an immediate source of glucose by glycogenolysis. The supply, however, lasts less than 1 day, and gluconeogenesis is stimulated using pyruvate, lactate and alanine as the main raw materials. After 2 or 3 days glyconeogenesis is more important than glycogenolytic activity. Protein provides the ultimate source for this, a fact reflected in the brisk rate of nitrogen excretion that occurs early in starvation.

In the resting state the major source of energy for muscular contraction is provided by the oxidation of fatty acids. During exercise the uptake of fatty acid is increased, but in addition there is a marked (up to 20-fold) increase in glucose uptake and oxidation. To compensate for this peripheral utilization, the liver releases glucose into the blood stream and the blood-glucose level shows little change. During short-term exercise the major source of this glucose is liver glycogen (glycogenolysis). During prolonged exercise glyconeogenesis plays an increasingly important role, because the liver's supply of glycogen is limited.

Secretion and actions of insulin

Insulin is synthetized in the B cells (β cells) of the islets of Langerhans as proinsulin, a polypeptide containing 81–86 amino-acid residues. The tail and head of this long polypeptide are joined by two disulphide bonds. By the action of peptidases the middle segment (termed the C peptide) is excised, leaving the two ends of the molecule to form the A (α) and B(β) chains of the insulin molecule; these remain united by the original disulphide bonds. The formation and excretion of C peptide has been used as a measure of the rate of insulin synthesis.

The major stimulus for both insulin synthesis and release is hyperglycaemia. Glucagon, gastrin, and other intestinal hormones also stimulate the islets of Langerhans, and the release of these hormones following oral administration of glucose plays a minor role in promoting insulin secretion.

The target cells of insulin are those of the adipose tissue and muscle, both of which have specific receptors: glucose transport into the cell is enhanced, and glycogen synthesis is increased.

Insulin promotes the synthesis of protein from amino acids; it inhibits the breakdown of neutral fat (*lipolysis*).

Furthermore, insulin has two important effects on the liver: *glycogenolysis is inhibited* by small increments in insulin secretion; larger increments *inhibit glyconeogenesis*. The net effect of insulin is to lower the blood-glucose level; since the half-life of the hormone is from 3 to 4 min, the continuous and varying secretion of insulin is the main regulatory mechanism whereby the blood-glucose level is normally maintained within narrow limits.

Other hormones affecting glucose metabolism

Several hormones affect glucose metabolism but their effect is less marked than that of insulin. *Glucagon* is the secretion of the A cells (α cells) of the islets of Langerhans and its main action is to promote glycogenolysis in the liver. The glucose so produced passes into the blood so that there is a rise in blood glucose. Lipolysis is also promoted. Glucagon therefore opposes the action of insulin and its secretion is stimulated by hypoglycaemia. *Pituitary growth hormone* also opposes the action of insulin. *Adrenaline* promotes glycogenolysis in the liver and also causes a rise in blood glucose. The *adrenal glucocorticoids* stimulate glyconeogenesis in the liver and diminish glucose utilization by muscle and fat cells. Hence these hormones cause a rise in the blood glucose level, an effect that is of importance in subjects who are diabetic.

DIABETES MELLITUS

The discovery of insulin by Banting and Best appeared to provide both an explanation of pathogenesis of diabetes mellitus and an effective treatment. Ironically, this outstanding discovery retarded further research into the true nature of the disease, so that even today its precise pathogenesis is not understood. It has become evident that insulin deficiency is only one factor in the disease. Many diabetic subjects need insulin in quantities far in excess of those required by a totally pancreatectomized individual. Some diabetics have a blood-insulin level that is normal or even above normal. Finally, insulin therapy can prolong the life of some diabetic subjects, but it fails to prevent premature death from the cardiovascular complications or the onset of blindness. The life expectancy of a diabetic patient is still below that of the normal individual.

Aetiology of diabetes mellitus

Diabetes mellitus may be regarded as a syndrome characterized by a relative or absolute deficiency of insulin. Three major types of the disease may be recognized.

Diabetes mellitus associated with other endocrine disorders. There are a number of diseases in which an overproduction of hormones that counter the actions of insulin can lead to a diabetic state. These include Cushing's syndrome, acromegaly and phaeochromocytoma.

Diabetes associated with pancreatic disease. Diabetes mellitus is occasionally encountered following total pancreatectomy, and in any disease in which there is extensive destruction of the pancreas, e.g. cystic fibrosis and chronic pancreatitis.

Spontaneous diabetes mellitus. This is the most common form of the syndrome and can be divided into two main types: type I, or insulin-dependent diabetes mellitus (IDDM); and type II, or non-insulin-dependent diabetes mellitus NIDDM.

Type I (insulin-dependent) diabetes mellitus. As its alternative name, juvenile diabetes mellitus, implies this type generally commences before the age of 30 years. The disease has an autoimmune basis and is associated with certain HLA haplotypes (DR3 and DR4); these are thought to predispose to islet cell damage, probably by a viral infection. Coxsackie virus has been best documented although some unknown poison has been postulated. Further damage is caused by the formation of auto-antibodies against islet cells.

IDDM generally begins abruptly with *thirst* (polydypsia), polyuria, and wasting. The islets show a lymphocytic infiltrate but are soon destroyed. Insulin production diminishes and the effects of the disease can be explained by the lack of insulin. Uptake of glucose by fat and muscle cells is low and yet the liver continues to manufacture glucose from glycogen and noncarbohydrate sources—chiefly amino acids derived from muscle. This explains the wasting that characterizes this form of diabetes. The blood glucose is high, and glycosuria results. In turn there is an osmotic diuresis that leads to water and electrolyte loss, and subsequently to *thirst*. An important effect of insulin deficiency is the accelerated release of fatty acids (lipolysis) from the adipose tissues. They are taken up by the liver and in the presence of a low level of insulin are converted into ketone bodies (β-hydroxybutyrate, aceto-acetate, and acetone). Ketosis and metabolic acidosis follows, and the combined effect is to cause *diabetic coma*; *death* results without insulin injections.

Type II (Non-insulin-independent diabetes mellitus (NIDDM). Also called maturity onset diabetes mellitus, this type generally commences insidi-ously in patients over the age of 40 years. Often the subjects are obese, and the disease is dis-covered on routine physical examination and urinalysis. The disease has a familial incidence but the exact mode of inheritance is unknown. There is no association with any HLA haplo-types. The islets of Langerhans are often nor-mal, at least in the early stages of the disease, and the blood-insulin levels may be low, normal or high. Hence islet destruction and an absolute lack of insulin do not seem to be the cause of this type of diabetes; the tissues seem to be resistant to the effects of insulin, possibly due to a lack of insulin receptors, the cause of which is not known. Obesity itself may be a factor because it causes insulin resistance. However, because patients with NIDDM have enough insulin to inhibit lipolysis in the tissues, the obesity may be an effect of the disease. Wasting and ketoacidotic coma are not features of NIDDM. The disease may often be managed with diet and weight reduction without resorting to insulin injections.

Complications of diabetes mellitus

Diabetic ketosis and coma

This is most common in IDDM, and may be precipitated by the patient's failure to administer his insulin. Vomiting and abdominal pain may be severe enough to simulate an abdominal emergency.

Hyperosmolar non-ketogenic coma

This condition is generally encountered in patients with NIDDM, and may be precipitated by an acute illness, such as an infection or a myocardial infarct. The plasma glucose level is very high and may exceed 55 mmol/L. The osmotic diuresis that this engenders leads to hypovolaemic shock. The effect of the dehydra-tion is most marked on the central nervous system—coma is characteristic, and seizures occur in about one-third of cases.

Cardiovascular disease

Diabetic subjects are more prone than normal people of the same age group to develop athero-sclerosis, peripheral vascular disease, gangrene of the toes and feet, and ischaemic heart disease. This tendency does not seem to be related to the severity of the diabetes nor to the efficiency of the treatment; indeed, treatment with oral hypogly-caemic drugs, may actually increase the mortality from cardiovascular disease.

Diabetic microangiopathy. A thickening of the basement membrane zone of capillaries has been described in many tissues. It is a com-ponent of peripheral vascular disease, and is particularly important in the pathogenesis of diabetic nephropathy and the changes in the eyes.

Diabetic nephropathy. In diabetic glomerulo-sclerosis there is thickening of the basement membrane of the glomerular vessels together with mesangial proliferation and an increase on the amount of basement-membrane-like material in the mesangium. Eventually the glomeruli are converted into functionless hyaline masses. Glomerulosclerosis leads to proteinuria, which may be severe enough to cause the nephrotic syndrome. Ultimately chronic renal failure ensues.

Urinary-tract infection is common in diabetic subjects, especially women, and papillary necrosis may occur; clinically this is characterized by haematuria and the rapid onset of renal failure.

Changes in the eye. The retinal microangiopathy causes ischaemic changes, microaneurysm formation, and bleeding (diabetic retinopathy). *Cataract formation* is another important complication of diabetes; it is little wonder that the disease is one of the leading causes of blindness in the world.

Diabetic neuropathy. Ischaemic damage to peripheral nerves leads to a variety of effects, e.g. pain, loss of sensation (stocking-and-glove distribution), and autonomic effects such as diarrhoea, difficulty in micturition, and impotence.

Liability to infection

Diabetic patients are susceptible to bacterial infections, especially of the skin, lungs, and urinary tract. The mechanism is incompletely understood, but abnormal polymorph function (chemotaxis and bactericidal action) may be of importance. Vaginal candidiasis is a troublesome complication in diabetic women.

GOUT

Gout is characterized by a high blood uric acid content (hyperuricaemia) and the deposition of monosodium urate crystals in the joints (causing arthritis), in the kidney, (causing stones and renal damage), and in the soft tissues of the skin (producing nodular masses called tophi).

Gout is divided into three phases. Initially there is *asymptomatic hyperuricaemia.* The second phase commences as an *acute sterile arthritis* affecting the metatarsal-phalangeal joint of the big toe. It is accompanied by rigors and fever. The pain can be extremely severe. The deposition of monosodium urate crystals in the joint cavity leads to their phagocytosis by neutrophils and the release of damaging lysosomal enzymes; acute inflammation and fever follow as a consequence. The arthritis subsides spontaneously over a few days. Colchicine usually provides rapid relief.

Further acute attacks tend to occur, affecting other joints. No joint is exempt, but the legs are affected more often than the arms and the distal joints more frequently than the proximal ones. Finally, the disease enters the third phase of *chronic arthritis*, and there is great deformity due to the nodular deposits of urates in and around the joints. Tophi occur in the cartilages of the ears, in bursae (especially the olecranon and prepatellar), in tendons, and in soft tissues.

The majority of patients with chronic gout develop some degree of renal damage, and renal failure was a cause of death in about 20% of patients before the advent of dialysis. In addition to direct renal parenchymal damage, uric acid stones form and indeed may be first indication of the disease. Hypertension is present in about one-third of patients.

Gout is now regarded as a symptom complex of multiple aetiology. In cases labelled *primary gout* there is sometimes a family history, while in others labelled *secondary gout* there is an obvious associated disease that appears to be the primary cause. In both types there is an upset in purine metabolism, either overproduction of uric acid or impaired excretion by the kidneys. Although a family tendency is well established in primary gout, the exact biochemical defect and mode of inheritance is not known, except in the case of a few rare syndromes. Primary gout is a heterogeneous group, and while the tendency to gout may be inherited the actual disease is precipitated by other factors. Obesity and overindulgence in alcohol are often incriminated. In the past, chronic lead poisoning may have been a factor and explains how the consumption of certain wines predisposes to the disease—in Roman times lead acetate was even added to wine!

Secondary gout may be due to increased cellular turnover, as occurs in leukaemias and other malignant diseases especially when treated with cytotoxic drugs. Alternatively there may be impaired urinary excretion due to renal disease; in this regard, chronic lead poisoning can be a factor. Certain drugs, chiefly thiazide diuretics, also impair renal excretion of uric acid.

GENERAL READING

Bogardus C, Lillioja S 1990 Where all the glucose doesn't go in non-insulin-dependent diabetes mellitus. New England Journal of Medicine 322:262

Eisenbarth G S 1986 Type 1 diabetes mellitus. New England Journal of Medicine 314: 1360

Foster D W, McGarry J D 1983 The metabolic derangement and treatment of diabetes ketoacidosis. New England Journal of Medicine 309: 159,

Leslie R D G 1983 Causes of insulin dependent diabetes. British Medical Journal 287: 5

Pak C Y et al 1988 Association of cytomegalovirus infection with autoimmune type 1 diabetes. Lancet 2:1

Stanbury J B, Wyngaarden J B, Fredrickson D S, Goldstein J L Brown M S (eds) 1983 The metabolic basis of inherited disease, 5th edn. McGraw-Hill, New York

Wolf E, Spencer K M, Cudworth A G 1983 The genetic susceptability to type 1 (insulin-dependent) diabetes: analysis of the HLA-DR association. Diabetologia 24: 224

18. Diseases of malnutrition

Maintenance of normal health demands that the body absorbs an adequate amount of food containing not only enough material for growth and ongoing energy production, but also essential vitamins and minerals. Diseases related to malnutrition can be divided into two groups—those caused by excessive food intake, and those caused by deficiencies due either to an inadequate diet or to defective absorption. Over-eating leads to obesity, under-eating and malabsorption lead to starvation and a myriad of disorders related to specific deficiencies. The effects of starvation will first be described.

STARVATION

During starvation the body's stores of energy are utilized to maintain energy requirements.

Energy stores

The body stores energy as neutral fat deposited in adipocytes. The glycogen of the liver and muscle (approximately 1 kg) is not used as an energy store but is used in metabolic pathways to maintain the blood-glucose level within normal limits. Likewise proteins are present within all tissues as essential cellular components.

With the onset of starvation the insulin-independent tissues, e.g. the brain, continue to utilize glucose as their major source of energy; indeed this is the brain's only source of energy under normal circumstances. The glycogen stores would be depleted within 24 h were it not for the formation of glucose from non-carbohydrate sources (gluconeogenesis). Initially proteins, chiefly from the muscles, are broken down, and the released amino acids (chiefly alanine) are transported to the liver and converted into glucose. Their released nitrogen is excreted as urea and the body develops a negative nitrogen balance. This is only a temporary mechanism for, as noted above, there are no large disposable stores of protein that can be used for metabolic purposes; after about a week protein catabolism and gluconeogenesis decline. Thereafter, energy is provided by neutral fat which is the body's major store of energy. The triacyl glycerols of depot fat are hydrolysed (lipolysis), and the glycerol and free fatty acids so formed are transported to the liver to be converted into glucose and ketone bodies. At this time the metabolism of the brain undergoes a change such that it can use ketone bodies, particularly β-hydroxybutyric acid instead of glucose. Starvation can now continue until the fat stores are exhausted. The individual becomes apathetic and loses weight as the fat deposits waste away. The laxity of the subcutaneous tissues combine with hypoalbuminaemia to cause oedema of the dependent parts. The starving person is particularly susceptible to infection, especially dysentery and tuberculosis.

The term *protein-calorie malnutrition* is applied to starvation in children. It may be precipitated when breast feeding is terminated by a further pregnancy. The term *marasmus* is used if there is lack of protein and calories in the diet; it resembles starvation in the adult, but in addition to the wasting there is striking lack of growth such that there may be dwarfism in those who survive. *Kwashiorkor* is a variant of starvation and is due to deficient protein intake in the face of an adequate supply of calories in the form of carbohydrate. It is encountered in African children between the ages of 1 and 3 years. A fatty liver, which does not predispose to cirrhosis, and marked oedema of the subcutaneous tissues are characteristic. There is deficient melanin formation which in black children causes the hair to become red and the skin to lighten in colour.

OBESITY

Obesity has been defined as an increase in body weight 20% or more over the norm taking into account, sex, age, and body frame. There is, however, no exact definition because what constitutes normality varies greatly depending on race and social custom. Witness the difference between Rubens' models of the last century and the model Twiggy in the 1960s.

The pathogenesis of obesity is poorly understood. The initial increase in weight is due to an excessive intake of food so that energy is stored as fat. When a constant, though excessive, weight is attained, energy output exactly matches energy intake as in the person of normal weight. How this balance is attained is not known, although some hormonal feedback mechanism has been postulated whereby messages are sent from the fat deposits to those hypothalamic centres that influence feeding and satiety. These centres are influenced by many known hormones. Thus noradrenaline and opioids stimulate appetite whilst dopamine, adrenaline, glucagon, cholecystokinin and other hormones are appetite inhibitors.

Obesity is associated with certain well-defined conditions. It is a feature of non-insulin-dependent diabetes mellitus, Cushing's disease, certain hypothalamic lesions, hypothyroidism and hypogonadism, but in the vast majority of cases there is no such obvious cause. It has been postulated that two main types of obesity occur. In one group the individuals are heavy in infancy and excess weight is a lifelong problem. The obesity tends to affect limbs and trunk. The *adipocyte hyperplasia theory* has been evoked to explain this. Adipocytes normally divide only during infancy and puberty. In this type of obesity the cells continue to divide throughout childhood and obesity is therefore related to the presence of too many adipocytes. In the second group of patients (with *adult-onset obesity*) the fat is deposited centrally and the limbs are spared. The condition is an extension of 'middle-age spread', and there is no adipocyte hyperplasia.

The pathogenesis of obesity must involve many factors. Heredity is clearly involved, and overweight families have their counterpart in the strain of rats that inevitably becomes obese. Social and racial customs seem to play a part, but, as with other complex multifactorial diseases, it is difficult to separate inherited traits from environmental influences.

Complications

Some complications of obesity are clearly mechanical—osteoarthritis of weight-bearing joints, intertrigo and hernias. Abdominal surgery is made more hazardous. Less easily explained but of great importance are systemic hypertension, atherosclerosis, diabetes mellitus of the non-insulin-dependent type, varicose veins and toxaemia of pregnancy.

ANOREXIA NERVOSA AND BULIMIA NERVOSA

In anorexia nervosa the subject, generally an adolescent female, undergoes self-imposed starvation in pursuit of attaining a slender figure. The subjects are nervous and aggressive; amenorrhoea is characteristic. In bulimia nervosa there is also an abnormal fear of fatness, and 'binge' eating is followed by drastic counteractive measures—induced vomiting, the use of diuretics or laxatives, strict diet or violent exercise. Both these abnormalities in appetite control are difficult to treat and have an appreciable mortality.

THE VITAMINS

The vitamins are a group of organic compounds required to maintain health and normal metabolism; the body cannot manufacture them. There are two groups—the fat-soluble and the water-soluble vitamins. Those presently recognized are listed in Table 18.1.

Table 18.1   The essential vitamins

Fat-soluble	Water-soluble
Vitamin A	Vitamin C
Vitamin D	Vitamin B complex:
Vitamin K	Thiamine
	Riboflavin
	Niacin
	Pyridoxine
	Cobalamin (B12)
	Folate

VITAMIN A

Vitamin A, a fat-soluble vitamin, is obtained from animal fats and dairy products in the diet. It can also be manufactured in the body from carotinoid pigments present in brightly coloured vegetables such as carrots, beetroot, etc. It is from the latter source that herbivorous animals obtain their supply of the vitamin. Vitamin A is necessary for the formation of rhodopsin, the pigment present in the retina and essential for the process whereby rods convert light into an electrical impulse. It is therefore not surprising that one of the first effects of vitamin-A deficiency is *night blindness*. Although an adequate supply of

vitamin A is required for the maintenance of good health, its other actions are less well defined. It is involved in the maintenance of the integrity of certain epithelial surfaces; in vitamin-A deficiency, the epithelia of the urinary tract, respiratory tract and conjunctiva undergo squamous metaplasia. This effect is very important in the eye because the conjunctiva becomes hyperkeratotic, dry, and cracked (*xerophthalmia*). Infection follows and can spread to the globe with subsequent perforation. Indeed, vitamin-A deficiency is one of the leading causes of blindness in the Third World, where vitamin-A deficiency is still common due to an inadequate dietary intake. It is rare in Europe and North America, but is occasionally encountered in patients with the malabsorption syndrome, particularly when the absorption of fat is impaired.

Vitamin-A toxicity

Large doses of vitamin A are toxic, causing acute increase in intracranial pressure, vomiting, drowsiness and diarrhoea. Chronic poisoning causes bone pains, headaches, dry skin, loss of hair and liver damage. These effects are occasionally seen accompanying food fads or following accidental poisoning. Similar effects are also encountered as complications of retinoid therapy. (The retinoids are synthetic derivatives of vitamin A and have been developed because of their effect on keratinization. Treatment with one of them, 13-*cis*-retinoic acid (Acutane), has greatly improved the outlook of severe acne vulgaris. An unfortunate complication is that this group of drugs is teratogenic.)

VITAMIN D

Vitamin D is present in animal fat; an important source is fish-liver oil. The vitamin is also synthesized in the skin by the action of ultraviolet light on 7-dehydrocholesterol. The important actions of this vitamin are on calcium metabolism and these are considered in Chapter 19.

VITAMIN E

The tocopherols that constitute vitamin E act as

antioxidants. Symptoms of deficiency have been described in infants and in subjects with severe malabsorption. The vitamin is avidly used by some enthusiasts who regard it as a panacea for many human ailments, but it is doubtful whether their hopes are ever realized.

VITAMIN C

Vitamin C is widely distributed in nature and is synthesized by many species. However, this does not include fish, some birds, bats and primates, including humans, and for them it is regarded as a vitamin. The main dietary sources of the vitamin are raw citrus fruits, berries, green vegetables and fruit. It is widely used as a food preservative and is therefore present in some commercially prepared food. After deprivation of the vitamin for several months, *scurvy* develops; the major defect is diminished collagen formation. Poor anchorage of blood vessels renders them fragile and liable to rupture, causing bleeding. Wound healing is greatly retarded.

Since ancient times scurvy was a problem in Northern Europe during winter, military campaigns and long sea-voyages when fresh vegetables were unavailable. In 1535–1536 James Lind, a naval surgeon, published his *Treatise on the Scurvey*, which showed that the disease resulted from a lack of fresh vegetables. By 1804 the Royal Navy had ordered lime-juice rations for all its crews, thereby giving the name 'limey' for British sailors and perhaps contributing to Nelson's victory over Napoleon!

Scurvy in infants and children

Milk, the main source of food, is a poor source of vitamin C. Hence if it is stored or processed, and no additional source of vitamin C is available, scurvy can develop in infants at about the age of 8 months. Infantile scurvy is characterized by the formation of very painful subperiosteal haematomas. Bleeding can occur anywhere, but gingival lesions, so characteristic of adult scurvy, are not found in infants unless the teeth have erupted.

Osseous lesions are also seen in infantile and early childhood scurvy, since there is an impaired formation of osteoid. An X-ray of a scorbutic bone shows generalized rarefaction due to osteoporosis, which is particularly well marked at the metaphyseal ends of the shaft. By contrast, the zones of provisional calcification are very dense; in the long bones this density appears as a transverse line at the junction between the epiphysis and the end of the shaft. There is heavy calcification of the cartilage with foci of fragmented spicules of calcified cartilage forming during the period of retarded longitudinal growth. The epiphysis may be fractured at the line of junction and undergo displacement and dislocation. Microscopically there is little evidence of bone formation either beneath the periosteum or at the margins of the calcified spicules of cartilage in the metaphyseal zone. Instead there is an accumulation of cells of fibroblast type embedded in a loose-textured, oedematous ground substance. These cells are in fact osteoblasts, and they start to lay down osteoid as soon as ascorbic acid is administered. The subperiosteal haemorrhages follow the disruption of the collagenous attachments (Sharpey's fibres) from the cortex of the bone. There is also an impairment in the formation of dentine, and the teeth may be loosened from the alveolar bone.

VITAMIN-B COMPLEX

The vitamin-B complex includes thiamine, riboflavine, niacin, and pyridoxine. They are all widely distributed in foodstuffs, and it is uncommon to encounter a patient with a pure deficiency of any one of them. In the Western World, multiple deficiencies are present in patients who are neglected or are chronic alcoholics. Hence preparations containing multiple vitamins are usually given.

Thiamine

Thiamine is synthesized by plants and certain microorganisms but not to any extent by animals; thus they must obtain their supply from the diet and, to a limited extent, from bacterial activity in the intestine. The vitamin is widely distributed in food, and it is especially rich in the outer layers of the grain. It is removed by mechanical milling; likewise highly polished rice is deficient, and this is the explanation of the prevalence of thiamine deficiency in the Far East where rice is the staple food. A diet high in carbohydrates increases the need for thiamine and, in addition, the diet may contain thiaminases that destroy the vitamin. In the developed countries, thiamine deficiency is occasionally encountered under unusual circumstances, e.g. in alcoholics or hunger strikers.

Thiamine diphosphate acts as a co-enzyme in various steps in carbohydrate metabolism and in its absence there is an increase in lactic and pyruvic acid which, instead of entering the Krebs cycle, accumulate in the blood. The impaired energy production and lack of ATP has been suggested as the cause of the neurological and cardiac malfunctions that characterize thiamine deficiency. However, this has not been confirmed, and the precise biochemical basis for the lesions remains unknown.

Beriberi

In humans, lack of thiamine causes *beriberi*, although there is some evidence that genetic factors are also involved. The early symptoms are vague, with loss of weight, oedema and paraesthesias; in due course one of the main types of the disease evolves, depending on whether the nervous system or cardiovascular system is involved.

Involvement of the nervous system. When the peripheral nervous system is involved there is a *peripheral neuropathy* with numbness, paraesthesia and paralysis—the condition is called *dry beriberi*. In the *cerebral form* (*Wernicke's encephalopathy*) there is paralysis of the extrinsic muscles of the eyes, and mental confusion that may progress to coma and death.

Involvement of the cardiovascular system. This type is called *wet beriberi* and is characterized by heart failure. In the *chronic form* the accumulation of lactic acid and other vasodilator chemical agents causes peripheral vasodilatation that leads to high-output heart failure. In addition there is bilateral ventricular enlargement and failure. The outstanding feature is extensive oedema with accumulation of fluid in the serous sacs. In the *acute form*, heart failure predominates and sudden death is common. This picture is similar to that of *infantile beriberi*, a condition that develops in infants of 2–6 months of age.

Riboflavine

Riboflavine is widely distributed in nature and is particularly abundant in yeast and green vegetables, but dairy products and meat are also valuable sources of the vitamin in the diet. The vitamin is a component of several enzymes that play an important part in metabolism. Pure riboflavine deficiency probably does not occur in humans except under experimental conditions.

Symptoms attributed to deficiency include angular stomatitis or perlèche, cheilosis and glossitis with a smooth sore tongue. A scaly dermatitis resembling seborrhoeic dermatitis affecting the face and scrotum or vulva has also been described.

Niacin

Niacin is a generic name that includes nicotinic acid and nicotinamide. As is the case for other components of the vitamin B complex, niacin is widely distributed in foodstuffs. In addition the body can manufacture it from tryphophane; strictly speaking, niacin is not a vitamin.

Niacin is an important component of several metabolic pathways. Deficiency causes *pellagra*, a disease that was once common in Spain, Italy and the southern states of the USA. It is associated with the consumption of maize, a cereal that does contain niacin but in a bound form that cannot be used. The presence of inhibitory factors and a diet low in tryptophane contributed to the condition. With the general improvement in socioeconomic conditions, pellagra is rarely encountered except under unusual conditions, e.g. in alcoholics.

The symptoms of pellagra are easily remembered as the three Ds: *dermatitis* that resembles a sunburn, *diarrhoea*, and *dementia*. Death is an occasional complication.

Vitamin B$_6$

This vitamin occurs in many foods, being particularly rich in meats, nuts and whole grain cereals. It occurs in several forms—pyridoxol (pyridoxine), peridoxal and pyridoxamine; 'pyridoxine' is commonly used as an inclusive term. It acts as a co-enzyme in many metabolic reactions, and deficiency results in anaemia, seizures, stomatitis, cheilosis, glossitis, and seborrhoeic dermatitis. So widespread is the distribution of the vitamin that clinical deficiency is only encountered under unusual conditions. Thus it is seen in infants fed on formulae which have been processed in a way that destroys the vitamin. Certain drugs antagonize the vitamin, e.g. isoniazid (an anticonvulsant drug) and cycloserine (used in the treatment of tuberculosis), cause deficiency.

The effects of pyridoxine deficiency are vague; dermatitis, cheilosis, angular stomatitis, and glossitis have all been noted. Thiamine, riboflavin, niacin, and pyridoxine are widely distributed in food and deficiencies are due to an unbalanced or inadequate diet. Multiple deficiencies are often present, and it is wise to administer a mixture of these members of the vitamin B complex.

Cobalamin (vitamin B_{12}) and folate

These vitamins are necessary for red-cell maturation. Their absence leads to a megaloblastic anaemia.

THE MALABSORPTION SYNDROME

The small intestine has two main functions: (1) the intraluminal digestion of food, mainly by the action of pancreatic enzymes aided by the bile salts, and (2) the absorption of nutrients, which is often aided by enzymes in the brush border of the absorptive cells that complete the process of digestion. A failure in the absorption of nutrients may be due to a derangement of either digestion or absorption. Three classes of disorder may be recognized:

1. The defect may be specific for a particular food component; this is usually associated with an enzyme defect, e.g. lactose intolerance due to lactase deficiency.

2. There may be a lack of major digestive fluid, e.g. the gastric juice following total gastrectomy, the pancreatic juice in pancreatic disease, or the bile in bile duct obstruction.

The gastric juice is not essential for digestion, apart from the secretion of intrinsic factor and its vital part in the absorption of vitamin B_{12}. Nevertheless, even a partial gastric resection leads to a degree of general malabsorption, because after gastrectomy there is a much more hurried passage of food in the intestine, and digestion is rendered less complete. Hence considerable loss of weight and an iron-deficiency anaemia are not uncommon.

3. There may be a gross abnormality of the small intestine itself such that many processes are affected.

In the last two groups there is a defective absorption of many food components, absorption of fat being particularly severely affected. Excess fat in the stools is termed *steatorrhoea*. The clinical state is that of the *malabsorption syndrome*.

SPECIFIC DEFECTS OF ABSORPTION

Carbohydrate maldigestion and malabsorption

The effects of a failure to digest and absorb carbohydrate are mainly attributable to the osmotic pressure exerted by the unabsorbed oligosaccharides or monosaccharides. Soon after ingesting the offending carbohydrate the patient feels bloated and the abdomen becomes distended. Furthermore, bacteria convert the carbohydrate to fatty acids, which appear to irritate the intestine; abdominal colic and diarrhoea may result.

Idiopathic lactase deficiency in adults

This is a common condition, its prevalence showing a racial incidence, being commonest in Oriental groups. The individual experiences no trouble during infancy or childhood, but later exhibits intolerance to milk, which is eliminated from the diet in order to avoid symptoms

Protein malabsorption

There are a number of inherited diseases in which there is a defective absorption of specific amino acids or groups of amino acids.

CAUSES OF THE MALABSORPTION SYNDROME

These may be either extrinsic or intrinsic. *Extrinsic causes* of malabsorption may be gastric, pancreatic, or biliary, and are related to impaired digestion of food products or intestinal hurry. *Intrinsic causes* are due primarily to defective intestinal function, and are related both to impaired absorption and disturbed enzyme action in the mucosal cells themselves.

Intrinsic disease of the intestine

Coeliac disease and tropical sprue will be described.

Coeliac disease

This disease results in a malabsorption disorder of the small intestine's mucosa, associated with the ingestion of gluten. For this reason it is sometimes referred to as gluten-sensitive enteropathy. The incidence in the UK is 1:3000, though it may be higher.

Symptoms of diarrhoea, weight loss, abdominal discomfort and nutritional deficiencies may occur in a baby with the introduction of solid foods. It is probably inherited as an autosomal dominant trait with incomplete expressivity. There is a high incidence of human leucocyte antigen HLA-B8 among coeliac sufferers.

Diagnosis is made by jejunal biopsy showing atrophy of the villi resulting in a flat mucosa.

Symptoms are relieved by a gluten-free diet, and the villi may return to normal. It is not known whether the gluten damages the small intestine by direct toxic action or by an immunological reaction. Apthous ulceration of the oral mucosa is common and responds to a gluten-free diet. The teeth developing at the time of introduction of solids may be hypoplastic (Fig. 18.1).

Tropical sprue

This disease is seen extensively in the Far East. It is not related to gluten sensitivity, but it often responds to oral antibiotics.

Malabsorption may also follow other diseases of the small intestine, for example lymphoma, congenital lymphangiectasia, amyloidosis, and ischaemia. The intestinal hurry associated with diabetes mellitus and the Zollinger–Ellison syndrome are other causes.

The blind loop syndrome

The blind loop syndrome, also called the *stagnant bowel syndrome*, may complicate any condition in which blind loops of bowel are found either as a result of disease (e.g. Crohn's disease) or surgical procedures.

It is generally accepted that the mechanism of malabsorption in this syndrome is an upset in the intestinal bacterial flora. Normally the small bowel is virtually sterile (p. 71). But blind loops, abnormalities in peristalsis, and gastro-colic fistulae all allow bacterial proliferation to occur.

Surgical resection of the small intestine

This, if extensive, leads to a serious reduction of the absorptive area. Such a resection may be necessitated by abdominal gunshot wounds, recurrent Crohn's disease, or massive intestinal infarction.

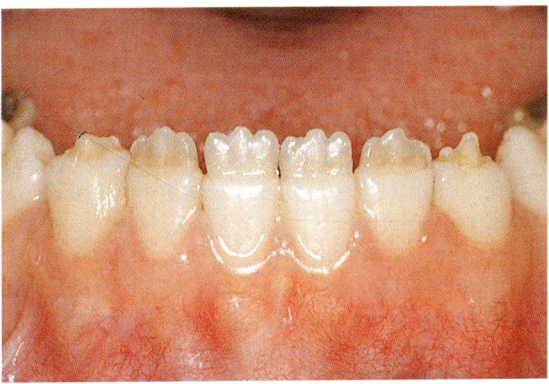

Fig. 18.1 Hypoplasia of the permanent mandibular incisor teeth in a child with coeliac disease. The hypoplasia corresponds to the age at which mixed feeding was introduced. The gluten in the diet resulted in a systemic disturbance. (Photograph by courtesy of Dr L Shaw, University of Birmingham. Previously published in Rock W P, Grundy M C, Shaw L Diagnostic picture tests in paediatric dentisry, Wolfe Medical Publications.)

EFFECTS OF MALABSORPTION

The effects of malabsorption may vary from sub-clinical disturbances to fatal malnutrition, depending on the portion of small bowel affected and the extent of the disease. The lack of absorption of essential nutrients may produce some effects similar to those of starvation, such as weight loss and generalized body atrophy.

Fat absorption is usually severely affected. If much fat—some of it undigested—is passed in the faeces, these will be pale and bulky.

Carbohydrate absorption is often affected, and the excess carbohydrate in the bowel is fermented by resident bacteria. The resulting gas renders the stool frothy and offensive.

Protein absorption is affected in intestinal and pancreatic steatorrhoea. If the hypoproteinaemia is severe enough to produce generalized oedema, an additional protein-losing gastroenteropathy should be suspected.

Vitamin absorption: the vitamin-B complex may be inadequately absorbed, producing effects already described. Vitamin C absorption is rarely impaired. The fat-soluble vitamins tend to be more severely affected, the lack of vitamins A and K producing characteristic effects. The malabsorption of vitamin D is aggravated by a concomitant binding of calcium to fatty acids in the bowel. Important effects of this dual interference with calcium absorption are a negative calcium balance, mild hypocalcaemia, a tendency to tetany, and in more prolonged cases osteomalacia. There may also be osteoporosis due to protein deficiency. Malabsorption of folic acid and vitamin B_{12} produces a megaloblastic type of anaemia.

Mineral absorption: an impaired absorption of iron is common, and this leads to hypochromic, microcytic anaemia. Other minerals that may be poorly absorbed are sodium, potassium, magnesium, and chloride (as well as calcium previously noted). Malabsorption may therefore be accompanied by symptoms of dehydration and muscular weakness.

It is evident that the effects of intestinal malabsorption are diverse, producing widespread disorder in many of the body's organs. This emphasizes the importance of the small intestine in the economy of the whole body.

CYSTIC FIBROSIS

An important cause of pancreatogenic malabsorption is *cystic fibrosis*, also called *fibrocystic disease of the pancreas* and *mucoviscidosis*. It is inherited as an autosomal recessive trait, and is one of the commonest hereditary diseases of white populations; by contrast it is very rare in blacks and almost unknown in Orientals. It is remarkable for the considerable variety of its presentations.

The *pancreas* is frequently involved: the gland secretes a thick mucus that obstructs the ducts, which dilate, and the gland undergoes atrophy. The disease sometimes develops in utero, when the absence of pancreatic enzymes leads to such viscosity of the intestinal contents (meconium) that intestinal obstruction (*meconum ileus*) and even perforation may ensue. More commonly the child later develops a chronic malabsorption syndrome which is often accompanied by constipation.

Pulmonary involvement is also common. The thick mucus blocking the bronchi is a powerful predisposing factor to infection and subsequent bronchopneumonia, which may become chronic and be complicated by bronchiectasis and lung abscesses. Indeed, chronic lung disease is a feature of most cases of cystic fibrosis that survive for several years.

Other organs affected include the *liver*, in which cirrhosis may later develop, the *salivary glands*, and the *cervix uteri*, resulting in infertility. Males are infertile. A remarkable feature is that the eccrine sweat glands secrete sweat with an abnormally high concentration of chloride; this forms the basis for a useful diagnostic test.

Treatment of cystic fibrosis is mainly palliative—special diets, physiotherapy for pulmonary involvement and antibiotics for infection.

GENERAL READING

Cahill G F 1970 Starvation in man. New England Journal of Medicine 282:668

Frommel D, et al 1984 Voluntary total fasting: a challenge for the medical community. Lancet 1:1451

Goldbloom D S, et al 1989 Anorexia nervosa and bulimia nervosa. Canadian Medical Association Journal 140: 1149

Leading Article 1982 Cardiovascular beriberi. Lancet 1: 1287

Leading article 1986 Vitamin E deficiency. Lancet 1:423

Machlin L J Ed 1984 Handbook of vitamins. Marcel Dekker Inc, New York

Tanaka K 1981 New light on biotin deficiency. New England Journal of Medicine 304:839

Trier J S 1988 Intestinal malabsorption: differentiation of cause. Hospital Practice 23:195

Truswell A S 1985 A B C of nutrition. Vitamins I and II British Medical Journal 291:1033, 1103

Van Itallie T B 1986 Bad news and good news about obesity. New England Journal of Medicine 314:239

19. Calcium metabolism and heterotopic calcification

In addition to providing rigidity to the bones, cacium ions play an important role in many physiological functions. The permeability of cell membranes is affected by the calcium ion concentration of the extracellular fluids: elevation of the calcium concentration reduces permeability. The calcium ion is important in regulating the electrical properties of membranes; thus, hypocalcaemia increases excitability (see tetany). Calcium plays an essential role in muscle contraction. It is involved in the release of preformed hormones from the endocrine glands, as well as playing a part in the formation of the cyclic AMP that is generated in target cells when acted upon by the relevant non-steroid hor-

mones. Finally, it will be recalled that calcium is important in many steps of blood clotting as well as in the activation of complement.

The total body content of calcium is about 1 kg. The average Western diet involves an intake of 600–1000 mg, and a rather similar quantity (about 600 mg) enters the gastrointestinal tract in the various digestive secretions. In all, about 800 mg of calcium is absorbed per day, and this involves a net gain of about 200 mg. This is approximately equal to the urinary loss, so that the individual is in calcium balance. Calcium is absorbed in the duodenum by an active transport mechanism, but the greatest amount is absorbed in the remainder of the small intestine. Its absorption is reduced in vitamin-D deficiency, uraemia, and in the malabsorption syndrome. The presence of phytic acid and an excess of unabsorbed fatty acids inhibit absorption.

Role of bone

Since bone constitutes the main repository for calcium it is not surprising that it plays a vital part in calcium metabolism and that upsets in calcium balance can cause severe bone disease.

The osteoid tissue of bone is manufactured by osteoblasts, and after a 5- to 10-day period of extracellular maturation this osteoid undergoes mineralization with the deposition of calcium salts in the form of hydroxyapatite. Bone salts are deposited first in the region of the gap between collagen molecules; their composition is not fixed, since ions other than calcium and phosphate are involved in their formation, e.g.

magnesium, sodium, potassium and fluoride. Initial mineralization of bone is a rapid process, about 70% of the total salts being deposited within a few hours. The remaining 30% are deposited slowly over a period of several weeks. The mechanism of normal mineralization of osteoid is not well understood. If the calcium–phosphate ion product of extracellular fluids is reduced, osteoid calcification does not take place normally and large amounts of osteoid remain unmineralized. This is the defect found in rickets and osteomalacia. As bone matures, so the osteoblasts become trapped within it and form osteocytes. These cells are not inactive, and are in communication with each other by means of delicate processes that lie in the canaliculi. The osteocytes are bathed in a fluid which is in equilibrium with the bone, but is separated from the general extracellular tissue fluids. The osteocytes play an important, though ill-defined, role in bone homeostasis: thus if they die the bone crumbles and is removed. There is considerable evidence that osteocytes are able to demineralize the bone adjacent to them and also remove its osteoid matrix. This process is called *osteolysis*, and is probably of great importance in the hour-to-hour regulation of the plasma calcium level. Having mobilized calcium by the process of osteolysis, the same cell can subsequently lay down more bone. It is generally agreed that the multinucleate osteoclast is capable of mobilizing calcium from bone by removing both the salts and the protein matrix. This destructive osteoclastic activity is probably of great importance in the general remodelling of bone that is continually taking place.

It is evident that the processes of osteolysis and osteoclastic resorption both involve the simultaneous removal of bone salts and bone matrix. The bone salts presumably enter the fluid surrounding the osteocytes and osteoclasts, but are not immediately able to diffuse into the plasma. Nevertheless, diffusion between this pericellular fluid and that of the extravascular extracellular space ultimately occurs, and the interchange of salts between bone and plasma is of vital importance in the regulation of plasma calcium levels. The mechanism involves three factors: parathyroid hormone, vitamin D, and calcitonin. The

actions of these substances is considered after a review of the normal plasma calcium levels.

Plasma calcium

The normal plasma calcium is remarkably constant in health and is about 2.4 mmol/L (9.5 mg/dl). It exists in three forms:

1. *Ionized calcium.* This component is diffusible and constitutes about 1.1 mmol/L (4.5 mg/dl). It is the most important fraction, and it is maintained at a constant level by the regulatory mechanisms to be described.
2. *Non-ionized, diffusible calcium.* This is the smallest fraction (0.25 mmol/L, or 1 mg/dl), and is present for the most part as citrate.
3. *Protein-bound calcium.* This component (1 mmol/L, or 4 mg/dl) is bound mostly to albumin and is therefore non-diffusible.

It is the total plasma calcium that is usually measured in clinical practice, and in the absence of a marked alteration of plasma proteins, it is a good guide to the level of the ionized fraction. The normal concentration lies between 2.3 and 2.6 mmol/L (9.2 and 10.4 mg/dl).

CALCIUM BALANCE

In spite of a varying diet, the amount of calcium absorbed from the intestine, the amount excreted in the urine, and the amount deposited or withdrawn from bone are so regulated that the level of plasma ionized calcium remains constant. The actions of parathyroid hormone, vitamin D, and calcitonin are vitally concerned in this homeostatic mechanism.

Parathyroid hormone

There is a continuous secretion of hormone from parathyroid glands, but the rate of secretion is influenced by the plasma ionized calcium level: a fall in calcium level stimulates parathyroid secretion, and a rise in calcium level inhibits it. The parathyroid hormone is a polypeptide containing 84 amino-acid residues; it acts on its target organs by activating cyclic AMP. Its major targets are bone, kidney, and intestine.

The effects of parathyroid hormone on bone. Parathyroid hormone promotes the resorption of bone by osteoclasts as well as promoting osteolysis by osteocytes; bone minerals are mobilized, and osteoid is removed. Osteoclasts appear to be directly stimulated so that their number increases (see hyperparathyroidism).

The initial action of parathyroid hormone on osteoblasts is to inhibit their action, but there is evidence that it can later stimulate them to produce bone. Hence the action of parathyroid hormone on bone is somewhat complex, although the overall picture is that of resorption.

Effects of parathyroid hormone on kidney. A characteristic effect of the hormone is to increase phosphate excretion. The result of this is that the plasma phosphate decreases in spite of the continued release of phosphate from the bone. The hormone, on the other hand, increases calcium reabsorption from the kidney, and this, together with the calcium released from the skeleton, results in a rise of plasma calcium. The increased level of ionized calcium leads to an increased glomerular load of calcium; the result is an increased quantity of calcium passed in the urine (*hypercalciuria*). Thus hyperparathyroidism is characterized by hypercalcaemia and an overall calcium loss from the body. Another important action of parathyroid hormone on the kidney is to increase the rate of synthesis of 1,25-dihydroxycholecalciferol, the active form of vitamin D (see later).

Effects of parathyroid hormone on intestine. The hormone increases the absorption of calcium from the intestine indirectly by augmenting the renal formation of 1,25-$(OH)_2D_3$, the active form of vitamin D.

Parathyroid hormone thus appears to be the major factor regulating the level of plasma ionized calcium. By its action it mobilizes calcium from the bone and it retards excretion in the urine. Parathyroid hormone secretion is regulated by the plasma ionic calcium level by a simple feedback mechanism.

Vitamin D

The two important forms of vitamin D are irradiated ergosterol (ergocalciferol), which is present in a diet containing artificially fortified foods and is also called vitamin D_2, and the natural vitamin D produced in the skin by ultraviolet radiation of 7-dehydrocholesterol, and called cholecalciferol or vitamin D_3. The originally described vitamin D_1 has been found to be a mixture.

The metabolism of both vitamins D_2 and D_3 is similar and only that for D_3 will be described. The vitamin is first hydroxylated in the liver to 25-hydroxycholecalciferol (25-OHD_3). The 25-HCC is further hydroxylated to 1,25-dihydroxycholecalciferol, 1,25-$(OH)_2D_3$ in the kidney. This is believed to be the final active metabolite. This final hydroxylation is promoted by low plasma levels of calcium or phosphate and by parathyroid hormone, prolactin, and possibly growth hormone.

1,25-$(OH)_2D_3$ is not the only active form of vitamin D. 25-OHD_3 is also hydroxylated to 24,25-$(OH)_2D_3$ in the kidney and elsewhere. The role of this form of the vitamin is not clear, but it probably plays a part in some cases of rickets and osteomalacia, in which the blood levels of 1,25-$(OH)_2D_3$ are normal or even raised.

The main action of vitamin D is to aid the absorption of calcium from the gut. There are several suggestions as to how this is mediated. It may be that the vitamin stimulates an active transport mechanism or that it promotes the formation of a calcium-binding protein in the intestinal wall. There is considerable confusion regarding the action of vitamin D on bone. In physiological concentrations vitamin D probably has no direct effect, but in pharmacological doses it exhibits a parathyroid-hormone-like action on bone.

Although parathyroid hormone and vitamin D both play important roles in maintaining calcium homeostasis, the action of vitamin D is the more vital. Patients with hypoparathyroidism can be maintained on vitamin-D therapy and additional calcium. On the other hand, the absence of vitamin D leads to severe skeletal disease.

Calcitonin

This hormone is a polypeptide containing 32 amino-acids residues and has the effect of lowering the plasma calcium level. It is secreted by the C cells of the thyroid gland, but the precise role of this hormone in calcium homeostasis is not known. Although tumours of C cells occur (medullary carcinoma of the thyroid) no upset in calcium metabolism has been described in the patients.

DISORDERS OF CALCIUM METABOLISM

Disorders of calcium metabolism form a complex group of topics, and will be described under five headings: vitamin D deficiency, hypoparathyroidism, hyperparathyroidism, hypocalcaemia, and hypercalcaemia. Some interrelationships between these conditions are depicted in Figure 19.1.

VITAMIN-D DEFICIENCY

The body obtains vitamin D from the food and by synthesis in the skin under the influence of ultraviolet light. An inadequate diet (particularly in those countries where there is not much sunlight) and the malabsorption syndrome will therefore lead to its deficiency.

A deficiency of vitamin D results in an impaired absorption of calcium from the intestine and consequent hypocalcaemia. There is a diminution, or even a complete cessation, of calcification of cartilage and osteoid.

Rickets

In the growing child calcification of the epiphyseal cartilage does not occur at the growing ends of the long bones. The cartilage therefore does not die and instead continues to grow, so that the epiphyses undergo enlargement at the bone ends with greatly delayed ossification.

Similarly, the costo-chondral junctions are enlarged, producing the clinical deformity called the 'rachitic rosary'. Growth of bone length is impaired, and the child is dwarfed. Even the

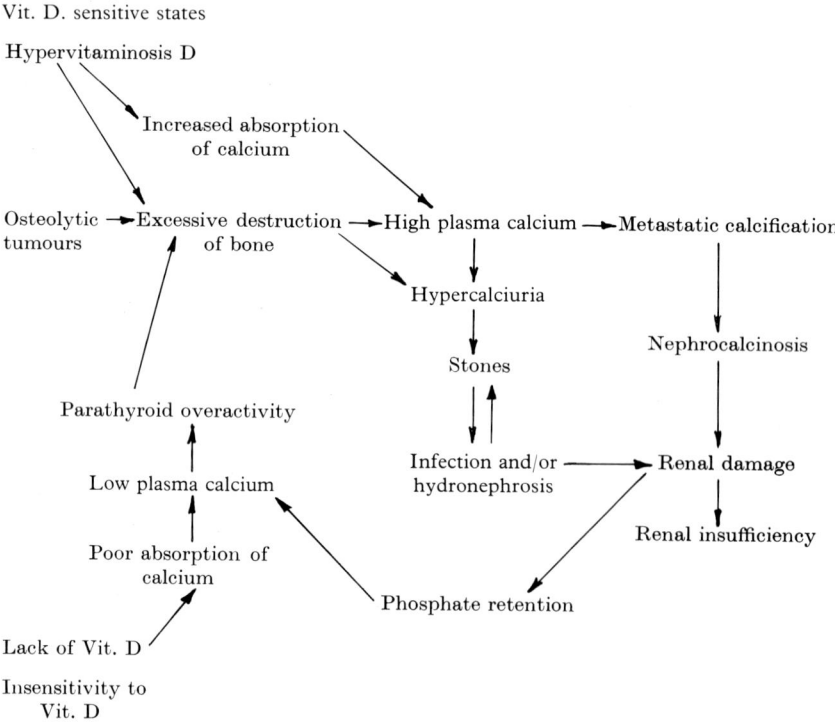

Fig. 19.1 Diagrammatic representation of the important effects of disturbed calcium metabolism. The effects of parathyroid hormone and dietary calcium intake on vitamin D are not shown (see pp. 216 and 217).

osteoid that is formed is poorly calcified, and the weakened bones are liable to deformities and fractures: knock-knees, kyphosis (forward curvature of the spine), and other deformities are common.

In infants there is a thickening of the frontal and parietal eminentia, and flattening and thinning of the occipital region (craniotabes), and there may be delayed eruption of the teeth. Fortunately, this florid picture of rickets is rare in the Western world.

In *vitamin-D resistant rickets* (familial hypophosphataemia) there is a renal defect that results in an excessive excretion of phosphate in the urine, and in a decreased hydroxylation of $25\text{-}OHD_3$.

Osteomalacia

The counterpart of rickets in the adult is osteomalacia. It is more common in women, because pregnancy imposes an additional drain on the supplies of calcium.

In the normal adult bone is continually being remodelled; it is removed by osteoclasts and replaced by osteoblasts laying down osteoid which promptly calcifies. If this calcification fails, the bones consist largely of osteoid and the result is osteomalacia: there is an abundance of osteoid but poor calcification, in contradistinction to osteoporosis, where the matrix is normally calcified but reduced in quantity.

All bones are affected, but it is the weight-bearing regions where the most severe effects are seen. Severe pelvic distortion may cause complications in subsequent pregnancies, and collapse of the vertebrae gives rise to pain due to compression of the spinal nerves in the intervertebral foramina.

HYPOPARATHYROIDISM

The most common cause of hypoparathyroidism is damage to the glands or their blood supply sustained during thyroid surgery.

Hypoparathyroidism is characterized by hypocalcaemia which causes tetany and convulsions and the other effects noted on page 220. Hyperphosphataemia is also present. These changes are also found in pseudohypoparathyroidism, a rare condition in which the parathyroids are normal but there is end-organ unresponsiveness to parathyroid hormone.

HYPERPARATHYROIDISM

Excessive secretion of the parathyroid glands may occur as a primary, secondary, or tertiary condition.

Primary hyperparathyroidism

The first account of this disease was published in 1743 by a Welshman, Sylvanus Bevan. It is generally due to idiopathic hyperplasia of the parathyroid glands, but sometimes an adenoma is responsible; rarely there is a parathyroid carcinoma.

Primary hyperparathyroidism can present in a variety of ways. The best known is classical *osteitis fibrosa cystica*, or *von Recklinghausen's disease of bone*, in which intense osteoclastic resorption leads to destructive cystic changes involving many bones. Bone pain is a prominent symptom, pathological fractures are common, and sometimes tumour-like masses of osteoclasts are formed.

These *brown tumours*, as they are called, closely resemble giant-cell tumours of bone (p. 413), and are seen typically at sites which normally contain haematopoietic tissue: the skull, jaw, ribs, and spine. Brown tumours are also found in the oral soft tissues, particularly the gingivae. The brown coloration is due to the content of haemosiderin.

Occasionally the first indication of hyperparathyroidism is a cyst-like lesion of the jaw. The radiographic description is of a 'ground-glass' appearance of the affected bone. There is resorption of bone, and although the lamina dura may be lost, the teeth are not usually resorbed. The diagnosis may be confirmed by finding the characteristic biochemical changes described below.

More commonly the bone resorption of hyperparathyroidism is generalized; the disorder is less conspicuous and presents as generalized osteoporosis. In these cases the hypercalcaemia causes the characteristic effects (p. 221). Death is due to renal failure. If the plasma calcium reaches very high levels (above 5 mmol/L, or 20 mg/dl), there may be a *hypercalcaemic crisis*. There is shock, haemoconcentration, anuria, and death preceded by confusion and coma.

Another well-known presentation of hyperparathyroidism is recurrent renal-calculus formation. These cases are usually of long standing, bone lesions may be inconspicuous, and the systemic effects of hypercalcaemia are often mild.

The biochemical changes of hyperparathyroidism are a raised level of plasma calcium (it may rise to 5.5 mmol/L, or 22 mg/dl), a lowered level of plasma phosphate, and an increased urinary output of calcium. The plasma alkaline phosphatase is usually considerably raised. Metastatic calcification in the usual sites is common, and is aggravated when renal failure develops. Often this renal failure is caused by metastatic calcification in the kidneys, so that a vicious circle is set up.

Secondary hyperparathyroidism

Hyperplasia of the parathyroids occurs as a result of hypocalcaemia in many types of osteomalacia and rickets. It is the hypocalcaemia that stimulates the glands into activity. In some cases the parathyroid hormone secretion is sufficiently marked to initiate osteoclastic activity in the bones, and therefore in addition to the changes or rickets or osteomalacia there develop those of osteitis fibrosa cystica. This type of response occurs only occasionally, and renal disease is the usual antecedent.

Renal osteodystrophy (renal rickets). Chronic renal disease, especially in young people, is sometimes attended by skeletal lesions which comprise a mixture of calcification defects—osteomalacia (or rickets according to age) and osteitis fibrosa cystica. Metastatic calcification affecting principally the kidneys, arteries, and subcutaneous tissues sometimes occurs.

Tertiary hyperparathyroidism

It is now recognized that some cases of longstanding parathyroid hyperplasia secondary to malabsorption or chronic renal failure may undergo adenomatous change. Hypercalcaemia then develops.

HYPOCALCAEMIA

Causes

The following are important causes of hypocalcaemia.

In association with hypoalbuminaemia. Since the ionized, diffusible calcium level is normal, tetany does not occur.

Hypoparathyroidism. This is described on page 219.

Renal failure. Phosphate retention leads to hyperphosphataemia and a reciprocal lowering of the plasma calcium. Another important factor is deficient hydroxylase activity in the kidney and reduced formation of $1,25(OH)_2D_3$, with a consequent impairment in the intestinal absorption of calcium.

Vitamin-D deficiency.

Widespread osteoplastic metastases. These may utilize so much calcium that hypocalcaemia results. The usual primary source of the tumour is the prostate.

Infantile hypocalcaemia. Neonatal tetany is well recognized and is due to functional immaturity of the parathyroid glands during the first 2 days of life.

Acute pancreatitis. Hypocalcaemia in this condition can be attributed partly to the deposition of calcium salts in the foci of fat necrosis (dystrophic calcification), and partly to the release of glucagon from the damaged pancreas.

Effects

1. Tetany and epileptiform convulsions. There may also be mental disturbances, especially states of depression and anxiety.

In milder hypocalcaemia, where there are no clinical symptoms, there are two simple manoeuvres which may elicit latent tetany: (a) *Trousseau's sign*, which is a spasm of the interossei and of the adductor and opponens muscles of the thumb following the inflation of a sphygmomanometer cuff on the upper arm to above the systolic blood pressure for up to 3 min, and (b) *Chvostek's sign*, which is a twitching of the muscles of that side of the face when the branches of the facial nerve in the parotid gland at the angle of the jaw are trapped. If Trousseau's sign takes more than 2 min to elicit, it is of doubtful significance. Chvostek's sign has been found in from 2 to 20% of normal people.

The actual manifestations of tetany usually commence with paraesthesiae of the hands and feet, and these are followed by classical carpopedal spasms. In severe cases there may also be spasms of the diaphragm, abdominal muscles and back. Spasm of the glottis in children leads to the alarming manifestation of *laryngismus stridulus*.

2. Abdominal pain of obscure origin. It may be due to smooth-muscle spasm.

3. Electrocardiographic changes: a prolonged QT interval principally in the ST segment.

4. A predisposition to eczema in chronic cases. There is also an increased incidence of *Candida albicans* infections of the skin.

5. Cataract, a well-known complication of chronic hypocalcaemia. The cause is uncertain.

HYPERCALCAEMIA

Causes

An increase in the level of plasma calcium occurs in the following conditions:

Primary hyperparathyroidism. This important condition is described on page 219.

Malignancy. In clinical practice malignancy is the most common cause of hypercalcaemia. Many factors have been incriminated. With extensive bone metastases (e.g. carcinoma of the breast) there may be a direct effect of bone destruction. Some tumours (e.g. multiple myeloma and some T-cell lymphomata) secrete an osteoclast stimulating factor. Secretion of prostaglandin E_2 is another factor. Others (e.g. squamous cell carcinoma of the lung and carcinoma of the kidney) form a parathyroid-hormone-like polypeptide.

Hypervitaminosis D. Excessive administration of vitamin D leads to hypercalcaemia and generalized metastatic calcification. The parathyroid-hormone-like activity of vitamin D potentiates this action.

Vitamin-D-sensitive states. Some cases of hypercalcaemia have been attributed, without good evidence, to an increased sensitivity to vitamin D. In *sarcoidosis* hypercalcaemia is common and has been related to hydroxylase activity of the epithelioid cells directly activating the vitamin.

Miscellaneous causes. *Prolonged immobilization, compulsive milk drinking,* and *hyperthyroidism* are occasionally associated with hypercalcaemia. In the rare *congenital hypophosphatasia,* hypercalcaemia and hypercalciuria are associated with low alkaline phosphatase level in the plasma and a clinical picture that resembles rickets.

Effects

1. Fatigue, lethargy, and muscle asthenia.

2. Anorexia, nausea and vomiting. Constipation is prominent, possibly due to the muscular hypotonia.

3. Pruritus, an unexplained symptom.

4. Psychotic manifestations.

5. Symptoms of progressive renal dysfunction: polyuria is the initial manifestation and is due to an unresponsiveness of the distal and collecting tubules to antidiuretic hormone. There is an accompanying thirst, which may also be due to the high plasma-calcium directly stimulating the hypothalamus. This is followed by disturbances in pH regulation and glomerular function, which terminate rapidly in renal failure. Indeed, the renal effects of hypercalcaemia are the most lethal aspect of the condition.

6. Electrocardiographic changes: a shortened QT interval and depressed T waves. These are seldom of diagnostic value.

7. Metastatic calcification.

8. Peptic ulceration. This is particularly common in primary hyperparathyroidism, but can occur in other types of hypercalcaemia also. The excess plasma calcium releases gastrin.

9. Pancreatitis, both acute and chronic. This again is seen most often in association with primary hyperparathyroidism, but can occur in other types of hypercalcaemia also. The mechanism is unknown (as indeed is that of pancreatitis generally); suggested factors include stones forming in the pancreatic ducts and the ionized calcium favouring the conversion of trypsinogen to trypsin in the pancreatic ducts.

HETEROTOPIC CALCIFICATION

It is convenient to conclude this account of calcium metabolism with a description of *heterotopic calcification*. This is defined as the deposition of calcium salts in tissues other than osteoid, dentine or enamel. Because calcium salts are radiopaque, their deposition is conspicuous on radiographs, and heterotopic calcification has therefore come to assume an importance in diagnostic radiology which far outweighs its pathological significance.

Microscopically calcium salts appear as granular deposits which stain a very deep blue colour with haematoxylin. Two quite distinct types of heterotopic calcification are recognized. *Dystrophic calcification* is the deposition of calcium salts in dead or degenerate tissue. The plasma levels of calcium and phosphate are normal and abnormal local conditions are the cause of the calcification. In *metastatic calcification* there is an upset in calcium metabolism and the calcification takes place in certain normal tissues.

DYSTROPHIC CALCIFICATION

The cause of dystrophic calcification can be considered under two headings: (1) calcification in dead tissue, and (2) calcification in degenerate tissue. Though the distinction between the two may be somewhat arbitrary, this forms a convenient division.

Calcification in dead tissue

Calcification is frequent in caseous tissue and remains as a permanent memorial to a previous tuberculous lesion, e.g. in the lung or hilar lymph nodes. Dead parasites (e.g. *Trichinella spiralis*), areas of fat necrosis (in pancreatitis), artheromatous material, and thrombi provide other examples of dead tissue that may calcify.

Calcification in degenerate tissue

Calcification is not uncommon in the fibrous tissue of scars or a chronic inflammatory lesion, e.g. in chronic tonsillitis or a treated lesion of bacterial endocarditis. Degenerate areas of tumour may calcify, and this forms the basis of *mammography*, in which radiographs of the female breast are examined as a means of detecting a carcinoma that cannot be felt.

METASTATIC CALCIFICATION

Metastatic calcification is caused by a disordered metabolism of calcium and phosphate, and although in the common type (following hyperparathyroidism) the calcium salts are truly metastatic, being derived from bone, there are other conditions in which the excess calcium is absorbed from the gut. Nevertheless, it is convenient in practice to use the term 'metastatic calcification' to cover both these varieties, and it will be used in this context in the account that follows.

Generalized metastatic calcification is usually due to hypercalcaemia, which has already been considered. Malignancy and hyperparathyroidism are important causes. Occasionally, as in renal osteodystrophy, a high plasma phosphate appears to be the precipitating factor. The bone salts are deposited in certain sites of election.

Sites involved

Kidney. This is the most frequent and important site. Deposition occurs especially around the tubules, where severe damage is produced. The condition is called *nephrocalcinosis*, and it may lead to renal failure (see Ch. 33). In addition, calculi often form in the pelvis and ureter, where they may predispose to infection and cause further renal damage. *Renal failure is therefore a prominent feature of generalized metastatic calcification whatever may be the primary cause.*

Lung, stomach, blood-vessel walls, and the cornea. These sites are sites frequently affected.

Causes of metastatic calcification

The following causes of metastatic calcification can be recognized:

Hyperparathyroidism. Primary hyperparathyroidism is due to parathyroid hyperplasia, adenoma, or rarely carcinoma. *Secondary hyperparthyroidism* is generally caused by renal failure.

Excessive absorption of calcium from the bowel. Hypervitaminosis D and vitamin-sensitive states, e.g. in sarcoidosis.

Destructive bone lesions. Widespread osteolytic metastatic carcinoma in bone and multiple myeloma are both sometimes complicated by metastatic calcification.

GENERAL READING

Audran M, Kumar R 1985 The physiology and pathophysiology of vitamin D. Mayo Clinic Proceedings 60:851

Heath D A 1989 Hypercalcaemia in malignancy. British Medical Journal 298:1468

Jamieson M J 1985 Hypercalcaemia. British Medical Journal 290:378

Schmidt N 1980 Hyperparathyroidism: a review. American Journal of Surgery 139:677

Leading article 1987 Vitamin D: new perspectives. Lancet 11:122

20. Disorders of development and growth

It is incredible that in the course of a few months, a single cell, the fertilized ovum, can proliferate and differentiate into the complex system of organs and tissues that constitute the mature organism. Errors in this remarkable process can produce severe effects and these will be discussed under the heading of *developmental anomalies*. However, cell division and differentiation do not end at birth, or even when the individual has attained maturity. All tissues, with the exception of neurons and most types of muscle cells, show a slow turnover of cells as mitosis compensates for cells that mature, die or desquamate. An upset in this steady state also leads to morphological abnormalities. These will be described in the second part of this chapter as *cellular adaptations*.

DEVELOPMENTAL ANOMALIES

Abnormalities of development range from the trivial to the lethal. Minor variations are so common that the differences which result are regarded as normal. More serious errors in development result in the production of various malformations which are usually apparent at birth, but which may develop at any time during the growing period of childhood and adolescence. Gross abnormalities may be incompatible with life, and these result in abortion, stillbirth, or neonatal death. Anencephaly, in which most of the brain is absent, is one such example.

CAUSES OF DEVELOPMENTAL ANOMALIES

Developmental anomalies may occur either as a result of genetic errors or be due to environmental factors.

Genetic errors

These have been described in Chapter 3. Chromosomal and genetic abnormalities should always be considered when developmental anomalies are present.

Environmental factors

It is becoming increasingly obvious that many external agents are capable of causing serious developmental anomalies. These are called *teratogenic agents* and have the most severe effects when they act in utero.

Infection

Transmission of infection from the mother to the fetus may cause severe damage. The first trimester of pregnancy is the most dangerous time, as it is during this period that rapid division and differentiation occur. Rubella has acquired a particularly evil reputation: deformities occur in as many as 25% of babies born to mothers who have had this infection during pregnancy.

Drugs

A notorious tragedy occurred around the period of 1960, when pregnant women who had taken the sedative thalidomide gave birth to grossly deformed babies. The drug thalidomide is dangerous during the crucial period from 37 to 54 days after the first day of the last menstrual period. The most common anomalies were absence of limbs or parts of limbs, haemangiomatosis of the upper lips and nose, and malformations of the alimentary tract, heart, and genito-urinary system. *Cytotoxic agents* also produce malformations, and the use of large doses of *progesterone* can produce genital deformities in female infants. *Isotretinoin* (Acutane), used in the treatment of severe acne vulgaris, is a potent teratogen and strict guidelines must be adhered to if the drug is given to female patients.

It is obviously wise to avoid the use of all drugs during pregnancy, especially during the first three months.

An even more serious hazard to fetal development is *maternal alcoholism*. Expectant mothers who consume large amounts of alcohol tend to give birth to babies that are below average weight and length. There is often hypoplasia of the maxilla with prominence of the forehead and lower jaw, short palpebral fissures, microcephaly, and mental retardation. Other defects are also described, and it is evident that excessive amounts of alcohol in the fetal blood constitute a very real teratogenic hazard.

Ionizing radiations

It is hoped that abnormalities due to external agents will become less frequent as knowledge about the factors involved is acquired.

TYPES OF MALFORMATION

Although it is a somewhat artificial subdivision, it is convenient to consider the types of malformation under separate headings.

Failure of development

There may be complete failure of development of a part (*agenesis*), or the part may remain rudimentary (*hypoplasia*) and never attain a full mature size. In the rare condition of anodontia there is agenesis of the dental lamina and complete absence of all the teeth. Congenital absence of a few teeth (partial anodontia or hypodontia) is more common (Fig. 20.1). Both these conditions may be associated with a general defect of ectodermal structures affecting the hair, nails, and sebaceous and sweat glands (ectodermal dysplasia) (Fig. 20.2).

Failure of fusion

During development many structures normally fuse, and a failure to do so results in an abnormality. A cleft of the lip and palate occurs as a result of failure of fusion of the globular portion of the median nasal process with the lateral nasal and maxillary processes.

Failure of separation

A good example of this is the webbing which may persist between the digits.

Failure of canalization (atresia)

Various channels in the body may fail to canalize, e.g. oesophageal atresia and imperforate anus.

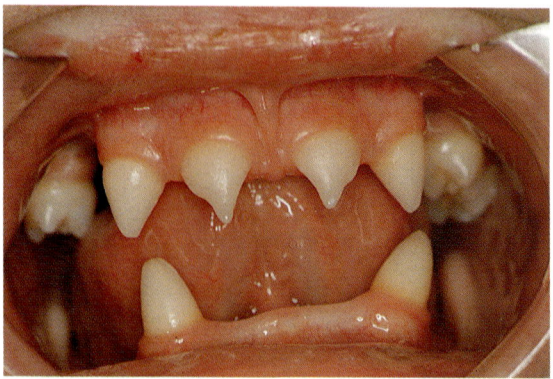

Fig. 20.1 Hypodontia. Many primary and permanent teeth failed to develop in this 8-year-old boy. The upper permanent incisors are conical in form. He also has ectodermal dysplasia (see Fig. 20.2.)

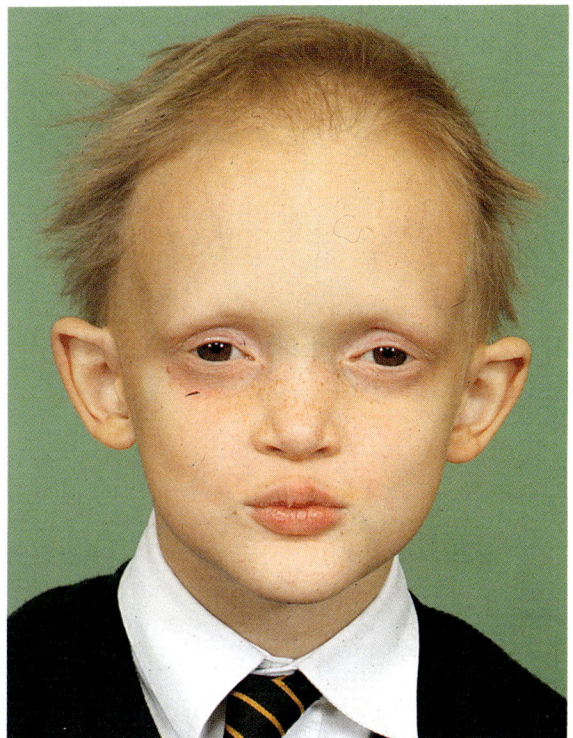

Fig. 20.2   This boy has ectodermal dysplasia (see also Fig. 20.1). He has sparse hair, lack of eyebrows, prominent ears, pigmentation around the eyes and everted lips.

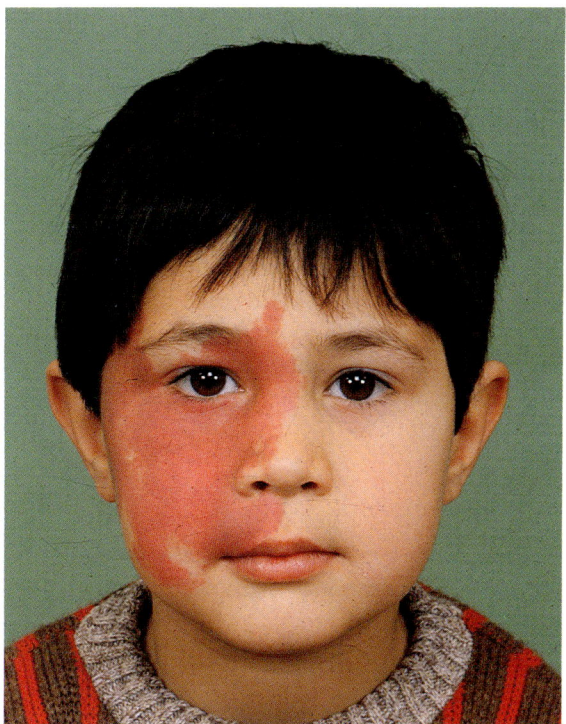

Fig. 20.3   Naevus flammeus affecting the right maxillary region. Note the clear line of demarcation. (Photograph by Department of Clinical Illustration, Birmingham Dental School. Previously published in Rock, W P, Grundy M C, Shaw L Diagnostic picture tests in paediatric dentistry. Wolfe Medical Publications, London.)

Ectopia

Sometimes organs and tissues are found in abnormal sites. This is called ectopia, heterotopia, or aberrance. Aberrant adrenal tissue may be found on the surface of the kidney and gonads, and an ectopic testis may be encountered in the abdominal cavity, the perineum, or the pubic area. Ectopic thyroid may be found in the tongue in the region of the foramen caecum, and in some cases no thyroid tissue may be present in its normal situation.

Heteroplasia

Sometimes there is an anomalous differentiation of a particular tissue in an organ. For instance, sebaceous glands may be found in the buccal mucosa (Fordyce spots). This is called heteroplasia, and must be distinguished from metaplasia, in which the alteration of the tissue occurs after normal differentiation has taken place.

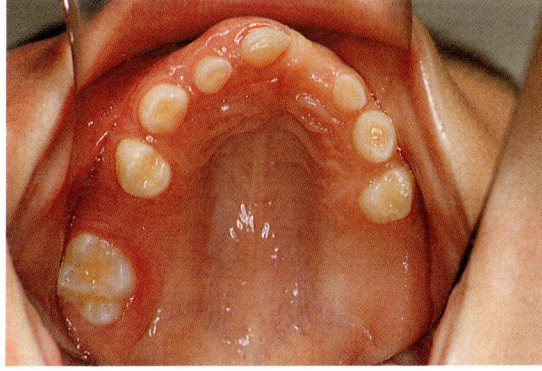

Fig. 20.4   Intra-oral view of the boy in Fig. 20.3 showing the increased vascularity of the maxillary region on the right side and early eruption of the first permanent molar in this 4-year-old boy. (Photograph by Department of Clinical Illustration, Birmingham Dental School. Previously published in Rock, W P, Grundy M C, Shaw L Diagnostic picture tests in paediatric dentistry. Wolfe Medical Publications, London.)

Heteroplasia implies that the abnormal differentiation is a primary affair.

Local gigantism

Sometimes there is simple overgrowth of an organ or tissue, e.g. an enlarged digit or limb in neurofibromatosis, and this is rather dubiously called 'hypertrophy'. It is in fact better called local gigantism, because the organ has never been normal in relation to the remainder of the body. In true hyperplasia and hypertrophy the part is initially normal in size and subsequently undergoes enlargement.

Supernumerary organs

Additional, or supernumerary, teeth may be present; likewise additional digits may occur (polydactyly).

Hamartomata

A hamartoma is a tumour-like malformation in which the tissues of a particular part of the body are arranged haphazardly, usually with an excess of one or more of its components. The term was coined by Albrecht in 1904, and is derived from the Greek word *hamartein*, a bodily defect. The concept it embodies is of great importance, for a large number of common lesions fall into the general category of hamartomata.

The best known hamartoma is the common 'mole' or melanocytic naevus which is described in Chapter 37. It is important to appreciate that a hamartoma is not true neoplasm from which it differs in many ways. A hamartoma grows pari passu with its surroundings and has no capsule. It contains only those tissues that are specific to the part from which it arises. Unfortunately many hamartomata have been given 'tumour sounding' names, e.g. haemangioma, osteochondroma, neurofibroma, etc. This is so ingrained in medical terminology that it is unlikely to change.

Vascular hamartomata. The very common haemangioma is a hamartomatous malformation and not a true neoplasm. The commonest site is the skin, where it forms a variety of *naevus*, a word used to describe any type of developmental blemish of the skin. A noteworthy feature of

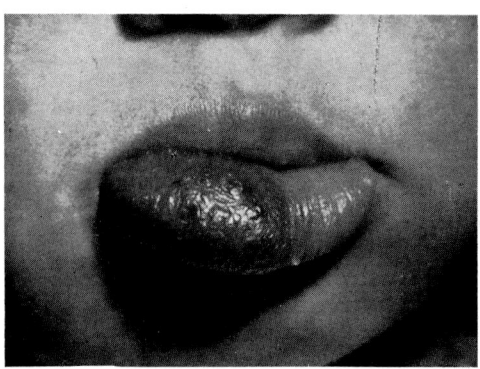

Fig. 20.5 Capillary haemangioma of lower lip. (Photograph supplied by Mr G.S. Hoggins.)

angiomata is their tendency towards multiplicity. They may be accompanied by angiomatous involvement of internal organs as well as being a component of a more generalized disorder. Several characteristic syndromes have been described, and since they involve the head and neck, they are of importance to the dentist.

Spider naevus. The characteristic morphology of the cutaneous spider naevus is due to the presence of a central pulsating arteriole which leads to a leash of radiating capillaries. The lesion blanches on pressure. Spider naevi may develop during childhood, but most commonly they occur in the course of chronic liver disease—usually cirrhosis. Spider naevi may also occur on the mucous membranes, but their 'spider' morphology is less evident than those on the skin.

Naevus flammeus or port wine stain. Persistent dilatation of the skin capillaries produces the characteristic *port-wine stain* Two types are recognized. *Medially located naevus flammeus* is a common lesion, usually overlying the occiput and therefore largely hidden by hair. It is of no importance. *Laterally located naevus flammeus* is generally evident at birth, and commonly affects the face and oral mucosa in the distribution of the trigeminal nerve. It is usually unilateral. Apart from its cosmetic significance, it may be associated with vascular anomalies of oral mucosa and early eruption of the teeth (Figs 20.3 and 20.4). There may be involvement of the meninges and eye; this is called *encephalo-trigeminal angiomatosis*, or the *Sturge–Weber syndrome*. Hemiparesis on the side opposite to the lesion, convulsions, and mental defect are due to hypoxia of the underlying cerebral cortex.

Capillary or strawberry haemangioma. This lesion is usually present at birth or during the first month of life as a well-defined lesion on the face (Fig. 20.5). It increases in size, often quite rapidly. Spontaneous regression with scarring usually occurs, but surgical treatment may be required for cosmetic reasons or for delayed regression. The strawberry naevus is predominantly composed of capillary-sized vessels, but it may be of mixed capillary-cavernous type.

Cavernous haemangiomata are less well circumscribed, and tend to extend more deeply into the subcutaneous tissues. They may occur on the lips, tongue, and bone.

Involvement of the bone by haemangiomata should be suspected if there is early eruption of the teeth in that area. Serious consequences may result from extraction of teeth in that region. (Fig 20.4.)

Hereditary haemorrhagic telangiectasia (Osler–Rendu–Weber disease). This disease is inherited as an autosomal dominant trait, and generally becomes apparent at puberty or somewhat later. Multiple telangiectases develop on the skin, being particularly conspicuous on the face and lips (Fig. 20.7). The mucous membranes are invariably involved, and bleeding can occur from any site; thus bleeding from the nose (epistaxis) may be the first symptom. Arteriovenous malformations may occur in the lungs and other internal organs.

Ataxia telangiectasia. This syndrome, which occurs in young children, is characterized by a complex immunological deficiency affecting both T and B cells, recurrent respiratory infections, cerebellar ataxia, and the presence of telangiectases first evident on the conjunctiva and later on the ears and the butterfly area of the face. The disease is inherited as an autosomal recessive trait, and death usually occurs by adolescence either from infection or a malignant lymphoma.

Microscopically haemangiomata consist of poorly demarcated, non-encapsulated masses and leashes of vascular channels, which are sometimes capacious, and described as *cavernous*, (Fig. 20.6), and at other times narrow and well formed (*capillary haemangioma*).

Another type of vascular hamartoma is the lymphangioma. A well-known example is the cystic hygroma of infancy, which forms a characteristic swelling in the neck. It infiltrates the vital surrounding structures so intimately that its complete removal is seldom possible.

Skeletal hamartoma. The common solitary exostosis or osteochondroma that grows from the epiphyseal cartilage of a long bone is a cartilaginous hamartoma. Growth stops after puberty, when it completely ossifies.

Dental hamartomata. An odontome is a malformation of all the dental tissues. As odontomes are composed of enamel, dentine, and cementum, they are termed composite, and there are several types. The compound odontome consists of a number of very small calcified structures which resemble teeth and are called denticles. The complex composite odontome consists of an irregular mass of calcified dental tissues. The odontome may replace a tooth in the arch, or it may be additional to the complete dentition having arisen from a supernumary anlage.

Neurofibromatosis (von Recklinghausen's disease). This is inherited as an autosomal dominant trait and is characterized by widespread hamartomatous overgrowth of nerve sheath tissue (Fig. 20.8). The nodules produced resemble the tumours called neurofibromata. Occasionally one

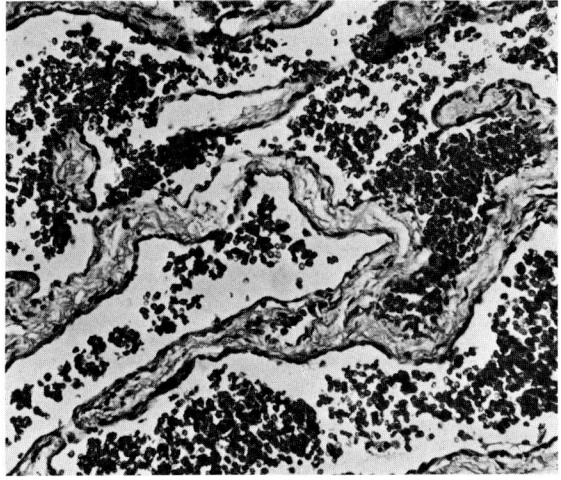

Fig. 20.6 Haemangioma. This is a cavernous haemangioma, and it consists of extensive vascular spaces enclosed in loose strands of endothelial-lined connective tissue. x 200.

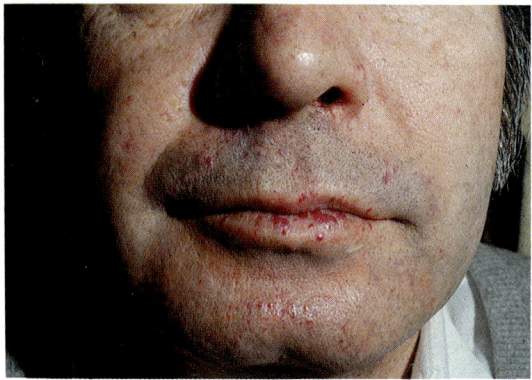

Fig. 20.7 Hereditary haemorrhagic telangiectasia (Osler–Weber–Rendu syndrome). Numerous telangiectatic vessels are present on the lips and surrounding skin.

undergoes sarcomatous change. There may be regional gigantism, which if on the face produces gross deformity. Café-au-lait lentigenes are present on the skin, and freckles in the axilla are characteristic.

Persistence of vestigial structures.

In the course of development many parts which are of importance to the embryo undergo obliteration by the time of birth. If this does not

happen, these normally vestigial structures persist and may lead to subsequent trouble. The two most important complications are *neoplasia* (see p. 259) and *cyst formation*.

CYSTS

It is appropriate to end this section with an account of the types of cyst, for many of them have a developmental basis.

The word *cyst*, derived from the Greek *kustis*, a bladder, means a *pathological fluid-filled sac bounded by a wall*. The fluid may be secreted by cells lining the wall or it may be derived from the tissue fluid of the area. It is often clear and colourless, but it may be turbid and thick, or contain shimmering crystals of cholesterol. By common usage a cyst does not contain frank pus or blood—in these circumstances the terms abscess or haematoma are employed.

Where the cyst wall is lined by an epithelium, this layer may be derived from developmental residues such as the epithelial rests of Malassez in the periodontal ligament or epithelial residues lying in planes of embryonic fusion. On the other hand it may arise from a normal anatomical structure, such as the cells lining the ducts and

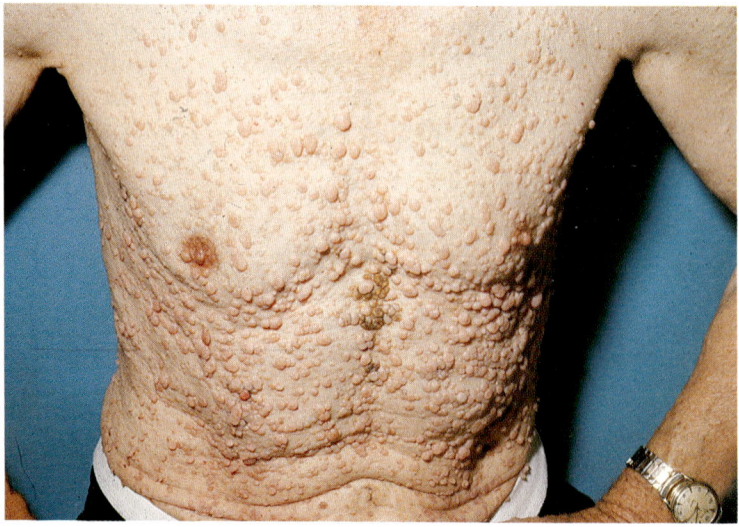

Fig. 20.8 Multiple neurofibromatosis (von Reckinghausen's disease). Numerous neurofibromata, many of them pedunculated, are present on the skin.

acini of an exocrine gland. Often the stimulus which provokes the epithelial proliferation is unknown, as for instance in cysts arising in planes of embryonic fusion like the globulo-maxillary cyst. Sometimes chronic inflammation is a factor, as in the development of the *apical* or *radicular cyst*, the commonest of the odontogenic cysts. Here the chronic inflammation in the periapical tissues of a non-vital tooth stimulates the epithelial rests of Malassez to proliferate and line the liquefied apical granuloma, thus forming part of the wall of the cyst, the contents of which are turbid and characteristically contain cholesterol crystals, which are a product of tissue breakdown.

The classification of cysts is difficult, but the most practical one is based on the pathogenesis of the lesion.

1. *Developmental*. See below.
2. *Inflammatory*, e.g. the *apical* cyst.
3. *Degenerative*, e.g. cystic changes in goitres, in solid tumours like the uterine myoma (fibroid), and in other pathological lesions like fibrous dysplasia of bone. The basic change is necrosis which is almost always ischaemic in origin. A degenerative cyst may occur in vascular disease, as in brain cysts following cerebral infarction, or in a tumour or other lesion with inadequate blood supply. The necrotic debris subsequently becomes liquefied.
4. *Retention*, e.g. a ranula, which is a cystic dilatation in the submandibular or sublingual gland formed as a result of obstruction of its duct. The name refers to the frog-like swelling produced—'ranula' is Latin for 'little frog'.
5. *Implantation*, e.g. epidermoid cyst following injury.
6. *Hydatid*, a parasitic cyst, found usually in the liver and lungs, due to the proliferation and expansion of the larval form of the canine tapeworm *Echinococcus granulosus*.
7. *Hyperplastic*, e.g. mammary dysplasia.
8. *Neoplastic*, e.g. cystadenoma of the ovary and cystic teratoma.

Developmental cysts

These may arise from ectopic tissues or from the persistence of vestigial remnants.

Ectopia of various tissues

In ectopia there is a dislocation of tissue into a neighbouring area, where it often becomes cystic. A good example is the dermoid cyst, which is due to the sequestration of a piece of skin beneath one of the lines of fusion of the various embryonic body processes. Dermoid cysts occur most commonly in the subcutaneous tissue of the face, usually near the angle of the orbit. Another site is under the tongue (sublingual dermoid). A dermoid cyst is lined by stratified squamous epithelium, and in its wall there are hair follicles, sebaceous glands, and sweat glands. It contains a thick, greasy material consisting of keratin produced by the epithelial lining and sebum secreted by the sebaceous glands. Matted hair is also often present. Unlike a teratoma, it does not include other tissues in its wall.

Persistence of vestigial remnants

Examples of this type are the branchial and thyroglossal cysts. A branchial cyst develops from a persisting portion of the cervical sinus; it is lined by stratified squamous epithelium and is surrounded by lymphoid tissue. Some odontogenic cysts are also due to the persistence of paradental remnants, e.g. the dentigerous cyst which surrounds the crown of an unerupted tooth. It is formed by the accumulation of fluid between the layers of the enamel epithelium or between the epithelium and the tooth crown.

DISORDERS OF CELLULAR ADAPTATION

This group of conditions affects individuals who have attained maturity when development is complete; nevertheless they can also occur in children. The factors that control the growth and differentiation of cells are largely unknown, although the recognition of growth factors, their receptors and the cyto-oncogenes that control them are being recognized. Nevertheless abnormalities in these two processes are frequent, and form an important aspect of many disease processes. They may be considered under three headings:

1. *Quantitative abnormalities of growth*
2. *Abnormalities of cellular differentiation*
3. *Neoplasia*, a topic so important that it is considered separately in the next chapter.

QUANTITATIVE ABNORMALITIES OF GROWTH

Excessive growth

Tissues composed of cells which can divide (labile and stable cells) respond to an increased demand for work primarily by multiplication. *Labile cells* are those that divide continuously during life, e.g. most covering epithelia. *Stable cells* divide occasionally but can be stimulated to do so, e.g. cells of the liver and most solid glandular tissue. *Permanent cells* which cannot divide either show no morphological change (neurons), or else only an increase in size (muscle). Even stable and labile cells usually show some increase in size. An increase in the cell number is called *hyperplasia*, and an increase in individual cell size is *hypertrophy*. Both are usually related to a tangible stimulus, which is often a basically physiological one acting to excess. The most important stimulus is an *increased demand for function*. As will be seen, this may take the form of increased muscular work in response to an abnormal load, an increased production of the blood cells in response to hypoxia or infection, a thickening of protective epithelium in response to external trauma, or an increased secretion of a gland in response to some external need.

Enlargements due to congestion, oedema, inflammation, amyloid infiltration, or tumour formation are excluded from the definition. The suffix—megaly is used to denote a large organ or tissue regardless of its cause, e.g. cardiomegaly is enlargement of the heart, splenomegaly is enlargement of the spleen, etc.

Hyperplasia

Hyperplasia is defined as an increase in size of an organ or tissue due to an increase in the number of its specialized constituent cells.

It is important to realize that those hyper-

plasias due to a specific stimulus exist only for so long as that stimulus is applied. When it is removed, the tissue tends to revert to its normal size.

Although the concept of hyperplasia is traditionally a morphological one, it must never be forgotten that the increase in size of the organ is accompanied by a corresponding increase in function. Nowhere is this more apparent than in hyperplasia of the endocrine glands.

Hyperplasia in the endocrine glands. In endocrine hyperplasias there is enlargement of the gland (or glands, as the case may be). Sometimes this enlargement is diffuse, but in many instances it is focal (Fig. 20.9). The nodules so formed are often labelled adenomata. In secreting epithelia generally the line of demarcation between hyperplasia and benign neoplasia is so tenuous that a distinction is often purely arbitrary.

Parathyroids. The parathyroid glands show hyperplasia in response to a persistent hypocalcaemia (see secondary hyperparathyroidism, p. 220). In primary hyperparathyroidism the stimulus for the hyperplasia is unknown.

Thyroid. Thyroid hyperplasia is rarely the result of prolonged stimulation by pituitary thyrotrophic hormone. As a primary idiopathic condition it occurs in primary hyperthyroidism (Graves' disease) (p. 435).

Hyperplasia of the endocrine glands is described in greater detail in Chapter 36.

Target organs of the endocrine glands. Hyperplasia of the epithelial tissue and surrounding specialized connective tissue is a normal feature of the female *breast* at puberty, during pregnancy and lactation, and to a lesser extent towards the end of each menstrual cycle.

In *cystic hyperplasia of the breast* (mammary dysplasia), there is considerable epithelial hyperplasia, and cysts often develop. It is a common condition, and causes discomfort as well as nodularity of the breast substance. Hormonal imbalance is presumed to be the cause, but its nature is obscure.

Senile enlargement of the *prostate* is due to epithelial hyperplasia as well as an increase in the fibromuscular element. The condition is common over the age of 60 years, and is erroneously called 'benign prostatic hypertrophy' or 'adenomatosis of the prostate'. It is an important cause of urinary obstruction, and surgical treatment is often necessary to relieve back-pressure effects on the bladder and kidneys. The cause is unknown, but is probably hormonal in nature.

Hyperplasia of skin and oral mucosa. This may be caused by constant rubbing as in lichen simplex chronicus. Likewise a jagged tooth or an ill-fitting denture causes thickening and orthokeratosis of the oral mucosa. Hyperplasia may be induced by viral infection, e.g. verruca vulgaris and condylomata acuminata and in fungal infections, e.g. blastomycosis.

Hyperplasia and bone marrow. Pronounced hyperplasia is seen in the haematopoietic tissue when there is a stimulus for blood cell production. The erythroid series is affected in hypoxia and in many types of anaemia, e.g. pernicious anaemia. In infection it is the white-cell precursors which are affected. The cellular marrow extends into the long bones of the adult (normally filled with fatty narrow), while in childhood extramedullary foci of haematopoiesis may occur in the liver, spleen and other organs.

Hyperplasia of the lymphoreticular tissue. Hyperplasia in chronic infection accounts for the enlargement of the spleen (*splenomegaly*) and lymph nodes (*lymphadenopathy*).

Hyperplasia in relationship to chronic inflammation. As noted previously hyperplasia is sometimes a feature of longstanding chronic inflammation (p. 102).

In the skin hyperplasia may affect the epithelium or the connective tissue. Epithelial hyperplasia may be seen in fungal granulomata or at the edge of chronic ulcers.

The granuloma pyogenicum is another curious skin lesion in which there is such a profuse proliferation of blood vessels and fibroblasts that the elevated nodule which is produced closely resembles a haemangioma. The lesion is misnamed, for it is not granulomatous nor is it inflamed unless as a secondary event following ulceration of the covering epidermis due to local trauma. Pyogenic granulomata often grow rapidly for a time and can easily be mistaken for a malignant tumour or a spindle-cell naevus. The pyogenic granuloma that arises from the gingiva is probably an exaggerated inflammatory

lesion (Fig. 20.10). Like its cutaneous counterpart, it is extremely vascular but it is always heavily infiltrated with polymorphs. The lesion is particularly common in pregnant women (*pregnancy tumour*).

In the oral mucosa chronic inflammation may likewise cause epithelial or connective tissue hyperplasia. Multiple warty epithelial overgrowths may occur, apparently as a result of the irritation from an ill-fitting denture (*papillomatosis*). Chronic inflammation may produce hyperplasia of the connective tissue so that fibrous nodules are formed. These are sometimes called 'fibromata', or if pedunculated, *fibro-epithelial polyps*. An *epulis* is a nodule on the gingiva, and most examples are due to connective-tissue hyperplasia induced by inflammation. Sometimes the fibrovascular proliferation and giant-cell formation is so marked that the lesion resembles a giant-cell tumour of bone. It is called the peripheral *giant-cell reparative granuloma* (*giant-cell epulis*) (Fig. 20.11).

Pseudoneoplastic hyperplasia. Reference has been made to the difficulties in distinguishing nodular hyperplasia from benign neoplasia, particularly in the endocrine glands, the prostate, and the breast. From a practical point of view the distinction is unimportant since both processes are benign. There are, however, many examples of hyperplasia in which the mass of cells produced closely resembles a malignant tumour. Experience has taught that they are benign, because they either resolve spontaneously or respond to simple treatment. Their importance lies in their recognition, for a mistaken diagnosis can result in grave therapeutic errors. Almost any tissue can show such lesions, and only a few examples will be described.

Pseudomalignant connective tissue hyperplasia. Pseudolymphoma of the skin appears as nodules of lymphoid tissue which histologically closely resemble the nodular type of lymphocytic lymphoma. Unlike the latter, however, the cutaneous lesion never becomes systematized nor develops into an overtly malignant process. Similar pseudolymphomata are described at other sites, e.g. orbit, rectum, and mediastinum. A persistent inflammatory reaction to an arthropod bite can closely mimic a cutaneous lymphoma.

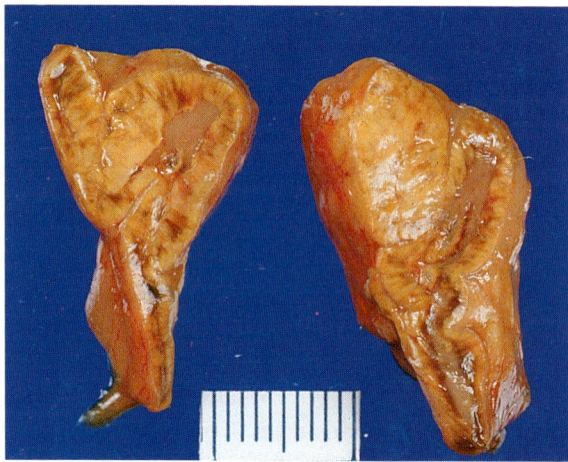

Fig. 20.9 Nodular hyperplasia of the adrenal cortex. Numerous ill-defined yellow nodules of hyperplastic cortical cells are present in the adrenal cortex.

Pseudosarcomatous nodular fasciitis affects the subcutaneous tissues, commonly of the arm. In children, the head and neck are the most frequently affected sites. Rarely, it affects the oral mucosa. There is rapid growth of a highly vascular mass which diffusely infiltrates the surrounding tissues. Many mitoses are present in its spindle-cell component, but in spite of the malignant microscopic appearance the lesion is benign in its behaviour.

Pseudomalignant epithelial hyperplasia. Marked hyperplasia of the epidermis which gives an appearance of dermal invasion by squamous cells is seen from time to time in a great variety of chronic skin lesions ranging from fungal granulomata and arthropod bites to basal cell carcinoma. The lesion is commonly called *pseudoepitheliomatous hyperplasia* and at times differentiation from squamous-cell carcinoma is not possible, especially when small biopsy specimens alone are available for study.

Pseudoepitheliomatous hyperplasia is well seen over a granular cell tumour, a somewhat controversial lesion found most often on the tongue and occasionally in the skin. It is composed of very large polygonal and strap-shaped cells, the cytoplasm of which contains coarse eosinophilic granules. The tumour was previously called a myoblastoma but is now thought to be derived from Schwann cells rather than muscle, and the cause of the overlying epithelial hyperplasia is unknown.

Keratoacanthoma may be regarded as a type of pseudoepitheliomatous hyperplasia. The lesion generally arises on the sun-exposed skin, grows rapidly and then undergoes spontaneous resolution leaving a scar. The lesion has a central keratin filled crater around which there is invading atypical squamous cells (Fig. 20.12). Morphologically it closely resembles a squamous cell carcinoma. Indeed sometimes if inadequate material is available for study distinction is not possible.

Hypertrophy

Hypertrophy is defined as an increase in size of an organ or tissue due to increase in size of its constituent specialized cells. Pure hypertrophy without accompanying hyperplasia occurs only in muscle, and the stimulus is almost always a mechanical one.

Hypertrophy of smooth muscle. Any obstruction to the outflow of the contents of a hollow muscular viscus results in hypertrophy of its muscle coat. It is seen in the *bladder* when there is prostatic hyperplasia, and in any part of the *gut* above an obstruction, e.g. a stricture or a carcinoma. The myometrium of the uterus shows tremendous hypertrophy during pregnancy, and the stimulus, although partly mechanical, is also a hormonal action of oestrogen.

Hypertrophy of cardiac muscle. Although the heart of the newborn child weighs only 30 g, it is believed that no further muscle cells are pro-

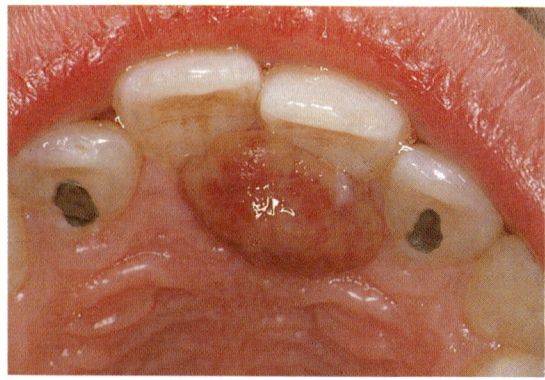

Fig. 20.10 Pyogenic granuloma which developed rapidly in 4 weeks, probably following trauma to the incisive papilla. Note the pronounced rougae in the palate.

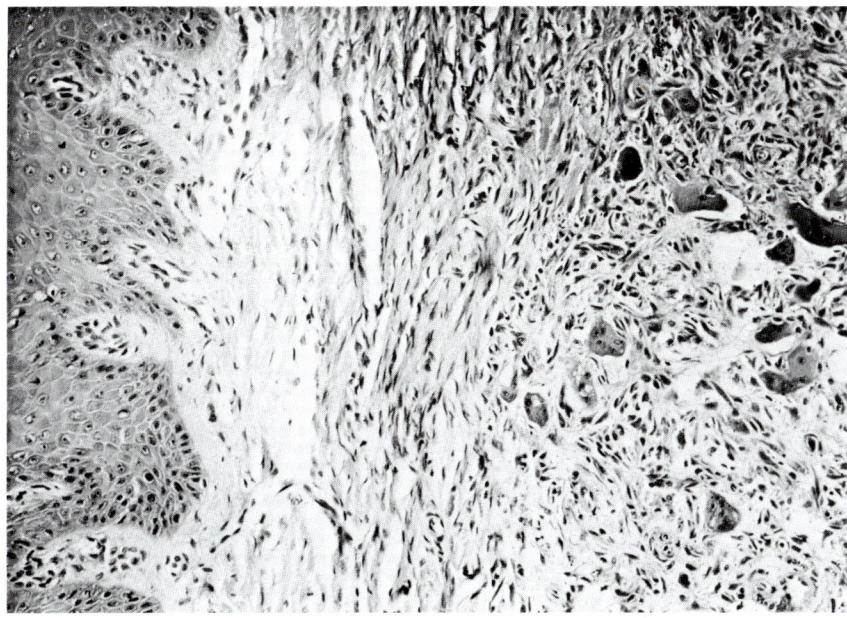

Fig. 20.11 Peripheral giant-cell reparative granuloma. There is a heavy infiltration of foreign-body giant cells in a stroma of collagen and spindle-shaped cells. This is situated in the subepithelial connective tissue of the gingiva, and is separated from the overlying epithelium by a narrow zone of fibrous tissue. × 100.

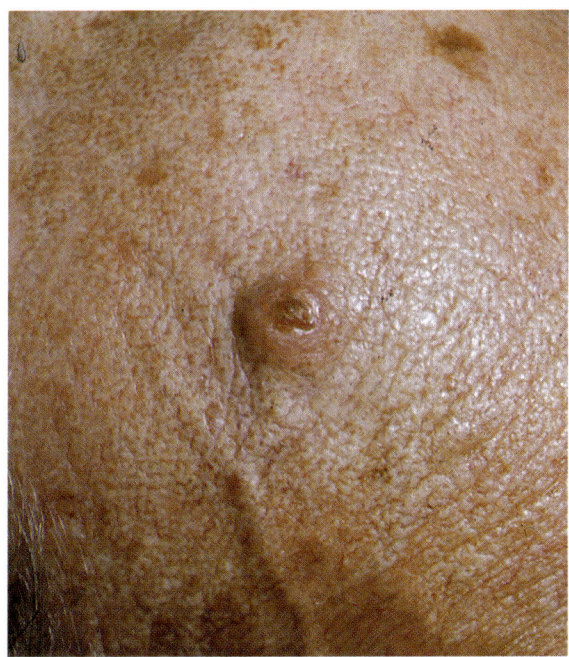

Fig. 20.12 Keratoacanthoma. The shape of the lesion resembles a volcano, being a elevated mass with a central keratin filled crater. The lesion is on the forehead of an elderly man. Note the multiple small yellow papules in the remainder of the skin; the appearance is caused by extensive solar elastosis.

duced. The fibres increase in size tenfold by the time adult life is reached. Any demand for an increased work-load leads to hypertrophy of the fibres of the chamber affected. The stimulus is probably the stretching which results from the additional strain, and the ability of the heart to respond in this way constitutes a part of the cardiac reserve (p. 361). Hypertrophy is best seen in the left ventricle (Fig. 20.13). Systemic hypertension, aortic valvular disease, and mitral regurgitation are the common causes.

Hypertrophy of skeletal muscle. The stimulus for hypertrophy is mechanical, as witnessed by the overdeveloped muscles of the trained athlete.

Diminished Growth

Atrophy is the acquired diminution in size of an organ due to a decrease in size or number of its constituent elements. Only in muscle is a decrease in size the major factor. In all other instances the number of cells is also reduced. This is brought about by the periodic destruction of some of the cells, but as the process occurs insidiously and sporadically, the actual necrosis is not apparent

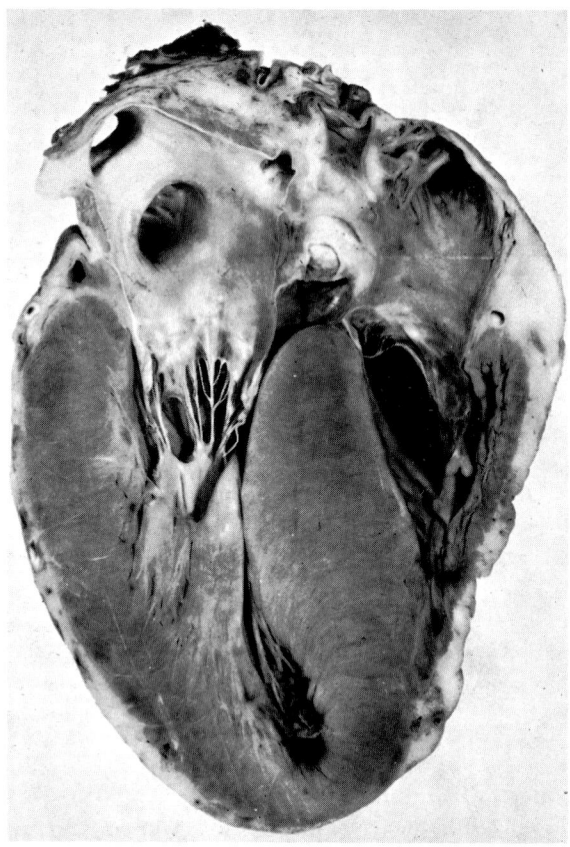

Fig. 20.13 Hypertrophy of the heart. The muscle of the left ventricle is greatly thickened. The cause of this hypertrophy is systemic hypertension. (C20.3. Reproduced by permission of the President and Council of the Royal College of Surgeons of England.)

(see below). A failure to replace lost cells is also a factor in the pathogenesis of atrophy in labile tissues, e.g. the bone marrow. By custom atrophy of the marrow is called *aplasia*, and if not too marked the word *hypoplasia* is used by some authorities. Unfortunately both these terms are used in a different connotation as noted above.

Atrophy

In tissues composed of labile cells, and to a lesser degree stable cells also, there is a constant loss of mature elements and their replacement by the mitotic activity of their fellows. Sometimes the mature cells are cast off from a surface but frequently they die and disappear by a process of

apoptosis. The cells condense, apparently due to loss of water, to form a pyknotic nuclear mass surrounded by a variable amount of cytoplasm in which, in the early stages, the organelles are still easily recognizable. This is called an *apoptotic body*; it may be cast off from a surface or phagocytosed by local histiocytes; it is incorporated in lysosomes and digested to form a small residual body.

Apoptosis is a normal process whereby unwanted or effete cells are removed. It is a feature of the normal process of cell turnover, and in tissues that are undergoing involution during development or in atrophy. It is a feature of malignant tumours and is seen in some types of therapeutically induced tumour regression. Unlike necrosis, apoptosis does not excite an inflammatory response.

Physiological atrophy. There are numerous examples of structures which are well developed at a certain period of life but which subsequently undergo atrophy or involution. Many *fetal structures*, e.g. the notochord, branchial clefts and thyroglossal duct, completely disappear before birth, while others, such as the ductus arteriosus, atrophy early in postuterine life. From adolescence onwards the lymphoid tissue in the body undergoes atrophy, and is partially replaced by fat. After the menopause and in old age there is atrophy of the gonads, and as age advances most tissues take part in a generalized atrophy.

Pathological atrophy. Pathological atrophy may be generalized or local.

Generalized. Starvation atrophy. All tissues of the body show atrophy during prolonged starvation. The *cachexia* of malignant disease is in many instances largely dependent upon an inadequate food intake.

Atrophy is most marked in the adipose tissues and in muscle. The brain is least affected. The heart in extreme cases may be reduced to a third of its normal size, and appear brown due to the lipofuscin in its fibres (*brown atrophy of the heart*).

Senile atrophy. This is the marked accentuation of the process of physiological atrophy of old age. Brown atrophy of the heart is especially prominent in senility, and other organs, e.g. the liver and spleen, may also show a lipofuscin accumulation in their cells. This substance, also called 'wear-and-tear pigment', is produced in the cells by the oxidation of lipids.

Endocrine atrophy. Hypopituitarism leads to atrophy of the thyroid, adrenal cortex, and gonads. Rarely the whole body becomes stunted and the patient cachetic (see Simmond's disease).

Atrophy of bone (osteoporosis) is described in Chapter 34.

Local. Ischaemic atrophy. This is a local form of tissue malnutrition in which hypoxia is super-imposed. With gradual vascular obstruction the parenchyma of many tissues undergoes atrophy, and this is followed by fibrous replacement. Cerebral atrophy is a feature of cerebral athero-sclerosis, and the subsequent neuronal loss with replacement gliosis plays an important part in the atrophy of the cortex and the intellectual impair-ment of old age.

Pressure atrophy. This is a variant of is-chaemic atrophy. It follows pressure on a solid organ, the vessels of which are progressively occluded by compression. It is the capillaries that suffer the most, and damage is caused both by malnutrition and hypoxia. In this way the capsule around a benign tumour or a cyst is formed (p. 242). Some of the best examples of pressure atrophy are seen in relation to bone.

Disuse atrophy. The best examples are encountered in the locomotor system and in the exocrine glands. The atrophy of bone, ligaments, and muscles that follows joint immobilization must always be borne in mind when limbs are encased in plaster. It also occurs when joints are ankylosed, or movement is prevented by pain; the atrophy around rheumatoid and tuberculous arthritis is particularly marked. Following the loss of teeth there is atrophy of the supporting alveolar bone.

When the duct of a secreting gland is suddenly and completely blocked, the parenchyma under-goes atrophy, e.g. after total obstruction of a ureter, a salivary duct, or the pancreatic duct. It is interesting to recall that it was this method of producing pancreatic atrophy which was employed by Banting and Best in the isolation of insulin.

Neuropathic atrophy. This term is loosely applied to the atrophy of a limb which follows nerve lesions. It has two components. Motor paralysis leads to atrophy of the muscles as well as to a more generalized disuse atrophy. Sensory loss may also prevent use of the limb, and lead to disuse atrophy. Direct damage due to unnoticed trauma and infection can sometimes be an ad-ditional factor.

Whether there is a specific 'neuropathic atrophy' of tissues that is unrelated to either disuse atrophy or direct trauma is disputed. In amphibia, the usual regeneration after an ampu-tation does not occur if the limb is first dener-vated. Indeed, the stump may be absorbed, so that amputation of even a digit may result in complete resorption of the limb. This nervous influence, whether for regeneration or for main-tenance of structural integrity, is called *trophic*, or more specifically, *neurotrophic*.

Idiopathic atrophy. There are examples of atrophy in which no cause is evident. In some instances, for example adrenal atrophy causing Addison's disease (p. 437), an autoimmune basis has been suggested. In other cases presenile change or inherited defect is possible.

ABNORMALITIES OF CELLULAR DIFFERENTIATION

Metaplasia

Metaplasia is a condition in which there is a change in one type of differentiated tissue to another type of similarly differentiated tissue. The importance of the word differentiated should be noted, because its use excludes tumour formation as a form of metaplasia. Metaplasia may occur in both epithelial and connective tissues.

Epithelial metaplasia

Squamous metaplasia. Many types of epi-thelium are capable of changing to a stratified squamous variety which may undergo keratin-ization. It often appears to be the result of chronic inflammation. For instance, squamous metaplasia may occur in the gallbladder and urinary bladder when these organs are chronically inflamed, especially if in addition stones (calculi) are present.

Keratinization and the formation of a granular layer may occur in the mobile oral mucous membrane if it is subjected to repeated trauma.* Such a white lesion must be distinguished from other white lesions in which dysplasia is a feature (p. 271).

While in these examples 'chronic irritation' appears to be the cause of the metaplasia, there is one condition in which squamous metaplasia is common, but in which irritation plays no part. This is *hypovitaminosis A*. Squamous metaplasia is widespread, being found in the nose, bronchi, and urinary tract. There is also conjunctival hyperkeratosis, or *xerophthalmia*, and this may be complicated by corneal ulceration and infection leading to loss of sight.

Columnar metaplasia. Squamous epithelium rarely shows metaplasia to a columnar type. It is occasionally seen in the lining of an apical cyst (p. 231).

Specialized columnar epithelium may change to a more simple type. The conversion of the pseudostratified columnar ciliated respiratory epithelium to a simple mucus-secreting columnar type is commonly seen in chronic bronchitis and bronchiectasis, and is a factor in predisposing patients with these conditions to bronchopneumonia.

Connective tissue metaplasia

Osseous metaplasia. Whether fibroblasts can produce osteoid tissue or not is largely a matter of how one defines 'fibroblast' and 'osteoblast'. The two cell types certainly exhibit great morphological similarity, and before the appearance of the intercellular substance, whether fibrous tissue or osteoid, they cannot be distinguished. 'Fibroblasts' do not normally produce osteoid, but under some conditions they may be regarded as undergoing metaplasia to 'osteoblasts'. Bone then makes its appearance. An alternative explanation is that the osteoblasts are derived from primitive stem cells.

Osseous metaplasia is occasionally seen in scars, and also in the fibrous tissue adjacent to any area

of dystrophic calcification—cystic goitres, caseous foci in the lung, etc.

Changes in mesothelium. The mesothelial cells lining the pleura and peritoneum may change to an epithelial type, columnar or even squamous. This is rare, but is important because such cells cast off into the pleural cavity may be mistaken by the unwary cytologist for cancer cells.

Tumour metaplasia. See p. 264.

Other cellular dystrophies

Dystrophy may be defined as a disorder, usually congenital, of the structure or function of an organ or tissue due to its perverted nutrition. In its widest sense it includes agenesis, atrophy, hypertrophy, and metaplasia, but in practice the term is usually applied to those disorders which do not readily fit into any of these other categories. The alternative term dysplasia* may also be used for such an abnormal development of tissue, although strictly it should be applied to developmental disorders only. Dyscrasia* literally means a bad mixture (of the four humours), and is now used by haematologists to describe any blood disorder of uncertain aetiology.

Many special dystrophies involving muscle, bone, cornea, retina, etc., have been described, but these are outside the scope of this book. It must be reiterated that the term dystrophy has no specific intrinsic meaning, but like dysplasia is used to describe a lesion whose nature is not understood and for which the author can find no other more appropriate name. In recent years dysplasia has acquired a specific meaning when applied to epithelium—most commonly that of the cervix uteri. It is used to describe a type of hyperplasia which is thought to progress to *carcinoma in situ* in some cases and later to invasive cancer. But dysplasia is also used in other instances, e.g. fibrous dysplasia of bone, mammary dysplasia and ectodermal dysplasia in which there is no suggestion of incipient neoplastic change.

In this chapter many different perversions of

---

*Keratinization is found normally in the attached gingiva and in the mucosa overlying the hard palate.

*The Greek derivation of these words is as follows: Dys—bad or difficult; Krasis—a mingling; Plasis—a forming.

cell growth have been described. The one thing they all have in common is that they are self-limiting. In the following chapter neoplasia is considered. Here the perversion of cell growth persists even when the stimulus that produced it is eradicated.

GENERAL READING

Clarren S K, Smith D W 1976 The fetal alcohol syndrome. New England Journal of Medicine 298:1063

Hill R M 1984 Isotretinoin teratogenicity. Lancet 1:1465

Rosa F W 1983 Teratogenicity of isotretinoin. Lancet 2:513

Searle J, et al 1982 Necrosis and apoptosis: distinct modes of cell death with fundamentally different significance. Pathology Annual 17(2):229

21. Tumours

The concept that tumour growth is a distinctive clinical and pathological entity has been evolving for many centuries. At first the term 'tumour' was applied to any swelling, and the use of the suffix -oma became established to denote such a lesion; even today this relic of the past persists in the use of names like haematoma, hamartoma, tuberculoma, and granuloma. In time the swellings of known aetiology, especially the infective ones, were excluded from the classification of tumours, and there was left a group of swellings of unknown cause apparently produced by the unrestrained growth of the individual's own cells. It appeared that these cells were no longer subject to the normal mechanisms controlling their growth, and had become independent. Recent knowledge of viral and cellular oncogenes has added weight to this concept.

The excessive proliferation of cells often produces a mass of tissue but this is not always the case. Sometimes the migration of cells outside the normal confining limits outweighs the bulk of the abnormal proliferation. In this case no 'tumour' as such exists—an excellent example is to be seen in the diffuse infiltrating carcinoma of the stomach. *Neoplasm*, which literally means new formation or new growth, is a more suitable term. It implies that there is an abnormal type of growth which may be evident not only in the intact animal but also when the cells are grown in culture.

CLASSIFICATION OF TUMOURS

The major grouping of tumours is related to their tissue of origin and to their behaviour.

Histogenetic classification

Since tumours are formed as a result of the overgrowth of cells, it is logical to name them according to the parent tissue of origin. The basic subdivision of the body into epithelium and connective tissue (mesenchyme) is reflected in the recognition of two major groups of tumours: those derived from epithelial cells and those derived from connective tissue. Furthermore, within each group there are as many subdivisions as there are different types of epithelium and connective tissue.

Behaviour

The second, equally important classification is based upon the behaviour of the tumour cells. In some neoplasms the cells always appear to maintain contact with one another, and never wander off into the surrounding tissues nor invade lymphatics or blood vessels. These tumours remain localized, never spread, and are therefore called *innocent*, or *benign*. This contrasts with *malignant* tumours, in which the neoplastic cells invade the surrounding tissues and enter natural tissue spaces such as the lumina of lymphatics and blood vessels. Frequently groups of tumour cells break off, and the resulting tumour emboli become lodged at some distant site, grow, and thereby produce *secondary deposits*, or *metastases*. Between these two extremes of behaviour there are tumours of intermediate malignancy. The classification currently used is shown in Table 21.1. Some difficulties are considered on p. 261.

BENIGN OR INNOCENT TUMOURS

General considerations and effects

The cells which constitute this type of tumour show no tendency to invade the surrounding tissues. Instead, the excessive accumulation of cells produces an expanding mass which causes two local effects:

Pressure atrophy. Adjacent parenchyma undergoes pressure atrophy while the more resistant connective tissue survives to form a fibrous *capsule.* The tumour is therefore *well-circumscribed,* and is not intimately connected with the surrounding tissue except for those points of entry of the vascular supply (Fig. 21.1). Benign tumours are fairly easy to excise surgically, and provided local removal is complete, they do not recur. A benign tumour within the skull or vertebral column can produce serious effects by pressure.

Obstruction. A benign tumour may obstruct a natural passage and produce serious effects. Obstruction of a bronchus leads to collapse of the lung and bronchopneumonia. A tumour of the intestine may produce intestinal obstruction.

Gross characteristics

Encapsulation. This is a characteristic feature when the tumour is situated in a solid organ or tissue (see above).

Shape. Benign tumours are usually rounded, but the shape may be moulded by the distribution of surrounding structures. A particular arrangement of fascia may make a tumour ovoid.

Size. Although benign tumours are usually smaller than their malignant counterparts, they may at times attain enormous proportions. The largest tumour in the museum of the Royal College of Surgeons of England is a fibroma of the kidney weighing 37 kg (82 lb)! A malignant tumour would have killed the patient long before reaching this size.

Ulceration and haemorrhage. These features are rare except in certain surface growths.

Rate of growth

The rate of growth of a benign tumour is generally slow. It is often erratic, and growth may cease after a period.

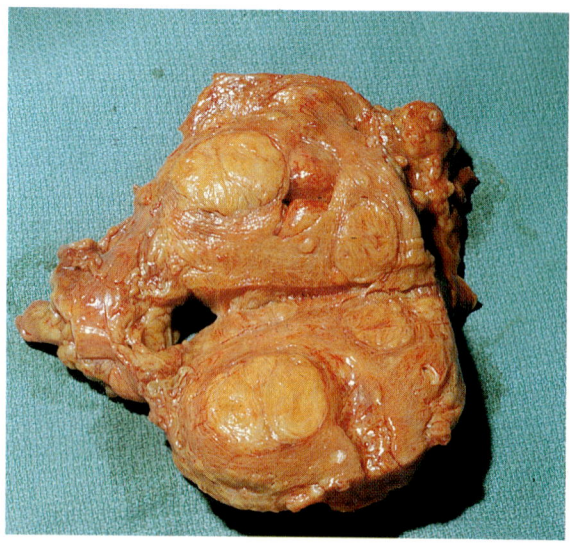

Fig. 21.1 Multiple fibromyomata of the uterus. The uterus has been opened to show several encapsulated 'fibroid' tumours in the myometrium.

Table 21.1   Classification of tumours

Tissue of origin	Benign	Intermediate	Malignant
Epithelium			
Covering and protective epithelium			
(a) Squamous	Squamous-cell papilloma	Basal-cell carcinoma	Squamous-cell carcinoma
(b) Transitional	Transitional-cell papilloma		Transitional-cell carcinoma
(c) Columnar	Columnar-cell papilloma		Adenocarcinoma
Compact secreting epithelium	Adenoma. If cystic, cystadenoma or papillary cystadenoma		Adenocarcinoma. If cystic, cystadenocarcinoma
Diffuse endocrine system		Carcinoid tumours	
Connective tissue			
Fibrous tissue	Fibroma		Fibrosarcoma
Nerve sheath	Neurofibroma		Neurofibrosarcoma
Fat	Lipoma		Liposarcoma
Smooth muscle	Leiomyoma		Leiomyosarcoma
Striated muscle	Rhabdomyoma		Rhabdomyosarcoma
Synovium	Synovioma		Malignant synovioma
Cartilage	Chondroma		Chondrosarcoma
Bone			
Osteoblast	Osteoma	Giant-cell tumour	Osteosarcoma
Mesothelium	Benign mesothelioma		Malignant mesothelioma
Blood vessels and lymphatics	Haemangioma and lymphangioma		Angiosarcoma
Meninges	Meningioma		Malignant meningioma
Specialized connective tissue			
Neuroglia and ependyma	Astrocytoma; oligodendroglioma; ependymoma*		
Chromaffin tissue	Carotid body tumour		Malignant carotid body tumour
Lymphoid and haematopoietic tissue	Pseudolymphoma		Malignant lymphoma Myeloproliferative disorders† Multiple myeloma Leukaemias
Melanocytes			Malignant melanoma
Fetal trophoblast	Hydatidiform mole		Choriocarcinoma
Germ cell			
(*Totipotential cell*)	Benign teratoma		Malignant teratoma and some ovarian and testicular tumours
Embryonic tissue			
(*Pluripotential cell*)			
Kidney			Nephroblastoma
(*Unipotential cell*)			
Retina			Retinoblastoma
Hind-brain			Medulloblastoma
Sympathetic ganglia and adrenal medulla	Ganglioneuroma		Neuroblastoma
Embryonic vestiges			
Notochord			Chordoma
Enamel organ		Ameloblastoma	
Parapituitary residues		Craniopharyngioma	
Hamartoma			
Melanotic			Malignant melanoma
'Exostoses' and 'ecchondroses'			Chondrosarcoma
Neurofibromatosis	Neurofibroma		Neurofibrosarcoma

Note. Any malignant tumour may be so poorly differentiated that it must be classified on a histological basis, e.g. carcinoma simplex, spindle-cell sarcoma, etc.

*These tumours are difficult to classify. The common types are locally malignant, but some also metastasize within the central nervous system. Rarely, and most often in children, they appear to be benign.

†These include polycythaemia vera, haemorrhagic thrombocythaemia, and myelosclerosis.

Hormonal effects

Benign tumours of endocrine tissue may produce excessive quantities of hormone which can have far-reaching and sometimes fatal effects. A tumour of the B or β cells of the islets of the pancreas may secrete so much insulin that the blood sugar level falls precipitously, and causes mental disturbances and seizures.

Microscopic appearance

The arrangement of the cells of a benign tumour closely resembles that of the parent tissue. The tumours are therefore described as being *well differentiated*. The cells themselves tend to be regular in size, staining, and shape. Mitotic figures are scanty, and when present are of normal type. The tumour cells are supported and nourished by a network of host connective tissue which consists predominantly of blood vessels, fibroblasts, and a varying amount of collagen. It is called the *stroma*, and although an intimate part of the tumour, it is not itself involved in the neoplastic change.

Benign epithelial tumours

These are of two main types. Benign neoplasia of a surface or lining epithelium produces a warty tumour, or *papilloma* (Fig. 21.2). In a compact gland (e.g. breast) the tumour is embedded in the tissue, and is called an *adenoma*.

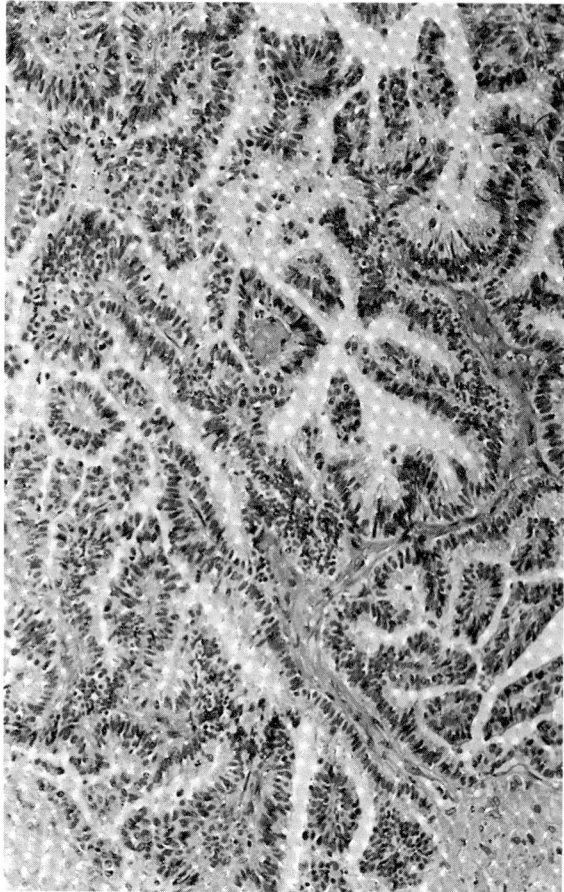

Fig. 21.2 Intraduct papilloma of the breast. The tumour is composed of fronds with a delicate fibrovascular core and a covering of neoplastic uniform columnar epithelium.

Papillomata

Papillomata may occur on any epithelial surface. Some have a broad base and are described as sessile, while others become pedunculated and form *polyps*, a morphological term applied to any pedunculated mass attached to a surface and not necessarily neoplastic (Fig. 21.3).

Papillomata are supplied by a core of connective tissue stroma containing blood vessels, lymphatics, and nerves. This is covered by a profuse neoplastic epithelium, composed of either stratified squamous, transitional, or columnal cells, according to that from which it has arisen. The cells show a regular arrangement, and the basement membrane zone is intact unless there is

distortion due to inflammation. The epithelial cells are entirely restricted to the surface, and do not show invasion.

Squamous-cell papilloma. Papillomata occur on the skin and other stratified squamous epithelial surfaces, e.g. the tongue and buccal mucosa. There is always *acanthosis*, i.e. a proliferation of the prickle-cell layer, and in the case of cutaneous papillomata there is often excessive keratin formation (*hyperkeratosis*) also. These lesions are described in greater detail in Chapter 37. Squamous-cell papilloma is a common tumour of the mouth, and is not infrequent in the larynx.

Transitional-cell 'papilloma'. This type of tumour occurs throughout the urinary passages, and has characteristic, delicate, finger-like

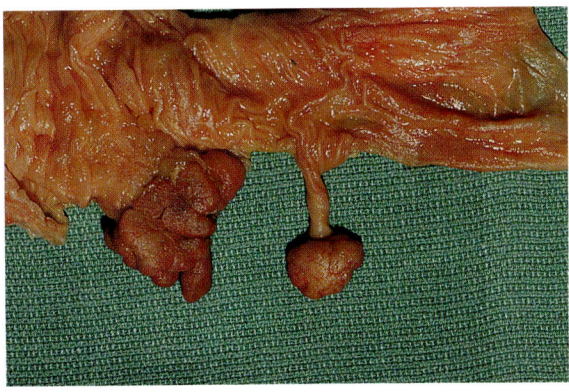

Fig. 21.3 Polypoid adenoma of the colon. The tumour is attached to the colonic mucosa by a long stalk. Adjacent to it is a sessile mass that histologically proved to be an invasive adenocarcinoma.

processes, or fronds, which give it the appearance of a sea anemone. Bleeding is quite common and leads to haematuria. Multiple lesions are the rule. These tumours present problems in classification for although they are histologically benign, the frequency with which they recur has led most pathologists to regard them as of low-grade malignancy.

Columnar-cell papilloma. This tumour occurs on any surface covered by columnar epithelium, for example in the colon. Papillomata are also to be found in cystic adenomata (see below).

Adenomata

Adenomata are composed of dense masses of epithelial cells, often forming acini lined by exuberant epithelium which may be columnar or cuboidal in shape. They occur in the salivary glands, pancreas, kidney, ovary, and the endocrine glands. They may also arise in the small glands which open on to epithelial surfaces; thus adenomata originate in sweat and sebaceous glands in the skin and the mucous glands of the mouth and respiratory tract.

Intestinal adenomata tend to become polypoid, and in familial *polyposis coli* thousands of tumours are present. Malignant change is

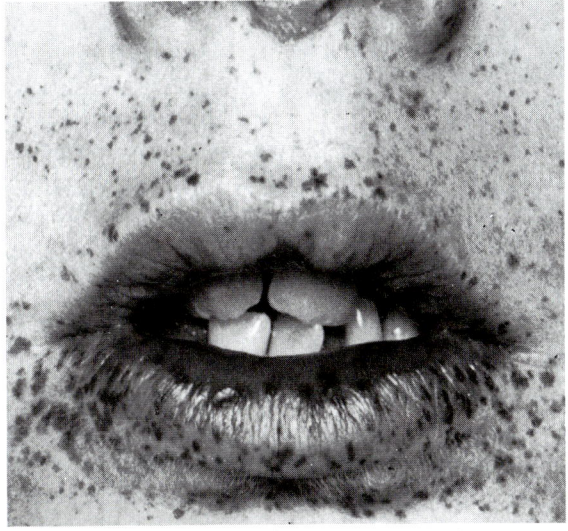

Fig. 21.4 Peutz–Jeghers syndrome. The multiple, circumoral, brown macules are well shown. The pigmentation is due to melanin. (From Sheward J D 1962 British Medical Journal 1:921.)

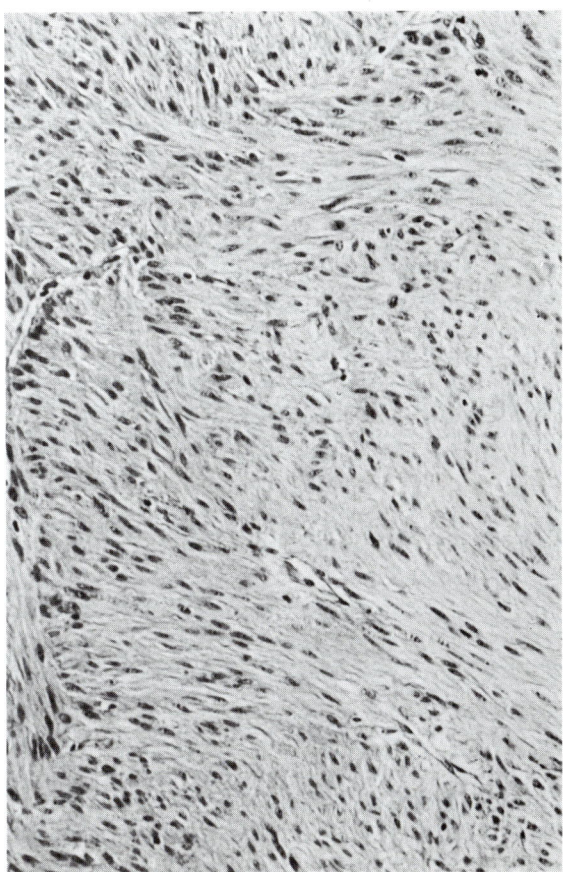

Fig. 21.5 Leiomyoma of stomach. The tumour consists of sheaves of elongated, spindle-shaped smooth-muscle cells arranged in interlacing whorls. × 100.

almost inevitable, and the patient dies of cancer of the colon. In a related condition, *Gardner's syndrome*, colonic polyposis is found in association with sebaceous cysts, osteomata of the face and skull, and multiple fibromata. This too is inherited as a dominant trait and terminates in colonic cancer.

A rather similar condition is the *Peutz–Jeghers syndrome*, in which multiple polyposis of the stomach and intestine (small and large) is associated with a brownish pigmentation peppered around the lips and mouth and sometimes in the skin elsewhere (Fig. 21.4). The polyps are not prone to become malignant, unlike those of polyposis coli; indeed, they are probably hamaetomatous rather than neoplastic.

Cystadenoma. Sometimes adenomata form elaborate spaces into which papillary ingrowths of neoplastic epithelium occur. These *papillary cystadenomata* are most common in the ovary, but may also be found in the salivary glands and kidneys.

Fibroadenoma. The common tumour in the breasts of young women is the fibroadenoma. It consists of epithelial and connective tissue elements, both of which are considered to be neoplastic.

Benign connective tissue tumours

Benign tumours of connective tissue are usually composed of cells which closely resemble the parent tissue. They are supported by an excellent stroma from the adjacent connective tissues, and there is a characteristic tendency to merge with this stroma. The neoplastic cells are not nearly so well demarcated from the stroma as are those of epithelial tumours. The tumours are named according to the cell of origin, e.g. fibroma from fibroblast, osteoma from osteoblast, myoma from muscle, etc.

Fibroma

Fibromata are not very common tumours. They consist of circumscribed collections of fibroblasts between which there is a variable amount of collagen. Hard fibromata have much collagen, whereas the softer variety is predominantly cellu-

lar. They are found in many sites, e.g. stomach, ovary, gingiva, etc.

There are a number of curious proliferative conditions of fibrous tissue, grouped as the *fibromatoses*, in which histological assessment of malignancy is difficult. One type of fibromatosis, known as a *desmoid tumour*, occurs in the abdominal wall. It usually affects young women either during pregnancy or shortly following childbirth. It is locally aggressive and tends to recur unless widely excised. A more common example is palmar fibromatosis, better known as *Dupuytren's contracture*. This disease affects elderly men and produces a cord like thickening of the palm associated with flexion deformity of the fourth and fifth fingers. It progresses very slowly over the years.

Pseudosarcomatous nodular fasciitis, also known as nodular fasciitis, described on p. 234, is related to the fibromatoses.

Myxoma

This is an uncommon tumour of connective tissue consisting of scattered stellate cells disposed in an expanse of connective-tissue mucin in which there is a network of reticulin fibres.

The myxoma may be found in the jaw (where it is probably of odontogenic origin) and arising from the interatrial wall of the heart and from soft tissues, usually in association with striated muscle and neighbouring tissues. In appearance it is well circumscribed, oval or spherical, and of translucent grey colour. Its cut surface is glistening and slimy, and it may exude a mucoid material. It probably arises from a fibroblastic cell that has not differentiated enough to produce collagen but is capable of forming acid mucopolysaccharides. Alternatively it may be of primitive mesenchymal origin.

Myoma

Tumours of muscle are of two types: from smooth muscle (leiomyoma) and striated muscle (rhabdomyoma).

Leiomyoma. This is the commonest of all tumours, being found in the uteri of about 20% of women over 30 years of age. Leiomyomata of the skin, stomach, and intestine are also not uncommon. Usually they are small and often multiple. A leiomyoma is composed of whorls of smooth muscle cells interspersed among which there is a variable amount of fibrous tissue (Fig. 21.5). The muscle element may be replaced by fibrous tissue, and the *fibroleiomyoma* (or fibroid) is produced. Such a tumour may undergo cystic change, or calcify. On section the whorled interlacing pattern of glistening white fibres resembling watered-silk is characteristic.

Rhabdomyoma. Benign rhabdomyomata are exceedingly uncommon.

Neurofibroma

The neurofibroma is derived from Schwann cells. It causes a diffuse, fusiform enlargement of a nerve, and is composed of spindle cells arranged in flowing streams with a varying amount of intervening collagen. Nerve fibres pass through the tumour, and myxomatous change is not infrequently present. The tumours may be solitary, and can occur on a spinal nerve root or a peripheral nerve. When multiple, they constitute a major feature of von Recklinghausen's disease. Whether all the nodules in this disease are true neoplasms is debatable—it may be more reasonable to regard them as hamartomatous in origin (see p. 229).

Neurilemmoma (Schwannoma)

This tumour is usually solitary, and may arise from any cranial or peripheral nerve. It is encapsulated and appears to arise focally on a nerve trunk, so that the nerve itself is stretched over the tumour rather than running through it, as in the neurofibroma. A common site for schwannomata is the auditory nerve, and they may be bilateral. Microscopically, the tumour is composed of spindle cells which are often palisaded so that all the nuclei are aligned in one strip and the clear cytoplasm of the cells in an adjacent strip (Fig. 21.6).

Lipoma

This common tumour is composed of adult adipose tissue. It is usually subcutaneous, but

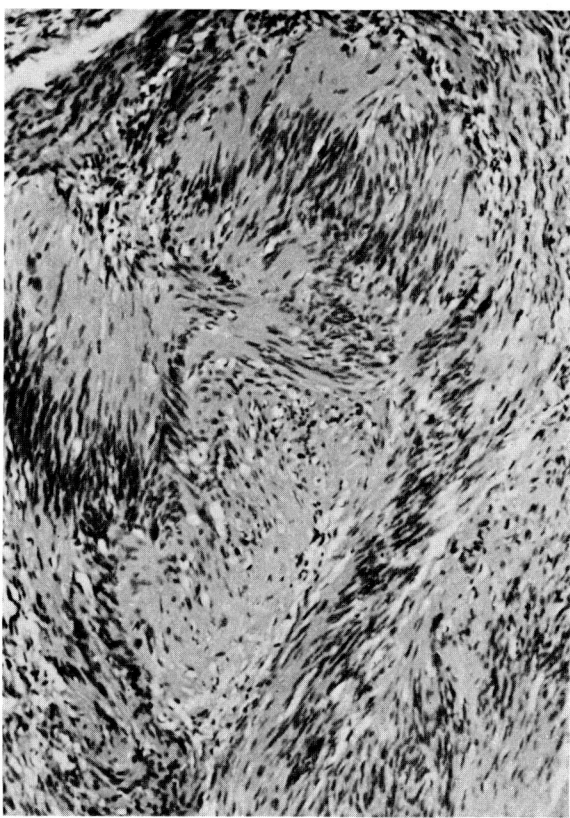

Fig. 21.6   Schwannoma. Note the palisaded, or regimented, appearance of the long, spindle-shaped cells; their nuclei form a continuous sinuous column, and on each side there is a similar column composed of clear cytoplasm. × 200.

may be retroperitoneal or subserosal. Oral lipomata are uncommon.

Chondroma and osteoma.

These are considered in Chapter 34.

MALIGNANT TUMOURS

The cells of a malignant tumour infiltrate the surrounding tissue. Normal cells are enveloped and destroyed, and the tumour edge is therefore ill-defined. Complete excision by surgery is correspondingly difficult, and even if the tumour is removed with much surrounding normal tissue, malignant cells often remain behind, and their continued growth results in a *local recurrence*. In malignant tumours the invading cells spread in the planes of least resistance: finger-like processes extend outwards from the main tumour mass, and this growth produces a fanciful resemblance to the silhouette of a crab, hence the term *cancer*, which is derived from the Latin word meaning a crab. The term is used by the layman to include all malignant tumours, but most physicians equate it with carcinoma. *A carcinoma is a malignant tumour of epithelial cells, while a sarcoma is one derived from connective tissue.*

Embolic spread of tumour cells is responsible for the production of distant metastases. *Local invasion and embolic spread are the two characteristics of malignant tumours.* Both are probably related to the reduced cell adhesiveness which is a fundamental characteristic of cancer cells, and is evident not only in vivo but also in tissue culture—the cells growing out of the explant do not resist mechanical separation as well as do those of normal tissue. The power to invade and spread combined with the capacity for progressive growth make the term malignant particularly suitable for this type of tumour. Death is inevitable in untreated cases, except for those very rare, though well-documented, cases of *spontaneous regression,* in which proven cancers have disappeared of their own accord.

Gross characteristics

Lack of encapsulation. Malignant tumours have no limiting capsule, because the cells actively infiltrate the adjacent tissues. In certain rapidly growing tumours (e.g. metastases in the liver) cell division exceeds infiltration, and the tumour by its expansive growth may give a false impression of encapsulation. Microscopy, however, always reveals infiltration.

Shape. This is irregular in outline and diffuse in definition.

Size. Malignant tumours are usually larger than their benign counterparts.

Ulceration and haemorrhage. As would be expected from the destructive property of cancer, these are common features. *Any ulcer which fails to heal within a few weeks without obvious cause should always be regarded as malignant until proved otherwise* (Fig. 21.7). In the mouth exfoliative

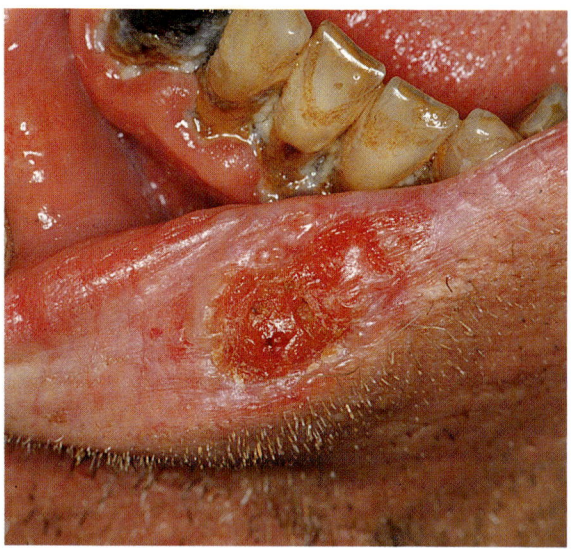

Fig. 21.7 Carcinoma of the lower lip with persistent firm ulceration in a 67-year-old man. (Photograph courtesy of Mr J. Hamburger, University of Birmingham.)

cytology may be used to aid in the diagnosis of suspicious lesions (p. 271).

Rate of growth

Malignant tumours usually increase in size steadily. This can be of diagnostic importance; for example, if a shadow on a lung or bone radiograph is known to have remained stationary in size for several years, it is unlikely to be due to a malignant tumour.

Microscopic features

Microscopically several important features should be noted. The tumour tissue may resemble the parent tissue to a considerable extent, but the similarity is not as great as with benign tumours (Fig. 21.8). Differentiation is not so well developed, and recognition of the tissue of origin is difficult or even impossible. Such tumours are called poorly differentiated.

Malignant tumours usually show much mitotic activity. The synthesis of DNA prior to division results in nuclear enlargement and hyperchromatism. This together with the formation of cells with abnormal numbers of chromosomes

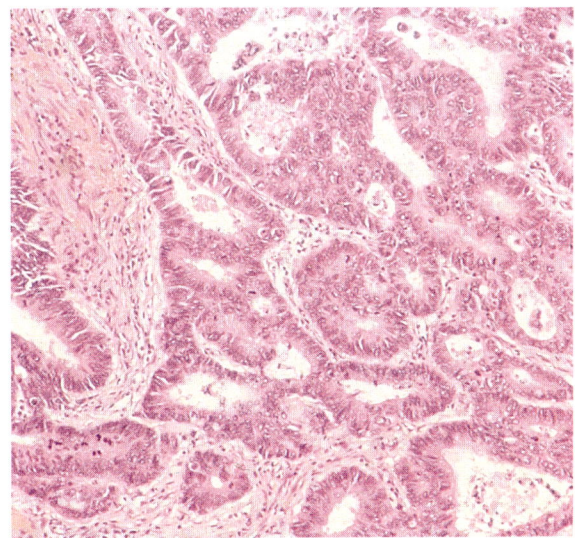

Fig. 21.8 Adenocarcinoma of the colon. The tumour shows well-marked differentiation into glandular structures.

accounts for the irregularity in size and shape (*pleomorphism*) and staining which is so characteristic of malignant tumours. Mitoses are not only numerous, but sometimes also abnormal, and the number of chromosomes may diverge from the normal 46. Tripolar mitoses with the formation of three daughter cells are particularly characteristic of malignancy. No single, constant change in chromosome form or number is characteristic of malignancy. However, in some tumour types an abnormality of a particular chromosome has been reported. The best-known example is the Philadelphia chromosome that is found in chronic myeloid leukaemia.

Anaplasia is a term which was introduced to describe new cells which deviated from the normal and resembled those of embryonic tissue. It is now generally restricted to those cellular changes which are found in malignant tumours. Thus a tumour which shows a high degree of anaplasia is poorly differentiated, and has frequent and bizarre mitoses and cells that are pleomorphic and have prominent nucleoli.

Stromal reaction in carcinoma

The reaction of the invaded tissue to carcinoma cells varies; its growth may be so stimulated that a hard, fibrotic desmoplastic or *scirrhous* type of tumour is produced. Most breast cancers are of this type. The dense fibrosis appears to be associated with a contracting tendency, which is ill understood. In the breast there is an accompanying retraction of the nipple and dimpling of the skin. Eventually a stony fixation to the chest wall ensues.

Scirrhous tumours are also commonly found in the stomach and colon. The contraction causes a 'purse-string' deformity, and obstruction of the lumen follows.

When a tumour has little stroma in relation to cell bulk it is soft or brain-like, and is described as *medullary*, or *encephaloid*. Some cancers of the stomach and colon are of this type, and ulceration and bleeding occur rather than early intestinal obstruction.

Effects of malignant tumours

Malignant tumours produce their ill-effects in a large number of ways:

Mechanical pressure and obstruction. Like benign tumours, malignant growths press on adjacent structures and cause obstruction to natural passages. A carcinoma of the colon soon leads to intestinal obstruction. Collapse of a lung and bronchopneumonia are often the features which first call attention to a carcinoma of the bronchus.

Destruction of tissue. In addition, malignant tumours, both primary and secondary, infiltrate and destroy tissue. This is well illustrated in bone where destruction may be so marked that pathological fractures occur, and replacement of the marrow results in anaemia.

Haemorrhage. Malignant tumours which involve any surface usually ulcerate and bleed. Repeated bleeding causes anaemia, and occasionally the erosion of a large artery leads to a massive fatal haemorrhage. This may happen when a carcinoma of the tongue involves the lingual artery. *Clinically unexplained bleeding from any site should be treated seriously, as it is a common symptom of cancer.* Haemoptysis is common in lung cancer, haematuria in urinary tract cancer, and vaginal bleeding, especially after intercourse, in cervical cancer.

Infection. All ulcerative cancers are bound to undergo secondary bacterial infection, and this aggravates the clinical condition. Infection also follows obstruction to the urinary or respiratory passages, e.g. bronchopneumonia occurs in lung cancer, and cystitis and pyelonephritis in cancer of the prostate. Cancer of the mouth interferes so much with swallowing that in due course there is inhalation of food and saliva into the respiratory passages. It is not surprising that suppurative bronchopneumonia is the commonest cause of death in this condition.

Starvation. In cancers of the mouth, oesophagus, and stomach there may be a direct nutritional effect due to the failure of food intake.

Pain. In advanced malignancy, particularly if there are spinal metastases, pain may be severe. It occasions anxiety and leads to insomnia.

Anaemia. Anaemia is common and may be due to chronic blood loss, malabsorption of essential dietary components, or bone-marrow replacement. Often, however, the cause is obscure.

Cachexia. The emaciated appearance of patients with advanced cancer is characteristic, but it is not uncommon for patients to remain obese. The cause of the loss of weight and the generalized body atrophy in cancer has given rise to much speculation. Cachexin, a polypeptide released by activated macrophages, may be a factor. Fat is mobilized from the fat deposits and, like interleukin I, it acts on the hypothalamus to cause fever. Nevertheless the present tendency is to attribute cachexia to secondary factors, e.g. starvation, haemorrhage, infection, liver damage, etc.

Hormonal effects. Malignant tumours of the endocrine glands occasionally produce effects due to an excessive production of hormones. This is less common than with benign tumours.

Carcinomatous syndromes. A variety of syndromes occur in association with neoplasms that are not explicable in terms of infiltration by the primary tumour or its metastases. *Dermatomyositis*, a wide variety of *skin eruptions* and the *nephrotic syndrome* are examples. Sometimes a patient exhibits signs and symptoms referable to the *nervous system*, such as peripheral neuritis or cerebellar degeneration. *Thrombophlebitis migrans* is a well-known association with carcinoma of the pancreas. *Pulmonary osteoarthropathy*, with clubbing of the fingers, sometimes with pain and swelling of the joints, is associated with lung cancer.

The pathogenesis of most of these intriguing syndromes is not known but possibly some secretion by the tumour is responsible. Thus the nephrotic syndrome is probably mediated by immune complexes formed by tumour antigen and specific antibody. Some tumours secrete substances not formed by their parent tissue. Presumably genes normally repressed are activated. As might be expected, such ectopic secretions are commonly polypeptides. The secretion may be a hormone or hormone-like substance. Cancer of the lung, particularly the oat-cell variety, is particularly adept at doing this. Examples of the effects of such ectopic hormone secretion include *Cushing's syndrome* due to ACTH production by a carcinoma of the lung, *thyrotoxicosis* in choriocarcinoma and hydatidiform mole, *hyponataemia and water retention* associated with antidiuretic hormone secretion by carcinoma of the lung, and *polycythaemia* due to erythropoietin production by renal-cell carcinoma. The tumour secretion may not be a normal hormone; as an example some tumours secrete an osteoclast-stimulating factor that leads to *hypercalcaemia*. The tumour secretion may have no obvious biological function but its detection in the blood can act as a marker for that particular tumour. Thus α_1-fetoprotein is secreted by some hepatomata and germ-cell tumours, and carcino-embryonic antigen (CEA) is secreted by a number of carcinomata, especially of the gastrointestinal tract. These markers are not specific enough for the diagnosis of a particular tumour. However, they can be used to monitor patients following treatment. A rise in the blood level may be the first herald of a recurrence, and give the clinician the chance to give treatment while the recurrence is still small.

Spread of malignant tumours

Direct invasion and embolization are the two methods of spread and must be examined in detail.

Direct spread. The direct infiltration of the surrounding tissues means that the microscopic edge of the tumour extends beyond what is macroscopically apparent. Infiltration along tissue planes and septa is well shown in cancer of the breast, and in this way the tumour becomes *attached to the skin and deep fascia*. Evidence of local invasion of a tumour is an important clinical sign, for it is tantamount to a diagnosis of malignancy.

Invasion of lymphatics. Carcinoma, but not sarcoma, shows a particular tendency to invade lymphatic vessels at an early stage, and the cells may grow as a long, ever-extending cord (Fig. 21.9). The process is called *lymphatic permeation*, and the lymphatic obstruction which it produces can cause lymphatic oedema.

Invasion of arteries and veins. This is a common event, and may lead to thrombosis and obstruction. It is frequent in lung cancer because so many large vessels are readily accessible to the tumour.

Spread by metastases. Groups of cells may become detached, travel in some natural passage to a distant site, become implanted, and finally grow to produce secondary deposits, or *metastases*. Spread via the lymphatics, blood vessels, and serous cavities are the most important examples.

Lymphatic spread. Detached groups of tumour cells in an invaded lymphatic are swept into the draining regional lymph nodes. If the cells survive and grow, the node soon becomes replaced by the tumour, and further spread occurs to the next group of nodes by way of the efferent channel. This is a familiar event in the course of carcinoma and melanoma, but is rare in sarcoma. A blockage of lymphatics results in a reversal of lymph flow in other vessels, and metastases may appear in unexpected lymph nodes. This is known as *retrograde embolism*, and the best-known example is the involvement of the left cervical nodes in gastric cancer. This is due to obstruction of the thoracic duct near its entry into the left subclavian vein, so that lymph is diverted up to the neck.

Blood spread. The occurrence of blood-borne metastases is the feature of malignant disease which is responsible for death in most cases. It is also the factor which limits the surgical and radiotherapeutic treatment of cancer.

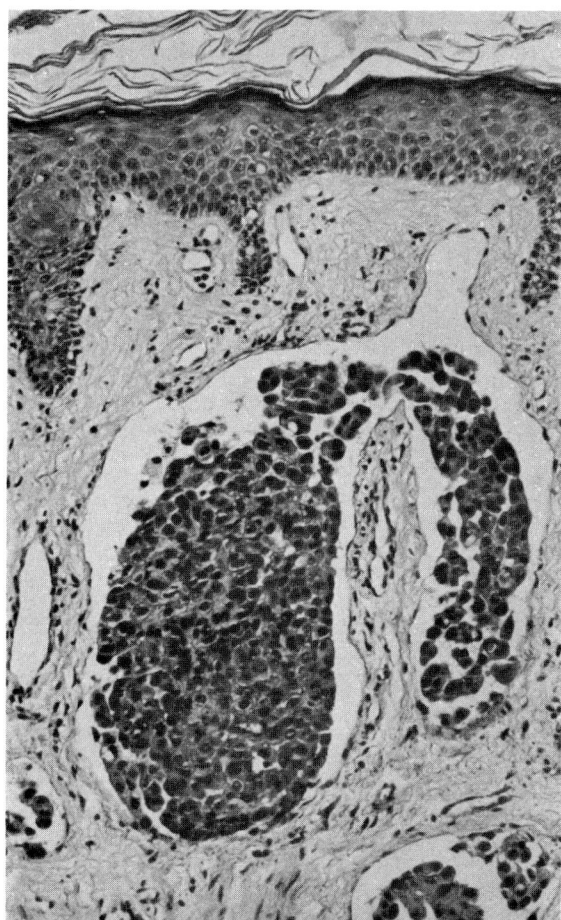

Fig. 21.9 Lymphatic permeation of cancer. This is a section of skin showing dilated lymphatic vessels filled with carcinoma cells arranged in solid cords. There was an advanced carcinoma of the breast. × 200. (From Walter J B (1992) An introduction to the principles of disease, 3rd edn, W B Saunders, Philadelphia.)

At first sight the mode of production of secondary tumours is easy to understand. Malignant cells invade small venules, become detached, and are then carried by the blood stream to some distant site where they reach a capillary network. There the emboli become impacted, and the cells proliferate and develop into secondary tumours. A second method of blood-borne metastasis is by way of the lymphatics, for all the lymph eventually drains into the venous circulation.

As would be expected, one of the commonest sites of metastasis for most tumours is the lung. Likewise, primary tumours arising from an area drained by the portal vein regularly metastasize to the liver (Fig. 21.10). Purely mechanical factors would appear to account for this distribution, but closer examination makes such an explanation inadequate.

Many tumours, e.g. of the breast and kidney, give rise to metastases not only in the lungs, but also in the liver, bones, and other organs, and such systemic metastases sometimes occur in the absence of apparent lung deposits.

The distribution of secondary tumours might be expected to be related to the blood supply, but this is not the case. Cardiac and skeletal muscle have an abundant blood supply, and yet are rarely the site of metastases. The spleen likewise is not commonly involved. The liver, on the other hand, is frequently studded with secondary tumours regardless of the site of the primary.

There is considerable evidence that malignant cells often reach the blood stream but that most of them die. Only a selected few are able to take root to grow into secondary deposits. What factors govern this are poorly understood. The 'seed' may be widespread, but only where the 'soil' is suitable does growth occur. Some examples of this *selective metastasis* must now be examined.

1. *Liver*. The commonest organ in which blood-borne metastases occur is the liver, for this organ appears to afford an excellent environment for the growth of tumour cells.

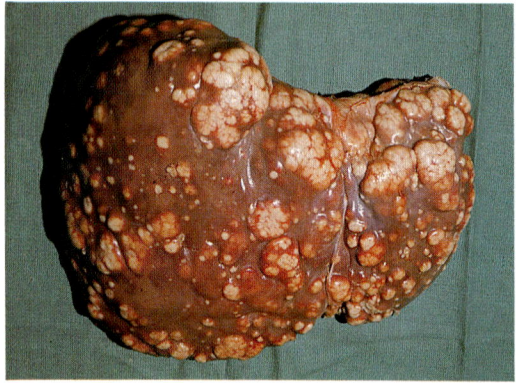

Fig. 21.10   Metastases in the liver. There are numerous nodules of metastatic carcinoma in the liver. The primary tumour was in the stomach.

2. *Lung*. This is the next most common site for metastases.

3. *Bone*. Carcinomata of the breast, lung, prostate, kidney, and thyroid quite frequently produce bone metastases (Fig. 21.11).

4. *Brain*. Carcinoma of the lung is notorious for the frequency with which it metastasizes to the brain.

5. *Adrenal glands*. These are frequently the site of secondary deposits of cancer of the lung and breast.

Experimental work on mice suggests that selective metastasis is related to the nature of the tumour cells rather than to the soil. The transplantable B16 melanoma metastasizes to many organs, including the lungs. If a metastatic lung tumour is grown in tissue culture, harvested, and reinjected intravenously into a group of mice, an increased number of lung metastases is obtained. Repetition of the cycle—lung metastasis, tissue

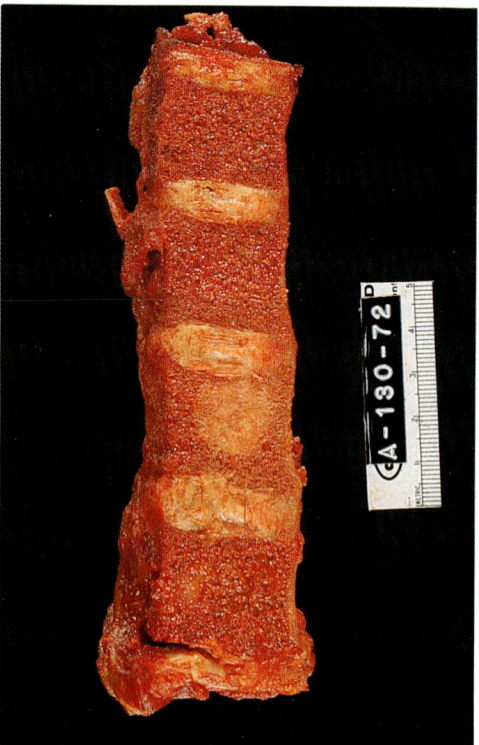

Fig. 21.11   Metastases in the spine. A mass of metastatic carcinoma is present in one vertebral body. the primary tumour was a carcinoma of the lung.

cuture, reinjection into mouse, lung colonization, etc.—results in a strain of B16 melanoma that forms significantly more lung metastases than the original tumour. A strain of melanoma that metastasizes to the brain can be obtained by a similar procedure. Hence it appears that the original tumour is heterogeneous and contains subpopulations of cells, each differing in their potential to form metastases in a particular environment. This conclusion has been confirmed in another way. Clones of the original tumour can be obtained by tissue culture derived from single cells. When injected into groups of mice, each clone gives rise to widely different numbers of metastases in various organs, indicating that the original uncloned tumour contains subpopulations, each differing with regard to malignancy and metastatic potential. Thus the behaviour of a particular human tumour may in part be related to the time taken for a particular malignant clone to become the dominant tumour cell.

Transcoelomic spread. When a malignant tumour invades the serosal layer of a viscus it causes a local acute inflammatory response. This results in the formation of a serous exudate into the cavity. Haemorrhage into the fluid is common, and therefore *the presence of a blood-stained effusion into a serous cavity should always raise the possibility of malignancy.* Tumour cells may break off and float free in the fluid, where they can be detected by the cytologist. They may alight on to other sites in the cavity and form the basis of secondary seedling growths. Such transcoelomic spread is seen in the pleural cavity with cancer of the lung, and in the peritoneum with cancer of the stomach and ovaries.

Staging and grading of tumours

The size of an individual tumour and extent to which it has spread is used to stage the tumour. In the commonly used *TNM staging* procedure the size is denoted T1–4; N1–4 indicates the extent of lymph-node involvement, while M describes the extent of metastases. The details of the procedure are defined for each type of tumour. The method is useful for assessing prognosis for a particular patient and for statistical purposes

when trying to compare the results of different treatments and treatments at different centres. Staging denotes the extent to which a tumour has grown and spread and therefore, being based on past behaviour gives some indication of future behaviour.

The *grading* of tumours is done by examining histological sections of the tumour and assessing the extent and degree of differentiation, pleomorphism and number of mitoses. The assessment is subjective and therefore open to error. Three grades are usually defined. Grade 1 is a well-differentiated tumour, while grade 3 is poorly differentiated. Although there are many exceptions, the higher the grade the worse is the prognosis and the more radio-sensitive is the tumour. Grading is an attempt to guess the future progress of the disease by detailed microscopical examination.

Dormant cancer

A difficulty about staging is the tendency for some metastases to appear many years after the primary tumour has been successfully removed. Such patients may remain well for 10–25 years, and then suddenly develop multiple secondary

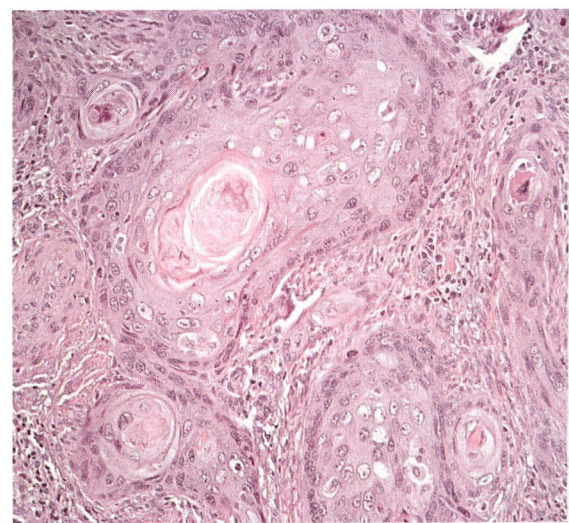

Fig. 21.12 A cell nest or epithelial pearl. This is group of cells from a well differentiated squamous-cell carcinoma. In the centre of the group the cells have differentiated so well that they resemble stratum corneum with keratin in the midst. × 380.

deposits, despite the absence of a local recurrence. It is assumed that the tumour cells were present in the body during the entire period, but for unknown reasons remained dormant. Factors that predispose to the phase of renewed growth after a period of dormancy are intercurrent illness, psychological trauma, and physical injuries. Carcinoma of the breast and kidney and melanoma of the eye are tumours notorious for this tendency towards dormant metastases.

Malignant epithelial tumours

These are called carcinomata, and are the commonest of all malignant tumours. This is probably because epithelium is a much more labile tissue than connective tissue (p. 232). Three types of carcinoma may be recognized:

1. *Squamous-cell carcinoma*
2. *Carcinoma of glandular epithelium*
3. *Transitional-cell carcinoma.*

Squamous-cell carcinoma

These tumours arise at any site normally covered by stratified squamous epithelium—skin, mouth, oesophagus, etc. They account for 90% of all malignant oral tumours. At other sites, e.g. lung, they may occur in an area of atypia or squamous cell carcinoma-in-situ, or sometimes as a result of tumour metaplasia.

Macroscopic types. Two are usually described:

The papillary (or exophytic) carcinoma appears as a warty outgrowth with an infiltrating base.

The nodular (or endophytic) type produces a hard, nodular mass beneath the surface, and shows more rapid infiltration and dissemination. Both types usually ulcerate to form a typical *carcinomatous ulcer*. This has a raised, craggy, rolled edge which is fixed to surrounding skin and deeper structures. The base is composed of white necrotic tissue, which is usually friable and bleeds easily.

Histological type. In considering the histological structure of a squamous-cell carcinoma it is necessary first to understand its formation (Fig. 21.13).

Formation. When epithelium shows malignant

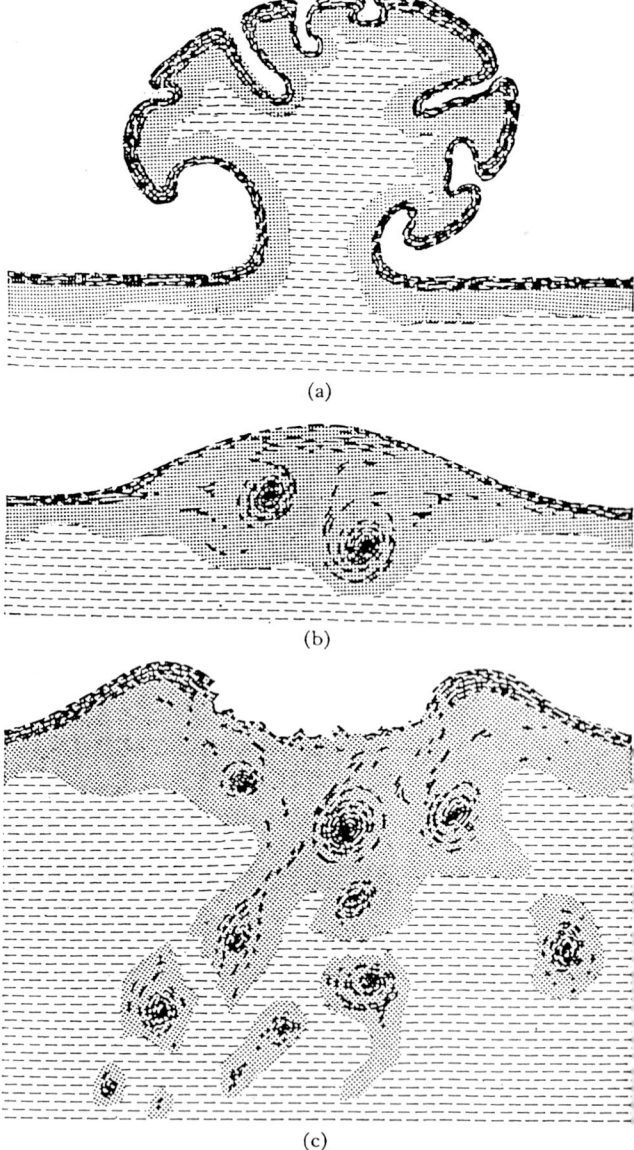

(a)

(b)

(c)

Fig. 21.13 Three types of neoplasia of a keratinizing squamous stratified epithelium, e.g. epidermis.
(A) Benign neoplasia results in an excessive production of regular epithelium, which is thrown into a complicated, folded structure in order to be accommodated. This formation is called a *papilloma*. The epidermal cells mature in an orderly way from the basal cells to the superficial squames.
(B) In *carcinoma-in-situ* there is excessive growth of epithelium, which thereby becomes thickened (acanthosis). Maturation of the cells is disorderly; foci of keratinization are found within the epidermis instead of being present only in the surface (dyskeratosis).
(C) In *carcinoma* the atypical epithelial cells break through the basement membrane and invade the underlying tissues.
(Drawings by Margot Mackay, University of Toronto.)

propensities, there is proliferation of the prickle-cell layer. This is sometimes so irregular that, even before the cells actually break through the basement membrane, they have the microscopic features of malignancy. To this condition the name *carcinoma-in-situ* is applied (p. 270–271).

The criterion of truly invasive carcinoma is the destruction of the basement membrane by masses of malignant cells, which then stream down into the deeper connective tissue and muscle. As they proceed they tend to break up into separate groups or columns. These clumps may comprise hundreds of cancer cells, or else only a few. In the most anaplastic tumours there may be no attempt at any splitting up, and the tumour mass proceeds in one diffuse sheet.

As the tumour infiltrates it destroys the tissue with which it comes in contact, and this is replaced by a fibrous stroma.

Nearly all malignant tumours excite an inflammatory reaction around them; lymphocytes are particularly numerous. Probably they play a part in restricting invasion. Once ulceration of the surface occurs, there is a more acute type of response due to secondary bacterial infection.

In those carcinomata which break up into discrete columns, each individual clump may then differentiate partly or completely to resemble the normal epithelium from which it has arisen.

Differentiation. Squamous-cell carcinomata vary considerably in the degree of differentiation which they show. When differentiation is good, *epithelial pearls* (also called *keratin,* or *horn, pearls*), or *cell nests,* are formed: these are groups of cells, which by differentiating produce a central whorl of keratin (Fig. 21.13). Surrounding this there are prickle cells, and sometimes a stratum granulosum is recognizable. A basal-cell layer is not well formed. In this way there is a fairly accurate reproduction of the upper layers of normal keratinizing stratified squamous epithelium. The cells are usually fairly uniform in size and shape, their nuclei are evenly staining, and mitoses are scanty. On the whole spread is slow. The skin is the commonest site, but sometimes well-differentiated cancers occur in the oral cavity and bronchus.

The more undifferentiated tumours contain no keratin, although groups of prickle cells may still be recognizable.

Poorly differentiated, or anaplastic, tumours show no attempt at prickle-cell formation. There is a diffuse sheet of neoplastic cells supported by a scanty, vascular stroma. No attempt at forming groups of cells is recognizable. The cells themselves show great pleomorphism, and mitotic figures abound— some of these are bizarre. Tumour giant cells may be present. It may be impossible to distinguish the tumour from a sarcoma. This type of tumour is usually found in the mouth, bronchus, and cervix. One variant of anaplastic squamous-cell carcinoma is spindle-cell carcinoma. It is highly malignant and usually arises in an area of radiodermatitis.

Verrucous carcinoma. This type of squamous-cell carcinoma forms a bulky papillomatous mass that histologically is extremely well differentiated. It occurs in the mouth and larynx, also penis, vulva and anal region where it is called a giant condyloma. The tumour is of intermediate malignancy, invading locally but rarely metastasising.

Carcinoma of glandular epithelium

These tumours arise from surface, secreting epithelia as well as from underlying glands. The pattern of invasion of neoplastic epithelium beneath the basement membrane into the deeper tissue is similar to that already described; in this case the groups of cancer cells, instead of producing keratin, tend to arrange themselves into acinar structures containing a central lumen into which secretion pours. The cells surrounding this lumen may be columnar, cuboidal, polygonal, or spheroidal (Fig. 21.14).

The well-differentiated cancers show excellent acinus formation, which mimics normal glandular structure. These tumours are called *adenocarcinomata* (Fig. 21.8).

In less well-differentiated tumours there are merely clumps of cells surrounded by a stroma, and no attempt at central cavitation to produce acini. To this type of cancer the names *carcinoma simplex*, spheroidal-cell or polygonal-cell carcinoma are applied. It is seen most commonly in the

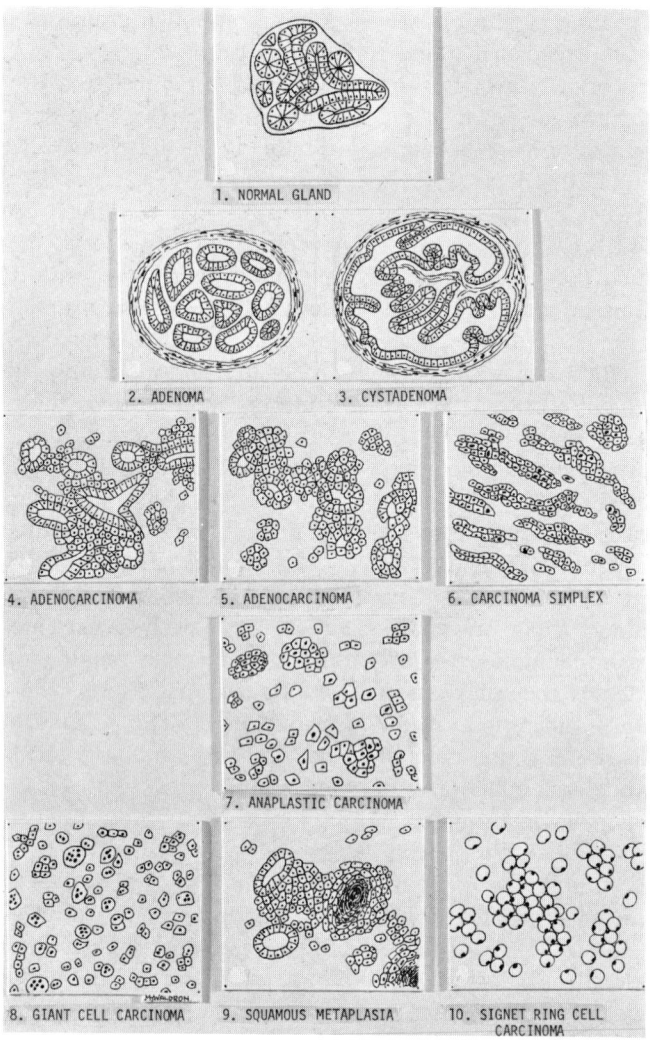

Fig. 21.14 Tumours derived from glandular epithelium. The normal gland (1) is contained within a sheath of connective tissue. Benign neoplasia results in the formation of an adenoma (2) with well-differentiated structure and encapsulation. Cystic dilatation of acini and complicated infolding of the epithelium produce a cystadenoma (3). The remainder of the tumours are malignant. The adenocarcinomata show some tubular differentiation which may be good (4) or poor (5). Lack of differentiation results in a carcinoma simplex (6). The most anaplastic tumours form a sheet of loosely attached cells (7). Giant-cell forms may predominate (8). These anaplastic tumours may be difficult to distinguish from sarcomata, melanomata, and tumours of squamous epithelial origin. Abnormal differentiation results in squamous metaplasia (9) or the formation of signet-ring cell carcinoma (10).

breast, where the cancer clumps are often surrounded by a dense fibrous stroma. Often there is acinus formation elsewhere in the tumour.

The most undifferentiated tumours have diffuse, sheet-like arrangements typical of anaplasia.

Mucoid cancer. The cells of a carcinoma

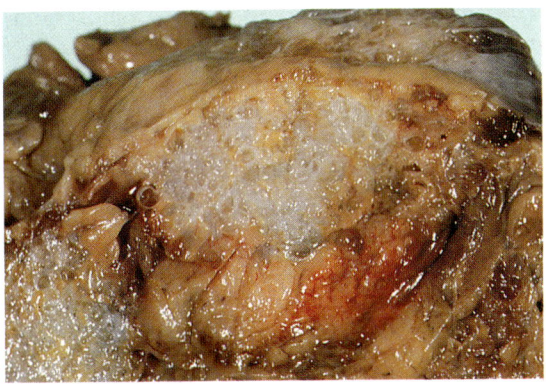

Fig. 21.15   Mucoid carcinoma. A section through an abdominal mass of metastatic carcinoma; it has the translucent appearance characteristic of mucoid carcinoma. The primary tumour was in the stomach.

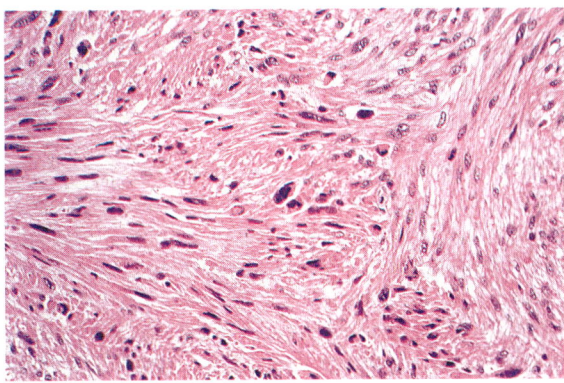

Fig. 21.16   Leiomyosarcoma. The tumour is composed of spindle cells showing marked nuclear pleomorphism.

derived from glandular epithelium may contain demonstrable mucus. Sometimes there is so large an accumulation of mucus in the cytoplasm that the nucleus is compressed on to the cell wall. This type of cell is called a *signet-ring cell*. If mucus secretion is marked, the tumour is called a mucoid cancer (Fig. 21.15). Often the stroma contains large lakes of mucus in which there are disintegrating malignant cells.

Transitional-cell carcinoma

These tumours occur in the renal pelvis, ureter, and bladder. They are often papillomatous in appearance, but differ from papillomata in having a broader base and showing invasion.

Malignant connective tissue tumours

These are called *sarcomata*. They are much less common than carcinomata, and unlike them, they occur at all ages. While carcinomata tend to be arranged in discrete cellular clumps surrounded by a variable amount of stroma, sarcomata are always disposed in diffuse sheets, in which the neoplastic cells merge inseparably into the stroma.

On the whole sarcomata spread more rapidly than carcinomata, and the prognosis is correspondingly more grave. Early blood-borne metastases are the rule, and the lungs are often riddled with secondary deposits. Lymphatic involvement is very much less common than with carcinoma.

Haemorrhage and necrosis are common features of most sarcomata, because the stroma is delicate and the vascular supply inadequate to meet the demands of the tumour.

Fibrosarcoma

Fibrosarcomata, derived from fibroblasts, are not encapsulated and show varying degrees of differentiation. Well-differentiated tumours show considerable collagen formation while with a poorly differentiated tumour, collagen formation is minimal but cellular pleomorphism and mitotic activity are greater.

Malignant fibrous histiocytoma

This is the most common type of soft-tissue sarcoma. It is composed of pleomorphic fibroblast-like cells, giant cells, and histiocytic-type cells often containing lipid. The cell of origin has been much debated and is undecided. Originally it was thought to arise from histocytes but such cells of bone-marrow origin are not now thought to be capable of forming collagen. In the past many tumours in this group were diagnosed as fibrosarcoma, liposarcoma, etc.

Osteosarcoma

This is a common form of sarcoma, and is

described in connexion with the section on bone (p. 412).

Liposarcoma

This is one of the commoner types of sarcoma. It arises usually from the deeper connective-tissue planes of the limbs, especially the thighs, and has considerable invasive potentialities. It metastasizes rather late. Histologically it consists of malignant lipoblasts which may assume giant proportions. A conspicuous tendency is the production of myxomatous tissue, which may overshadow the lipomatous element of the tumour.

Leiomyosarcoma

Leiomyosarcoma is an uncommon tumour usually found in the retroperitoneal tissues, less frequently in skin or myometrium. It is composed of spindle cells often arranged in interlacing fascicles (Fig. 21.16).

Malignant tumours of blood vessels

Angiosarcoma is a rare tumour which usually arises in the soft tissues including those of the oral cavity, and consists microscopically of poorly formed vascular channels lined by atypical endothelial cells. The histological appearances and behaviour depend on the site of the tumour. Angiosarcoma of the sun-exposed face (often called malignant angioendothelioma) has a poor prognosis, while Kaposi's sarcoma is a type of malignant blood-vessel tumour that varies in prognosis according to type.

Tumours of the lymphoreticular system

Neoplasms of the lymphoreticular system are the lymphomas and tumours of the haematopoietic system. The latter includes the leukaemias (see Ch. 26), and multiple myeloma (see Ch. 34).

The lymphomata

The lymphomata are malignant tumors of the lymphoreticular system. Hodgkin's disease is the most common, and the remainder are now classified as the non-Hodgkin's lymphomata.

Hodgkin's disease. This disease is most common in young and middle-aged adults. The first manifestation is enlargement of a group of lymph nodes, commonly in the neck or mediastinum. Fever may be present and in time the disease spreads to involve other lymph nodes and the spleen as well as other internal organs. Severe itching of the skin is a well-known but unexplained symptom. The affected nodes are replaced by a pleomorphic mass of cells. The most characteristic are Reed–Sternberg cells, the precise origin of which is undecided. They are multinucleate, have abundant cytoplasm, and large nuclei with prominent nucleoli. A characteristic cell has two nuclei which appear to be the mirror image of each other (Fig. 21.17). Mononuclear variants are called Hodgkin's cells. In addition there is a varying admixture of lymphocytes, histiocytes, neutrophils and eosinophils.

The prognosis in Hodgkin's disease is related to the histological appearances. Thus if there is lymphocyte predominance the prognosis is good. In the lymphocyte-depleted type the prognosis is poor. The prognosis is also related to the extent of the disease and a system of staging has been evolved. It ranges from stage I, where there is involvement of lymph nodes confined to one region, to stage IV, in which there is widespread disease.

Non-Hodgkin's lymphomas. This group of tumours arises from the cells of the lymph nodes, and it is the complexity of these cells that has caused the problems in classifying this group of lymphomas. Electron microscopy and immunochemistry have revealed that there are many types of cells involved—e.g. B lymphocytes, T cells, follicular centre cells, etc.—but on routine H. & E. microscopy they appear very similar if not identical. Cells thought to be reticulum cells turned out to be lymphocytes! From this confusion and with the aid of specific cell markers, several new classifications emerged. The best known are those of Lukes and Collins, and Lennert (Kiel classification); the reader should consult specialized texts for details. However, certain points should be noted. Most of the B-cell lymphomata are derived from germinal centre cells. 'Histiocytic lymphomata' of previous classifications do not have histiocyte markers and are follicular centre cell lymphomata (Fig. 21.18). Tumours with a follicular pattern have a better prognosis than those that have a diffuse pattern. In clinical practice, lymphomata are classified according to a 'working formulation for clinical usage' devised by a study initiated by the National Cancer Institute of the USA. On the basis of clinical features, the lymphomata are divided into three groups: *low-grade*, *intermediate-grade*, and *high-grade*. Individual types are classified histologically.

Clinically the various lymphomata appear as a mass arising in a lymph node or some extranodal site. If lymph nodes are involved there is often spread to internal organs such as spleen or liver. Invasion of the lymphoma cells into the blood stream adds an additional leukaemic element. In some instances secretion of B cells leads to characteristic clinical syndromes. One such is *Waldenström's macroglobulinaemia*. The tumour cells secrete abundant IgM that leads to hypergammaglobulinaemia. The immunoglobulin is homogenous, indicating that the secreting tumour cells are monoclonal. In this respect it resembles multiple myelomatosis, and both are examples of a *monoclonal gammopathy* and contrast with the hypergammaglobulinaemia of non-neoplastic diseases, i.e. the *polyclonal gammopathy* of systemic lupus erythematosus or chronic infection. Waldenström's macroglobulinaemia runs a prolonged course and is characterized by anaemia, a high ESR, and haemorrhages from the mucous membranes, especially the gingivae, either spontaneously or following dental extraction.

Extranodal lymphoma may occur at any site where lymphoid tissue is present.

With one exception lymphomata are uncommon in the oral cavity. The exception is the Burkitt's tumour. It is a high-grade B-cell lymphoma occurring in low-lying, moist regions of Central and West Africa and associated with infection by Epstein–Barr virus (p. 195). It is peculiar in being almost exclusively confined to children between the ages of 2 and 14 years, and affecting the jaws (especially the maxilla), ovaries, retroperitoneal lymph nodes, and kidneys. The usual presentation is as an enormous facial swelling with loosening of neighbouring teeth. A histo-logically similar type of tumour has been described in other areas (non-endemic Burkitt's lymphoma), but its clinical features differ somewhat; thus the jaws are infrequently affected.

Tumours of embryonic tissues

Tumours may arise from tissue that is normally present only during embryonic life but which persists into postnatal life. These tumours are generally malignant and occur during infancy or childhood. For example nephroblasts normally differentiate to form renal tissue, both epithelial and connective tissue, but may occasionally persist and become malignant. The tumour is the *nephroblastoma* (Wilms's tumour). It is usually poorly differentiated and composed of small darkly staining cells, but sometimes the malignant nephroblasts differentiate into tubular structures as well as forming recognizable connective tissue elements. This is an example of a *mixed tumour*. Other tumours of this type arise from the retina (*retinoblastoma*), the hind brain (*medulloblastoma*), and adrenal medulla and sympathetic ganglia (*neuroblastoma*).

Tumours may also arise from vestigial remnants. For example the *ameloblastoma* arises from remnants of the enamel organ. This is a cystic tumour of the jaws which grows slowly and is locally malignant. Both in behaviour and in structure it resembles the common basal-cell carcinoma quite closely. It usually occurs in the mandible, and is seen most often in young adults. It consists of round or angulated clumps of epithelial cells. In the centre of these aggregations there is often an open meshwork resembling the stellate reticulum of the enamel organ. Between the cells there is an accumulation of fluid which gives rise to the cystic appearance typical of this tumour (Fig. 21.19). Other tumours in this group are rare. The *chordoma* arising from the notochord and the *craniopharyngioma* arising from residues of Rathke's pouch may be cited as examples.

Tumours of germ cell origin

The germ cells first appear in the embryo in the wall of the yolk sac, from where they migrate to the genital ridge on the posterior abdominal wall. They become incorporated into the developing gonad, but it is believed that some cells remain

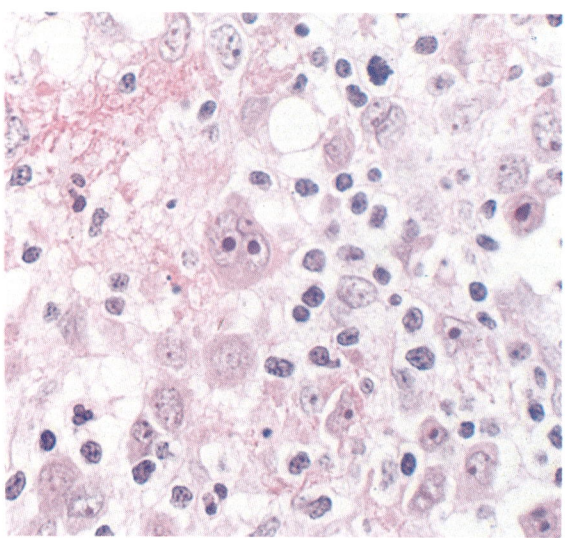

Fig. 21.17   Hodgkin's disease. The cells in the centre is a Reed–Sternberg cell; it has two large nuclei, each with large nucleoli surrounded by a pale halo.

behind or stray from their final path, and come to rest at various sites along the posterior wall of the embryo near the midline. If these cells remain viable they later give rise to tumours in just these situations. Hence, germ-cell tumours are found in the retroperitoneal area, the sacral region, and

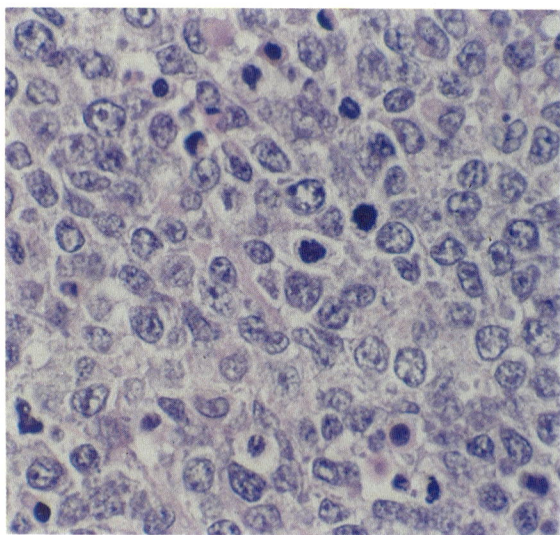

Fig. 21.18   Non-Hodgkin's lymphoma. The malignant cells in this lymphoma are derived from follicle-centre cells.

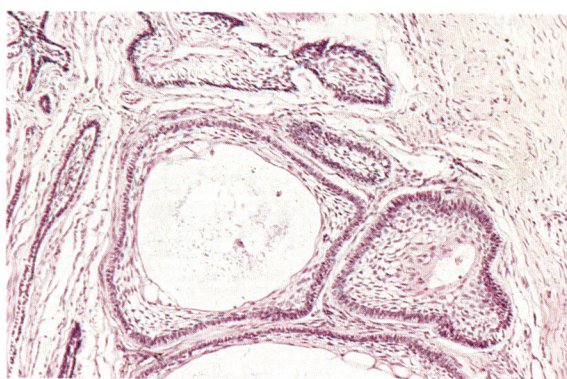

Fig. 21.19   Ameloblastoma. The tumour consists of aggregations of small epithelial cells, the outer layers of which form a palisade as is found in the basal-cell carcinoma. In the centre of the clumps there is an open meshwork reminiscent of the stellate reticulum of the developing tooth germ ('enamel organ'). Degeneration of these cells has led to the formation of a small cyst in parts of the tumour. (Photograph courtesy of Dr J W Rippin.)

the mediastinum, and around the pineal gland; the greatest number, of course, are in the gonads.

The germ cells are totipotent and able to form any tissue found normally in the body. The common germ-cell tumour is the *teratoma*, a

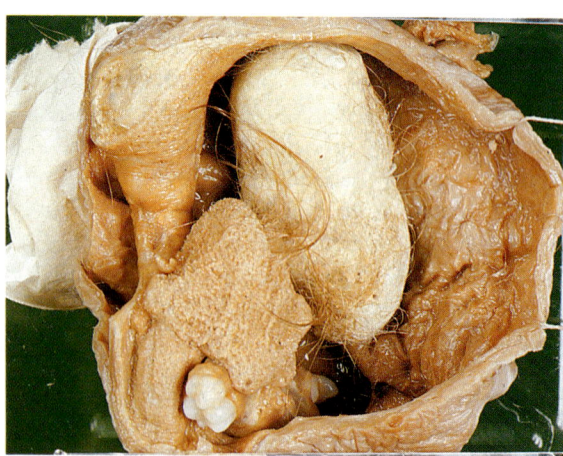

Fig. 21.20   Teratoma of the ovary. This tumour had caused episodes of abdominal pain in a 32-year-old for about 5 years. When she experienced a particularly severe attack a laporotomy was performed and a cystic ovarian tumour was removed. The specimen shows the cyst cut open. It is lined by skin containing numerous sebaceous glands and a tuft of hair. There is also bone present with a number of teeth partially embedded, one of which can be clearly seen. (Photograph of specimen by courtesy of the Boyd Museum, University of Toronto.)

tumour that contains structures derived from the three primitive germinal cell layers. In the ovary the tumour is well differentiated and benign; it is encountered in women between the ages of 20 and 30 years. Ovarian teratomata are usually cystic, with a wall formed by tissue resembling normal skin including the presence of pilosebaceous follicles (Fig. 21.20). The cyst is therefore filled with hair matted together with greasy sebaceous material. The lesion is commonly called a 'dermoid cyst' but is really a mixed tumour; there is a nodule in the wall of the cyst which contains a variety of structures such as bone, teeth, thyroid, and brain, structures never found in a true dermoid cyst.

Teratomata of the testis are nearly always malignant. They are composed of cystic spaces lined by a variety of different types of epithelium and a connective tissue element containing primitive mesenchyme, cartilage, muscle, etc. The tumour, together with other testicular tumours thought to be of germ-cell origin (e.g. seminoma), form the foremost malignant tumour of males between the ages of 15 and 35 years. Similar tumours occur in the ovary.

Tumours of chorionic tissue

Tumours derived from placental tissue may be benign (hydatidiform mole) or malignant (choriocarcinoma) and they complicate pregnancy; occasionally they arise from germ cells.

DIFFICULTIES IN TUMOUR CLASSIFICATION

Tumour classification is based on histogenesis and behaviour. In both areas there are some difficulties.

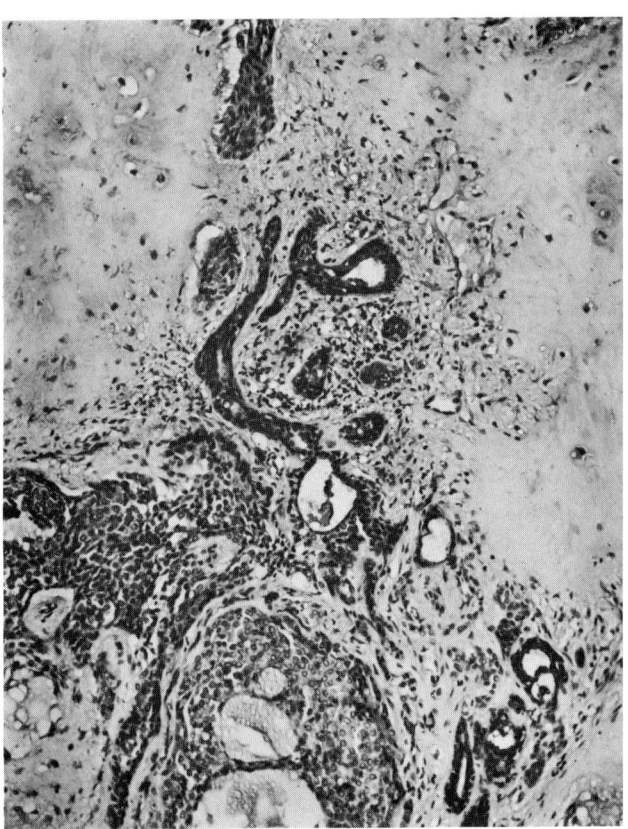

Fig. 21.21 Pleomorphic salivary gland tumour ('adenoma'). There are columns of epithelial cells, some arranged in ductules, surrounded by a dense rather acellular stroma which resembles hyaline cartilage. × 110.

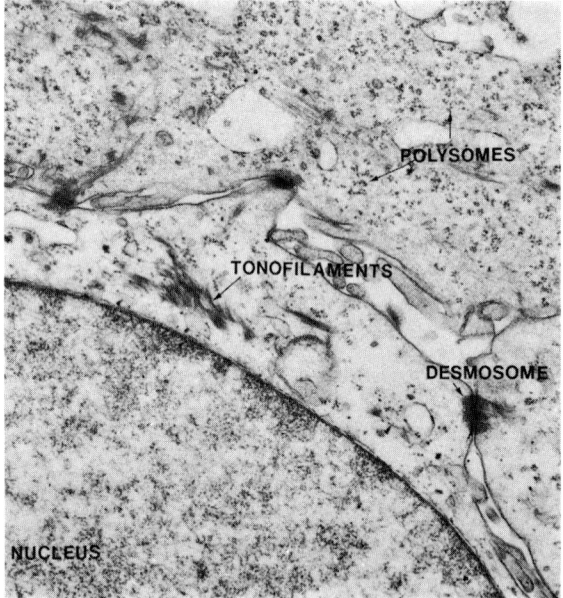

Fig. 21.22 Squamous-cell carcinoma of nose. A 50-year-old man developed a polypoid lesion of the nose. This was excised, and the specimen reported as consisting of inflammatory tissue. However, the lesion recurred, and a biopsy revealed a vascular lesion with many spindle cells consistent with a diagnosis of spindle-cell sarcoma. Electron microscopy showed typical features of an epithelial tumour. The figure shows several tight junctions with desmosome formation. In the cytoplasm tonofilaments are present as well as numerous free ribosomes, which are grouped as polysomes. The tumour was therefore regarded as a spindle-cell squamous-cell carcinoma. × 27 500. (Photography by courtesy of Dr Y C Bedard, New Mount Sinai Hospital, Toronto.)

Difficulties related to histogenesis

The precise origin of certain tumours is difficult to decide; four examples will be described.

Pleomorphic salivary gland tumour. These tumours are found most commonly in the parotid gland, but may arise from other salivary glands and also the mucous glands of the oral mucosa, trachea, and bronchi. They consist of acini, cords, and thin strands of epithelial cells suspended in a stroma which often has a myxomatous appearance (Fig. 21.21). This was at one time regarded as true cartilage, and the tumour was called a 'mixed parotid tumour'. It is now realized that the mucoid appearance is due to a sero-mucinous secretion from the tumour cells into the stroma. True cartilage is very rarely found, and when it is present it is due to chondral metaplasia of the stroma.

The tumour may appear well encapsulated, but the capsule is often infiltrated by lateral extensions of growth. Simple enucleation is likely to be followed by recurrence. Furthermore, obvious local invasion may sometimes occur. Occasionally distant blood-borne metastases are encountered, even in tumours which appear 'benign' microscopically.

Endothelium and mesothelium. The flattened lining cells of the serous spaces, like the pleural cavity, synovium and the endothelial cells of blood vessels are sometimes regarded as epithelial, but in fact the tumours which are derived from them usually behave as connective-tissue tumours, and are commonly classified as such.

Poorly differentiated tumours. A second difficulty in the histogenetic classification is the occurrence of tumours so poorly differentiated

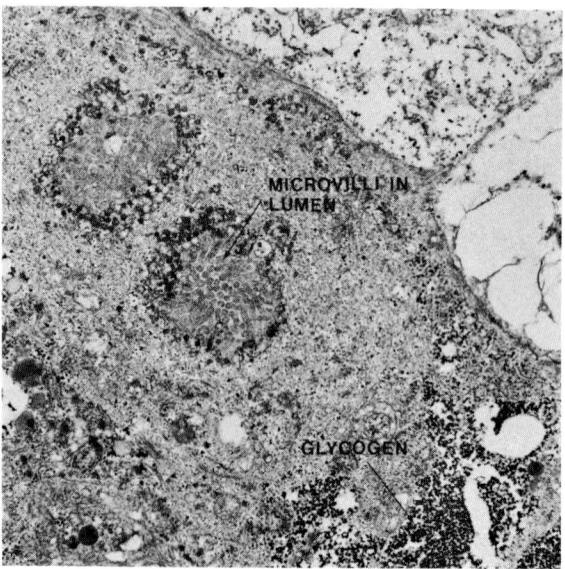

Fig. 21.23 Carcinoma of the breast. A 65-year-old woman developed enlarged axillary lymph nodes, and biopsy revealed an anaplastic tumour. Lymphoma was considered to be the most likely diagnosis, but electron microscopy revealed intracellular lumina with microvilli. This is a feature of poorly-differentiated glandular carcinoma. A blind biopsy of the ipsilateral breast of this patient showed infiltrating lobular carcinoma. Note the presence of numerous glycogen granules. × 14 000 (Photograph by courtesy of Dr Y C Bedard, New Mount Sinai Hospital, Toronto.)

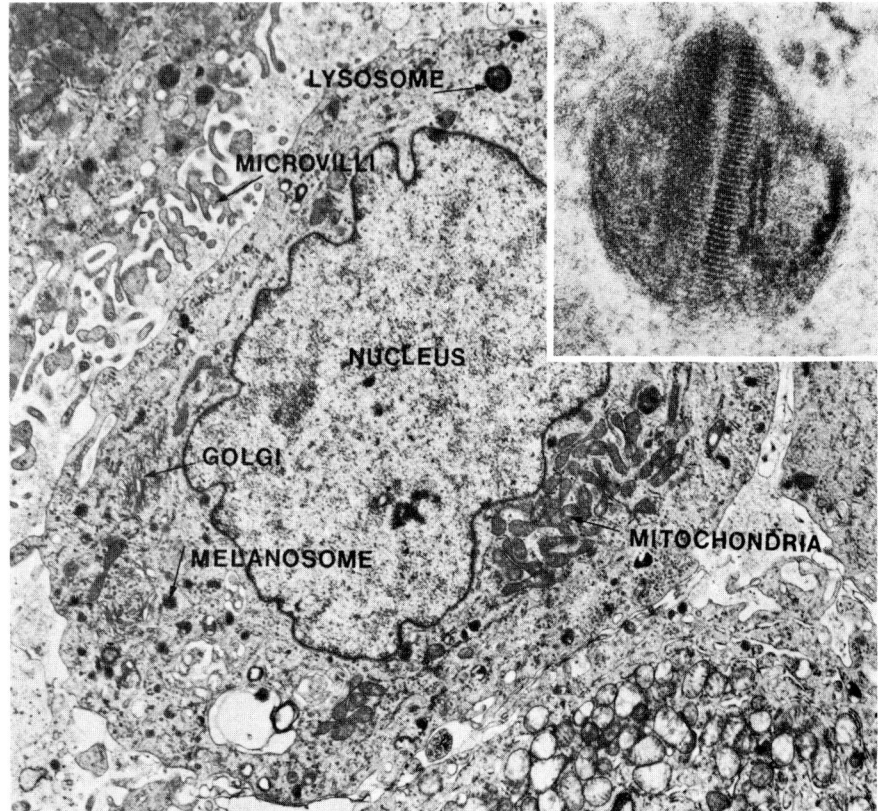

Fig. 21.24 Malignant melanoma. A 16-year-old boy developed enlargement of the inguinal lymph nodes, and biopsy revealed an anaplastic tumour consistent with anaplastic carcinoma, lymphoma, or malignant melanoma. No melanin could be demonstrated by silver staining. Electron microscopy revealed cytoplasmic structures (mel), which on high magnification (inset) show the characteristic banding of melanosomes that is visible before the extensive deposition of melanin obscures this detail. On reviewing the patient's history it was found that a 'mole' had been removed from the leg two years previously. This had been reported as a benign naevus, but in fact was a malignant melanoma. × 11 000. Insert × 143 000. (Photograph by courtesy of Dr Y C Bedard, New Mount Sinai Hospital, Toronto.)

that their cell of origin is difficult to determine. Such tumours have been given descriptive names, e.g. small anaplastic cell carcinoma, spindle-cell sarcoma, etc. Two techniques are now available for investigating the possible nature and the origin of anaplastic tumours.

Electron microscopy. The fine structure of tumour cells may give a hint as to its origin or type of differentiation. Thus the presence of desmosomes and the formation of a basement membrane adjacent to cells indicates an epithelial origin (Fig. 21.22). The formation of intracellular lumina suggests a glandular origin (Fig. 21.23). The presence of melanosomes indicates

that an anaplastic tumour is a malignant melanoma (Fig. 21.24). On the other hand, the presence of neurosecretory granules points to an origin from cells of the diffuse endocrine system (Fig. 21.25).

Tumour markers. The development of tagged monoclonal antibodies against cell components has been a great step forward in the recognition of tumour types. Immunofluorescent or immunoperoxidase techniques can be used. Some examples will be cited, but the list of antibodies available is rapidly increasing.

The presence of cytokeratin is a feature of epithelial cells, vimentin of connective tissue cells,

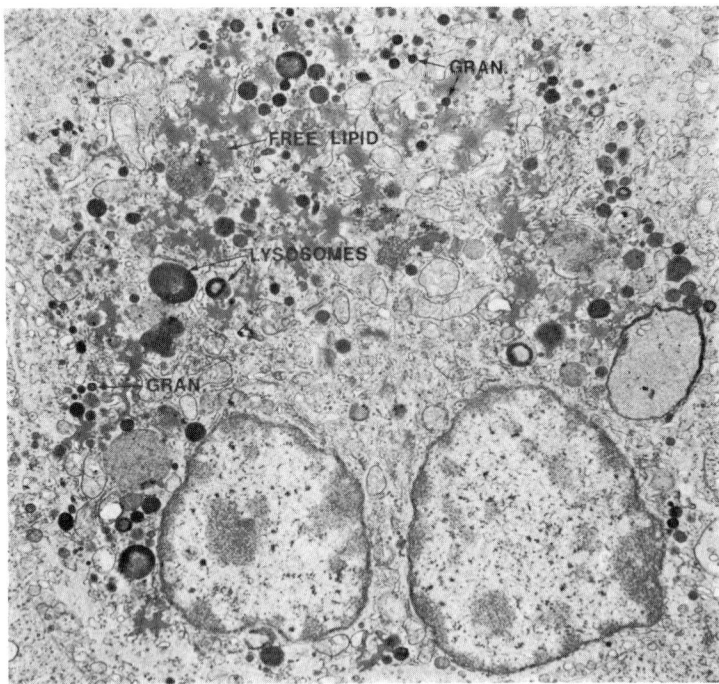

Fig. 21.25 Oat-cell carcinoma of the lung. A 45-year-old woman developed features of Cushing's syndrome, and a scalene lymph-node biopsy revealed an anaplastic tumour consistent with the diagnosis of oat-cell carcinoma of the lung. The electron micrograph of the tumour shows typical neurosecretory granules. Note also the presence of free lipid and lysosomes, some of which contain myelin figures. × 14 000. (Photograph by courtesy of Dr Y C Bedard, New Mount Sinai Hospital, Toronto.)

desmin detects muscle and some endothelia, and S100 is positive for Schwann cells and melanocytes. α_1-fetoprotein is present in yolk-sac tumours and hepatomata, while factor VIII related protein can be detected in endothelial cells. A large number of markers is available for the various subsets of lymphocytes.

Tumour metaplasia. A further difficulty arises when tumour cells differentiate in a direction other than that of the parent tissue; thus sometimes a tumour of glandular epithelium shows differentiation towards a keratinizing squamous-cell type. Such a tumour would be called a squamous-cell carcinoma, although it is of glandular origin (see carcinoma of lung, p. 373).

Melanoma. A fourth difficulty is the histogenetic classification of tumours arising from cells whose precise origin is disputed. The best example of this is the *melanoma* of the skin (p. 454).

Difficulties related to behaviour

The behaviour of a number of tumours is neither benign nor malignant as previously described. In one group, called *locally malignant tumours,* there is local invasion and yet distant metastases almost never occur. The basal cell carcinoma of the skin (see Chapter 37) and the ameloblastoma (see p. 259) are good examples. Some tumours are somewhat more aggressive and distant metastases do occur, although they are often small and do not shorten life. Such tumours are now put into a group of *tumours of intermediate malignancy.* A good example is the carcinoid tumour derived from the diffuse endocrine cells (see Chapter 36). Carcinoid tumours of the appendix invade but do not metastasize, whereas tumours of the small intestine metastasize to the lymph nodes and occasionally to the liver. It will be appreciated that as regards behaviour there exists a range of tumours, from those that may be called completely benign, which never invade and never metastasize, to those that are called malignant and always invade and always metastasize.

An outline of the present classification of tumours is shown in Table 21.1.

AETIOLOGY OF TUMOURS

Careful observation of the incidence of tumours has indicated that particular tumours are more frequent in certain groups of people. An association with occupation or environment has identified various external agents that are responsible. These chemical and physical carcinogenic agents have been extensively investigated. Clustering of cases in a family has indicated that hereditary factors are operating. Experimental work has identified the involvement of hormonal factors, and, finally, that some tumours appear to be caused by viruses. Each of these possible causes of cancer will be examined in detail.

The current evidence suggests that most tumours arise from a *single clone of cells*, or perhaps only a few such clones, that have undergone malignant transformation. This evidence is derived from the following sources:

(1) In the monoclonal gammopathies, of which Waldenström's macroglobulinaemia and multiple myeloma are the typical examples, there is good evidence that a single clone of B lymphocytes (which have developed into plasma cells in the case of multiple myeloma) have become malignant, and by metastatic spread as well as local proliferation have crowded out the many normal clones of immunoglobulin-forming B lymphocytes. These neoplastic cells produce only one type of immunoglobulin molecule, and so can be easily identified.

The same argument applies to those tumours of B lymphocyte origin which, although not producing a circulating immunoglobulin, nevertheless have a specific cell-surface immunoglobulin. Chronic lymphatic leukaemia is a good example.

(2) According to the Lyon hypothesis, one of the X chromosomes in each cell of a female becomes inactivated early in fetal life.* This random inactivation may affect either the maternal or paternal X chromosome, and the progeny of the cell inherits this change. The enzyme glucose 6-phosphate dehydrogenase (G6PD) is coded for by a gene on the X chromosome, and in black populations two allelic forms, called A and B, are commonly found. Some 40% of black females are heterozygous, so that extracts of blood, skin, and other tissues contain a mixture of enzyme types A and B. It is apparent that if only one type of enzyme, whether A or B, is found in an extract of a tumour from a person whose normal tissues contains both types, the inference is that the tumour arose from a single clone of cells.

On the basis of G6PD typing a clonal origin has been demonstrated for many tumours both benign and malignant.

This emphasis on a clonal derivation does not mean that tumours develop from a transforming event affecting only a single cell. It is probable that successive waves of clones emerge during the course of the evolution of malignancy, and that the formation of a tumour is a multi-step process (see p. 266).

FACTORS KNOWN TO PRODUCE CANCER

The three factors generally recognized as causes of human neoplasia are:

External carcinogenic agents—chemical and physical agents.
Hereditary predisposition.
Chronic disease, usually of an inflammatory nature.

Two additional factors have to be considered, *hormones* and *viruses.*

---

* This hypothesis was put forward by Mary Lyon, and it is called *lyonization of the X chromosome.* The inactivated chromosome replicates later than the other chromosomes during the mitotic cycle, and its descendants follow the same pattern. Since the two chromosomes may carry different sets of X-linked genes, there may be patchiness of a visible characteristic transmitted thus, e.g. coat colour in an animal. Women heterozygous for glucose 6-phosphate dehydrogenase deficiency, an X-linked dominant characteristic, possess two races of red cells, one normal and the other enzyme deficient, and it is the latter that undergo haemolysis.

External carcinogenic agents

Chemical carcinogens

It has been known since the eighteenth century that those people whose occupation brings them into contact with coal tar or mineral oil are liable to develop carcinoma of the skin. The chemical carcinogens involved are aromatic polycyclic hydrocarbons; *1:2:5:6-dibenzanthracene*, *methylcholanthrene* and *3:4-benzpyrene*, and many more have been identified. They are produced by heating organic material to destruction and are found in smoke from wood and coal fires, car exhaust fumes, cigarette smoke, food and coal tar products. Since the discovery of the aromatic amines, many other examples of carcinogenic chemical have been discovered. Some are *direct-acting carcinogens*. These are in a reactive electrophilic form and require no activation. They are weak carcinogens—such as some cytotoxic drugs used in the treatment of cancer. Other carcinogens (termed *procarcinogens*) do not act directly but must first be metabolized to strongly positively-charged electrophilic reactants termed ultimate carcinogens. The microsomal mixed-function oxidase group of enzymes are necessary for this conversion. They are present in many tissues, and the ultimate carcinogen can act at the site of its formation. However, the liver is the most important site for the formation of the ultimate carcinogens, and these may act on the liver or elsewhere at some distant site.

Important groups of carcinogens include:

Aromatic amines. These include napthylamine and benzidine used in the rubber industry. They are converted into an ultimate carcinogen in the liver and released conjugated with glycuronic acid. Excretion occurs in the urine, but the urinary bladder of humans contains an enzyme (β-glycuronidase) that releases the free ultimate carcinogen. Carcinoma of the bladder results.

Nitrosamines. These carcinogens have been suggested as a cause of cancer of the stomach. They are formed in the alimentary tract from nitrates and nitrites in the diet, e.g. in processed meats. The decline in the incidence of cancer of the stomach has been attributed to the increased use of the refrigerator as a means of preserving meat.

Vinyl chloride. Industrial exposure is associated with hepatic cholangiocarcinoma.

Aflatoxin. This carcinogen causes liver cancer and is produced by the fungus *Aspergillus flavus*, which contaminates groundnut meal. This probably explains the frequency of the cancer in Africa and Southeast Asia.

Other carcinogens. Public awareness of the possible carcinogenicity of food additives, drugs, industrial effluents, and other chemicals in the environment, has led to the identification of many examples. Scarcely a week passes that some new agent is not incriminated—dioxan, formaldehyde, saccharine, to mention but a few. Some carcinogens have been identified by noting a high incidence of cancer in workers in certain occupations, thus, asbestos, nickel, chromium and arsenic have been incriminated.

Initiation and promotion. When a carcinogen is applied to a tissue it binds to cells and causes a change that can be reversed. However, if the cell undergoes proliferation the change, termed *initiation*, can become fixed. Morphologically no change can be detected, but if the tissue is irritated by some relatively non-specific agent termed a *promoter*, a malignant tumour develops. It follows that all complete carcinogens are both initiators and promoters. Carcinogenesis has therefore been regarded as a two-phase phenomenon, but further work has indicated that in fact it is a *multi-step process*. Following the action of a carcinogen, foci of hyperplasia develop, to be followed by cellular atypia, in situ carcinoma, invasive carcinoma of low malignancy and finally carcinoma of high malignancy. This evolution is termed *tumour progression*. The concept of initiation and promotion has important implications in human disease. Thus if a tissue is exposed to a carcinogen, the necessary promoter may not be applied until years later. This could explain why cancer due to an industrial chemical could evolve years after leaving the employment.

Numerous chemicals are now known to be carcinogenic to animals and the testing of new substances, particularly industrial chemicals, drugs and food additives, is a major business. Animal testing is expensive, time-consuming and to many people morally unacceptable. Also there is great difference in susceptibility of different animal species to the carcinogenic effect of an agent. Since most carcinogens are mutagens, the agent can be tested for its ability to produce a mutation in a bacterium. This is the basis of the *Ames test*. Nevertheless, the only way to assess whether a chemical is carcinogenic to humans is to observe the effect of giving it to humans.

Physical carcinogenic agents

The important relationship between ionizing radiation and cancer is considered in detail in Chapter 22. Ultraviolet radiation exerts its harmful effect in the form of strong sunlight. Melanin in the skin affords considerable protection, but individuals of North European descent who live in sunny places— Australia, South Africa and North America—are at great risk if their occupation or pleasures involve being out of doors. In later life, *actinic* or *solar keratoses* develop, and a number evolve into *squamous-cell carcinoma. Basal-cell carcinoma* and *malignant melanoma* are other penalties of unprotected exposure to the sun.

Hereditary predisposition

There are a number of malignant human tumours that are inherited. Retinoblastoma, particularly if bilateral, is inherited as a dominant trait. Cancer of the breast is more common in relatives of affected women than in the population at large. Cancer of the ovary is common in certain families. However, for most other malignant tumours there is little evidence of an inherited cause.

There are, nevertheless, a number of uncommon traits that may predispose to malignancy.

The trait of *familial polyposis coli* is transmitted as an autosomal dominant. Multiple adenomata of the colon usually first manifest themselves at puberty. They are not present at birth. By the time the patient reaches the age of 30 years, multiple colonic cancers appear. Life is seldom prolonged over the age of 40 years. Gardner's syndrome is also associated with an increased incidence of colonic carcinoma (p. 246).

Xeroderma pigmentosum is inherited as an autosomal recessive trait. The skin is abnormally susceptible to the effects of sunlight, and multiple squamous-cell and basal-cell carcinomata develop on the exposed parts. Death usually occurs within the first decade. The mechanism of xeroderma pigmentosum has now been elucidated. Ultraviolet light gives rise to dimer formation between neighbouring thymidine radicles in DNA, and when such DNA replicates, the dimer causes a mutation. In normal cells there are enzymes that can excise the dimer and replace it by the correct nitrogen bases. In xeroderma pigmentosum one such enzyme is lacking, and the disease is an inborn error of metabolism.

The inherited susceptibility to the action of carcinogen in experimental work has been mentioned previously.

Chronic disease as a cause of cancer

Chronic irritation. Although once cited as a cause of cancer, a concept of chronic irritation is too vague to have much meaning nowadays. It is extremely doubtful whether physical irritation acting alone can ever produce cancer, though it may certainly promote a tumour in a field already initiated by a carcinogenic substance. There are, however, a number of chronic diseases which may from time to time be complicated by malignancy.

Chronic ulcers. The sinuses of chronic osteomyelitis, and old burn scars occasionally give rise to squamous-cell carcinoma.

Syphilitic glossitis. This has been regarded as an important precursor of oral cancer. The glossitis was often associated with dysplastic leucoplakia on the tongue and elsewhere in the mouth, and this condition often proceeds to malignancy. But whether the leucoplakia was due to syphilis, or whether the syphilis was merely a coincidental lesion is not certain. Syphilitic glossitis, like many other tertiary lesions of this infection, is now so rarely encountered that the controversy is unlikely to be settled.

Ulcerative colitis. About 4% of all cases eventually develop carcinoma.

Cirrhosis of the liver. Primary liver-cell cancer is usually superimposed on a previous cirrhosis. Liver cancer is extremely prevalent in African races and also among the Chinese and Japanese. This is undoubtedly due to the high incidence of cirrhosis, and is not dependent upon racial factors.

The Plummer–Vinson syndrome. This is associated with postcricoid carcinoma (pp. 307).

Paget's disease of bone. Occasionally this is complicated by osteosarcoma.

Malformations. There are a number of *hamartomatous lesions* which occasionally become malignant, for example neurofibromatosis. A *congenitally abnormal organ*, e.g. an imperfectly descended testis, is more liable to malignancy than is a normal one.

Hormones and neoplasia

The early observations that oestrogens were a factor in the causation of cancer of the breast in mice led to widespread speculation that such a mechanism was applicable to the human being. However, it soon became evident that the operative factor was the presence of the oncogenic Bittner virus. The oestrogens acted by producing breast development in the male mice. A somewhat similar event has been encountered in humans when males have developed breast cancer following castration and oestrogen administration as part of a 'sex-change' procedure. A somewhat similar event occurred when pregnant women were given diethylstilboestrol during pregnancy. Female children showed a high incidence of carcinoma of the vagina, a tumour that is otherwise rare. The tumour arises in vestigial remnants. Oestrogen administered to menopausal women has been incriminated as a factor in endometrial cancer.

Hormone-dependent tumours. If hormones cannot be directly incriminated in the aetiology of human cancer, they are undoubtedly of great importance in maintaining the growth of some tumours. These are called the *hormone-dependent tumours*, and the best example is *carcinoma of the prostate.*

Both the normal prostatic epithelium and the carcinomata derived from it are dependent for their integrity upon a supply of testosterone. If patients with carcinoma of the prostate are castrated, there is often a dramatic relief of symptoms and regression of the tumour and its

metastases. Nowadays stilboestrol is administered and has a similar effect. The relief may last for at least 5 years, and, as many of the patients are over 70 years of age, some succumb to intercurrent illness before the cancer loses its hormone dependency and once more pursues its progressive course.

Carcinoma of the breast is another tumour which manifests hormone dependence in some patients. The picture is, however, complicated, because the tumour may depend upon ovarian, adrenal, or pituitary hormones. Nevertheless, in some patients the removal of the ovaries, adrenals or pituitary produces a marked but temporary remission. In other cases the administration of oestrogens or testosterone may have an ameliorative effect.

Oncogenic viruses

Tumour-producing (oncogenic) viruses have been demonstrated in many species including humans. Ellerman and Bang (1908) were the first to show that a fowl leukaemia was caused by a virus, and shortly after, Rouse (1911) described virus induced fowl sarcoma. Since then many other examples have been discovered. One of the most interesting is the agent described by Bittner as causing mammary carcinoma in mice. Initially the tumour appeared to be inherited, but in fact the disease is caused by a RNA retrovirus that is transmitted from the mother to her offspring in her milk. The tumour does not develop in female mice until they attain maturity because oestrogens must first act to produce breast development.

Oncogenic viruses may contain either DNA or RNA, and have the ability to integrate their DNA, or proviral DNA in the case of RNA viruses, into the host DNA. This integration of viral material into the host cell causes the cell to undergo *transformation.* This is evident as abnormal proliferation in tissue culture and the ability to form a tumour if injected into a suitable animal.

The DNA oncogenic viruses

Cells transformed by a DNA virus have viral DNA incorporated into the cell's genome; mRNA of viral type is produced, and subsequently viral-type protein is synthesized by the cell. One early product is the *T-antigen*, which is found in the nucleus of infected cells. It is an important marker because the segment of DNA that encodes for it also contains the transforming genes. Two such genes must be present; one gives the infected cell the property of immortality, the other completes transformation into a malignant cell. Another viral gene product is the *tumour-specific transplantation antigen*, which is present on the cell's surface.

The DNA viruses that may be involved in human carcinogenesis fall into two groups: the herpesviruses and the papovaviruses.

Oncogenic herpesviruses. The Epstein–Barr virus (EBV), is a herpesvirus associated with Burkett's lymphoma in Africa. The virus also causes *infectious mononucleosis* in healthy young adults in North American and European societies. This is a self-limiting disease characterized by fever, sore throat, lymphadenopathy, and a leucocytosis due to overproduction of B lymphocytes. It is not known why the virus causes a benign infection in some patients and a malignant tumour in others. Possibly the virus becomes oncogenic in cooperation with chronic infection, particularly with malaria. This suggestion would explain the geographical distribution of the tumour.

Herpes simplex virus. Genital infection with the herpes simplex virus type 2 virus (HSV-2) is associated with an increased incidence of carcinoma of the cervix uteri.

Oncogenic papovaviruses. This group of viruses derives its name from its three subgroups: *the papilloma viruses*, which causes warts, the *polyoma viruses*, and the *vacuolating viruses*. The polyoma viruses cause a variety of tumours in animals but, like the vacuolating viruses, have not been incriminated in human disease.

Human papilloma viruses (HPV). This is a large group of viruses that cause human warts. The common wart is a squamous-cell papilloma that usually resolves either spontaneously or with treatment. It rarely becomes malignant. However, certain types (HPV-16 and HPV-18) cause genital warts, and are associated with a variety of dysplastic lesions of the vulva, vagina and cervix uteri. These may progress to carcinoma particularly in the cervix. As with HSV-2 infection, the exact role of the viral infection is not clear. Subjects who have many sexual partners are more prone to develop cervical carcinoma, and are also more liable to acquire infection with these sexually transmitted viruses.

The RNA oncoviruses (oncornaviruses)

The *oncornaviruses* are one of three genera within the family of retroviruses. These are double-stranded RNA-containing, enveloped viruses that are characterized by containing the enzyme RNA-dependent DNA polymerase, also called reverse transcriptase, within the virion. The enzyme transcribes the viral RNA into DNA *provirus*, which is then integrated into the DNA of the host cell's nucleus. This process is of great interest because it is a reversal of the usual sequence of transcription of DNA to RNA. The provirus encodes for further RNA, and free viral particles are released from an infected cell. The cell may become malignant if the infecting virus contains an *oncogene*. The genetic structure of the retroviruses is relatively simple (they contain only three genes, *gag*, *pol*, and *env*). The oncogene may be in addition or it may replace one of these genes. The viral oncogenes (termed v-*onc*) have been identified using the new methods of DNA methodology and named according to their virus of origin, e.g. v-*ras* is derived from a rat sarcoma virus, v-*myc* is from a myeloproliferative disorder of chickens. In all, about 30 viral oncogenes have been recognized. They encode for proteins that are an abnormal form of the factors produced by their normal counterpart (cellular oncogenes (see below).

Specific DNA probes have now been developed by which oncogenes can be identified in a cell. Remarkably similar oncogenes can be identified in normal cells. These are termed proto-oncogenes or *cellular oncogenes* (c-*onc*). The normal role of these cellular oncogenes is the production of growth factors, growth-factor receptors, membrane-associated protein kinases and other factors that are involved in gene transcription. They are therefore involved in the normal cell growth and replication.

The DNA of human tumours can be split into fragments by the action of bacterial endo-

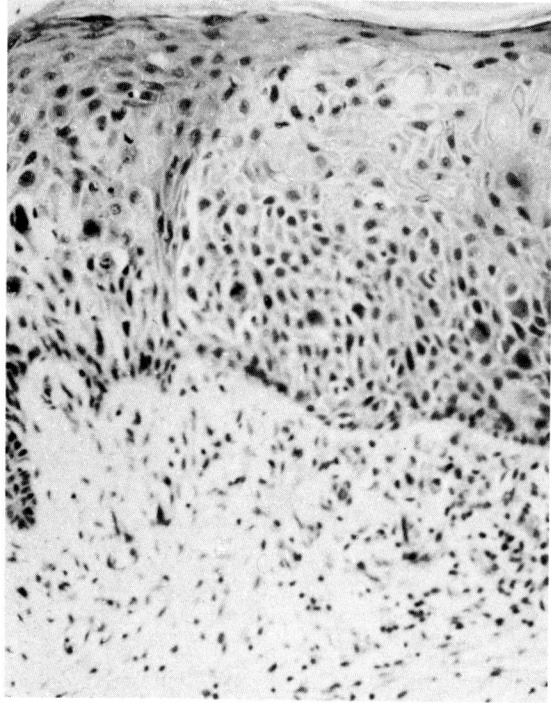

Fig. 21.26 A carcinoma-in-situ. This is a skin biopsy from a case of Bowen's disease. The cells are pleomorphic, and the orderly arrangement of the upper layers of the prickle-cell layer is disrupted. A number of cells have large, darkly-staining nuclei, and elsewhere in the section there were mitotic figures. There is a heavy lymphocytic infiltration in the dermis. Serial sections of the block failed to show any evidence of invasion. × 200.

amplification has been observed in some tumours —that is, the tumour cells contain multiple copies of the oncogene. Possibly the effect of a oncogene is quantitative rather than qualitative, and due to an increased dosage of the gene product. Another possibility is that viral oncogenes are mutated cellular oncogenes. For instance, the genetic change responsible for the activation of the oncogene in human T24 human bladder cancer is a point mutation of guanosine into thymidine. Another possibility is the activation of cellular oncogene by a translocation. As an example, in chronic myeloid leukaemia there is a 9–22 translocation. The translocated part of the short arm of 9 contains the oncogene c-*abl*, and in its new position on 22 it is close to a locus known as the breakpoint cluster region *bcr*. The combination of c-*abl/bcr* is somehow related to the development of leukaemia. A similar mechanism may explain how DNA viruses or RNA viruses, while not containing an oncogene, might by integrating into the cell's DNA activate an adjacent oncogene already present in the cell. The presence of *anti-oncogenes*, the action of which is to inhibit an oncogene, may also be important.

The only human retrovirus so far incriminated as a cause of human cancer is the human T-lymphotropic virus 1 (HTLV-1) isolated from cases of adult T-cell lymphoma. A related virus HTLV-2 may be involved in hairy-cell leukaemia.

nucleases. Some of these fragments, when mixed with a culture of a suitable strain of mouse fibro-blasts, become incorporated into the genome of the cell by a process known as *transfection*. If the DNA contains an oncogene then the cell culture shows transformation and the cells develop into tumours if injected into a suitable mouse. Using this technique it has been shown that oncogenes derived from human tumours can transform a mouse cell into a malignant cell. The genes involved are mostly of the *ras* family.

The precise role of oncogenes in the genesis of tumours is not clear, for viral oncogenesis is probably not a simple one-step process, but rather a multi-step phenomenon, possibly involving several oncogenes. Various models for viral oncogenesis have been proposed. Thus *gene*

EARLY MALIGNANT LESIONS

In the human subject the question of early malignant change is of great importance, for it is at this stage that complete eradication of the disease is easiest. In recent years a number of interesting lesions involving epithelial surfaces has been recognized. In these areas there is atypical epithelial proliferation with the cells showing the microscopical changes usually associated with malignancy. They vary in size and shape, have large, darkly-stained nuclei, and show an increased amount of mitotic activity. The cells tend to lose their polarity, and lie haphazardly in relationship to one another. In stratified squamous epithelium there may be foci of abnormal keratinization within the area of cell proliferation, and this is called *malignant dyskeratosis.* Cellular pleomorphism, atypical mitotic activity, and other features of *dysplasia* may become so marked that the epithelium gives the impression of malignancy even though the cells have not broken through the basement membrane and invaded the underlying tissues. To this condition the names *carcinoma-in-situ* or *intra-epithelial carcinoma* are applied (Fig. 21.26).

Carcinoma-in-situ has been described in most epithelia, and it is encountered most typically in the stratified squamous covering epithelium of the skin, mouth, and cervix. Some clinical examples are worth noting:

Bowen's disease of the skin

This occurs in the middle-aged and elderly, and appears as discrete, red plaques which are sometimes mistaken for superficial basal-cell carcinoma, or resistant chronic dermatitis or psoriasis. Any area of the skin may be implicated. Invasive carcinoma may finally ensue, sometimes after many years.

Actinic, or solar, keratosis

All gradations of changes are seen varying from mild atypicality of the epithelial cells to *carcinoma-in-situ* and on occasions invasive squamous-cell carcinoma. This rarely metastasizes, but it is advisable to treat all solar keratoses.

Erythroplasia of Queyrat

This is a rare condition which usually involves the penis and appears as a red, velvety plaque of *in-situ* carcinoma. It can also occur in the oral mucosa.

Leucoplakia with dysplasia *

This appears as dead-white shiny plaques on a mucous membrane. The mouth and tongue are

---

* The term leucoplakia is often used clinically in its literal sense to describe any white plaque on a mucosal surface. This may include candidiasis, epithelial naevi, simple keratosis due to trauma, dysplasia, carcinoma, and lichen planus, as well as other less common conditions. To some pathologists the term implies a dysplastic condition that will in due course progress to invasive cancer. Hence the term should never be used without qualification.

commonly affected, and the vulva is another favourite site. Microscopically the epithelium shows all degrees of cellular atypicality ranging from mild dysplasia to *carcinoma-in-situ.* Invasive squamous-cell carcinoma may develop, especially in the vulva.

Dysplasia of the cervix uteri

Dysplasia of the cervical epithelium is common, and may vary from mild atypicality to *carcinoma-in-situ.* The study of this condition has been greatly aided by the technique of exfoliative cytology.

EXFOLIATIVE CYTOLOGY

When cancer involves a lining epithelium, some of the neoplastic cells are shed on to the surrounding surface. If the surface is internal these cells are trapped in the secretions of the part, and are ultimately discharged to the exterior. Bronchial carcinoma cells may be coughed up in the sputum, gastric carcinoma cells may be aspirated in the gastric juice, and cervical carcinoma cells may be shed into the vaginal secretions. In recent years much progress has been made in recognizing clumps of cancer cells in such secretions, and sometimes this allows the early diagnosis of malignant disease. The technique was pioneered by Papanicolaou, and has been applied especially to the study of cervical cancer ('Pap smear').

It is often assumed that the onset of malignant change is a sudden event, but exfoliative cytology has shown that in the case of the cervix uteri this is certainly not so. There is considerable evidence that the first change in the epithelium involves certain cellular abnormalities which have been called *dysplasia.* The nuclei are enlarged, show variation in size and shape, and are hyperchromatic (*dyskaryosis*). The epithelium is not as abnormal as has been described in *carcinoma-in-situ.* Nevertheless, a dysplastic epithelium is thought to progress to a state of *carcinoma-in-situ* and finally to one of true invasive squamous-cell carcinoma. The whole process is apparently drawn out over a long period, probably in the order of 10 years. Routine cytological examinations will detect early lesions, which although not cancerous themselves, are thought to progress to invasive, killing cancer. The same situation applies in the mouth. All suggestive or atypical lesions should be smeared to detect the presence of abnormal cells. If these are found, biopsy should be carried out. Dysplastic epithelium may be watched and treated, but if *carcinoma-in-situ* is present, excision of the whole lesion is indicated.

NATURE OF NEOPLASTIC CELLS

It is generally accepted that the essential basis for cancer is a change in the character of its cells. Apart from their property of unrestrained growth in their host, tumour cells exhibit uncontrolled growth in vitro, indicating that they have attained immortality because unlike normal cells they can be grown indefinitely if subcultured at suitable times into an appropriate medium (see HeLa cells, Chapter 1). Furthermore, their cultural characteristics are different from normal cells. They are termed *transformed cells* and show *loss of anchorage dependence*, meaning that they grow more easily in fluid or semi-fluid medium. They require lower concentrations of serum, and when cultured on a glass surface show decreased sensitivity to both *contact inhibition* and *density-dependent inhibition of growth* (p. 98).

There has been a great deal of research into morphology and behaviour of neoplastic cells in the hope that this would give some insight into the essential difference between them and normal cells. The pleomorphic and bizarre appearances of malignant cells have already been described. The loss of surface fibronectin, release of plasminogen activator and secretion of hyaluronidase may be correlated with the lack of cell adhesion and possibly the invasive tendency of malignant cells. Other changes include increased surface mobility of cell receptors and increase in number of receptors to growth factors.

In the early days of cancer research it was hoped that some *biochemical change* would provide a clue as to the nature of malignancy. The results have been disappointing, and no specific change has been identified that could be used in the detection of cancer, nor in the understanding of its essential nature. Some tumours produce enzymes or hormones that their parent cells were incapable of producing, e.g. chorioembryonic antigen or ectopic hormones. Sometimes the detection of these abnormal products is useful in clinical diagnosis or in the detection of metastases following removal of the primary growth. However, there is no specific change indicative of malignancy, and the changes described all appear to be differences from the normal quantitatively but not qualitatively.

Subjects with immunodeficiency have an increased incidence of certain neoplasms. Skin malignancies and lymphoma are especially common, but not the tumours that usually occur in otherwise normal people. It has been proposed that the immune reaction is important in maintaining tissue surveillance and that loss of this *immunological surveillance* plays an important part in holding tumours in check. Changes in the antigenicity of tumour cells have therefore been studied. Some tumours appear to lose tissue-specific antigens, perhaps because of their poor differentiation, and it has been proposed that they thereby escape the immunological surveillance activity of lymphocytes. Nevertheless, some tumours develop new antigens: the most important are tumour-specific transplantation antigens. These may be individual for the particular tumour (e.g. tumours produced by chemical carcinogens), or they may be shared by all tumours produced by the same virus in the case of experimental animal tumours. Possibly the heavy lymphocytic infiltrate around some tumours is indicative of a cell-mediated immune response, but it is not known whether it plays a part in limiting the growth or spread of these tumours. Attempts to cure cancer by stimulating the immune response, e.g. by administration of BCG, have been disappointing. Another approach has been to use interleukin-2 and lymphokine-activated killer (LAK) cells. Some tumour regression may occur, but the treatment needs further assessment. Whether the effect is a direct influence on the malignant cells or, more likely, mediated by some immune response is not known. One must conclude that a breakdown in immunological surveillance may play a part in the evolution of a tumour, but it does not seem to play a critical role and may indeed play only a minor part. For instance, immunoglobulin production against tumour antigens has been suggested as the basis for certain immune-complex manifestations—such as the nephrotic syndrome, arthralgia and skin eruptions—that are encountered in patients with malignant disease.

The study of oncogenes in relation to carcinogenesis has revealed that they may, by replacing or modifying normal cellular oncogenes, be involved in cell transformation. Changes in the karyotype of malignant cells are well established. A great variety of chromosomal abnormalities in regard to number (aneuploidy), translocations, ring chromosomes, etc., have been described. High-resolution banding techniques have revealed even more subtle chromosomal abnormalities in neoplastic disease. The best known variation is the Philadelphia chromosome found in most cases of chronic myelogenous leukaemia: here there is a balanced reciprocal translocation between the short arms of chromosomes 22 and 9. Likewise, in Burkitt's lymphoma, there is a translocation between chromosomes 8 and 14. In some instances several different patterns have been found in one disease, e.g. in acute non-lymphocytic leukaemia there are 17. In Burkitt's lymphoma three translocations can be found, all involving the long arm of chromosome 8 at the site of the *myc* oncogene.

Evidence using the X-linked marker glucose 6-phosphate dehydrogenase suggests that tumours are clonal (see the Lyon hypothesis). It is postulated that during the development of a tumour new clones evolve, each showing changes that enable it to replace its predecessors. Cancer is a disease that evolves slowly, and it is not surprising that in those sites that have been intensively studied a sequence of premalignant changes can be found that ultimately progress through varying grades of atypia (dysplasia) to malignant tumour formation; at first in-situ, and later invasive.

The fundamental change in the cancer cell still eludes us. Possibly there is some genetic change, either due to mutation or the introduction of new genetic material by viral infection. This has been called the *genetic theory*. In the alternative *epigenetic theory* the neoplastic cell is assumed to show aberrant differentiation due to some abnormality in the expression of its genetic material, the defect lying anywhere from the transcription of DNA in the nucleus, to the translation of the messenger RNA at the cytoplasmic level. Support for the theory that malignant tumours possess a normal genome but that differentiation is at fault is the observation that occasionally a neuroblastoma (a highly malignant tumour derived from primitive neuroblasts) differentiates into a benign ganglioneuroma containing mature neurons. Sometimes the tumour even shows spontaneous regression and self-cure. If this process could be encouraged it would provide a treatment that would be vastly superior to those at present in vogue.

Although the genetic and epigenetic theories seem far apart, it is likely that there is truth in both approaches. The difference between 'normal' DNA and 'abnormal' DNA is probably more apparent than real. Chemical carcinogens, viral infections and genetic rearrangement could all lead to the expression of a gene that hitherto had been repressed.

GENERAL READING

Ames B N 1983 Dietary carcinogenes and anticarcinogens. Science 221:1256

Bos J L 1989 *ras* oncogenes in human cancer: a review. Cancer Research 49:49

Broder J E 1979 Hormone production by bronchiogenic carcinoma. A review. Pathobiology Annual 9:205

Chan V T W, MacGee J O D 1987 Cellular oncogenes in neoplasia. Journal of Clinical Pathology 40:1055

Durant J R 1987 Immunotherapy of cancer. New England Journal of Medicine 316:939

Farber E 1981 Chemical carcinogenesis. New England Journal of Medicine 305:1379

Failkow P J 1974 The origin and development of human tumours studied with cell markers. New England Journal of Medicine 291:26

Hart I R, Fidler I J 1980 Cancer invasion and metastasis. Quarterly Review of Biology 55:121

Howley P M 1986 On human papillomavirus. New England Journal of Medicine 315:1089

Kaplan H S 1984 The search for retroviruses in human leukaemias and lymphomas. Progress in Medical Virology 30:139

Knudsor A G 1985 Hereditary cancer, oncogenes and antioncogenes. Cancer Research 45:1437

Krontiris T G 1983 The emerging genetics of human cancer. New England Journal of Medicine 309:404

Leading Article 1983 Reversal of cancer. Lancet 1:799

Leading Article 1986 Molecular mechanisms of tumour evolution. Lancet 1:780

Leading Article 1987 Gene amplification in malignancy. Lancet 1:839

Leading Article 1986 Growth factor and malignancy. Lancet 2:317

Leading Article 1980 Multistage carcinogenesis. Lancet 1:395

Lebovitz R M 1986 Oncogenes as mediators of cell growth and differentiation. Lab Invest 55:249

Melnick S, et al 1987 Rates and risks of diethylstilbestrol-related clear-cell adenocarcinoma of the vagina and cervix. New England Journal of Medicine 316:514

Mundy G R, et al 1984 The hypercalcaemia of cancer. New England Journal of Medicine 310:1718

Sukumar S 1989 *ras* Oncogenes in chemical carcinogenesis. In:Vogt V K (ed.), Current topics in microbiology and immunology; oncogenes and retroviruses. Springer-Verlag Berlin, p 93–114

Weber J, McClure M 1987 Oncogenes and cancer. British Medical Journal 294:1246

22. The effects of ionizing radiation

The ever-increasing use of radioactive substances in both industry and medicine has made the study of radiation damage of great practical importance. On the human body the effects of radiation vary from local tissue necrosis to genetic damage, cancer, and death. With such a perplexing array of effects it is little wonder that ionizing radiations are regarded with a fear and amazement that has been fully justified by the effects of dropping the atomic bombs on Hiroshima and Nagasaki, and the accident at Chernobyl in the USSR.

The basic action of ionizing radiations is to produce changes in the structure of the atoms through which they pass. Such changes in turn lead to secondary events in molecules, cells, tissues, and finally in the individual as a whole. These events will be examined in turn, but with so many steps it is not surprising that there are many gaps in our knowledge of the pathogenesis of radiation damage.

MECHANISMS OF RADIATION DAMAGE

PHYSICAL AND CHEMICAL CONSIDERATIONS

The energy of the absorbed radiation gives rise to the following changes:

1. Ions and free radicles are formed
2. There is excitation of molecules
3. Secondary electrons are generated, and these produce changes similar to (1) and (2) in adjacent areas.

The net effect is that molecules become more reactive and chemical changes ensue. Large biological molecules like DNA and proteins could be affected by two separate processes:

Direct action

Energy absorbed in the molecule itself may lead to chemical change, e.g. denaturation of a protein.

Indirect action

Alternatively chemical change may be induced in a large molecule as a result of the action of an adjacent ion or radicle, e.g. $OH^{\cdot}$ and $HO_2^{\cdot}$ radicles are formed from water. Powerful oxidizing agents, e.g. H_2O_2 are formed particularly when the radiation is performed in the presence of oxygen.

It is generally supposed that ionizing radiations produce a type of biochemical lesion, but if this is so its nature has so far eluded detection.

EFFECTS ON THE CELL

Although it would be desirable to explain the cellular damage in terms of the known physicochemical changes, it must be admitted that this is not yet possible. The effects of radiation on cells in culture may be summarized:

1. Immediate death of the cell occurs with very heavy dosage, i.e. 10 000r* or more. This effect occurs regardless of the stage of mitosis and is called *interphase death*. It is also seen in very sensitive cells, e.g. small lymphocytes with moderate dosage.

2. DNA synthesis is inhibited.

3. Mitosis is delayed, usually due to a prolongation of the G_2 phase (see p. 21).

4. DNA synthesis may occur unrelated to cell division so that giant-cell forms are produced. Giant fibroblasts are seen in irradiated skin.

5. When mitosis does occur in irradiated cells, abnormalities such as chromosome breaks may occur. At this stage the cell may die. Nevertheless, a cell may go through several mitotic cycles before death finally occurs.

6. The growth rate may be slowed down even in sublethally irradiated cells.

7. Fractionated doses of radiation do not produce a strictly cumulative effect. Hence there is an intracellular mechanism whereby radiation damage can be reversed or 'repaired'.

8. The sensitivity of cells to damage varies according to the stage in the cell cycle when the radiation is given. Maximum sensitivity occurs in most cell types during mitosis itself. Cells are relatively resistant during most of the G_1 phase, but radiosensitivity returns during the late G_1 and early synthetic (S) phases. They are most

---

*The letter r signifies roentgen, a commonly used measurement of radiation. One roentgen is that amount of radiation which under specified conditions produces in 1 ml of air at NTP, one electrostatic unit of electricity of either charge. A more recently introduced unit is the gray (gy); it equals 100 rads.

resistant during the late S and early G_2 phases.

Two main theories have been put forward to explain the cellular damage:

The target theory supposes that the injury is due to damage in some specific sensitive spot in the cell. Attractive as it may be to visualize a chromosome or an organelle as a target, there is in fact very little to support this theory.

The poison theory proposes that the ionization leads to the production of poisonous substances, usually powerful oxidizing agents, which then cause the damage. There is considerable evidence that oxidizing substances are formed in irradiated tissue. Thus chemicals with a reducing action (e.g. cysteine) will give some degree of protection against ionizing radiation. Furthermore, if cells are irradiated in the absence of oxygen, they are 2 to 3 times more resistant. This is probably because free oxygen is necessary for the production of oxidizing substances by ionizing radiation. This observation is of some importance in clinical radiotherapy, because many areas of a tumour are relatively hypoxic and might conceivably be less sensitive to damage during irradiation therapy.

EFFECTS ON THE INTACT ANIMAL

This most important aspect of radiobiology is also the most difficult. A feature which is outstanding is the remarkable *delay* in the appearance of radiation lesions. The actual damage caused by radiation must be almost instantaneous, and yet the effect may not be apparent for days, months, or even years. Experiments with amphibians help to explain this phenomenon. Frogs can be given a dose of radiation which will kill them within 6 weeks. If the irradiated animals are kept at 5°C, they remain alive for several months, but on being warmed up die within 6 weeks, like the control animals kept at normal temperature. The experiment indicates that radiation damage manifests itself only when cells are active. This lends strong support to the concept that a biochemical lesion is produced. Such a lesion is not in itself harmful, but produces effects when cellular activity commences. This goes some way in explaining two of the phenomena of radiation damage:

Relative sensitivity of cells

In the human the germinal cells of the ovary are the most sensitive. Then in sequence follow the seminiferous epithelium of the testis, lymphocytes, the erythropoietic and myeloid marrow cells, and the intestinal epithelium. Least sensitive are nerve cells and muscle cells. This order to some extent parallels the rate of cell division seen in the various tissues; thus neurons never divide, while epithelial tissue, especially that of the intestine, shows constant mitotic activity.

The chronic nature of radiation lesions

When tissue is irradiated, several phases of damage occur. This is probably because different tissues have different rates of division and metabolic activity, and therefore exhibit damage at different times. Hence an irradiated area shows changes which persist for many weeks or even months and have the characteristics of chronic inflammation, even after a single exposure.

When considering the action of radiation on any tissue, two main effects must be borne in mind.

The *primary effect* of radiation on the tissue concerned.

The *secondary effect*, which is due to damage to adjacent tissues. The most important example of this is the damage to vessels which, by causing thrombosis or endarteritis obliterans, leads to ischaemia. Some authorities attribute much of the beneficial effects of radiotherapy in cancer to this mechanism.

THE EFFECT OF IRRADIATION ON INDIVIDUAL TISSUES

SKIN

Following a single exposure to ionizing radiation, redness (erythema) appears after about 10 days, and the skin shows all the features of acute inflammation. Pigmentation is increased, giving the skin a red dusky colour. With heavy dosage necrosis occurs, and ulceration results. Healing is often very slow, and ulceration may recur; even when healed the scar may break down after trivial injury so that chronic ulceration with much surrounding fibrosis is frequent. With lower dosage the blood vessels show endarteritis obliterans. The hair follicles and accessory glands are much more sensitive to radiation than is the less active surface epithelium. With a dosage of above 700 r these structures undergo necrosis, and do not regenerate. The delaying effect on wound healing is described in Chapter 8. Chronic radiodermatitis is a late effect of radiation. There is atrophy, irregular pigmentation, and telangiectasia—a triad that constitutes poikiloderma.

GONADS

The ovary and testis are particularly susceptible, and with a dosage of over 500 r the germinal cells are destroyed and permanent sterility results.

LUNGS

Irradiation of the lungs produces acute alveolar damage (acute interstitial pneumonitis) which, if marked, progresses to interstitial fibrosis. This is sometimes seen as a complication of radiotherapy for lung, breast, and oesophageal cancers.

BONE

Irradiation of bone produces inflammatory changes which may persist for years, and are punctuated by episodes of painful radionecrosis. If the jaw is involved, radionecrosis is often precipitated by the extraction of teeth and complicated by infection. Doses of over 1000 r inhibit growth at the epiphysis, an effect of importance in children. Thus the coincidental irradiation of the mandibular condyle during the ill-advised treatment of an angiomatous hamartoma may lead to cessation of growth with consequent hypoplasia of the mandible.

TOTAL BODY IRRADIATION

The effects of total body irradiation depend on the dosage, and have been studied in people involved in atomic explosions. It is convenient to describe the effects of total body irradiation under two headings—those occurring during the first two months (immediate), and those occurring later.

IMMEDIATE EFFECTS

Although no hard-and-fast rules can be given, three groups of cases may be recognized:

Very heavy dosage (over 5000 r single exposure) produces severe effects due apparently to direct damage to the brain. Death occurs within a day or two following shock, convulsions, and coma.

Moderate dosage, 800–5000 r single exposure. Loss of appetite, nausea, and vomiting develop soon after irradiation, the reasons for which are not known. The symptoms usually abate, only to recur some 2–3 days later with intractable severity. This latter episode of vomiting is accompanied by severe diarrhoea due to necrosis of the intestinal epithelium. This is called the *gastrointestinal syndrome*, and usually results in death from dehydration and shock.

Low dosage, under 800 r single exposure. Initial nausea and vomiting are less severe, and the subject may then appear to make a complete recovery. Two or three weeks later the results of bone-marrow aplasia become apparent. The serious effects of irradiation during the *haematological phase* are due to damage to the haematopoietic tissues.

HAEMATOLOGICAL EFFECTS

Lymphocytes. Lymphopenia is the earliest blood change of total body irradiation, and is most marked after a day or two.

Granulocytes. The total granulocyte count falls after about a week, and may reach very low levels by the second to sixth weeks. This predisposes to infection, e.g. of the mouth and lungs.

Platelets. After a few days the number of platelets drops dramatically, and is very low by 4 weeks. This leads to a haemorrhagic tendency which may manifest itself either as trivial petechial haemorrhages into the skin or other organs, or as severe, possibly fatal, intestinal or pulmonary bleeding.

Red cells. Because the primitive, or erythroblastic, cells are highly radiosensitive and the mature red cells are resistant, the effect of bone-marrow aplasia on the peripheral count is delayed. The anaemia is of gradual onset and maximal at 6–8 weeks.

LATE EFFECTS

Those exposed to a sublethal dose may show the following after-effects:

The carcinogenic effect

It has been realized since the beginning of the century that tumours may develop after the application of ionizing radiation. The first case, a carcinoma of the skin, was reported in 1902, and subsequently *squamous-cell cancers of the skin* of the hands have been frequently seen in X-ray workers. This also occurred in dental surgeons who held films in position in the mouth. It is important for all those who use X-rays to avoid unnecessary exposure to radiation.

Another danger of exposure to ionizing radiation is the development of *leukaemia*. A high incidence of this disease has been recorded in the survivors of the Nagasaki and Hiroshima atomic explosions and in patients with ankylosing spondylitis treated with radiotherapy. However, the hazard of modern diagnostic radiology is slight.

Osteosarcoma has been reported to follow local irradiation years after the treatment of benign or inflammatory bone lesions. The tumour has also followed the injection or ingestion of radioactive substances, such as radium and mesothorium, which are stored in the bones.

Genetic effects

The ability of ionizing radiation to increase the rate of mutation is well established in micro organisms, plants, and animals. In somatic cells this effect is probably not important, but in the germ cells it is of potential significance, since the new factor is handed down to subsequent generations. It may have a profoundly deleterious effect, since most mutations are harmful.

Protective lead covering should always be used in dental radiography.

RADIOTHERAPY

The destructive effects of ionizing radiation on living cells, particularly those in an active state, have led to their widespread use in the treatment of malignant disease. Nowadays radiotherapy plays an important part in the curative treatment of some primary cancers, as well as in the palliation of those which have already metastasized, and are beyond the scope of surgical excision.

FACTORS INFLUENCING RESPONSE

Tumours differ widely in their reaction to radiotherapy, and it is only after treatment has been commenced that the response can be assessed. However, some guide to the probable local results of treatment may be given by consideration of the following factors:

Tissue of origin

The relative sensitivities of normal tissues are often reflected in the radiosensitivities of the tumours derived from them. Thus lymphomata, like the parent lymphoreticular cells, are very radiosensitive. Fibrosarcoma, however, like the fibroblasts from which it is derived, is radioresistant.

Degree of differentiation and mitotic activity

It is generally taught that within any tumour group the most poorly differentiated tumours are also the most radiosensitive. As a generalization this is true, but nevertheless it is found that the histological appearances of an individual tumour are no sure guide to the results obtained in practice. It is found, for instance, that well-differentiated squamous-cell carcinomata of the skin and tongue frequently respond very well.

The tumour bed

The nature of the stroma supporting a tumour is probably important. If it is avascular as the result of previous irradiation, the tumour is more resistant. This may well be attributable to hypoxia. Some authorities maintain that connective tissues have a restraining effect on the growth of the tumour. If excessive irradiation is given, the results are said to be much worse than if a modest dose is given, because under these circumstances the tumour bed itself is destroyed. It seems quite certain that all tumour cells are not destroyed by radiotherapy, and that the cure of the patient is related to some other destructive mechanism on the growth of the tumour.

Nature of the individual tumour

Certain tumours respond extremely well, for example most basal-cell and squamous-cell carcinomata of the skin. On the other hand, squamous-cell carcinoma of the lung generally responds poorly. It is evident that tumours of similar histological appearance in different organs may react very differently to irradiation. The reason for this is not known.

CURE RATE

The *cure rate* to be expected from radiotherapy must, as with surgical treatment, be considered in relation to the general properties of the tumour. Many malignant conditions, for example lymphoma, cannot be considered as local diseases, and although a tumour mass may respond remarkably well to treatment, the disease progresses sooner or later to its inevitable end. Oat-cell carcinoma of the lung is a similar example.

Radiotherapy is often effective as a palliative treatment. It can reduce the size of a tumour mass and produce relief of symptoms. This is well seen in mediastinal tumours producing obstruction to the great vessels. Radiotherapy may also control haemorrhage from a bleeding tumour, and help to clear up a fungating carcinoma of the breast. Pain from bone metastases may be alleviated. Slowly-growing tumours, like cancer of the breast and Hodgkin's disease, can sometimes be held in check for long periods, and the patient given several years of useful life. It may well be that radiotherapy and surgery are both forms of palliation which allow the body to retard the growth of the tumour. Depending on whether the malignant cells stay dormant for a short or long period, one may speak of a 5-year cure, 10-year cure, etc. There is increasing evidence, however, that on some occasions a thorough eradication of malignant cells is effected by the combined action of therapeutic measures, whether surgical excision, ionizing radiation, or cytotoxic drugs, on the one hand, and the natural defences of the body on the other. In these cases the patient's life-span is no shorter than that of a healthy control and we may speak with growing confidence of a complete cure.

GENERAL READING

Finch S C 1979 The study of atomic bomb survivors. American Journal of Medicine 66:899

Pizzarello D J, Witcofski R L (eds) 1982 Medical radiation biology, 2nd edn. Lea & Febiger, Philadelphia

23. Temperature regulation: fever and hypothermia

THE NORMAL BODY TEMPERATURE
TEMPERATURE REGULATION
FEVER
HYPOTHERMIA

One of the most important developments in the higher animals is the evolution of mechanisms whereby a constant environment is maintained for its constituent cells. This fixity of the internal environment has been well recognized since the time of Claude Bernard. Temperature regulation is an important aspect of homeostasis, which in the case of the human being and other warm-blooded mammals has attained a high degree of efficiency. Cellular activity, involving as it does numerous chemical reactions largely dependent upon enzymatic activity, is very susceptible to changes in temperature. On the other hand, some of the energy released during cell metabolism is emitted as heat. Indeed, the temperature of highly active organs, like the brain and heart, would rise were it not for the cooling effect of the blood stream which carries away the excess heat, and distributes it to those areas where it can be dissipated to the atmosphere, viz. the skin and the mucosa of the upper respiratory tract.

It is probable that the development of a reliable temperature-regulating mechanism has contributed considerably to the biological supremacy of the warm-blooded group of animals.

THE NORMAL BODY TEMPERATURE

Methods of measuring. Body temperature is commonly measured with the thermometer placed under the tongue. It is sometimes necessary to measure the rectal temperature, which is about 0.3°C (1°F) higher than the arterial temperature but is less responsive to changes in the arterial temperature. Thus, if warm saline is infused into a vein, the rise in blood temperature is reflected in an elevation of the sublingual temperature but not that of the rectum. The sublingual temperature taken with the lips closed is therefore held to be the most reliable guide to the arterial temperature.

Normal variation. The normal temperature taken in this way is 36.8°C (98.4°F), with a range of 36.1–37.4°C (97.0–99.3°F). The maximum temperature is generally attained at about 18.00 h, while it is at its lowest at about 03.00 h. In women there is an elevation of the temperature during the middle of the menstrual cycle; its onset is thought to herald ovulation and is probably caused by the action of certain steroid hormones.

TEMPERATURE REGULATION

The constancy of the body's temperature is maintained by balancing the amount of heat gained with that lost.

Sources of heat. The major source of heat is from the body's metabolic activity. Heat production under fasting conditions with the individual at complete mental and physical rest is called the *basal metabolic rate* (BMR). This ranges from 1400 to 1800 kcal per day. Under active conditions additional heat is produced by *exercise* and the *ingestion of food*, especially protein. Fever itself affects the BMR, a rise of 1°C in body temperature increasing it by about 10 %.

Sources of heat loss. Heat is lost from the blood as it perfuses the skin—evaporation of sweat, conduction, and convection all play a part. Since

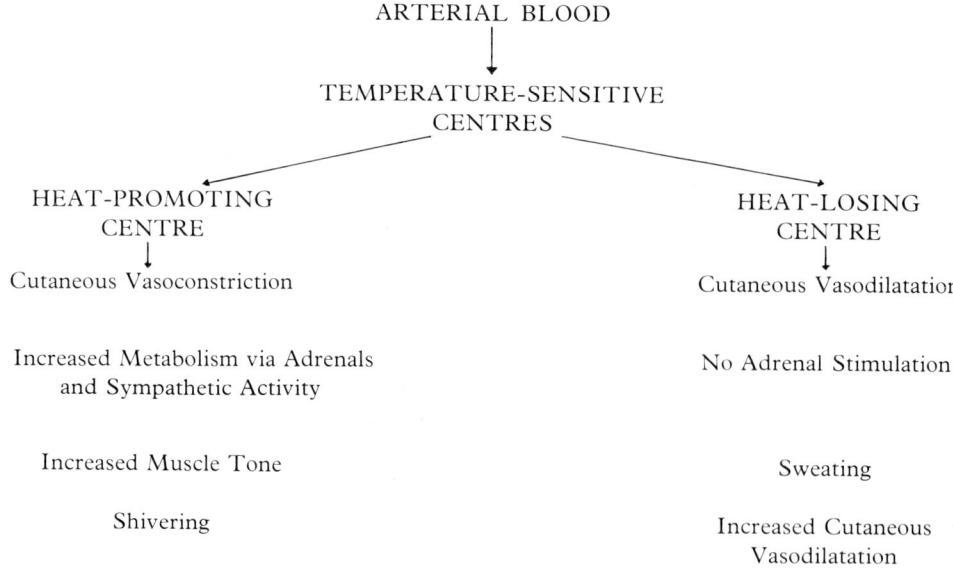

Fig. 23.1   Diagram to illustrate the principal heat-regulating mechanisms

the blood supply to the skin is regulated by the autonomic nervous system, the latter plays a dominant role in the maintenance of a constant body temperature. Some heat is also lost from the respiratory tract, and in animals this can be increased by panting.

Mechanisms are present for both increasing and decreasing the body's temperature. These come into play in response to impulses from the temperature-sensitive receptors. These receptors are situated both centrally within the hypothalmus and peripherally, mainly in the skin. A change of as little as 0.2°C can activate the compensatory mechanisms.

The central temperature receptor. There is a group of cells in the pre-optic area of the hypothalamus that are sensitive to the temperature of the arterial blood reaching them. With fluctuations of blood temperature, impulses pass to other parts of the hypothalamus. There are two main areas: (1) an anterior *heat-losing centre*, which when stimulated leads to changes in the remainder of the body, causing increased heat loss, and (2) a posterior *heat-promoting centre*, which when stimulated leads to increased heat conservation and heat production (Fig. 23.1).

Peripheral temperature receptors. These are situated mainly in the skin and are of greatest

importance when the body's temperature falls. Impulses then pass to the posterior centre in the hypothalamus and lead to conservation of heat.

Mechanism for decreasing body temperature

When the body's temperature tends to rise, there is a withdrawal of sympathetic vasoconstriction activity, the skin becomes warm, and heat is lost. The subject feels hot and may remove clothing, retire to the shade, or take other appropriate action. If this regulating mechanism does not suffice, the heat-losing centre initiates *sweating*. Evaporation of this fluid requires heat, but further heat is lost as a result of cutaneous vasodilatation induced by the release of bradykinin that results from sweating.

Mechanism for increasing body temperature

The heat-promoting centre acts mainly through the autonomic nervous system. Cutaneous vasoconstriction reduces the amount of heat lost from the skin, and blood diverted to the internal organs is insulated from the exterior by the subcutaneous fat. Furthermore, as the skin becomes cooler, the subject feels cold and may take appropriate voluntary action such as putting on extra clothing.

An important effect of increased sympathetic activity is generalized *increase in muscle tone*. This alone can increase heat production by 50 per cent: the mechanism appears to be related to a partial uncoupling of oxidative phosphorylation. The increased sympathetic outflow causes an increased output of adrenaline and nor-adrenaline from the adrenal glands. Together with the increased sympathetic tone, these hormones increase the metabolic rate of cells by a mechanism that is not well understood. The increase in muscle tone may reach a point at which stretch reflexes are elicited and *shivering* commences. This muscular activity greatly increases heat production.

FEVER

Fever, also called *pyrexia*, may be defined as an elevation of the body's temperature consequent upon a disturbance of the regulating mechanism. When the temperature reaches or exceeds 40.5°C (104°F) the condition is called *hyperpyrexia*. Fever occurs under the conditions given below.

Causes of fever

Heat pyrexia. A rise in body temperature normally occurs during severe exercise when the heat-eliminating mechanisms cannot keep pace with the excessive heat production in the muscles. When the environment is hot and humid, even mild exercise may cause a marked rise in body temperature. This in turn increases the metabolic rate. Sometimes the heat-regulating mechanism breaks down under these circumstances, and the temperature rises to 41°C (106°F) or more. This is 'heatstroke', or 'sunstroke', and unless treated promptly the temperature may continue to rise, reaching 43°C (109°F) or more, a level at which the patient becomes comatose, and permanent brain damage ensues. Death is not uncommon.

Infection. Fever is a frequent accompaniment of infection by viruses, bacteria, and larger parasites. The pattern of the pyrexia is often characteristic of particular diseases, e.g. the sudden onset in influenza and the step-ladder rise in typhoid fever (Fig. 7.1).

Infarction. Fever is often seen in patients with myocardial infarction.

Tumours. Some tumours are particularly liable to produce pyrexia, e.g. Ewing's tumour of bone, renal-cell carcinoma, and Hodgkin's disease.

Haemorrhage. This may be followed by fever, especially when it occurs into the gastrointestinal tract or the pleural or peritoneal cavities.

Brain damage. Cerebral haemorrhage and other intracranial lesions may disturb the central regulating mechanism.

Following injury. Fever occurs during the catabolic phase of convalescence.

Fulminating or malignant hyperthermia. Although rare, this is one of the most common causes of anaesthetic-induced deaths. Most of the reported cases have followed the administration of halothane or suxamethonium. The pyrexia develops extremely rapidly, and unless vigorous cooling is employed, the temperature rises to very high levels, e.g. 43 to 44°C, and death occurs from cardiac arrest. In most cases the skeletal muscles develop increased tone, and this is believed to be the source of the increased heat production. A predisposition to develop malignant hyperpyrexia is inherited in some families, and can be detected by finding an increased blood level of creatine phosphokinase (CPK).

Miscellaneous conditions. Fever is a prominent feature of many other conditions. Acute rheumatic fever, serum sickness, and gout may be cited as examples. Release of interleukin-1 and other pyrogens from cells in the inflammatory exudate of the lesions is the presumed pathogenesis.

Clinical features

Of all the causes of pyrexia, infection is by far the most important. The development of fever in an acute illness like lobar pneumonia or malaria has been the object of most study. Three stages are described:

The cold stage. At the onset of illness there is a feeling of intense cold, peripheral vasoconstriction is manifested by pallor, and the patient starts to shiver. Chattering of the teeth completes this picture of the familiar *rigor*. The temperature rises, as does the blood pressure. There is usually a rise in pulse rate of 18 beats/min for each 1°C rise of temperature (10 per 1°F).

The hot stage. As the temperature approaches its peak, the peripheral vasoconstriction relaxes and the patient feels dry and warm. Heat loss now balances heat gain, and the temperature remains constant. The 'thermostat' of the heat-regulating mechanism is still in control, but is geared to maintain the temperature at a level higher than normal. The extra heat produced is due to the raised metabolic rate caused by the fever. Should hyperpyrexia occur, this regulation may fail. During this phase the blood pressure falls.

The sweating phase. The temperature begins to fall, and the patient soon experiences a sensation of intense heat. Bedclothes are thrown off, sweating becomes profuse, and the temperature returns to normal. This is described as termination by *crisis*. If the pyrexia subsides slowly, as in typhoid fever, the termination is described as *lysis*.

The pathogenesis of fever

The intravenous injection of Gram-negative coliform organisms, which contain a lipopolysaccharide substance called bacterial pyrogen, causes a sharp rise in body temperature. The pyrogen does not act directly but causes white cells, particularly macrophages, to release endogenous pyrogens. The most important is *interleukin-1* which acts on muscle to increase protein catabolism and on the central heat-regulating centre in the hypothalamus to cause an increase in body temperature. The action is not direct. Interleukin-1 acts by stimulating the formation of prostaglandin E_2. It is understandable that cycloxygenase inhibitors, such as aspirin and indomethacin, act as antipyretic drugs by blocking prostaglandin formation from arachidonic acid. Another cytokine, *cachexin* (also known as tumour necrosis factor-alpha, TNF-α) also acts as an endogenous pyrogen, but its major action is to increase lipolysis in the adipose tissues.

White cells also release endogenous pyrogens during phagocytosis; polymorphs release some pyrogen but the major source is the macrophages and other cells of the MPS. It is therefore not surprising that fever is a feature of non-infective inflammatory conditions, for example acute gout and lupus erythematosus.

The bacterial pyrogens are heat-stable and are of importance because they can produce febrile reactions if present in the fluids used in intravenous therapy, which, though sterile, may still cause a sharp rigor on intravenous injection. Fluids used for injection purposes must be carefully prepared by distillation to insure the exclusion of all bacterial products. Such pyrogen-free fluids must always be used. Other agents that cause a rise in temperature are certain steroid hormones, e.g. aetiocholanolone. It is believed that the release of progesterone is responsible for the temperature rise that occurs in women at the time of ovulation. Disturbances of the nervous system can also affect the body's temperature. Emotions can raise it, and periodic fever, a cyclical fever of unknown origin, has been linked to cerebral dysfunction, perhaps with excessive aetiocholanolone formation.

The heat-regulating mechanism is in abeyance during deep anaesthesia and the body therefore becomes poikilothermic (like the body of an amphibian) and equates with the temperature of the surrounding atmosphere. The patient must therefore be protected against changes in temperature, either hypothermia or hyperpyrexia.

Although recent work has shed some light on the mystery of fever, much has yet to be learned. It would be satisfying to believe that a rise in temperature in infection is a beneficial reaction designed to aid the body's defences. In viral infections this may be so, because fever stimulates the production of interferon. However, with most infections there is little evidence that fever is beneficial. For the present we must regard the maintenance of normal temperature as an important homeostatic mechanism for the proper functioning of the body. Any departure from the normal is usually deleterious to well-being and can, if marked, be fatal.

HYPOTHERMIA

Hypothermia may be defined as a body temperature below 35°C. It is an important cause of death in cold climates, and can easily be overlooked both in infancy and the elderly unless clinical thermometers that register as low as 24°C (75°F) are used when the possibility of hypothermia exists. Hypothermia has been utilized as an adjunct to anaesthesia.

Hypothermia in infants

Newborn infants are particularly susceptible to cold, because of the relatively high ratio of surface area to body mass, the paucity of subcutaneous fat, and the low production of heat by physical means because of the inability to exercise or shiver. Furthermore, the thermoregulatory mechanism is relatively inefficient at birth and remains so for several hours.

During the first few weeks of life, infants need constant warmth, especially when ill. In cold countries open windows, lukewarm baths, and power cuts can precipitate hypothermia.

The early signs of cold injury are lethargy and difficulty in feeding. Indeed, the child has a still, serene appearance and the cheeks, nose, and extremities have a flush that deludes the onlooker into believing all is well. The cry is like a whimper, and the body feels cold. Later, bradycardia and oedema of the eyelids and extemities occur. Pulmonary haemorrhages and hardening of the subcutaneous fat occur in the worst cases.

Hypothermia in adults

Hypothermia can occur in adults in a number of circumstances. Immersion hypothermia is one of the lethal factors in shipwreck. Hypothermia is an important complication of myxoedema and hypopituitarism, and it also occurs in patients with widespread eczema and generalized erythroderma. In widespread skin disease, the passive diffusion of water through the epidermis is greatly increased, and heat is lost both by evaporation and convection.

Spontaneous hypothermia is a well-recognized occurrence in old people—usually women—who live alone in poorly heated rooms and are poorly clothed. Undernutrition is an additional factor for persons who are in both calorie- and protein-deficient states, the basal metabolic rate is decreased. Hypothermia in the aged is sometimes a complication of senile dementia, or the effects of depressant drugs like alcohol and chlorpromazine that have dulled the mind. There is sometimes a severe precipitating infection such as pneumonia.

The patient with hypothermia looks ill. There is a corpse-like chill of the body, and the rectal temperature can be as low as 21°C (70°F). The skin is pale, and the subcutaneous tissue is pliant and doughy. The patient remains still; muscles are rigid, and shivering is absent. The tendon reflexes are sluggish, and there is bradycardia, sometimes with atrial fibrillation. Since peripheral oedema and puffiness of the eyelids are common, myxoedema may be simulated. Oliguria (diminished urine output) is common, respiration is depressed, and death often occurs from cardiac arrest.

Induced hypothermia

Hibernation in a state of hypothermia has been evolved by some animals as an adjunct to survival in winter. From experimental work carried out on small animals, it has been found that they can be cooled below 0°C (32°F) if they are made first to ingest propylene glycol. Mice can be kept in suspended animation for about 1h and then reanimated by artificial respiration and microwave diathermy. Larger animals do not tolerate this treatment so well and usually die within a few days. A lesser degree of hypothermia has been used as an adjunct to cardiac surgery. If the body's temperature is lowered, cardiac arrest can be tolerated for about 1 h. Extracorporeal circulations are now so efficient that hypothermia is less commonly used or is merely used as an adjunct to this procedure.

Local hypothermia.

Much damage can be inflicted on tissues if they are subjected to extreme cold. The condition arises accidentally in frost bite when exposed parts—hands, feet, nose and ears—are affected. Capillary damage and occlusion add to the tissue damage produced directly by the cold. When the affected area is warmed the necrotic tissue leads to a surrounding inflammatory response. In cryotherapy tissue is deliberately damaged by freezing.

Solid carbon dioxide or more usually liquid nitrogen are used. The method is useful for the destruction of superficial skin tumours, e.g. warts, seborrhoeic keratoses and superficial basal cell carcinomata. With suitable refrigerated probes deeper lesions can be treated.

GENERAL READING

Guyton A C 1981 Textbook of medical physiology, 6th edn. Saunders, Philadelphia, see in particular ch 72

Nelson T E, Flewellen E H 1983 The malignant hyperthermia syndrome. New England Journal of Medicine 309:416

Dinerello C A, Wolff S M 1978 Pathogenesis of fever in man. New England Journal of Medicine 298:607

Beisel W R 1983 Mediators of fever and muscle proteolysis. New England Journal of Medicine 308:586

24. Amyloidosis (beta fibrillosis)

Amyloid tissue consists of a group of fibrillar proteins having in common a β-pleated structure. They are composed of polypeptide chains derived by digestion of precursor protein. Usually this is either the λ light chains of immunoglobulin, serum amyloid A (SAA, an acute phase reactant) or transthyretin. The amyloid is insoluble and found deposited at various sites. When the deposits are widespread the condition is called generalized *amyloidosis*; the precursor proteins are in the blood, broken down by proteolytic enzymes, and the polypeptide chains so formed condense to produce amyloid fibrils which are deposited at various sites. In the localized type of amyloidosis, amyloid is usually formed from local proteins and synthesis occurs locally.

In H.&E. sections amyloid appears as a hyaline, eosinophilic, structureless extracellular material. Methyl violet and congo red are empirical stains by which it may be recognized:

Methyl violet. This is a metachromatic histological stain; the amyloid changes the methyl violet from a violet to a rose-pink colour.

Congo red. This dye is soluble in amyloid, and stains it an orange colour; when the stained slide is viewed in a polarizing microscope a characteristic green birefringence is imparted. Apart from electron microscopy, this is the most reliable method of identifying amyloid, because it is dependent on characteristic β-pleated structure of amyloid.

Immunohistological stains. Immunofluorescence and immunoperoxidase methods using anti-AA (anti-amyloid-A) and anti-AL can be used to distinguish between the two common types of amyloid (see later).

TYPES OF AMYLOIDOSIS

Currently amyloidosis is classified on the basis of its composition and clinical features. Four main types are recognized.

Immunocyte-derived systemic amyloidosis (AL amyloidosis)
Reactive systemic amyloidosis (AA amyloidosis)
Heredofamilial amyloidosis
Localized amyloidosis.

IMMUNOCYTE-DERIVED SYSTEMIC AMYLOIDOSIS

This type may occur as a primary disease, or in association with multiple myelomatosis. The amyloid is derived from the light chains of immunoglobulin.

Primary system amyloidosis

Primary amyloidosis is a disease of the elderly, the patients generally die from renal failure within a year of diagnosis. Weakness, loss of weight, ankle oedema, dyspnoea, paraesthesiae and purpura are common manifestations. Organs involved include the myocardium, tongue, oesophagus, skin and nerves.

Amyloidosis associated with multiple myelomatosis

In multiple myelomatosis there is clonal expansion of immunocytes producing light chains, and in about 10% of cases generalized amyloidosis develops, the amyloid being derived from the light chains. An excess of these light chains is usually present in the blood and is found in the urine as 'Bence–Jones protein'. This type of amyloidosis closely resembles primary systemic amyloidosis described above. Indeed, it is probable that the primary type is associated with an early manifestation of a B-cell dyscrasia. However, the prognosis of primary amyloidosis is so poor that there is insufficient time for the disease to progress to obvious malignancy.

REACTIVE SYSTEMIC AMYLOIDOSIS (SECONDARY AMYLOIDOSIS)

This is the commonest type of generalized amyloid disease. It is associated with certain chronic diseases, e.g. chronic osteomyelitis, empyema, tertiary syphilis and chronic pulmonary tuberculosis. These conditions are now uncommon and it is most often encountered in lepromatous leprosy, rheumatoid arthritis, Crohn's disease, ankylosing spondylitis, chronic decubitus ulceration and in malignant disease, particularly Hodgkin's disease.

The amyloid deposits in reactive systemic amyloidosis are widely distributed and affect particularly the kidneys, liver, spleen, lymph nodes and intestine. The fibrils that make up the bulk of the deposits in this type of amyloidosis consists of amyloid A (AA), a protein of molecular weight 8000–14 000 daltons. This has an amino-acid sequence in common with part of a serum protein (serum amyloid-A or SAA), which has a molecular weight of about 180 000 daltons. The amyloid is thought to be derived from it by proteolytic cleavage—perhaps by the activity of macrophages or polymorph proteinases. SAA is an apolipoprotein of high density lipoprotein and like C-reactive protein is greatly elevated in the acute phase reaction.

The SAA levels in the blood are greatly elevated in those chronic conditions associated with a long lasting acute phase reaction in which amyloidosis is common (e.g. rheumatoid arthritis and Crohn's disease), but not in those in which amyloidosis is unusual (e.g. chronic ulcerative colitis and systemic lupus erythematosus).

HEREDOFAMILIAL AMYLOIDOSIS

Many hereditary syndromes associated with deposits of amyloid have been described but they are uncommon. A single organ, e.g. the cornea or heart, may be affected, or the amyloid may be deposited in the blood-vessel walls of many tissues. Involvement of the nerves is common in some types. The type of amyloid varies from one syndrome to another. It may be of AA type or derived from transthyretin of the blood. In most cases the nature of the amyloid is unknown.

LOCALIZED AMYLOID DEPOSITS

Deposits of amyloid may occur in the form of localized masses. These cases are uncommon and deposits are generally found in the bladder, tongue, larynx, or bronchi. Amyloid may be found in the stroma of a tumour, e.g. basal-cell carcinoma of the skin and calcifying epithelial odontogenic tumour. Extensive deposition of amyloid in the stroma of medullary carcinoma of the thyroid is characteristic. It is derived from calcitonin produced by this tumour.

Amyloid, derived from insulin or its prohormone, is common in the islets of Langerhans in association with diabetes mellitus in advancing age, and it is also found in the stroma of some islet cell tumours.

Senile amyloidosis

Deposits of amyloid are common in the aged and are found in the heart. They form senile plaques in the brain and here the precursor protein is pre-albumin.

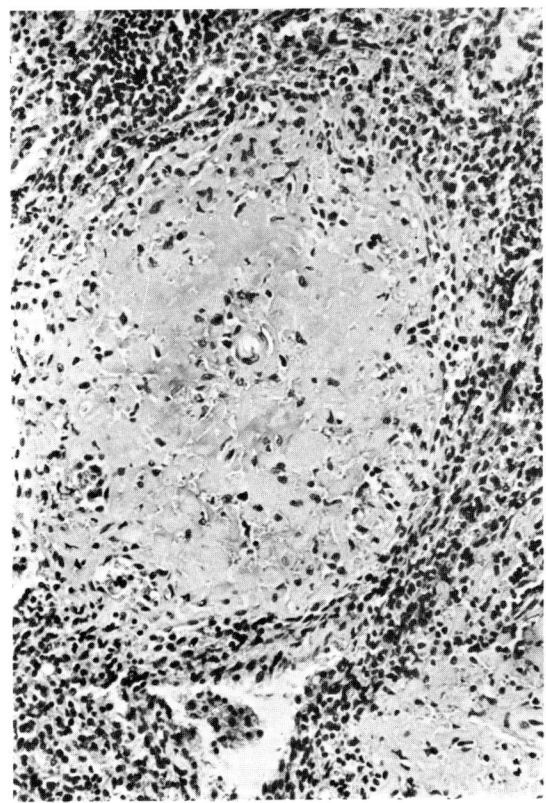

Fig. 24.1   Amyloidosis of spleen. The malpighian body is grossly enlarged, and is replaced by a mass of acellular amyloid. × 160.

ORGAN INVOLVEMENT IN AMYLOIDOSIS

Spleen. Amyloid is laid down in the walls of the malpighian arterioles, and the cut surface therefore presents a characteristic appearance of *sago spleen* with numerous scattered firm translucent nodules (Fig. 24.1). A diffuse type of amyloid spleen is also recognized, in which the amyloid is laid down in the walls of the sinuses.

Liver. The organ is enlarged, heavy, pale, and firm. The amyloid is laid down in the walls of the sinuses between the endothelium and the liver cells (Fig. 24.2).

Kidney. The organ is large and pale. The amyloid appears in the glomeruli, which may eventually be converted into hyaline masses. Proteinuria is severe, and the nephrotic syndrome follows.

Other sites. Adrenals, lymph nodes, lung, and gut may all be affected. Deposits in the intestine may cause diarrhoea, and biopsy of the rectum is sometimes used as a diagnostic procedure. Amyloid is also laid down in the gingiva, and again biopsy may be employed to facilitate diagnosis.

EFFECTS OF AMYLOID

The deposition of amyloid generally excites no inflammatory reaction, but there is atrophy of the parenchyma. In an organ with an abundant reserve, like the liver, this is of little functional significance, but in other situations, for example nerves and kidneys, the effects may be severe. Renal involvement leads to the nephrotic syndrome and later renal failure; this is common terminal manifestation of amyloidosis. An affected organ becomes rigid and this is important if it has a mechanical function to perform, e.g. the heart and tongue. Affected vessels tend to bleed

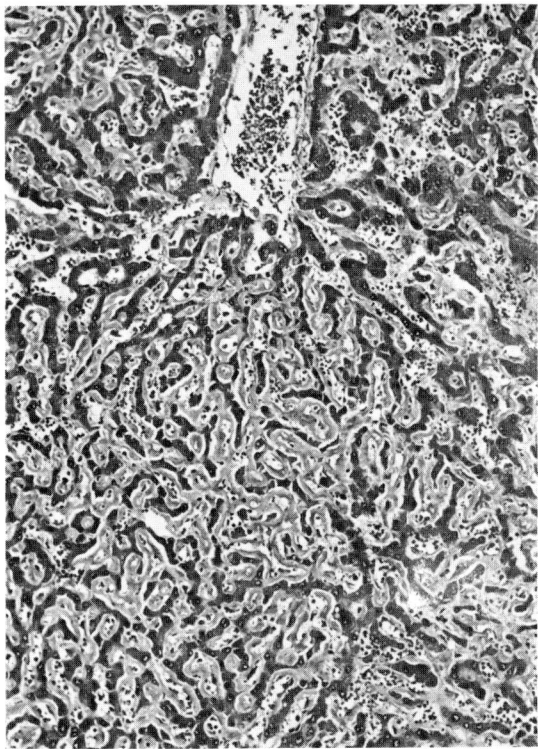

Fig. 24.2   Amyloidosis of liver. The amyloid is deposited in the space of Disse surrounding the sinusoids of the liver lobules. The liver cells adjacent to the amyloid are compressed, and show pronounced atrophy. × 120.

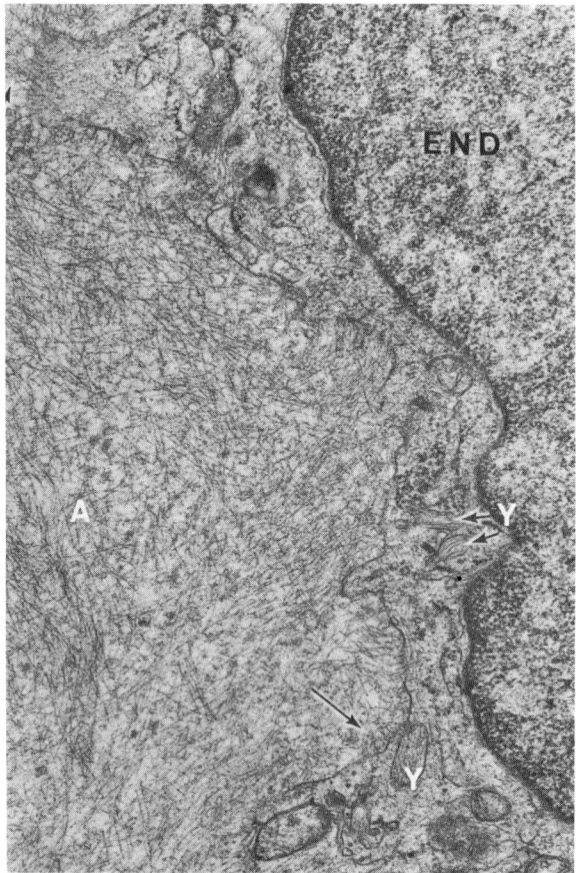

Fig. 24.3 Amyloid-laden rabbit spleen. The amyloid fibrils (A) fill most of the space near the endothelial cell (END), whose plasma membrane bears an intricate relationship to the fibrils, especially in the areas marked by arrows. In several areas (Y) fibrils appear to be intracellular. Osmium-fixed, Epon-embedded tissue, stained with lead citrate. × 24 000. (From Cohen A S 1965 In: Richter G W, Epstein M A (eds) International review of experimental pathology, vol. 4. Academic Press, New York, p 159.)

easily, and therefore repeated haemorrhages are to be expected. Since almost any tissue can be involved in amyloidosis, the clinical picture may be extremely varied and the diagnosis should always be kept in mind whenever one is confronted with an unusual case.

THE NATURE AND PATHOGENESIS OF AMYLOIDOSIS

Electron microscopy has revealed that amyloid material contains two components. The *major*

component consists of a felt-like mass of 7.5–10.0 nm rigid, non-branching, aggregated fibrils (Fig. 24.3). These fibrils have a characteristic β-pleated configuration and are responsible for the unique staining and biological properties of amyloid. Most research has centred on the nature and formation of these fibrils.

The *minor component* of amyloid consists of rod-shaped structures that are made up of pentagonal subunits (P components) having the same chemical composition as a normal α_1 serum glycoprotein closely related to C-reactive protein (L300). The relationship of the P component to the major fibrillary part of amyloid is unknown but, being a glycoprotein, it is responsible for the variable positive staining with PAS.

Two major chemical types of amyloid fibrils have been identified.

Amyloid of light-chain origin (AL)

The amyloid of immunocyte-derived systemic amyloidosis consists of one of the light chains of immunoglobulin, or part of the light chain. Fibres with identical appearance and staining properties to that of native amyloid can be produced in vitro by limited proteolytic digestion (by pepsin) of Bence–Jones protein—particularly of the L type. The plasma of patients with primary amyloidosis or mutiple myeloma contains monoclonal protein (M-protein) with identical amino-acid sequences to those of the amyloid deposits in that particular patient. It should be noted that in amyloidosis of any type, all the deposits of amyloid present in an individual patient have the same chemical composition, but differ from the amyloid found in other patients.

Amyloid of unknown origin (AA)

The amyloid of reactive systemic amyloidosis (secondary amyloidosis) is of unknown origin. In any individual case there is a circulating plasma component, termed SAA, which is related in composition to the amyloid itself. This SAA is thought to be a circulating precursor of the amyloid fibrils, and is found in all patients with amyloidosis. Indeed, it is found in all normal adults, but its concentration increases with age and also in some chronic diseases, for example tuberculosis, rheumatoid arthritis, and cancer; its level rises following stress, and it has been regarded as an acute-phase protein similar to C-reactive protein.

Amyloid derived from other proteins

The amyloid found in some types of heredofamilial amyloidosis is derived from pre-albumin. In localized deposits the amyloid is often derived from some local protein, e.g. calcitonin, insulin, keratin, etc. It has been found that the peptic digestion of many proteins—immunoglobulin, insulin, calcitonin, etc.—may yield products that in vitro will form typical amyloid fibrils. It is therefore probable that amyloid fibrils can be

formed in vivo from a variety of polypeptide fragments, derived either from a circulating protein such as immunoglobulin, SAA or pre-albumin, or from a local protein. In localized amyloidosis the site of proteolysis appears to be in macrophages. In generalized amyloidosis it is possible that the precursor protein is taken up by cells of the mononuclear phagocyte system so that the polypeptides can be released to form the amyloid fibrils with their characteristic β-pleating. Some polypeptide fragments are more amyloidogenic than others, and as noted previously, the L light chains form amyloid fibrils more readily than do the K chains. It is still not clear why amyloid deposition occurs in some patients and not in others, nor why it occurs in some sites and not in others.

GENERAL READING

Cohen A S, Sipe J D, Skinner M 1983 Amyloid proteins, precursors, mediator, and enhancer. Laboratory Investigation 48:1
Glenner G G 1980 Amyloid deposits and amyloidosis: the β-fibrilloses. New England Journal of Medicine 302:1283, 1333
Kyle R A 1982 Amyloidosis. Clinical Haematology 11:151
Levo Y, Livni N, Laufer A 1982 Diagnosis and classification of amyloidosis by an immune–histological method. Pathology Research and Practice (Stuttgart) 175:373

25.   The general reaction to trauma: haemorrhage and shock

Following major trauma there ensues a complex series of changes from which scarcely any tissue of the body escapes. The nervous system responds promptly with an increased outflow of autonomic impulses. There is an immediate outpouring of catecholamines from the adrenal medulla, while the other endocrine glands respond more slowly: stimulation of the hypothalamus leads to an increase in the secretion of ACTH from the pituitary gland, which in turn results in adrenocortical overactivity. These changes assist the injured animal to withstand trauma; in fact, there is little doubt that the adrenalectomized animal is less equipped to withstand infection and trauma than is the normal.

One very obvious early effect of trauma involves the circulatory system. When the trauma is severe, a state develops from which recovery may not occur; this is called *shock*, and is characterized by inadequate perfusion of the tissues, hypotension, and depression of general metabolic activity.

If the patient survives, there ensue metabolic changes that terminate in complete recovery. This is called the period of *convalescence*.

For descriptive purposes therefore it is convenient to consider the response to injury under three headings:

The metabolic changes
The circulatory changes
Shock.

THE METABOLIC CHANGES

These changes may be considered under the following headings;

The early, or ebb, phase
Convalescence: (a) Catabolic phase
*   (b) Anabolic phase.*

THE EARLY OR EBB PHASE

The early response to injury is termed the low flow, or ebb, phase. After severe injury it is an accompaniment of the state of shock. It is characterized by a reduction in the metabolic rate, a reduced body temperature, and an increased output of catecholamines from the adrenal medulla (see Table 25.1). The increased blood-level of catecholamines has several effects:

1. There is increased glycolysis in the liver.
2. Lactic acid is released from the muscles and is converted into glucose in the liver (Cori cycle). The result of all this is hyperglycaemia and possibly glycosuria.
3. A reduction in insulin secretion promotes gluconeogenesis in the liver, and this contributes to the hyperglycaemia.

Table 25.1 Metabolic changes following injury*

	Low-flow phase	High-flow phase
Metabolic rate	↓	↑
Body temperature	↓	↑
Catecholamine output	↑	Normal or slightly↑
Blood insulin level	↓	↑
Blood glucose	↑	Normal or slightly↑
Blood lactate	↑	Normal or slightly↑
Blood fatty acid	↑	↓

*Modified from Ryan N T 1976 Metabolic adaptations for energy production during trauma and sepsis. Surgical Clinics of North America 56:1073

4. Catecholamines have a lipolytic effect, and fatty acids are released from the adipose tissues. The blood level of fatty acids is therefore raised. The metabolic acidosis that accompanies this ebb phase in shocked patients is considered on page 298.

CONVALESCENCE

Assuming that the patient survives the initial phase and does not die of shock, there ensues a period of metabolic upset that has been termed the *high-flow phase*, or simply the *flow phase*. This has two components: (a) a *catabolic phase*, which is characterized by excessive protein breakdown and a negative nitrogen balance, followed by (b) an *anabolic phase*, during which the body's stores are replenished. These important metabolic changes are highly complex and are incompletely understood. They have been studied extensively both in animals and the human subject.

The catabolic phase

During the catabolic phase there is increased glucose production in the liver (Table 25.1). This gluconeogenesis is fed by lactate, pyruvate, and alanine and other animo acids derived from muscle, which are used as substrates. The breakdown of muscle components, particularly the proteins, for use in energy generation leads to muscular atrophy and a consequent loss of weight. The nitrogen of the metabolized amino acids is excreted as urea, and the body enters a phase of negative nitrogen balance. The duration of this nitrogen loss varies with the extent of the trauma: after a minor surgical procedure it may last only a day or two, but with severe burns it can continue for 10 days or more. Fractures cause more disturbance than might be supposed from the clinical condition; suppuration may prolong the catabolic state for weeks. During this catabolic phase there is a marked loss of weight. A moderate *pyrexia* is invariable, and is not due to concomitant infection.

The *haematological changes* are a moderate neutrophilia accompanied by a lymphopenia and eosinopenia. There is also a thrombocytosis (see p. 332). An interesting feature of severe trauma is the development of a progressive normocytic, normochromic anaemia. This is not due to iron deficiency; it may be that there is deficient haemoglobin synthesis during a period of general protein breakdown. Sludging may accentuate this anaemia (see p. 298).

The anabolic phase

The final stage of convalescence is characterized by a positive nitrogen balance and a resynthesis of muscle protein. The changes noted during the catabolic phase are reversed, and the body returns to normal.

THE CIRCULATORY CHANGES

The changes in the circulation are seen to their best advantage following acute haemorrhage; this will therefore be described first.

HAEMORRHAGE

Haemorrhage is defined as the escape of blood from the vascular system. The extravasated blood may escape to the exterior or it may remain internal.

Types of haemorrhage

External

Blood may be coughed up (*haemoptysis*), passed in the urine (*haematuria*), vomited (*haematemesis*), or be passed in the faeces either as fresh blood or, if from higher up in the intestinal tract, as a black, partially digested mass (*melaena*).

Internal

Small flat haemorrhages, less than 2 mm in diameter, are called *petechiae*, or *purpuric spots;* they are usually found in the skin and mucous membranes. A larger, more diffuse, haemorrhagic area is called an *ecchymosis*. A *haematoma* is a discrete pool of blood, usually clotted, in a tissue. Collections of blood in natural spaces are named anatomically, e.g. *haemothorax* (in the pleural cavity), *haemopericardium*, *haemoperitoneum*, *haemarthrosis* (in a joint cavity), etc.

Causes of acute haemorrhage

Haemorrhage may result from direct physical violence to a vessel as with a stab wound, or it may occur spontaneously. Weakening of the wall is a common cause and in the arteries atherosclerosis, arteritis and aneurysm provide examples. Increased intraluminal pressure may cause a normal vessel to rupture or contribute to bleeding from a weakened vessel. Systemic hypertension predisposes to haemorrhage from a cerebral artery, and portal hypertension is an important cause of bleeding from varicose oesophageal veins.

Effects of acute haemorrhage

The vascular system contains about 5 litres of blood, which is kept in motion by the action of the heart so that all the tissues are adequately perfused. The amount of blood reaching any area is determined by two factors—the *calibre of the arterioles supplying it* and the *blood pressure*.

The capacious venous system acts as a reservoir for the blood, and therefore when a small quantity is lost, an increase in venous tone reduces the capacity of the circulatory system, so that there is no reduction in the volume of blood reaching the heart (the venous return). Therefore there is no reduction in the cardiac output. When a larger volume of blood is suddenly withdrawn, this reserve mechanism is inadequate. The venous return is diminished, the cardiac output falls, and with it the amount of blood available for perfusing the organs. It is therefore not surprising that the next response to haemorrhage is a series of reactions designed to restore the blood pressure.

Restoration of blood pressure and redistribution of blood

The fall in blood pressure is detected by the pressure-sensitive carotid sinus and the other baroreceptors, and these reflexly initiate a sympathetic outflow from the central nervous system (Fig. 25.1). The effect is a *vasoconstriction* of the arterioles of the *skin*, *kidneys*, and *splanchnic area* by direct action, as well as indirectly via the adrenal medulla, which is stimulated to secrete adrenaline and noradrenaline. The lowered blood pressure acts on the juxtaglomerular apparatus and causes the kidney to release renin (p. 326). There is therefore an overall increase in the peripheral resistance. The blood pressure is restored, and the blood flow to the brain, heart, and respiratory muscles remains almost unaltered. However, the areas affected by arteriolar vasoconstriction tend to suffer; for example the *skin* is cold and pale, the *kidneys* show a reduced urinary output (oliguria), and the *salivary glands* cease to secrete. Thus the vasomotor response to acute haemorrhage causes a *redistribution of blood,* a mechanism which may be regarded as an emergency measure designed to keep the essential organs supplied.

Restoration of blood volume

During the first few hours after a haemorrhage extravascular fluids pass into the blood stream,

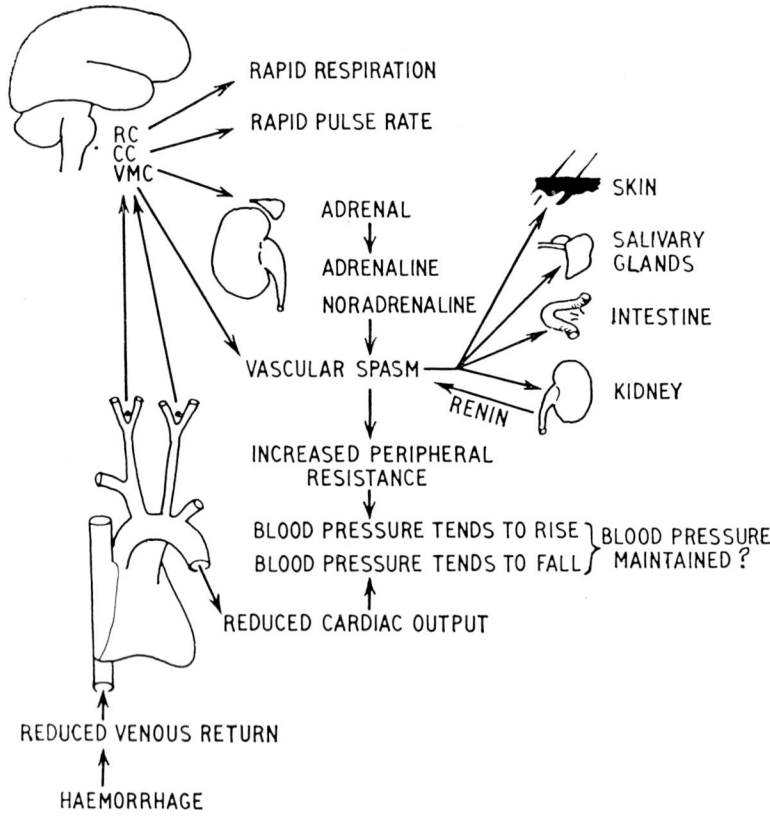

Fig. 25.1 The cardiovascular of sudden haemorrhage. RC (Respiratory Centre). CC (Cardiac Centre). VMC (Vasomotor Centre).

the volume of which is thereby restored. This is easily demonstrated by following the haemoglobin level. Immediately after a sudden haemorrhage the *haemoglobin level is normal.* During the next 8 h it falls as dilution occurs, and this process is largely complete by the end of 48 h. At this stage therefore the haemoglobin level is a good guide to the extent of the previous blood loss. This transfer of extracellular fluid to the blood stream appears to be the result of the reduced capillary hydrostatic pressure which follows the arteriolar vasoconstriction. The osmotic pressure of the plasma due to its protein content is now greater than the hydrostatic pressure, and fluid is drawn into the blood until a balance is achieved (p. 327). Complete restoration of the plasma volume is dependent upon replacement of the lost plasma proteins. These enter the circulation

via the thoracic duct, and are primarily contributed by the liver.

Changes in the blood

Within a few minutes of bleeding the clotting time is considerably decreased, and during the next few hours there is a considerable increase in the level of platelets and neutrophils, which persists for several days. The restoration of the red-cell count is a much slower process, since the body has virtually no reserve store of erythrocytes. New red cells have to be manufactured, and a normal count is not attained until 4–6 weeks later.

The effects of acute haemorrhage depend upon both the volume and the speed with which the blood is lost. The normal adult can donate one pint (approx. 500 ml, or 10% of the blood volume) with little discomfort. A sudden loss of

30–50% may well be fatal; however, if spread over a day or so it can be tolerated. If the haemorrhage is so severe that the compensatory mechanisms are inadequate to maintain an adequate blood flow to vital organs, death ensues. This constitutes one variety of *shock*, a subject which will now be considered.

SHOCK

Shock is the name given to a clinical state in which the patient has tachycardia (an increased heart rate), and is pale, ashen, and sweating. Two quite separate conditions have been included:

VASOVAGAL ATTACK, PRIMARY SHOCK, OR SYNCOPE

Immediately following injury or loss of blood, a patient may feel nauseated, become giddy, and finally lose consciousness. Convulsions occasionally occur. The attack rarely lasts more than a few minutes, and causes no permanent damage. It is sometimes seen after quite trivial injury, e.g. the insertion of a needle, or even, in nervous individuals, at the suggestion of injury. The attack appears to be mediated by a vasomotor imbalance so that widespread vasodilatation occurs in the skeletal muscles. The blood pressure drops, the heart rate slows, and the cerebral blood flow diminishes so that consciousness is lost. If the patient is laid horizontally, or attains that position spontaneously, recovery soon occurs. In rare cases death may occur—at least this is one suggestion for the rare cases of sudden death which occur unexpectedly, e.g. when introducing a needle into the pleural cavity or during an attempted abortion. It has been reported that syncope occurring during the induction of anaesthesia may be fatal if the anaesthetic is administered with the patient in the upright position, e.g. in a dental chair.

SECONDARY SHOCK

This is a much more important condition, and it is best to restrict the unqualified term 'shock' to it. The important factor in shock is circulatory failure leading to inadequate perfusion of tissues. This leads to metabolic acidosis, because lactic acid is produced in the presence of inadequate oxygen. Clinical features depend on the tissues involved; lung, kidney, liver and heart are common victims.

Shock can complicate any condition in which the volume of the circulating blood is diminished (hypovolaemic shock). Examples include haemorrhage, loss of plasma due to the formation of an acute inflammatory exudate as may occur with an extensive burn or a severe infection such as gasgangrene, or loss of fluid and electrolytes as may occur with severe diarrhoea or vomiting.

Shock may occur in the presence of a normal blood volume if there is peripheral vasodilatation and pooling of the circulating blood, usually in the splanchnic area. This is termed *peripheral circulatory failure*. This is an important component of the shock that accompanies severe infection.

Shock may be due to sudden low cardiac output (*cardiogenic shock*). This can occur following a large myocardial infarct, with a sudden dysrhythmia or with acute cardiac tamponade.

Finally, shock may follow trauma (*traumatic shock*). This important topic will be considered in more detail.

Haemorrhagic shock

If following a large haemorrhage the compensatory mechanisms described on p. 295 fail to maintain the blood pressure, either as a result of their own inefficiency, or the excessive load placed upon them by a large haemorrhage, the patient enters into a state of shock. Recovery may occur spontaneously, or as a result of efficient treatment, e.g. transfusion; such shock is therefore said to be *reversible*. It sometimes happens that in spite of vigorous and efficient treatment the blood pressure continues to fall, the patient's clinical condition deteriorates, and death ensues. This is *irreversible shock*.

Traumatic shock

The circulatory changes which follow trauma are very similar to those following haemorrhage. Initial *syncope* may occur, to be followed shortly by secondary shock. The possible causes of the latter are:

Haemorrhage. It is often not appreciated that injury, apart from causing external bleeding, leads to an extensive blood loss into the tissues. Thus in a closed fracture of the femur, 4 pints of blood may be lost. It is obvious that the swelling of injured parts is produced either by extravasated blood or by inflammatory exudate, i.e. plasma.

In surgical operations it is very important to estimate the amount of blood lost so that it can be replaced. The amount on swabs can be estimated by weighing, or by extracting the haemoglobin and measuring it colorimetrically.

Toxins. Toxins from damaged tissue have been postulated, but their importance has never been substantiated.

Infection of the wound. There is little doubt that the powerful exotoxins of the pathogenic clostridia exert a profound effect on the circulation. Gas-gangrene even in the absence of substantial traumatic damage causes a shock-like state which may result in death.

Endotoxic factor. Since the generalized Shwartzman phenomenon resembles shock, it has been suggested that following trauma the intestinal coliform organisms or their endotoxins enter the blood stream and cause a similar reaction. Nevertheless, this has not been substantiated as an important cause of human traumatic shock, although it is probably important in the severe shock which develops in patients with Gram-negative septicaemia (see below).

In summary, it seems that *blood loss is the most important factor in traumatic shock.*

Shock in infection

Shock is seen in a variety of infections. It is prominent in infections with toxic organisms, e.g. diphtheria and gas-gangrene, but it is also a feature of many other severe infections—pneumonia, peritonitis, etc. In recent years a new syndrome, *endotoxic shock* (bacteraemic or Gram-negative shock), has been recognized, and is caused by the sudden entry of Gram-negative organisms into the circulation. It is a complication of any coliform infection, but is usually seen as a sequel to urinary infection. There is a sudden onset of profound shock, and

unless treated expeditiously this carries a high mortality. The condition bears some resemblance to the shock seen in the generalized Shwartzman reaction.

The pathogenesis of shock in infections is complex. There may be hypovolaemia due to loss of protein-containing exudate in acute inflammatory exudate, as with an infected wound or gas-gangrene. Circulatory failure with pooling of blood in the splanchnic area is a feature of some infections, particularly if there is endotoxic shock. Heart failure is an additional factor when the myocardium is damaged by bacterial toxins, for instance in diphtheria.

Anaphylactic shock

This is discussed in Chapter 13.

The metabolic upset during shock

A patient in shock shows a profound *reduction in metabolic rate*, the nature of which is not well understood; it appears that there is a block in carbohydrate utilization. In spite of cutaneous vasoconstriction, and therefore a reduction in heat loss, *the body's temperature falls*. An important effect of shock is that the under-perfusion of tissues results in anaerobic glycolysis with the release of pyruvic and lactic acids into the circulation. There is therefore often a severe *metabolic acidosis*. It is evident that an important aspect of shock is that tissues are underperfused with blood. Indeed, it has been stated that 'shock is not merely a problem of blood volume, blood pressure, and anaemia, but essentially a problem of flow'. A factor to be considered in this respect is sludging.

Sludging

If the flowing blood of a shocked patient is observed, it will be seen that the red cells are clumped together. This differs from true agglutination in that the masses can be broken up, though with some difficulty. The original description of the phenomenon described the blood as being converted into a 'muck-like sludge' —hence the name *sludging*. The *cause* of this is an increase

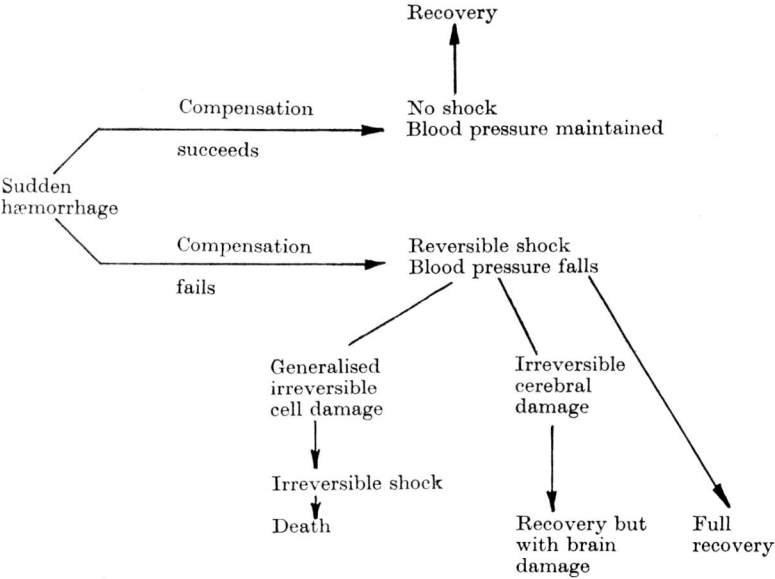

Fig. 25.2 The possible end-results of a sudden haemorrhage.

in the level of high-molecular-weight substances (e.g. fibrinogen) in the plasma and a reduction in the low-molecular-weight albumin, as occurs in the acute-phase response (p. 300). The *effect* is to impede the blood flow through the tissues. Sludging can be prevented or reversed by the infusion of low-molecular-weight substances; for example dextran (40 000 daltons) has been used.

Irreversible shock

Some patients with shock recover either spontaneously or as a result of treatment. Others steadily deteriorate in spite of all efforts to save them and there has arisen a concept that there exists a stage from which recovery is impossible. This is called *irreversible shock* (Fig. 25.2).

The causes and the concept

Prolonged underperfusion of tissue. Although the selective vasoconstriction and redistribution of blood flow tide the patient over the initial period following injury, they may, if they persist, lead to permanent damage. The kidney is particularly sensitive to the effects of shock and acute tubular necrosis is common.

Patchy *myocardial necrosis* can lead to heart failure, a condition that, combined with the circulatory failure, leads to centrilobular hepatic necrosis. Ischaemia of the gastrointestinal tract can cause acute mucosal erosions that result in severe bleeding, either from the stomach (acute gastric erosions) or from lower down in the intestinal tract. Involvement of the lung leads to the *acute respiratory distress syndrome*. Also the *metabolic acidosis* may induce vasodilatation and further lower the blood pressure. Whatever the mechanism, there is little doubt that the longer a patient remains in shock, the less likely is he to recover.

Inefficient treatment. The patient in shock often requires large volumes of fluid. This must be adjusted to the clinical situation, depending on whether blood, plasma, fluid or electrolytes are required. Metabolic acidosis must be corrected. Depressant drugs such as morphine must be given with care, and because of the potentially toxic effects of high concentrations, pure oxygen must not be given. The advantages of the modern intensive-care units is that the many facets of shock can be monitored and treated.

Conclusion. There are many features about shock which we do not understand. Nevertheless, vigorous, well-designed treatment can save many cases. 'Shock' is not a diagnosis which should be accepted unqualified; it indicates that something is wrong—a low blood volume, metabolic acidosis, sludging, arterial desaturation, renal failure, pericardial haemorrhage, etc., all of which may be diagnosed and treated. With severe injury, in old age, and in the chronic sick, death may be inevitable, but the diagnosis of irreversible shock can be made only post mortem.

THE ACUTE-PHASE RESPONSE

The acute-phase response follows many acute inflammatory conditions and trauma. It involves an increase in the release of several proteins from the liver (fibrinogen, C-reactive protein and others) which combine to cause red cells to adhere to each other in rouleau formation. This is measured clinically by estimating the speed with which red cells sink when blood is mixed with anticoagulant and allowed to stand vertically, in vitro. The result is termed the *erythrocyte sedimentation rate* (ESR). The value is raised in the acute-phase response, and whenever there is an increase in the proportion of high-molecular-weight substances in the blood. It is therefore raised in multiple myeloma, when the macroglobulins are raised. The ESR is a useful clinical test because a raised level indicates that something is wrong. It is of no specific diagnostic value but can be used to follow the activity of a known disease, e.g. systemic lupus erythematosus or rheumatoid arthritis.

GENERAL READING

Kushner I 1982 The phenomenon of the acute phase response. Annals of the New York Academy of Sciences 389:39
Lefer A M (ed.) 1981 Advances in shock research, vol 5. Alan R. Liss, New York
Mizock B 1984 Septic shock—a metabolic perspective. Archives of Internal Medicine 144:579

PART 2

Diseases of individual systems and organs

26. Disorders of the blood

The formed elements of the blood are the red cells (*erythrocytes*), white cells (*leucocytes*), and *platelets*. In the fetus blood formation (*haematopoiesis*) occurs both in the bone marrow and in a few extramedullary sites such as the liver and spleen. After birth haematopoiesis is solely medullary.

All blood cells are derived from a totipotent haematopoietic stem cell, itself derived from the yolk sac of the developing embryo. In the bone marrow this cell gives rise to stem cells of more restrictive potential. These stem cells have been isolated by injecting marrow cells into lethally irradiated mice and analysing separate clonal colonies that appear in the spleen. They have been called *colony-forming units (CFU)*. One gives rise to the lymphoid cells, another to pleuripotent myeloid stem cells (CFU-S), which in turn give rise to further units of lesser potential, e.g. CFU-NM for neutrophil myelocytes and monocytes, CFU-EOS

for eosinophils, CFU-E for red cells and CFE-MEG for megakaryocytes. These stem cells divide both to replace themselves and to differentiate into cells that ultimately lead to the production of the mature blood cells. Specific growth factors are known that act on these stem cells.

THE RED CELL

The first recognizable red-cell precursor is the pronormoblast which has nucleoli, and has no haemoglobin in its cytoplasm. In the next cell type, the *normoblast*, nucleoli have been lost. Three stages are recognized—early, intermediate, and late—depending on the degree of haemoglobinization of the cytoplasm and the pyknosis of the nucleus (Fig. 26.1). Eventually the nucleus is extruded, and a mature red cell is left.

The mature cell

The red cell is a biconcave disc, and in blood films appears as a roughly circular cell. It stains red with the Romanowsky dyes used in haematology.* When young it contains rough endoplasmic reticulum, and this imparts a bluish tint to the cell. This is called *polychromasia*. If such a cell is stained supravitally with brilliant cresyl blue, the RNA stands out as a network, or reticulum, of fine blue strands, and the cell is called a *reticulocyte*. The proportion of reticulocytes to older red cells gives an indication of the

---

* These include stains such as Leishman, Jenner, and Giemsa, and consist of a blended mixture of methylene blue and eosin.

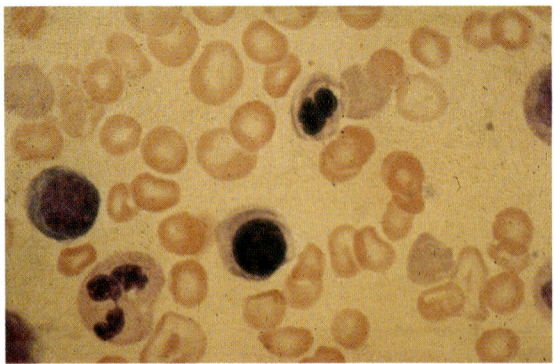

Fig. 26.1 Normoblasts in peripheral blood. The patient was an infant with haemolytic disease of the newborn due to rhesus incompatibility. Several normoblasts and one neutrophil polymorph are shown. × 960.

activity of erythropoiesis. The *reticulocyte count* is normally 0.8–2.5% in males, and 0.8–4.1% in females. A rise in the reticulocyte count indicates increased red-cell formation and occurs after haemorrhage, haemolysis or the successful treatment of an anaemia. When erythropoiesis is much increased, nucleated forms also appear in the circulation. A good example is haemolytic disease of the newborn (Fig. 26.1).

Examination of the red cell. The normal red cell count is 4.6–6.2×10^{12}/L in males, and the normal haemoglobin content is 140–180 g/L. In females the red cell count is 0.5×10^{12}/L and the haemoglobin level 20 g/L lower. The red cell count is high at birth, but drops precipitously within the first few months.

A haemoglobin estimation is an essential examination to assess the presence and degree of anaemia. The normal value is 140–180 g/L. Another useful investigation is the *haematocrit* reading, or *packed cell volume*. In this test a thin, cylindrical, graduated tube is filled with blood and centrifuged for half an hour at 3000 revolutions per minute. In the adult male 40–50% of the volume consists of red cells.

The experienced haematologist derives the most information about the red cell by inspecting a well-made, well-stained blood film. The normal red cell is described as *normocytic* and *normochromic*. If smaller than normal it is *microcytic*, and if larger, *macrocytic*. A cell cannot be over-haemoglobinized, and so there cannot be hyperchromia. If cells are poorly haemoglobinized, they look pale and are described as *hypochromic;* in a stained film they are easily recognized by their colourless centres, which may be so extensive that only a narrow rim of haemoglobin is left around them peripherally. In addition the cells may contain a small central aggregation of haemoglobin surrounded by the extensive colourless zone; these are called *target cells. Spherocytes* are almost spherical in shape and therefore appear as small dark-staining cells. *Burr cells,* or *acanthocytes,* are mature red cells which possess one or more spiky projections on their periphery. Burr cells are characteristic of those haemolytic anaemias in which mechanical trauma is believed to damage the red cells, e.g. microangiopathic haemolytic anaemia. They are also found in uraemia.

Marked variation in size of the population of red cells is called *anisocytosis,* and a marked variation in shape, *poikilocytosis.*

Haemoglobin. Haemoglobin is a conjugated protein. The molecule consists of four haem groups attached to the protein globin which in turn is composed of two pairs of polypeptide chains. Six types of chain are known—α, β, γ, δ, ε and ζ. In haemoglobin A (Hb-A) the normal major component of adult human blood, the globin consists of two α chains and two β chains

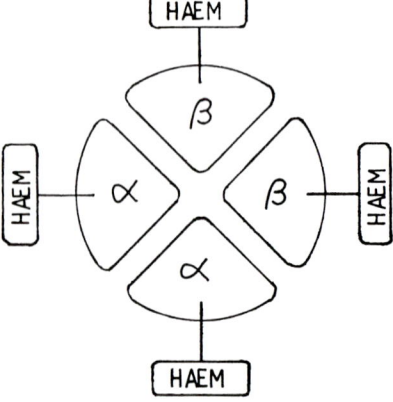

Fig. 26.2 Diagrammatic representation of haemoglobin. The four polypeptide chains of globin are labelled α and β. (After Wintrobe M M 1967 Fig. 3.7 in *Clinical Hematology*, 6th edn Lea & Febiger, p 139.)

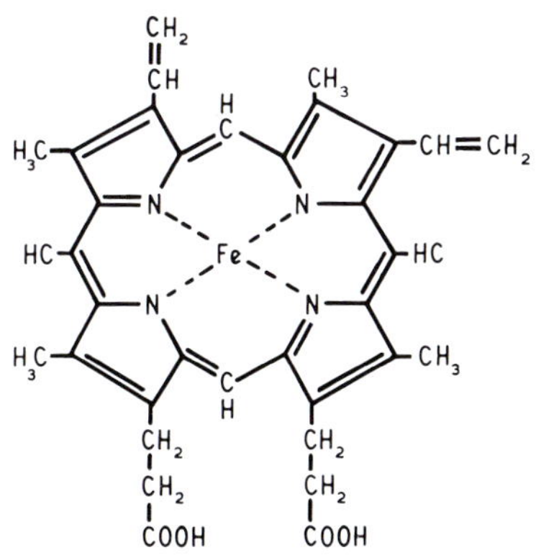

Fig. 26.3 The structural formula of haem. Note the protoporphyrin ring structure which is composed of four pyrrole rings joined by methene (=CH–) bridges.

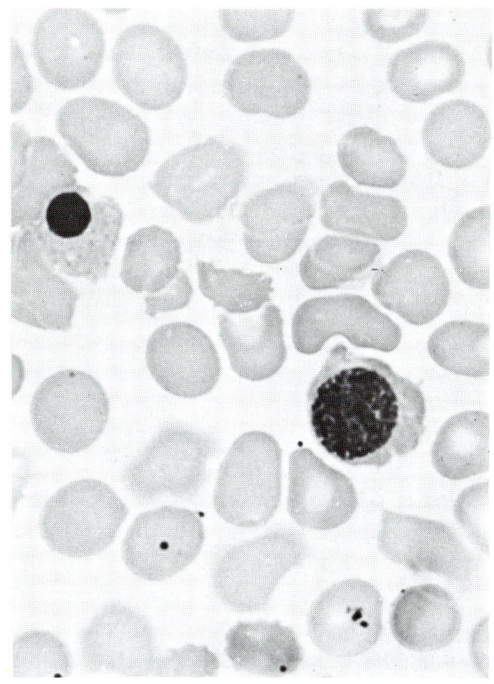

Fig. 26.4 A megaloblast. Note the large size of the cell and its stippled nuclear chromatin as compared with the much smaller normoblast and its pyknotic nucleus. The smear is from the marrow of a patient with pernicious anaemia. × 960.

(Fig. 26.2). Fetal haemoglobin (Hb-F) is the type found in the fetus and during early infancy but not in the normal adult; it consists of two α chains and two γ chains. In a group of conditions known as the *thalassemia syndromes*, the fetal or embryonic haemoglobins may be formed at the expense of normal haemoglobin and be present in the adult red cell.

There is a second group of conditions, called the *haemoglobinopathies*, in which an abnormal form of haemoglobin is present. There is an abnormal sequence of amino acids in either the α or β chain of HbA due to a genetic abnormality. Sickle-cell anaemia (due to the formation of HbS) is the most important example of this type of defect.

Requirements for red-cell formation. Apart from protein, which forms part of haemoglobin, the most important requirements are iron, folic acid, and vitamin B_{12}.

Iron. In its ferrous form (Fe^{2+}) iron is an integral part of haemoglobin. As seen in Fig. 26.3 the iron atom lies in the centre of the porphyrin structure composed of four pyrrole rings. Iron is absorbed from the food in an ionic form by the mucosal cells of the duodenum and upper small bowel. Here it combines, in ferric form (Fe^{3+}), with the iron-free protein *apoferritin* to form *ferritin*, the storage form of iron in the body. Ferric iron is absorbed as required into the blood stream and carried in combination with a globulin called *iron-binding protein, transferrin,* or

siderophilin. The concentration of transferrin in the plasma is 1.2 g per litre, but more commonly transferrin is quantitated in terms of the total iron it will bind, the *total iron-binding capacity (TIBC) of the plasma,* which is normally 45–70 μmol/L (250–400 μg per dl): the plasma is normally one-third saturated with iron. Iron is used for the synthesis of haemoglobin and myoglobin; it is stored in the MP system as ferritin.

Vitamins. The important group belong to the B complex—folic acid and vitamin B_{12}. Both are necessary for the proper development of the normoblast; without either (or both) the cell undergoes a perversion of development, remaining large, and retaining a delicate stippled pattern of chromatin instead of showing the nuclear pyknosis of a maturing normoblast. Such a cell is called a *megaloblast* (Fig. 26.4). Both vitamins are present in the diet and absorbed in the small bowel, but whereas folic acid is directly taken up, vitamin B_{12} cannot be absorbed unless bound to a complex mucoprotein secreted by the gastric mucosa. This substance is called *intrinsic factor*. It follows that the gastric secretion is essential for the absorption of vitamin B_{12}. Both vitamins are stored in the liver, where stores of vitamin B_{12} are so great that they can last for several years before deficiency becomes apparent. Folic acid stores on the other hand suffice for 2–4 months.

Other substances are required but their role is less well understood; they include copper, cobalt, and hormones, such as thyroxine, adrenal cortical hormones, sex hormones and *erythropoietin* (a glycoprotein growth factor manufactured in the kidney and to a lesser extent elsewhere, that is responsible for stimulation of red cell production in hypoxia).

Disposal of the red cell. The normal lifespan of the red cell is about 120 days. The manner in which the effete red cells are destroyed is still uncertain. The process of ageing precedes and is responsible for eventual destruction, and it is possible that the cell undergoes fragmentation in the circulation prior to its ultimate removal by the MP cells of the liver, bone marrow, and spleen. In these cells the haemoglobin is broken down. The globin portion is released, degraded, and returned to the body's pool of amino acids. The iron portion of the haemoglobin is stored in the MP cells as ferritin, while the porphyrin nucleus is broken down to bilirubin which is excreted by the liver. Normally there is a mere trace of free haemoglobin in the plasma—any that does appear is immediately removed by combination with a globulin component of the plasma proteins called *haptoglobin*. If haemoglobin in excess of the haptoglobin binding capacity of the plasma is released, the free haemoglobin in the plasma is readily oxidized to methaemoglobin, which dissociates into haem and globin. The haem combines with *haemopexin*, a normal β-globulin of the plasma, and when this binding protein is exhausted its place is taken by albumin, which binds haem to form *methaemalbumin*. The haptoglobin, haemopexin, and albumin complexes are all metabolized in the MPS, principally in the liver, and none escapes into the urine. It is only when all these binding proteins are consumed that free haemoglobin appears in the blood (*haemoglobinaemia*) and urine (*haemoglobinuria*).

THE ANAEMIAS

Anaemia is defined as a condition in which there is a fall in the quantity of either red cells or haemoglobin in a unit volume of blood in the presence of a low or normal total blood volume. The normal blood volume is 5 litres, of which 2.8 litres is plasma and 2.2 litres red-cell mass. It might be expected that the blood volume would be reduced in anaemia owing to the decreased number of red cells, but in fact it is little altered as there is a compensatory rise in plasma volume.

The classification of the anaemias is controversial, and the following scheme is recommended:

1. Acute posthaemorrhagic anaemia, which has been described on page 296
2. Iron-deficiency anaemia
3. Megaloblastic anaemia
4. Haemolytic anaemia
5. Anaemia of bone-marrow inadequacy.

The effects of anaemia are attributable to cellular hypoxia.

The main clinico-pathological features are as follows:

Pallor, best detected in the conjunctiva, nail bed, or oral mucous membrane. Skin pallor, particularly of the face, is a deceptive sign. It may be absent in some patients with anaemia, and yet present in many pale-skinned healthy people.

Tiredness, easy fatiguability, and *generalized muscular weakness* are common symptoms; their pathogenesis, however, is not clear. Such symptoms are also common in psychoneurotic patients who are not anaemic.

Shortness of breath, and *palpitations* are common. They are related to tissue *hypoxia* and an increased cardiac output. *Heart failure* can occur.

Angina pectoris, intermittent claudication, and *giddiness* are due to tissue hypoxia in organs in which the blood supply is already impaired by arterial disease.

The basal metabolic rate is raised, and in severe degrees of anaemia *pyrexia* is quite common. The cause of this is unclear.

Table 26.1 The normal white-cell count

	%	per litre	per µl
Neutrophil polymorphonuclears	40–75	2.0 to 7.5 × 10^9	2000–7500
Eosinophil polymorphonuclears	1–5	0.05 to 0.4 × 10^9	50–400
Basophil polymorphonuclears	0–1	up to 0.1 × 10^9	up to 100
Lymphocytes	20–45	1.5 to 4 × 10^9	1500–4000
Monocytes	3–7	0.2 to 0.8 × 109	200–800

quantity of red cells is raised in a unit volume of blood in the presence of an increased total blood volume. It must be distinguished from haemo-concentration following plasma or fluid loss, in which the blood volume is reduced.

Polycythaemia may be *secondary* to chronic hypoxia, e.g. living at very great altitudes, chronic pulmonary disease, and cyanotic congenital heart disease. It is seen occasionally in patients with malignant disease, especially renal-cell carcinoma due to the secretion of erythropoietin by the tumour cells.

As a primary condition (*polycythaemia vera*) it is a neoplastic proliferation of the normoblastic element of the marrow. The red cell count may be increased to 10 × 10^{12}/L. There is usually a considerable increase in the white-cell and platelet counts, a change not occurring in secondary polycythaemia. The disease is best classified as a myeloproliferative disorder; it may terminate in acute myeloblastic leukaemia or myelofibrosis. These patients are usually middle-aged or elderly, of florid complexion, with enlarged spleens and livers, and are liable to succumb to thrombotic complications, e.g. mesenteric venous thrombosis, coronary thrombosis, etc. Peptic ulcer is another common complication.

THE WHITE CELLS

Stem cells of the CFU-NM form cells that are destined to differentiate into neutrophils and monocytes.

The precursor cell of the granulocyte series is the *myeloblast,* which resembles the pronor-moblast. As it matures it loses its nucleoli, and is then termed a *promyelocyte.* When specific neutrophil cytoplasmic granules appear, the cell is called a neutrophil *myelocyte.* The nucleus becomes indented to form a *metamyelocyte,* and is ultimately drawn out into two or three discrete lobes joined by fine chromatin threads. This is the mature granulocyte, often called a *neutrophil polymorphonuclear leucocyte* (or polymorph) because of the shape of the nucleus.

Eosinophils and basophils develop along parallel lines. Monocytes develop from precursor monoblasts.

The normal white-cell count and its variations

The total white-cell count in the blood is 4.0–11.0 × 10^9/L. The range of the differential count is given in Table 26.1.

The suffix -cytosis implies an excess of cells, e.g. *leucocytosis* indicates an increased white cell count, and *lymphocytosis* indicates an increase in the number of lymphocytes. The suffix -penia means a decrease in the relevant cells, e.g. *leucopenia* means a decrease in the number of white cells, and *lymphopenia* is a decrease in the number of lymphocytes. *Neutrophilia* is sometimes used as an alternative to neutrophil leucocytosis. Likewise *neutropenia* denotes a reduction in the total number of neutrophil polymorphs, and the term *agranulocytosis* is commonly used as a synonym. The number per litre in Table 26.1 gives the absolute number of cells present. This is a more useful figure than the percentage. Thus, if there is a drop in the number of neutrophils, the percentage of lymphocytes increases—the condition called a *relative lymphocytosis.* The term, however, is misleading, since the actual number of lymphocytes can remain unchanged. The main variations in the white cell count are as follows:

Neutrophil leucocytosis (neutrophilia). This common condition is usually due *to infection by* *pyogenic organisms*, e.g. staphylococcal, pneumococcal, coliform, etc. Some non-pyogenic infections can also lead to a neutrophilia, e.g. plague, diphtheria, and anthrax.

Strenuous exercise, anaesthetics, and emotional stress all produce a transient rise in the number of neutrophils.

Other important causes are *massive tissue necrosis*, as following a myocardial infarct, *uraemia, acute gout*, following severe haemorrhage and haemolysis, *rapidly growing malignant tumours*, and *neoplastic disease of the marrow*, e.g. chronic myeloid leukaemia and polycythaemia vera.

At one time a classification of the maturity of neutrophils based on their nuclear segmentation was very much in vogue. Results were expressed in tabular form with the left-hand side of the page listing the most primitive cells and the more mature cells being on the right-hand side. Although this detailed counting is now obsolete, the term 'a shift to the left' is still useful in denoting an increase in the blood of young forms of polymorphs. In most of the causes of neutrophil leucocytosis listed above there is a shift to the left, and in extreme cases metamyelocytes and even myelocytes may enter the blood. This *leukemoid blood picture* can sometimes closely mimic leukaemia itself.

Neutropenia. This may occur in certain *infections*, such as typhoid fever and brucellosis. It is common during the prodromal period of viral disease and in chronic protozoal infection, e.g. malaria. Overwhelming infection of whatever cause also lowers the neutrophil count.

Other causes of neutropenia are some diseases associated with splenomegaly (*hypersplenism*), and also *pernicious anaemia, bone-marrow aplasia*, and *acute leukaemia*.

Regulation of the neutrophil count. The neutrophil count can be altered by two regulatory mechanisms:

1. Release of neutrophils from the reserves. Of the neutrophils in the blood stream, over half are in a 'marginated pool' adherent to the walls of blood vessels, particularly in the lungs. These can be released rapidly; their release accounts for the leucocytosis occurring during exercise and following the administration of adrenaline. The second reserve is in the bone marrow, where the number of neutrophils sequestered is about 10 times the total of the cells present in the blood. The mechanism of their release is poorly understood, but various neutrophil-releasing factors have been described.

2. Increased production of neutrophils in the bone marrow. Various *colony-stimulating substances* have been isolated from macrophages, and lymphocytes. However, the role, if any, of these agents in the regulation of the neutrophil count in health or disease is not clear.

Lymphocytosis. An absolute lymphocytosis is not common. It is seen in *whooping-cough* and *infectious mononucleosis (glandular fever)*. In the latter disease the lymphocytes are atypical. The disease is caused by the Epstein–Barr virus (EBV). It is an important cause of prolonged fever, and is not uncommon in young adults. An interesting feature is the presence in the serum of antibodies which agglutinate sheep red cells to high titre (*Paul–Bunnell test*). There are other types of infectious mononucleosis that are part of cytomegalic inclusion disease and toxoplasmosis, and in these the Paul–Bunnell test is negative.

Another important cause of lymphocytosis is *chronic lymphocytic leukaemia.*

Monocytosis. A rise in the monocyte count is seen typically in *protozoal diseases*, such as malaria, trypanosomiasis, and leishmaniasis. It may occasionally occur in *chronic bacterial infections* also, e.g. tuberculosis and *S. viridans* endocarditis. Another cause is *monocytic leukaemia.*

Eosinophilia. An eosinophilia is encountered in some *hypersensitivities of atopic type*, e.g. bronchial asthma, hay-fever, and urticaria, and in *helminthic infections*, especially when the parasites are migrating through the tissues.

Eosinophilia is also seen in some skin diseases, e.g. pemphigus vulgaris and exfoliative dermatitis.

THE LEUKAEMIAS

Leukaemia is a condition in which there is a widespread proliferation of the leucocytes and their precursors throughout the tissues of the body, with a variable circulating component. Radiation and certain drugs, e.g. the alkylating

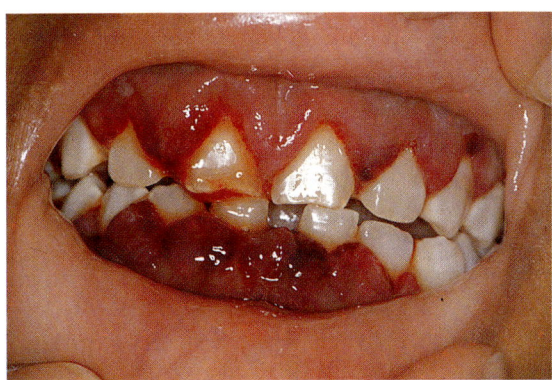

Fig. 26.7 Spontaneous haemorrhage and gross gingival enlargement due to leukaemic infiltration. The presenting symptoms in this case of acute myeloid leukaemia. (Previously published in Rock W P, Grundy M C, Shaw L Diagnostic picture tests in paediatric dentistry, Wolfe Medical Publications, London.)

agents melphalan and chlorambucil, predispose to the development of leukaemia, but for the most part the cause of human leukaemia remains an enigma. In birds and mice leukaemia has been shown to be due to a retrovirus infection, but, with two exceptions, no virus has been found in humans: human T-cell lymphoma virus (*HTLV-I*) has been implicated in a T-cell lymphoma with a leukaemic component, and *HTLV-II* has been associated with a few cases of hairy cell leukaemia. Oncogenes have been incriminated, e.g. the characteristic 9–22 translocation in most cases of chronic myeloid leukaemia involves the oncogene c-*abl*. The significance of this association remains to be assessed.

The classification of leukaemia is based on the rapidity of the disease and the type of cell involved. The following outline is used but it will become apparent that subsections of each type are known:

Chronic leukaemia — chronic myeloid leukaemia (CML)
— chronic lymphocytic leukaemia (CLL)
Acute leukaemia — acute myeloid leukaemia (AML)
— acute lymphoblastic leukaemia (ALL).

Chronic myeloid leukaemia. This is a disease usually of middle life. The outstanding hae-matological finding is an enormous leucocytosis, even up to 1000×10^9/L. Nearly all of these are neutrophil polymorphs, metamyelocytes, and myelocytes, but there is also a significant increase in the eosinophils and basophils and their precursors. In most cases of chronic myeloid leukaemia (CML) the affected white cells have a short or abnormal chromosome 22 with the characteristic reciprocal translation between chromosomes 9 and 22 (the Philadelphia chromosome, Ph'). There is a slowly progressive normocytic, normochromic anaemia and a gradual fall in platelet count. The bone marrow shows marked proliferation of the myeloid series of cells.

Clinically the patient has immense enlargement of the spleen and a lesser enlargement of the liver. Death usually occurs within 3–5 years, and may be heralded by an *accelerated phase* in which symptoms and leukocytosis increase rapidly. The blood may be flooded by blasts (*blast crisis*).

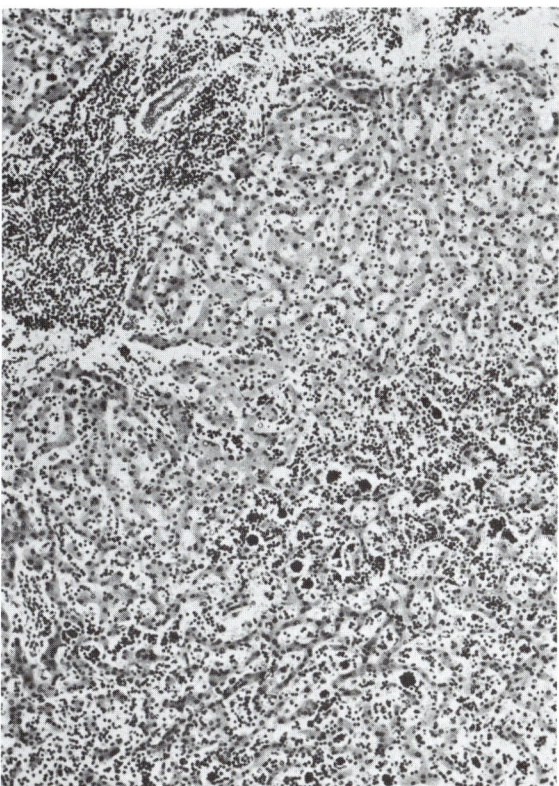

Fig. 26.8 Chronic lymphoblastic leukaemia. Note the dense infiltration of leukaemic cells especially in the portal tracts. There is a less dense infiltration in the sinusoids. × 100.

Chronic lymphocytic leukaemia. This is usually a disease of later life. There is marked lymphocytosis varying from $20–250 \times 10^9$/L. Most of these lymphocytes are mature, and any number of lymphoblasts in the blood is unusual. In a few cases with chronic lymphocytic leukaemia (CLL) the lymphocytes have T-cell markers, but in the majority the lymphocytes are of B-cell type; a subset of these is the uncommon *hairy-cell leukaemia*. There is a progressive nor-mocytic, normochromic anaemia, thrombocyto-penia and neutropenia. The marrow is less affected than in myeloid leukaemia, and it may show no changes at all initially. Later it becomes replaced by lymphocytes.

The condition affects the lymph nodes pri-marily, and the patient usually presents with a generalized lymphadenopathy. Sometimes the tonsils are conspicuously affected, and occasion-ally there is bilateral salivary-gland enlargement. The spleen and liver are enlarged, but to a lesser extent than in myeloid leukaemia. Death usually occurs in 4–6 years, and is due to anaemia and secondary infection.

Acute leukaemia. The various types of acute leukaemia are best considered together, because it is often very difficult to distinguish between them either haematologically or clinically. In acute leukaemia the white-cell count can vary from less than 1×10^9/L up to 100×10^9/L. When there is a raised count the blood is flooded with primitive 'blast' cells.

It is often difficult to identify myeloblasts from lymphoblasts but they can be distinguished by special stains. Furthermore, in some cases of acute myeloblastic leukaemia (AML) some or all of the cells are monoblasts (acute myelomonocytic or acute monocytic leukaemia). Occasionally some or all the cells are erythroblasts (acute erythro-leukaemia or acute erythraemic myelosis). The existance of these many subtypes of AML is a reflection of the common cell origin of the blood cells. The *French–American–British* (FAB) system of classification is based on the cell type involved.

Acute lymphoblastic leukaemia (ALL) can be subdivided on the basis of marker studies. The common type (C-ALL) has pre-B markers, while others have B, T or no (nul) markers.

In cases where the white cell count is very low,

nearly all the circulating leucocytic elements are primitive blast cells. This type of leukaemia may be called 'subleukaemic'. A frankly 'aleukaemic leukaemia', in which there are absolutely no blast cells present in the blood, does occur but is very uncommon.

In acute leukaemia there is a rapidly progressive normocytic, normochromic anaemia and a severe thrombocytopenia. No matter how low the peri-pheral blood count, the marrow is crowded out with 'blast' cells except, of course, during a remission.

Acute leukaemia occurs at all ages, ALL being most common in children and AML in adults. The monocytic variant of AML is a disease of middle age. It is not possible to distinguish clini-cally between these types.

The onset of acute leukaemia is usually sudden, though there may have been a period of preceding malaise with obscure anaemia. The main features are high fever, a generalized bleed-ing tendency due to the thrombocytopenia, progressive anaemia, and necrotic infective lesions which are the result of the poor body resistance accruing from the absence of mature polymorphs (*agranulocytosis*). Oral and faucial lesions are prominent, and sometimes are the first symptoms which bring the patient for treatment. There is painful confluent ulcerative pharyngitis, sto-matitis, and gingivitis (Fig. 26.7). Gross gingival enlargement due to leukaemic infiltration is said to be particularly characteristic of the monocytic variant of acute myeloid leukaemia, but it can occur in the other varieties also.

Most untreated patients die within 3–6 months, usually as a result of infection or bleeding into vital areas such as the central nervous system. Intensive modern therapy has increased the average survival period considerably. As many as 50% of patients may survive 5 years, and perhaps one-third of children with acute lymphoblastic leukaemia can now be cured.

The morbid anatomy of leukaemia

There is a monotonous infiltration of leukaemia cells into numerous organs, which are enlarged, soft, and pale in colour. The lymph nodes, spleen, and bone marrow are particularly likely to be crowded out with the responsible cells. The liver is diffusely infiltrated throughout its sinusoids in chronic myeloid leukaemia, while in the lymphocytic type it is the portal tracts which are mostly involved (Fig. 26.8). The bone marrow is pinkish-grey in colour, and extends down the shafts of the long bones. No organ is exempt, and massive local infiltrations are characteristic of the acute leukaemias. The other changes are those of diffuse haemorrhage and secondary infection.

MULTIPLE MYELOMA (MYELOMATOSIS)

Multiple myeloma is a condition in which a neoplastic proliferation of plasma-cell series occurs in the marrow. It is considered in Chapter 34.

BONE-MARROW APLASIA

When the marrow ceases to release mature elements into the circulation, there is a serious drop in the blood count and the condition is described as *aplasia of the bone marrow*. Sometimes the failure of division occurs at the 'blast' stage, in which case no mature elements are present, but sometimes the failure in division occurs at the later stage of haematopoiesis. In this case the marrow is crowded with maturing cells, but few enter the peripheral blood. This is called 'maturation arrest'.

Aplasia of the marrow may involve all three elements, when it leads to diminution of all the cells of the blood (*pancytopenia*), or it may affect only one of the elements. Pure red-cell aplasia is very uncommon, but aplasia of the granulocytes, or *agranulocytosis*, is an important condition. Pure platelet aplasia probably does not occur.

Pancytopenia

Aplasia affecting all the elements of the marrow (aplastic anaemia) is usually due to an external agent, e.g. *ionizing radiations* or *drugs*, of which the most important are cytotoxic agents used in cancer chemotherapy, gold salts, phenylbutazone and chloramphenicol. It is an occasional complication of *viral hepatitis*, and may be *idiopathic*, in which case it is important to rule out aleukaemic

leukaemia by a careful study of the bone marrow. An occasional cause is *splenic overactivity* (see below).

Haematologically there is a normocytic, normochromic anaemia without any evidence of regeneration in the form of reticulocytes, a leucopenia with neutropenia and a thrombocytopenia. The marrow is usually severely hypocellular, and those cells present are mostly lymphocytes. The prognosis is bad, and most cases die of infection or intractable haemorrhage. In maturation arrest the cellularity may be normal or even increased, and in these cases spontaneous recovery may occur.

Agranulocytosis

Aplasia of the white cells is a very serious complication of certain *drugs*, namely amidopyrine (an analgesic), thiouracil, phenylbutazone, chlorpromazine (a tranquillizer), sulphonamides, pyribenzamine (an antihistamine), and trimethadione (an anticonvulsant). It may follow ionizing radiation and cancer chemotherapy also, but is here part of a more widespread aplasia. Some cases are associated with splenic overactivity, and some are apparently idiopathic.

There is a profound leucopenia, and nearly all the white cells in the blood are lymphocytes. Red cells and platelets are unaffected. The marrow shows inhibition of white-cell production. The leucopenia leads to a serious deficiency in the body's defence mechanism, and ulcerative, infective lesions occur in the mouth and throat, lungs, gastrointestinal tract, and vagina. Death soon occurs from overwhelming infection, and the lesions all show a virtual absence of polymorphs. The cellular infiltration consists of lymphocytes and plasma cells.

Relation of the spleen to blood cells

The spleen is able to modify or remove and destroy defective cells in the circulation. Following a splenectomy abnormal red cells may be found in the peripheral circulation. Other functions are less clear. In some cases of splenomegaly (e.g. secondary to cirrhosis of the liver or Gaucher's disease) there is either a haemolytic anaemia or a drop in the number of blood cells. This has given rise to the concept of *hypersplenism*. Whether it ever occurs as a primary event is very doubtful.

THE SYNDROME OF BONE-MARROW REPLACEMENT

The normal bone marrow is sometimes crowded out by foreign elements. The commonest is *tumour tissue* from skeletal metastases in cancer of the lung, breast, or prostate, or in cases of multiple myeloma. Sometimes the element is a *lipid-filled marcophage*, as in Gaucher's disease, *fibrous tissue* (myelosclerosis), or even *bone*, as in marble-bone disease of childhood, where there is a failure of replacement of osseous tissue by marrow spaces.

Bone-marrow replacement gives a typical blood picture of *leucoerythroblastic anaemia*. This consists of a normocytic, normochromic anaemia in which there are many nucleated red cells (normoblasts) in the blood. There is a moderate to considerable polymorph leucocytosis, and many myelocytes and metamyelocytes are also present in the blood. The main feature of this type of blood picture is thus the presence of both immature red and white cells in the circulation. The platelets may be reduced in number, and giant forms are sometimes present.

THE PLATELETS AND CLOTTING FACTORS

The normal platelet

The platelets are small discs, devoid of a nucleus but with fine intracellular granules. They are derived from the large polyploid *megakaryocytes* by a process of fragmentation of their cytoplasm.

The platelets are important in haemostasis because they readily adhere to damaged vessel walls and thereby prevent haemorrhage. Platelets thus adhere to surfaces and stick to each other, and these properties of *adhesiveness* and *aggregation* have been the subjects of much research because of their possible bearing on the cause of thrombosis (p. 332). Platelets synthesize a variety of prostaglandins, and they play a part in acute inflammation (p. 64) and in thrombosis.

Platelet aggregation

Platelets aggregate immediately in the presence of adenosine diphosphate (ADP). This may be demonstrated in vitro by the addition of ADP to a platelet-rich preparation of plasma which is kept agitated. The aggregation can be detected by measuring the ensuing decrease in optical density. Adrenaline, noradrenaline, and 5-HT have a similar effect. *Thrombin* leads to aggregation, but only after a delay of 5–10 s. It probably acts by converting platelet adenosine triphosphate (ATP) to ADP.

Platelet adhesiveness

Platelets adhere to a variety of foreign surfaces, and the drop in platelet count when blood is passed through a column of glass beads has been used as an in vitro method of measuring platelet adhesiveness. Platelets will also adhere to vascular endothelium if it is damaged mechanically, and to collagen, but not to pure fibrin.

Adherent platelets swell and release a variety of chemicals (*platelet release reaction*), including phospholipid (platelet factor 3, which plays a part in clotting), heparin neutralizing substance (platelet factor 4), 5-HT, and ADP. The last causes platelet aggregation and a small platelet thrombus is built up. This is unstable, and in vivo the platelets may break off and be released into the circulation as small emboli. Though clotting is not involved in the mechanism of platelet adhesiveness, the clotting system is soon activated by platelet factor 3, and by the activation of factor XII. Fibrin is formed, and this stabilizes the platelet thrombus.

Thus following injury, whether extensive or that caused by a pin-prick, the injured vessels are sealed by a mass known as a *haemostatic plug*. At first this consists of platelets, but soon this is consolidated by fibrin formation. Finally the entire aggregate contracts, probably due to the contractile protein in the platelets called *thrombosthenin*. Thrombin released during clotting causes further platelet deposition as well as fibrin formation. Defects in the intrinsic system of blood clotting, such as in haemophilia, do not prevent the formation of a haemostatic plug, and therefore the bleeding time is normal (p. 319).

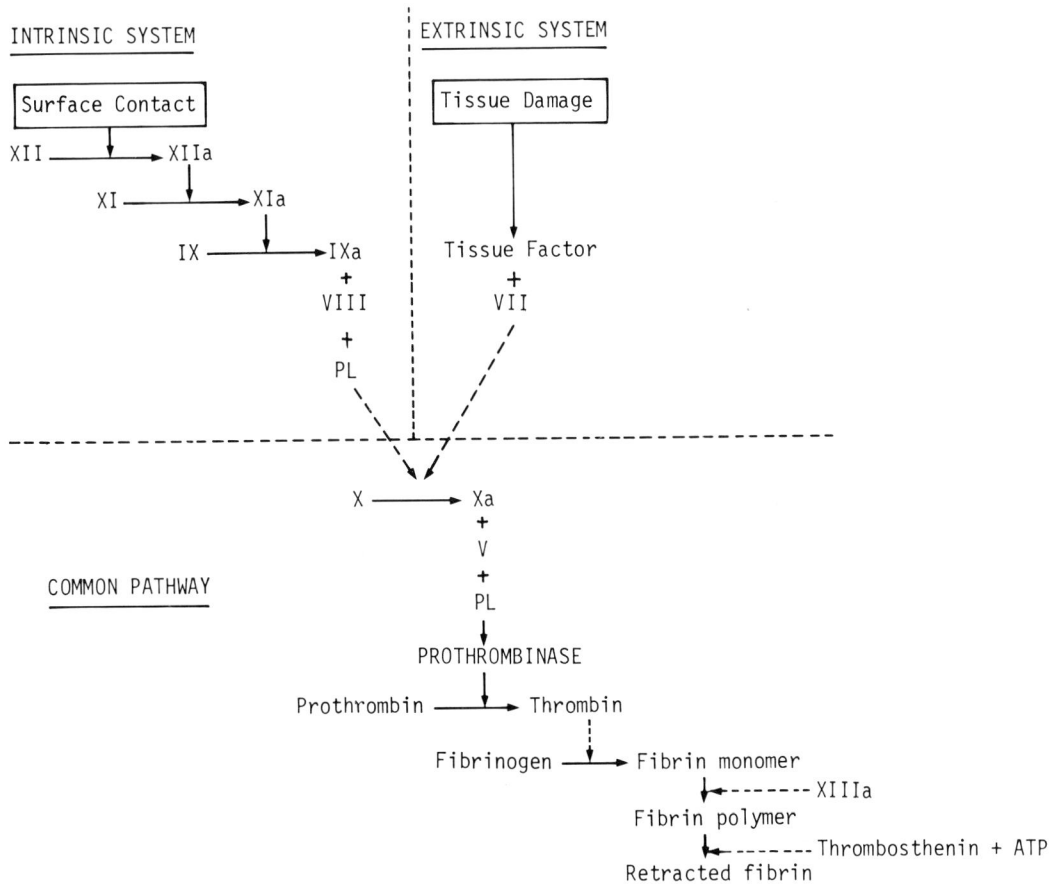

INTRINSIC SYSTEM

Surface Contact

XII ────→ XIIa

XI ────→ XIa

IX ────→ IXa
              +
             VIII
              +
             PL

EXTRINSIC SYSTEM

Tissue Damage

Tissue Factor
      +
     VII

COMMON PATHWAY

X ────→ Xa
          +
          V
          +
          PL
          ↓
     PROTHROMBINASE

Prothrombin ────→ Thrombin

Fibrinogen ────→ Fibrin monomer
                       ←------- XIIIa
                 Fibrin polymer
                       ←------- Thrombosthenin + ATP
                 Retracted fibrin

Fig. 26.9 A simplified diagrammatic representation of the blood clotting mechanism. The three pathways are separated by interrupted lines. Solid arrows indicate transformation, interrupted arrows denote actions. PL denotes platelet factor 3. There is evidence that platelets in conjunction with Factor XII can form a platelet 'tissue-factor' and thereby initiate the extrinsic system. The importance of this in vivo is debatable. Not shown in the diagram is the calcium which is required for most of the steps shown. (After Marcus A J 1969 *New England Journal of Medicine* 280:1213.)

However, the plug is not stable and rebleeding occurs later. Serious bleeding can therefore follow the infliction of a wound such as that caused by dental extraction.

It can be readily understood why a deficiency in platelets or in the clotting mechanism can lead to a bleeding tendency. The normal platelet count is 150 to 440×10^9/L, with an average of 250×10^9/L. It is raised after injuries and operations (especially splenectomy). A count below 100×10^9/L is designated *thrombocytopenia*.

The clotting mechanism

Blood clotting itself is a very complex mechanism

(Fig. 26.9). In essence it consists of a conversion of *fibrinogen (Factor I)* to fibrin by the action of thrombin. This enzyme exists normally as an inert precursor *prothrombin (Factor II)*, which is activated to thrombin by *prothrombinase* which itself is generated by the interaction of activated Factor X (designated Factor Xa) with Factor V, platelet factor 3, and calcium ions (Factor IV). This sequence is called the *common pathway*, and can be initiated by two completely separate mechanisms, the *intrinsic (blood) system* and the *extrinsic (tissue) system* (Figs 26.9 and 26.10).

The intrinsic system. In the *intrinsic (blood) system*, contact with an abnormal surface leads to the activation of Factor XII to Factor XIIa. This

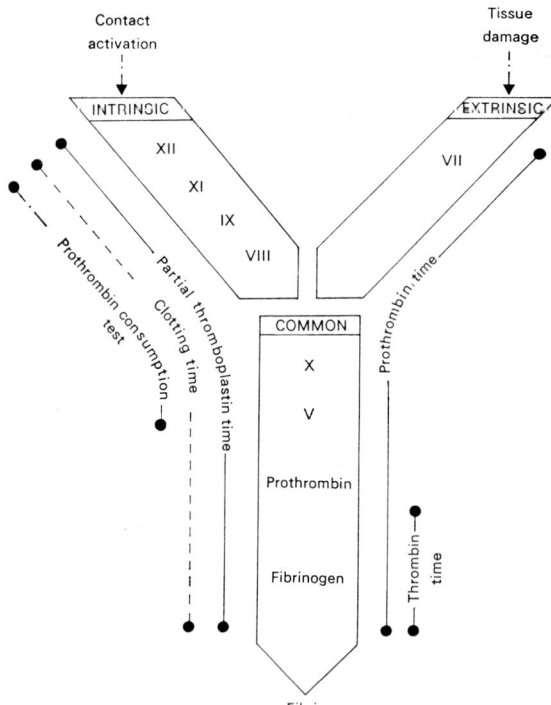

Fig. 26.10 The interpretation of screening tests of blood clotting. (From Bithell T C, Wintrobe M M 1970 In Harrison's Principles of Internal Medicine, 6th edn Fig 62.3. McGraw-Hill, New York, p 323.)

activates Factor XI, and Factor XIa activates Factor IX. Factor IXa in conjunction with Factor VIII and platelet phospholipid, activates Factor X.

The extrinsic system. In the *extrinsic (tissue) system*, tissue damage results in the release of a tissue factor rich in phospholipid. It is called Factor III. This in conjunction with Factor VII activates Factor X, which, as already described, is involved in the production of prothrombinase via the common pathway.

The two pathways of blood clotting are both important, for a derangement of either leads to a serious defect in haemostasis. The intrinsic system develops much more slowly than the extrinsic one, but both are initiated by tissue damage, either by releasing tissue factor or providing an abnormal surface. In both systems there is activation of Factor X, and from then on there is a final common pathway involving Factor V, platelet factor 3, calcium ions, prothrombin, and fibrinogen.

It should be noted that Factors II, VII, IX, X, XI, XII, and XIII are all enzymes; they are of a class called *serine esterases*. Digestive enzymes and complement enzymes are also members of this class. Characteristically they are all stored as an inactive precursor, activated by a given stimulus, and then undergo a cascade-like activation. Thus the activation of the various factors involved in clotting is believed to follow a *cascade sequence*, many of the factors being substrates that are activated by a preceding enzyme.

The earliest phase of the intrinsic system is slow, but once thrombin is formed the process is greatly accelerated—indeed, there is a real cascade, for thrombin potentiates the activity of Factors V and VIII. It also causes platelets to aggregate and so increase the amount of lipid factor 3. This is called the *autocatalytic action of thrombin*. Interestingly, thrombin also destroys Factors V and VIII after potentiating their reactivity; in this way fibrin formation is stopped when a high concentration of thrombin has been achieved.

It should be noted that the plasma clotting factors (all globulins) are given Roman numerals. They are also given alternative names: Factor V is *labile factor*; Factor VII is *stable factor*; Factor VIII is *antihaemophilic factor*; Factor IX is *Christmas factor*; Factor X is *Stuart–Prower factor*; Factor XI is *plasma thromboplastin antecedent*; Factor XII is *Hageman factor*. The personal names refer to the surnames of the patients in whom a deficiency of the particular factor was first described. The latest factor described is Factor XIII (*fibrin-stabilizing factor*), which converts soluble fibrin into insoluble, or stabilized, fibrin.

In order to prevent spontaneous intravascular clotting there are also natural anticoagulant mechanisms. The first natural mode of inhibition of intravascular clotting is the slowness of thrombin formation due to the exclusion of tissue factor and the almost complete absence of prothrominase, which is attributable to the stability of the various clotting factors. Once the vascular endothelium is damaged, there is tendency for intravascular clotting to occur. This is counteracted by the presence of antithrombins which are described below. Fibrin once formed can be removed by the fibrinolytic system.

Antithrombins

Fibrin. At one time fibrin was called antithrombin I. It is an antithrombin in that thrombin is adsorbed by the fibrin fibres.

Antithrombin III. This is by far the most important natural constraint to coagulation. It combines with, and inactivates, most serine esterases. This combination is enhanced by heparin. In fact, antithrombin III is the factor through which heparin exerts its effects, and for this reason is called the *heparin cofactor.*

Heparin. Heparin is a sulphated mucopolysaccharide found in the granules of the mast cells. Its anticoagulant effects involve a preliminary interaction with plasma proteins called *heparin cofactors.* The most important of these is antithrombin III.

Fibrinopeptides (p. 62). These also act as antithrombins.

Protein C. This is an anticoagulant that antagonizes factors V and VIII. It is manufactured in the liver. Protein S is its cofactor.

The fibrinolytic system

Plasminogen is a normal plasma protein that can be activated in a variety of ways to produce the active fibrinolytic enzyme *plasmin.* The major activator of plasminogen is thought to be *kallikrein,* an enzyme that is itself present as an inert precursor form called *prekallikrein.* The fibrinolytic system is activated under a wide range of conditions, e.g. exercise, stress, anaphylaxis, shock, as well as locally whenever fibrin is formed. One may indeed postulate that the fibrinolytic system balances the effects of the clotting system. An imbalance leads to intravascular coagulation on the one hand and afibrinogenaemia on the other (see p. 322).

TESTS OF IMPORTANCE IN THE BLEEDING DISEASES

Platelet count.

Bleeding time. This is the time taken for a small skin puncture to stop bleeding. It varies from 1 to 9 min, and is prolonged when there is a lack of platelets, which, as has been described, are essential for haemostasis.

Clotting time. The time taken for a specimen of whole blood to clot is, at 37°C, about 5–15 min. The clotting time is prolonged if there is a deficiency of any of the factors concerned in the *intrinsic clotting system* or in the *common pathway* (Fig. 26.10). The test is insensitive, and a normal result can be obtained even in the presence of a very low level of some clotting factors. The test is not affected by the level of Factor VII (extrinsic system), but is prolonged when a circulating anticoagulant such as heparin is present in excess. The clotting time is widely used to control heparin therapy. Thrombocytopenia does not increase the clotting time, because only a trace of the platelet lipid factor is necessary for the formation of prothrombinase.

Prothrombin consumption test. The clotting time can be normal even though small amounts of prothrombinase are produced (see above). However, much unused prothrombin will remain, and this can be measured in the prothrombin consumption test. The test measures only those factors required for prothrombin production via the intrinsic system and is more sensitive than the clotting time (Fig. 26.10).

Partial thromboplastin time (PTT). This is the time taken for plasma to clot under the following three conditions:

1. The test is carried out in a glass tube—the surface activates Factor XII
2. A fraction of brain extract called 'cephalin' is added. This provides excess phospholipid and makes the test independent of the platelet count
3. Calcium chloride is added.

The PTT is a sensitive measure of the factors concerned in the *intrinsic* and *common pathways.*

Prothrombin time. In this test equal amounts of brain extract (containing tissue factor), calcium chloride solution, and test plasma are incubated and the time taken for clotting to occur is recorded. A control must be put up at the same time, and this should clot in 10–16 s. The prothrombin time is a measure of the factors concerned in the *extrinsic system* and in the *common pathway.* The intrinsic system is by-passed.

Capillary fragility test. This is performed by inflating the cuff of a blood-pressure manometer to a pressure between the diastolic and systolic for five minutes. If positive, the arm and forearm below the cuff show a petechial eruption. This occurs in platelet deficiency, because normally the platelets seal off any defects caused by a sudden rise in blood pressure. The test is also positive if the vessels themselves are abnormal, e.g. in scurvy.

The four tests which can most easily be carried out as an initial investigation of a patient with a bleeding disease are: the *platelet count*, the *bleeding time*, the *partial thromboplastin time* (PTT) and the *prothrombin time* (PT). If both PTT and PT are normal, the defect is probably in the vessels or the platelets. If either PTT and PT is prolonged, there is probably a defect in the clotting system. If both PTT and PT are abnormal, the defect is most likely in the common pathway. If the PTT is prolonged and the PT is normal, it is the intrinsic system which is most likely at fault. A prolonged PT and a normal PTT is rare, and indicates a deficiency of Factor VII.

In practice, complex defects in haemostasis are best investigated in specialized centres where the activity of each individual factor can be assessed.

THE HAEMORRHAGIC DISEASES

These manifest themselves as bleeding into the tissues. *Petechial haemorrhages* are smaller than 2 mm, *ecchymoses* are larger and flat, while *haematomata* are large and produce a swelling. Petechial haemorrhages into the skin or mucous membranes is called *purpura*. The three factors to be considered in a bleeding disease are the *blood vessels*, the *platelets*, and the *clotting factors*.

Bleeding due to vascular disease

Bleeding may be due to local cause or be a component of a generalized disorder. Lack of vascular support due to dermal atrophy is a common local cause. This is the mechanism of senile purpura, and the ecchymoses that complicate dermal atrophy produced by local or systemic administration of potent steroids. Scurvy is another example.

Generalized purpura due to vascular damage is seen in many severe infections, e.g. scarlet fever, typhus and the haemorrhagic viral fevers. Drugs can cause endothelial damage either directly or by an immune mechanism. *Vasculitis* is an important cause and, because the lesions can be felt due to the inflammatory swelling, the condition is called *palpable purpura*. This may be a component of a drug rash and is probably immune complex mediated. It is sometimes a feature of the collagen vascular disease. Often the cause is not found.

Bleeding due to platelet abnormality

The number of platelets may be decreased (*thrombocytopenia*) or they may be abnormal functionally (*thrombocytopathia*). Manifestations are purpura, but deep haematomata and haemarthroses are not a feature; bleeding from the gingiva, nose and other mucous membranes is common, e.g. causing haematemesis and haematuria; sometimes there is fatal bleeding into internal viscera, especially the brain. Prolonged postoperative bleeding is another danger, but serious bleeding after relatively minor trauma, such as dental extraction, is uncommon. The bleeding time is prolonged, but the clotting time and PTT are normal. The capillary fragility is strongly positive and clot retraction is impaired.

Thrombocytopenia. Thrombocytopenia is a feature of many conditions including aplastic anaemia, leukaemia, drug toxicity, and disseminated intravascular coagulation. In *immune thrombocytopenic purpura (ITP)* there is increased platelet destruction secondary to an autoimmune reaction with the production of IgG anti-platelet antibodies. The sensitized platelets are sequestered and then destroyed in the spleen. The disease occurs as an acute self-limiting disease in young children, and as a more chronic condition in older children and young adults. Other causes of immunological platelet destruction are systemic lupus erythematosus, and some drug-induced thrombocytopenias.

Thrombocyopathia. In thrombocytopathia there is defective platelet function but a normal platelet count. Thrombocytopathia is a feature of several uncommon inherited conditions which will not be considered here. Additionally, there are a number of acquired conditions in which the platelet function is abnormal. Thus the drugs aspirin and indomethacin impair the release reaction and inhibit the production of prostaglandins by platelets. Another important example is uraemia. In all these conditions purpura develops in the face of a normal platelet count but with a prolonged bleeding time.

Bleeding due to defects in the clotting mechanism

Defects in the clotting mechanism are accompanied by extensive bleeding into the joints and deep tissues. Purpura is unusual and initial bleeding from superficial wounds is minimal, but delayed and intractable bleeding is characteristic. Hence serious and even fatal bleeding can occur after dental extraction. The partial thromboplastin time is prolonged, and if the defect is severe, so also is the less sensitive clotting time.

The clotting disorders may be inherited or acquired.

Inherited defects.

Haemophilia A. This disease is due to a deficiency of a component, termed Factor VIIIc, in the larger more complex Factor VIII. It is the classical example of a sex linked recessive trait affecting males only but being carried by unaffected females. However, the disease is more heterogeneous than is commonly supposed, and the severity of the disease varies considerably depending on the plasma Factor-VIIIc level. Within one family, the manifestations are relatively uniform, and sometimes female carriers also have a bleeding tendency.

Haemophilia A is characterized by bleeding from mucous membranes and the formation of deep haematomata, e.g. in the retroperitoneal space, muscles and sometimes within the brain. Bleeding into large joints is characteristic (*haemarthroses*) and eventually the joint spaces are obliterated by fibrous tissue or even bone.

The use of preparations of human Factor VIII has been of great value in the treatment of haemophilia A, but unfortunately the available material was often contaminated with the AIDS virus, and many haemophiliacs were infected.

Current preparations have been rendered safe but this is too late for many sufferers.

Haemophilia B (Christmas disease). This disease is due to a deficiency of Factor IX. Its mode of inheritance and clinical manifestations are indistinguishable from those of haemophilia A. Only by specialized tests can they be separated.

Although the bleeding time is normal in both Haemophilia A and Christmas disease, the haemostatic plug which is formed in injured vessels is not stabilized by fibrin, and continued oozing and rebleeding is characteristic. Any fibrin which is formed tends to be removed by the activation of plasmin.

von Willibrand's disease. This is probably the second most common of the hereditary clotting disorders, but its precise incidence is not known because there are no established criteria for its diagnosis. The clotting disorder is complex and is not completely understood. The disease has features of a combined platelet and clotting-factor defect. Thus mucosal bleeding from the nose and gastrointestinal tract is considerably more common than in haemophilia, but cutaneous petechiae are rare. In severe cases haemarthroses and intramuscular haematomata occur. Posttraumatic and postoperative bleeding is an important feature.

Other bleeding diseases. There are a considerable number of rare inherited bleeding disorders which may manifest as postoperative bleeding. The treatment of all these conditions is basically similar. The deficient factor is replaced by either fresh plasma or some suitable concentrate.

Acquired clotting disorders.
The acquired clotting disorders are not only common but complex because many factors are often involved.

Deficiencies of vitamin-K-dependent factors. Vitamin K is necessary for the synthesis of prothrombin and other clotting factors in the liver. Deficiency may occur through malabsorption particularly in obstructive jaundice. It is also encountered in the newborn particularly of mothers who themselves were deficient. The condition is called *haemorrhagic disease of the newborn.*

Anticoagulants such as dicoumarin are antagonists of vitamin K and are used therapeutically to lessen the chance of intravascular clotting.

Liver disease. A bleeding disorder in liver disease is common and many factors contribute. These include lack of clotting factors manufactured in the liver, increased fibrinolytic activity in the blood, and thrombocytopenia associated with splenomegaly.

Disseminated intravascular coagulation (DIC). Widespread endothelial damage and the entry of coagulation factors into the blood can both initiate intravascular clotting with obstruction of many small vessels and lead to microinfarcts. This can occur as a complication of severe injury and fat embolism. It is a hazard of major surgery particularly if involving the lung or heart. It is a feature of some severe infections especially those due to Gram-negative organisms.

The entry of tissue activators into the circulation can activate the plasmin system. Not only is fibrin digested but so also are fibrinogen and other clotting factors. The blood becomes incoagulable, and bleeding such as from a surgical wound results. The condition is called the *fibrinolytic syndrome* and can occur under a variety of circumstances—following major surgery, in liver disease and as a complication of pregnancy. DIC and the fibrinolytic syndrome have much in common and both may occur together with evidence of vascular obstruction combined with a bleeding disorder. The term *consumptive coagulopathy* is sometimes used as an alternative to DIC since it embodies the concept that many clotting factors are consumed.

BLOOD GROUPS

The red cells contain many antigens, but for practical purposes those concerned with the ABO and Rhesus blood groups are the most important.

The ABO system. The antigens concerned are glycoproteins. The basic antigen is called the H substance. Under the influence of the *A* and *B* genes, it is converted into A and B substances, depending on the presence of either or both genes. At birth there are no corresponding antibodies in the plasma, but within 3–6 months the antibodies corresponding to the antigen *not present* make their appearance. These are called *alloantibodies*, and are capable of agglutinating the red cells of normal people who are of a different blood group, but not those of the same blood group as that of the individual.

The following table describes the distribution of ABO antigens and antibodies:

Blood group	Antibody normally present in plasma
A	anti-B
B	anti-A
AB	none
O	anti-A and anti-B

Why these antibodies develop is not certain. It is known that many Gram-negative intestinal bacilli have high concentrations of blood-group specific substances, and it is possible that the infant forms antibodies against those to which it is not immunologically tolerant.

To perform a blood grouping it is necessary to treat a suspension of red cells with 'anti-A' and 'anti-B' serum (derived from a donor with a high titre of these antibodies). If 'anti-A' serum causes agglutination of the cells, they are group A; if 'anti-B' does it, they are group B. If they are agglutinated by both, they are group AB, and if by neither, they are group O. Although group-O cells contain H substance, anti-H is rarely present in the plasma of group-A and group-B subjects in sufficient strength to cause a significant reaction in the body. It will be noted that the naturally-occurring ABO antibodies are of the IgM class and 'complete', i.e. they agglutinate red cells in saline suspension (p. 309).

The Rhesus system. About 85% of the white population of the world have a red-cell antigen which was first noted in Rhesus-monkey red cells. It is called the *Rh antigen*, and cells that contain it are described as Rh-positive. Rh-negative individuals do not normally have Rh antibodies in their plasma (cf. the ABO system), but if they are immunized by Rh-positive red cells, they form antibodies very easily. Such immunization may follow a mismatched blood transfusion, or occur after the pregnancy of a Rh-negative woman bearing a Rh-positive fetus (p. 309).

Rh-grouping is done by suspending the red cells in serum obtained from a pregnant woman with a high titre of complete Rh antibody. Rh-positive cells undergo agglutination.

BLOOD TRANSFUSION

Indications

Blood transfusion is an essential procedure in clinical practice. Not only is it mandatory for restoring the blood volume after *severe haemorrhage*, but it is also used extensively in *major operative procedures*. The administration of packed red cells plays a part in the treatment of *severe anaemia* of whatever cause, but if possible this should be treated with the specific agent, e.g. iron, vitamin B_{12}, etc., unless the patient's life is in danger. Various blood components are available from transfusion centres, and these are useful in *restoring deficient clotting factors*, such as Factor VIII, prothrombin, and fibrinogen. Platelet and granulocyte transfusions are used in specialized centres only.

Storage of blood

Blood is collected aseptically from a healthy donor into a plastic bag in which there is an anticoagulant. The one most used is ACD, a mixture of citric **a**cid, trisodium **c**itrate, and **d**extrose. Blood is stored at 4°C, and must not be allowed to freeze or to exceed 10°C. It can be stored for periods up to 3 weeks. Up to this time most of the red cells survive in the recipient as well as do fresh cells.

Cross-matching

The important elements are the donor's red cells and the recipient's plasma. With rare exceptions the donor's plasma is not important, because the antibodies it contains are so diluted by the recipient's plasma that they are not likely to react with the recipient's cells. It is always preferable to use blood of exactly the same ABO and Rhesus groups as those of the recipient, but group-O blood can be used if necessary, provided it is properly cross-matched. Group O is called the 'universal donor', because it is not normally agglutinated by any serum. In extreme emergencies, where delay might lead to death from exsanguination, it is permissible to use uncross-matched group-O Rh-negative blood, but otherwise cross-matching is essential, because (1) there may be an error in sample identification, and (2) the recipient's serum may contain antibodies other than anti-A, anti-B, and anti-Rhesus.

Technique of cross-matching. (1) Mix a 2% suspension of donor cells and recipient serum at room temperature for 1 h. Absence of agglutination rules out a 'complete' antibody. (2) Mix the cells and serum at 37°C for 1 h. Then centrifuge the cells, wash them three times in saline, and suspend them in an antiglobulin serum (indirect antiglobulin or Coomb's test). Absence of agglutination rules out an 'incomplete' antibody.

Hazards of blood transfusion

Haemolytic transfusion reactions are usually due to the rapid destruction of the donor red cells by antibodies in the recipient's plasma, and are generally the result of transfusion of ABO incompatible blood, for example group A red cells into a group O recipient. *These mishaps are almost always due to an error in the identification of the patient, a specimen, or the unit of blood, rather than a technical failure to detect incompatibility.* The antigen–antibody reaction leads to the release of vasoconstrictor substances from the red cells, which cause widespread vascular phenomena. There is initial pain along the vein, and this is followed by facial flushing, headache, a sensation of constriction around the chest, and backache. A danger is severe renal arterial spasm with ischaemia of the kidneys. Free haemoglobin in the plasma causes mild renal vasoconstriction, and the presence of vasoconstrictor substances (as well as the original condition that necessitated transfusion) accentuates this markedly. ABO incompatibility leads to much more severe renal effects than does Rh incompatibility, and death from uraemia may occur.

Bacterial contamination of the blood due to the adventitious introduction of coliform organisms leads to fatal septicaemia.

Diseases introduced from the donor, the most important of which are AIDS, viral hepatitis (B and non-A, non-B) and syphilis.

Febrile reactions are usually due to the presence of white-cell antibodies formed by the recipient as a result of previous transfusions or pregnancy. Another cause is pyrogens present in the bottles, tubing, or anticoagulant fluid. The fever is sharp, but usually lasts only a few hours.

Allergic reactions, usually urticarial are not uncommon, and are due to some antigen in the donor's plasma to which the recipient is hypersensitive. Life-threatening acute anaphylaxis is rare. Allergic reactions may also be due to the presence of IgE in the plasma of the donor.

Overloading of the circulation, leading to heart failure.

Air embolism is very rare with modern equipment.

Thrombophlebitis following the local irritation of the vein by the needle.

Transfusional haemosiderosis occurs when repeated transfusions are given frequently over a long period of time. There is a gradual accumulation of iron pigment which is not used in erythropoiesis, and it is deposited in the tissues (particularly the liver), where it may set up fibrosis.

Sensitization: the transfusion of blood carrying antigens not present in the recipient's cells may stimulate the production of alloantibodies directed against the foreign antigen. These alloantibodies to red-cell, white-cell, platelet, or plasma-protein antigens may complicate future transfusions or pregnancies.

In modern centres blood transfusion is lifesaving procedure. However, the possible complications are numerous, and except under emergency conditions, transfusion should never be attempted without expert supervision.

GENERAL READING

Clark S C, Kamen R 1987 The human hematopoietic colony-stimulating factors. Science 236:1229

Quesenberry P, Levitt L 1979 Hematopoietic stem cells. New England Journal of Medicine 301:755, 819, 868

Winlow R M, Anderson W F 1983 The hemoglobinopathies. In: Stanbury JB, et al (eds), The metabolic basis of inherited disease, 5th edn. McGraw Hill, New York

Wintrobe M M, et al 1981 Clinical hematology, 8th edn Lea and Febiger, Philadelphia

27. Disorders of the circulation

The function of the circulatory system is the maintenance of adequate perfusion of blood to all the tissues of the body. Each ventricular contraction ejects a quantity of blood into the arterial system, and in the systemic system the expansion of the elastic arteries prevents an undue rise in pressure. Nevertheless, the arterial pressure rises to a maximum (normally 120–150 mmHg), and during the subsequent diastole it falls steadily as blood flows away through the arterioles to the various vascular beds. The lowest pressure (diastolic pressure) reached is generally 60–90 mmHg. The major resistance encountered by the blood is in the arterioles, so that by the time the capillaries are reached, the pressure is about 30 mmHg. The blood flow in the major arteries is pulsatile. The elasticity of the major vessels and the high resistance provided by the arterioles reduce this pulsation, so that in the capillaries and veins the blood flow is constant. It follows that whereas blood escapes from capillaries and veins in a constant ooze, it spurts out when an artery is cut.

Disorders of the circulation will be considered under two headings: those that involve changes in the circulation as a whole, and those where the changes and effects are local.

CHANGES IN THE CIRCULATION AS A WHOLE

These changes can be considered under three headings: hypertension, the general reaction to trauma including the effects of haemorrhage, and shock—these have been considered in Chapter 25—and changes which involve the body's fluids and their distribution between the circulating blood and the extravascular tissues.

HYPERTENSION

The physiological mechanisms involved in maintaining the blood pressure will not be described in detail. In the main they involve the regulation of arteriolar tone by the autonomic division of the nervous system in response to stimuli from the aortic and carotid baroreceptors.

A considerable rise in the blood pressure in the system circulation is a normal response to emotional and physical stimulation. A persistent or recurrent elevation of the blood pressure at rest is abnormal, and is termed *hypertension*. Two types are recognized.

Primary, or essential, hypertension

This is the common form of high blood pressure, and its cause is unknown. It is a condition that is more common in women than in men, and is especially prevalent in North American blacks. Primary renal or adrenal abnormalities have been postulated but never proven.

Secondary hypertension

Hypertension is characteristic of phaeochromocytoma, where it is due to the effects of adrenaline and noradrenaline produced by the tumour (p. 437). Hypertension is also seen in some adrenal cortical tumours, and is an accompaniment of both Conn's and Cushing's syndromes (p. 437). The most common cause of secondary hypertension is renal disease.

The classical experiments of Goldblatt proved that in the dog an obstruction to the renal arterial blood flow could produce hypertension. This is due to the release from the kidney of the proteolytic enzyme *renin*, which acts on a plasma globulin, *angiotensinogen,* converting it into *angiotensin I*, and this in turn is converted into *angiotensin II*. These angiotensins are vasoconstrictors and also stimulate aldosterone secretion with its attendant retention of salt and water.

In the human, hypertension sometimes, but not always, occurs in acute and chronic glomerulonephritis, pyelonephritis, and other renal diseases. It is not certain whether the mechanism of its production is similar to that of the Goldblatt experiments; present evidence is against such a pathogenesis. Hypertension in unilateral renal lesions is sometimes relieved by nephrectomy, but unfortunately this is not always so.

Effects and complications of hypertension

Haemorrhage. Weakened blood vessels tend to rupture more commonly in the hypertensive subject than in the normal; dissecting aneurysm of the aorta, ruptured berry aneurysms of the circle of Willis, and cerebral haemorrhage are all more common in the hypertensive subject.

Atherosclerosis. Systemic hypertension is an important contributing factor in the production of atherosclerosis with all its attendant complications.

Arteriolosclerosis. The small arteries and arterioles of many organs show thickening of their walls, particularly the tunica intima, with hyaline material. The afferent arterioles of the kidney are commonly affected and the glomeruli are slowly destroyed—the result is *benign nephrosclerosis.* When the retinal vessels are affected ischaemic changes lead to *hypertensive retinopathy.*

Heart failure. Systemic hypertension causes left ventricular hypertrophy and ultimately left ventricular failure.

Malignant hypertension

Hypertension, whether primary or secondary, may occasionally evolve into a malignant phase. The blood pressure becomes very high, causing necrosis of the arteriolar walls (*malignant arteriolosclerosis*). The kidneys and the brain are the two organs most severely affected. In the kidney glomerular destruction causes haemorrhage and culminates in uraemia (*malignant nephrosclerosis*). In the brain the changes cause haemorrhage and oedema. Swelling of the optic discs (*papilloedema*) is a useful sign of raised intracranial pressure; symptoms include mental confusion and seizures. The syndrome of malignant hypertension usually progresses rapidly over a period of weeks, and unless treated expeditiously results in death from uraemia, heart failure, or an intracranial vascular accident.

CHANGES IN THE BODY'S FLUIDS

About 72% of the lean body weight consists of water. It amounts to 42 litres in a normal adult man weighing 70 kg, and of this two-thirds (28 litres) are intracellular, and the remaining third (14 litres) extracellular. The latter has two components: the extravascular *interstitial fluid* which comprises 11.2 litres, and the *plasma volume* which is 2.8 litres.

Fluid balance

The total water content of the body is maintained by balancing the fluid output with the intake.

This important homeostatic mechanism is not completely understood, and a textbook of physiology should be consulted for the details. It may, however, be noted that fluid balance is controlled by three factors:

1. Indirectly, by the mechanisms that regulate sodium balance. Sodium cannot be retained without water. *Aldosterone* secreted by the adrenal cortex has the effect of increasing sodium reabsorption by the distal tubule of the kidney, and thereby causes water retention. Sodium reabsorption from the proximal tubule is dependent to a large extent on the total glomerular filtrate. When the volume is reduced, as in shock and heart failure, sodium absorption is more complete, and water is therefore also retained.

2. The mechanisms that regulate the output of water by the kidney. The antidiuretic hormone (ADH) from the posterior lobe of the pituitary is important in this connexion. It acts by increasing water absorption from the collecting tubules of the kidney.

3. Regulation of the water intake by the sensation of thirst.

Water is freely diffusible across the barriers which separate the various compartments (Fig. 27.1). The volume in each is preserved by the osmotic, electrochemical, and hydrostatic forces which are acting upon it. As far as osmosis is concerned potassium, phosphate, and protein are important in the intracellular compartment, while in the interstitial and intravascular spaces sodium, chloride, and bicarbonate have the greatest influence.

Water and sodium metabolism are so closely interrelated that it is convenient to consider them together.

Disturbances in water and sodium balance

Pure water deficiency. This follows the deprivation of water, e.g. in people who cannot swallow because of oesophageal obstruction or coma, and during enforced starvation. It is also seen in *diabetes insipidus*, which is due to a lack of ADH. Patients with this disease pass enormous quantities of urine, e.g. 20 litres per day instead of the normal 1 to 1.5 litres.

Effects. Since water can cross the membranes which separate the fluid compartments, they are all depleted. The largest compartment, the intracellular space, is the most severely affected, and the cellular dehydration causes intense thirst and eventually death.

Pure water excess. The converse condition, water intoxication, or cellular oedema, occurs when excess water is absorbed and retained. This may be seen in patients to whom too much water is given intravenously (as glucose solution), a situation particularly liable to arise during the postoperative period when water excretion is impaired and in acute renal failure (p. 394.). The effects of water excess are serious. There is vomiting, muscle cramps, headache, convulsions, and sometimes death.

Combined salt and water deficiency. Salt,

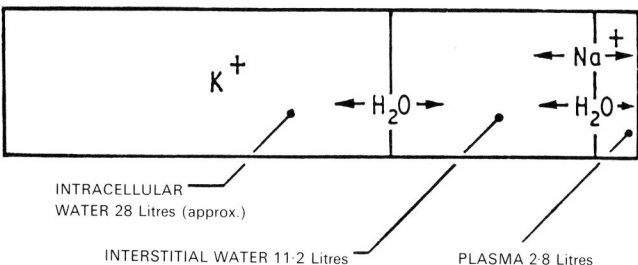

Fig. 27.1 Diagrammatic representation of the three compartments in which the body's water is accommodated. An excess or deficiency of water, which is freely diffusible, produces the greatest effects in the largest compartment, the intracellular one, whereas changes in sodium affect mainly the volume of the interstitial fluid.

or salt and water, deficiency is seen when there is loss from:

The gastrointestinal tract, e.g. severe vomiting or diarrhoea,

The skin, due to prolonged excessive sweating (heat-exhaustion),

The kidney, e.g. following prolonged administration of diuretics for chronic heart failure.

Effects. The effect of salt deficiency is the undermining of the osmotic support of the extracellular fluid. The interstitial fluid volume is reduced in amount, and therefore the patient shows *dehydration.* The eyeballs are sunken, the skin wrinkled, the tongue dry and the face haggard. Thirst is often absent. Despite a compensatory vasoconstriction, the blood pressure is low and the veins are poorly filled. Little urine is passed, and there is a reduction in the plasma volume, which is evidenced by a rise in the packed cell volume and haemoglobin concentration (haemoconcentration). Unless relieved the condition rapidly terminates in circulatory failure.

Combined salt and water excess. This is another artificially induced condition, and is seen in patients with defective renal function who are given excessive amounts of saline solution, e.g. during the early postoperative period, or during the course of acute renal failure.

Effects. The fluid is distributed evenly throughout the extracellular compartment which therefore becomes expanded. The manifestations are those of increased venous pressure and oedema, both systemic and pulmonary; in due course pulmonary oedema will kill the patient.

Oedema

Oedema may be defined as an excessive extravascular accumulation of fluid. In its usual context it is applied to the morbid accumulation of fluid in the interstitial tissues. It is particularly liable to occur in the various preformed serous sacs, giving rise to *ascites, hydrothorax,* and *hydropericardium,* as effusions into the peritoneal, pleural, and pericardial cavities are specifically called. When generalized, it is called *anasarca,* or *dropsy.* It is, of course, also possible to have intracellular

oedema as in hydropic degeneration and in pure water intoxication, but for the remainder of this discussion only the interstitial type will be considered. It is necessary first to understand the normal mechanisms which regulate the distribution of fluid in the body.

Mechanism of normal control in the systemic circulation

Starling postulated that the movement of fluid between vessels and the extravascular spaces was determined by the balance of the hydrostatic and osmotic forces acting upon it (Fig. 5.1).

The forces tending to move fluid out of the blood vessels. *The hydrostatic pressure in the vessels.* This is generally accepted as 32 mmHg at the arterial end of the capillary and 12 mmHg at the venous end in the skin of the human subject at heart level.

The colloidal osmotic pressure, also called the oncotic pressure, of the interstitial fluid. Since the vascular wall is completely permeable to water and crystalloids, the only effective osmotic forces are those due to the colloids, mainly proteins. The interstitial fluids normally have a low protein content, and this is therefore not an important factor in the formation of the extravascular fluids under normal conditions. Furthermore those proteins which do escape into the tissue spaces are normally removed by the lymphatics.

The forces moving fluid into the blood vessels. *The tissue tension.* This is low (3–4 mmHg). Tissue tension is important in relation to the distribution of oedema; for instance lax areas like the face, particularly around the eyelids, the ankles, sacrum, and scrotum, tend to accumulate fluid, while tense areas, like the palms and soles, are never the site of marked oedema. A rise in tissue tension is probably an important factor in limiting interstitial-tissue fluid formation in the legs under normal conditions and also in acutely inflamed parts.

The osmotic pressure (oncotic pressure) of the plasma proteins. The osmotic pressure of plasma proteins is about 25 mmHg, and is due largely to albumin. Since the plasma proteins cannot normally pass through the vessel walls, the vascular permeability is important in regulating the distribution of fluids between the intravascular and the extravascular compartments. In the event of an increase in permeability, an exudate is formed which is rich in protein, e.g. in acute inflammation.

There are indeed two types of oedema:

An exudate, the accumulation of fluid due to an increased vascular permeability, such as occurs in inflammation—the fluid contains a high percentage of protein due to the increased vascular permeability.

A transudate, the accumulation of fluid due to a hydrostatic imbalance between the intravascular and the extravascular compartments, despite normal vascular permeability. It has a low protein content.

The importance of the lymphatics should not be forgotten. They form an elaborate network in most tissues, and their function is to drain away fluid and protein. The lymph is of considerably higher protein content than is the interstitial fluid itself.

The various factors involved in Starling's hypothesis are depicted in Fig. 5.1 (p. 53). It must be realized, however, that this merely represents an average state of affairs found in many capillaries at the level of the heart. Pressures in individual vessels show considerable variation.

Types of oedema

When considering the cause of any type of oedema, it should be realized that the process is usually due to a combination of factors. Starling himself appreciated this, and stated that dropsy was probably never due to a derangement of a single mechanism acting alone.

Oedema can be classified into local and generalized (widespread) types. The local oedemas are the simplest ones to understand because there are usually fewer factors involved in their production.

Local oedema. Acute inflammatory oedema is covered elsewhere (p. 53).

Hypersensitivity (allergic oedema). Oedema due to an increase in vascular permeability is present in all lesions of anaphylactic and immune-complex hypersensitivity. The oedema of anaphylaxis is widespread. Oedema is also seen in the acute inflammatory response of type-IV hypersensitivity.

Venous obstruction. A rise in venous pressure leads to an increase in capillary pressure, and the result is the formation of a transudate. This is seen in the legs following thrombophlebitis.

Lymphatic oedema. Extensive lymphatic obstruction can produce an oedema of rather high protein content, although not nearly as high as that of an exudate. Chronic lymphatic oedema stimulates an overgrowth of fibrous tissue, and in due course there is fibrous tissue and epithelial hyperplasia so that the affected part becomes grossly enlarged. If marked this is called *elephantiasis*. It is seen in the leg in filariasis due to the obstruction of the lymphatics by a nematode worm. A similar effect is sometimes caused by recurrent bacterial lymphangitis. Lymphoedema may occur in the arm, when the lymphatics of the axilla are obstructed by cancer of the breast or by the fibrosis which may follow radiotherapy.

Primary lymphoedema is a special variety of lymphatic oedema due to a malformation of the lymphatics of the lower limbs. Women are usually the victims. One type of primary lymphoedema is hereditary and congenital, and is called *Milroy's disease*.

Generalized oedema. *Cardiac oedema.* In right-sided and congestive cardiac failure there is a retention of sodium and water by the body as evidenced by an increase in body weight. The distribution of this fluid is influenced by gravity. When the patient is ambulant the legs are affected first, and swelling of the ankles is often the initial symptom; when recumbent the oedema appears in the sacral and genital areas. The oedema readily pits on pressure.

Renal oedema. Acute glomerulonephritis. Oedema particularly affecting the face and eyelids is often the first symptom of this disease. It is due to water retention by the damaged kidney, but its facial distribution is unexplained

Nephrotic syndrome. The outstanding feature of this is proteinuria with hypoproteinaemia. On Starling's hypothesis the diminished osmotic pressure of the plasma proteins can easily explain the generalized oedema, and this is undoubtedly an important factor. However, there are other considerations. A salt-free diet reduces the oedema, especially if combined with diuretics. It seems likely that salt and water retention, perhaps due to an oversecretion of aldosterone, is also important.

Famine oedema (nutritional oedema). The oedema that is seen after prolonged starvation is usually confined to the legs. At first sight it would seem to be explicable in terms of the marked hypoalbuminaemia which is usually present, but there is no close correlation between the level of the plasma proteins and the presence of oedema. The true explanation of famine oedema is not known. An important factor appears to be the loss of compact tissue, mostly fat, and its replacement by a loose connective tissue in which fluid can accumulate without a rise in tissue tension.

Hypoalbuminaemic oedema. Oedema is a feature of severe hypoalbuminaenia (see kwashiorkor (p. 206)).

Generalized oedema and ascites in cirrhosis of the liver. These are considered in Chapter 32.

Unexplained oedema. Generalized oedema sometimes occurs in the absence of any known cause, and although such cases are uncommon, they indicate that factors other than those already discussed may operate even in the common types of oedema. A well-recognized condition is *cyclical,* or *periodic, oedema,* in which there are recurrent attacks of oedema involving skin, mucous membranes, joints, or even internal organs. If the skin and subcutaneous tissues are affected the condition is called *angio-oedema;* one variety is familial and is associated with a deficiency of the C1-esterase inhibitor of the complement system. How the attacks are precipitated is not clear but activation of the kinin system is probably involved. Apart from skin and gut lesions, acute oedema of the larynx may occur and threaten life. In the very common condition of *urticaria* or hives, there is oedema confined to a localized area of the dermis. Attacks may be immunologically mediated, but often no cause can be found.

Oedema associated with oestrogens. Administration of oestrogens is associated with retention of fluid and a similar event may be apparent in some women in the premenstrual period.

Pulmonary oedema. This is considered in Chapter 30.

Although dropsy has been recognized as a symptom of disease since the beginning of medical history, it is evident that the mode of its formation is complex. In patients under hypnosis it is sometimes possible by suggestion to produce oedema at the site of previous injury. The mechanism is completely unknown, and it is therefore no surprise to find that the mode of production of oedema in such simple conditions as acute inflammation and heart failure is incompletely understood.

LOCAL CIRCULATORY CHANGES

THROMBOSIS

In the vascular system the platelets and the clotting mechanism guard against the danger of haemorrhage. Minor degrees of injury are constantly being sustained by blood vessels, and a layer of platelets is soon laid down to prevent haemorrhage. Endothelial cells cover this platelet deposit so that the smooth lining of the vessel is restored, further deposition ceases, and the process is brought to an end. The presence of naturally occurring anticoagulant substances, like heparin and antithrombin III, and the constant bathing by the stream of blood, tend to prevent clotting. Nevertheless, small quantities of fibrin are probably formed even under normal conditions, and there exists a *fibrinolytic mechanism* for its removal (p. 319). The active agent *plasmin* is formed on the fibrin threads and leads to their dissolution. Thus, three mechanisms normally prevent the intravascular accumulation platelets and fibrin:

1. Endothelialization of both platelet deposits and areas of damage
2. The fibrinolytic system
3. Factors that limit the deposition of platelets (see below).

Under abnormal conditions an excessive deposit of platelets and fibrin may be formed, and this endangers the circulation by causing obstruction This is *thrombosis.*

Pathogenesis of thrombus formation

Thrombosis may be defined as the formation of a

solid mass in the circulation from the constituents of the streaming blood. The mass itself is
called a *thrombus*. Thrombosis involves two distinct processes:

***The deposition of platelets on a vascular
surface.*** This occurs under three circumstances:

1. When the endothelial lining is damaged or
   removed.
2. With vascular stasis, when the platelets fall
   out of the axial stream and impinge on the
   wall
3. In association with turbulence when eddy
   currents deflect the platelets on to the wall.

Whenever any of these three factors operates to
an excessive extent, an abnormal mass of platelets is formed. This is a *pale*, or *platelet, thrombus*.

Platelets do not adhere to a normal intact
endothelial surface; although this may be due to
the active blood flow sweeping them along, there
is also a possibility that a chemical mechanism is
involved. This involves the formation of thromboxane A_2 and prostacyclin, and is described
below together with the role of the prostaglandins
in thrombosis.

***The formation of a clot of fibrin in which
the blood cells are trapped.*** If the platelet
thrombus is not speedily endothelialized, or if
there is stasis, blood clot is formed, and in its
meshes are trapped the red and white cells.
Thrombin is potent in causing platelets to adhere
to each other, and its liberation during the process of coagulation readily leads to a further
deposition of platelets. In this way a large mass is
built up. When blood clot is the major component, it is called a *red*, or *coagulation, thrombus*.
Frequently the thrombosis is made up of both
red clot and pale platelet components, and is
then called a *mixed thrombus*.

The crucial feature of thrombosis is the deposition of platelets on a vascular surface. This can
occur only in the presence of a flowing stream,
and is therefore produced spontaneously only in
the living animal. The clotting is a secondary
phenomenon. It follows that the terms 'clot' and
'thrombus' are quite distinct; a thrombus contains a variable amount of clot, but the important
feature is a platelet scaffold which is lacking in a
clot; it can be formed only in vivo. Clotting, on

the other hand, may occur as part of thrombosis,
and is also seen in a column of static blood in
vivo or in vitro.

Since the cardinal process in thrombosis is the
deposition of platelets on an intimal surface, it is
evident that the integrity of the vascular system is
all-important in preventing it. The two factors are:

1. The smooth endothelial lining which diminishes frictional resistance between the wall and
   the circulating blood, and
2. the streamline of blood along the complex circulatory pathways, which results in the formed
   elements moving in a central axial stream (p.
   52).

The speed of flow prevents local stasis, and the
absence of irregularities in the walls avoids turbulence. The streamline of blood can be threatened
in a variety of ways, which are illustrated in Fig.
27.2. These lesions all lead to local stasis as well
as to the formation of eddy currents, and the
platelets that cover them are actually performing
a remedial function. They serve to smooth out
the contours of the wall and restore the streamline of blood in the vessel. The small amount of
clotting factors that they generate is dissipated in
the flowing blood, and they themselves are rapidly endothelialized. It is when this process is
retarded that the platelet mass grows, clotting
factors accumulate, much fibrin is produced, and
thrombosis proceeds even to the extent of oblit-
erating the vessel lumen.

Role of the vascular endothelium

Although traditionally the role of the endothelium has been related to its mechanical effect
of forming a smooth lining in the blood vessels, it
is now realized that endothelial cells play a much
more complex role in relation to the circulation.

The endothelium has a definite anticoagulant
function. Its cells secrete a heparin-like substance
which enhances the action of antithrombin III,
itself the most important anticoagulant in the
blood. Thrombomodulin is a cell-surface protein
found on endothelial cells. It binds thrombin and
accelerates the activation of protein C. Activated
protein C is a potent anticoagulant which acts by
proteolytic cleavage of factors V and VIII, and in

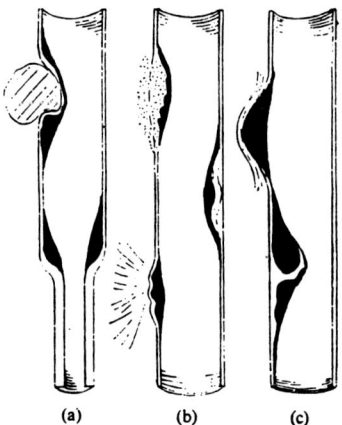

Fig. 27.2 This diagram shows seven different causes of a disruption of the normal streamlining of the blood flow, and the manner whereby platelets (shown in black) are laid down to restore the architecture. (a) Bulging due to external pressure and spasm. (b) Endothelial swelling and roughening due to inflammation, a plaque of thickening, e.g. atheroma, and corrugation due to adjacent cicatrization. (c) Aneurysm, and a hard sclerotic valve. (From Hadfield G 1950 *Annals of the Royal College of Surgeons of England* 6:219.)

addition stimulates the release of plasminogen from endothelial cells. Protein S, also secreted by endothelial cells, is its cofactor.

Endothelial cells secrete many other compounds related to the maintenance of the circulation, regulating vascular tone and prevention of thrombosis. These secretions include fibronectin, heparin sulphate, interleukin-1, tissue plasminogen activator which promotes fibrinolysis, various growth-promoting factors, platelet-activating factor, endothelin-1, *prostaglandins*, *endothelium-derived relaxing factors*, and *endothelium-derived contracting factors*. Imbalance between these various secretions is an important mechanism involved in the pathogenesis of diseases of the circulatory system. Three important members will be described.

Derivatives of arachidonic acid–prostaglandins. The prostaglandins are potent agents synthesized from *arachidonic acid* which is released from cell-membrane phospholipid by the action of phospholipase A_2. The enzyme cyclo-oxydase converts arachidonic acid into the two unstable *prostaglandin endoperoxides*, PGG_2 and PGH_2. In platelets these endoperoxides are converted into *thromboxane A_2* (TXA_2), which is a powerful agent that causes vasoconstriction and platelet aggregation (Fig. 27.3). (see also page 63.)

When platelets adhere to a vessel wall TXA_2 is formed, platelet aggregation is encouraged, and a platelet thrombus is formed. However, the endoperoxides formed by the platelets can also be used by cells of the vessel walls; these cells convert the endoperoxides into *prostacyclin* (PGI_2), which is a vasodilator and can inhibit platelet aggregation. A balance between the formation of thrombaxane A_2 by the platelets and prostacyclin by the vessel wall may well be an important factor in determining the extent of thrombus formation. Damage to a vessel wall may impede prostacyclin formation and thereby encourage thrombus formation.

The vessel wall synthetizes prostacyclin from its own precursors, as well as from endoperoxides released by platelets. Thus the continuous formation of prostacyclin may be an important homeostatic mechanism whereby platelets which are forced on to the vascular endothelium (or on areas of minimal damage) are prevented from building up an abnormal platelet thrombus. Prostacyclin in the circulation, partially derived from the lungs, appears to be an additional protective mechanism. When it is remembered that platelet deposition on arterial walls is thought to be a major factor in the pathogenisis of atherosclerosis, it will be readily understood why research into the formation and properties of the prostaglandins is currently so active.

Endothelium-derived relaxing factors (EDRF). Acetylcholine causes contractionof isolated blood vessel smooth muscle but it is a powerful vasodilator in the intact animal because it acts indirectly by causing the release of *endothelium-derived relaxing factor (EDRF)* from endothelial cells. This has now been identified as *nitric oxide*. EDRF is rapidly inactivated by haemoglobin and its action is therefore entirely a local or paracrine effect. By a similar action on platelets, EDRF also inhibits their aggregation and adhesion. Under normal conditions, the continual release of EDRF leads to a base-line vasodilatation; a breakdown in its production may be a factor in the pathogenesis of hypertension. As a matter of interest, it should be noted that the formation of nitric oxide from organic nitrates (such as nitroglycerine) is the probable mechanism of action of these time-honored medications for angina pectoris.

The capacity of the endothelium to generate

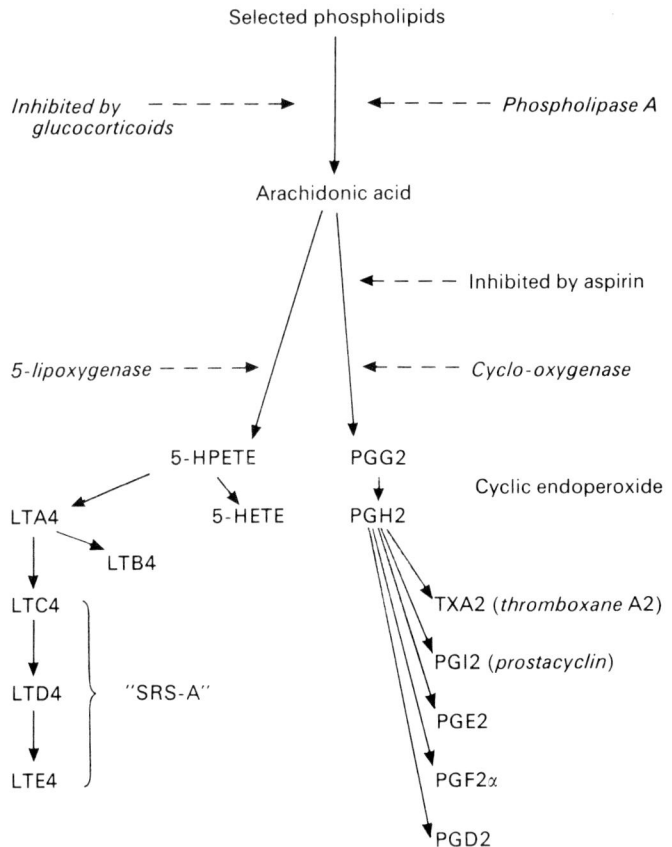

Selected phospholipids

Inhibited by — — — — — → ← — — — — Phospholipase A
glucocorticoids

Arachidonic acid

← — — — Inhibited by aspirin

5-lipoxygenase — — — → ← — — — Cyclo-oxygenase

5-HPETE   PGG2

Cyclic endoperoxide

LTA4   5-HETE   PGH2

LTB4

TXA2 (*thromboxane* A2)

LTC4

PGI2 (*prostacyclin*)

LTD4 } "SRS-A"

PGE2

LTE4

PGF2α

PGD2

Fig. 27.3 Arachidonic-acid derivatives. Cyclo-oxygenase acts on arachidonic acid to form two cyclic endoperoxides, PGG2 and PGH2. From these are formed PGI2 (*prostacyclin*) and TXA2 (*thromboxane A2*). The enzyme 5-lipoxygenase generates 5-hydroperoxyeicosatetraenoic acid (5-HPETE), and this, if directed along the SRS-A pathway, is converted into the leukotrienes LTC4, LTD4, LTE4. The product actually formed, whether along the 5-lipoxygenase or cyclo-oxygenase pathway, depends upon the cell type, the species, and the stimulus applied to the cell. (From Lewis R A, Austen K F 1981 Mediators of local homeostasis and inflammation by leukotrienes and other mast-cell-dependent compounds. Nature 293: 103–108.)

EDRF diminishes with age and is also impaired in diabetes mellitus, hypertension and atherosclerosis.

Endothelium-derived contracting factors. Endothelial cells can also produce factors that cause vasoconstriction. These include thromboxane A2, superoxide ions and the peptide endothelin-1. Endothelin-1 is slowly released by endothelial cells and causes intense vasoconstriction, especially well marked in the kidney. Its role in disease states is conjectural but it may be an important factor in the renal failure of shock and in the pathogenesis of hypertension.

Causes of thrombosis

Three factors (*Virchow's triad*) must be considered in regard to the mechanism of thrombosis:

The vessel wall. The various types of anatomical changes in the vessel wall which may lead to platelet deposition have already been depicted (Fig. 27.2). In general these abnormalities play an important part in thrombosis involving the heart and arteries. In the veins they are of less importance. The role of the endothelium has been discussed above.

The flow of blood. The importance of *eddy currents* has already been noted. These lead to platelet deposition, and the resulting thrombus is pale. This occurs in fast moving streams, e.g. over the heart valves and in arteries. *Stasis* is the most important cause of extensive thrombosis involving veins. It is also a factor in inducing thrombosis in the sac of an aneurysm.

The constituents of the blood. An increase in the platelet count, an increased tendency to platelet adhesion and aggregation, a decrease in the clotting time, and decreased antithrombin activity all contribute to thrombosis. The interaction of these factors is complex, but changes in them help to explain the thrombosis that occurs after parturition, splenectomy, trauma, and severe haemorrhage, and also the thromboses that complicate hyperlipidaemia and the administration of certain drugs, e.g. the birth-control pill.

It should be noted that usually more than one factor is implicated in causing thrombosis. For instance, there is regional stasis and a high platelet count after an operation, and atherosclerotic plaques act both by causing a loss of the endothelium and inducing eddy currents.

Thrombosis in arteries

In the high-velocity arterial system the most important cause of thrombosis is disease or spasm of the arterial wall itself. Intimal involvement leads to deposition of platelets, and atheromatous plaques or aneurysm lead to turbulence.

Thrombosis in the heart

Thrombosis in the atria is generally due to stasis as can occur in heart failure particularly if there is fibrillation. The situation is analogous to phlebothrombosis in veins. The thrombi generally form in the auricular appendages and may become detached to form emboli in either the systemic or pulmonary circulation depending on which atrium is involved.

Thrombosis in the left ventricle commonly complicates a myocardial infarct or a ventricular aneurysm.

Coiled thrombi are found in the pulmonary trunk and right ventricle in massive pulmonary embolism. These should not be confused with post-mortem clots. The latter are formed after death, and their shape conforms to that of the cavity in which they are formed. They are shiny and elastic, and never exhibit the lines of Zahn which are characteristic of thrombi. Furthermore, in conditions accompanied by a high ESR the blood may separate before it clots, so that there is an upper portion consisting largely of coagulated plasma. This is pale yellow, and is usually called the 'chicken-fat clot', while the clot underneath contains sedimented red cells. This is the so-called 'red-currant-jelly clot'.

Thrombi on the heart valves are called vegetations and form a ready source of emboli (see Chapter 29).

Thrombosis in veins

This is described in Chapter 28.

Fate of thrombi

Figure 27.4 summarizes the possible fate of a thrombus.

1. Many thrombi undergo lysis, and leave no trace of their previous existence. The fibrinolytic mechanism is of importance (p. 319).

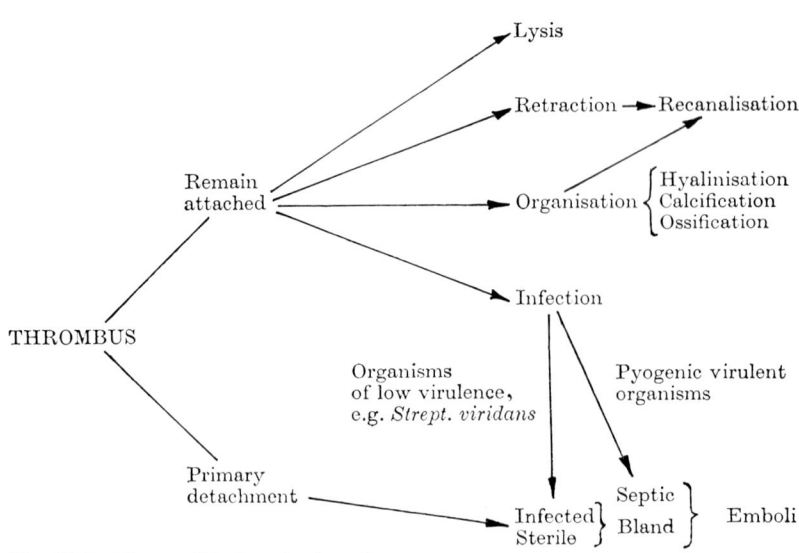

Fig. 27.4 The possible fate of a thrombus.

2. If an occluding thrombus in an artery or vein contains much clot, it retracts sufficiently for blood to pass by. In this way a new channel is formed. Endothelium quickly lines this passage, and recanalization occurs. In the pulmonary arteries a thin web of connective tissue may be all that remains of a previous life-threatening thrombo-embolism.

3. A thrombus which is not removed may become organized. In veins the granulation tissue invades it from the mural aspect, and endothelium grows over the thrombus from the adjacent intima. In large, elastic arteries the vasa vasorum from the adventitia do not penetrate as far as the intima, organization is therefore impaired and the thrombus remains as a degenerate mass for many months or years.

4. Organized thrombi may become hyalinized and calcified. This is common in the pelvic veins, and the *phleboliths* so produced may be seen on radiographic examination.

5. Thrombi may become detached to form emboli.

EMBOLISM

An *embolus* is an abnormal mass of undissolved material which is transported from one part of the circulation to another. The most satisfactory classification is based upon its composition. Five categories may be recognized: *thrombi and clot* (bland or infected), *gas* (air and nitrogen), *fat, tumour, miscellaneous.*

Emboli composed of thrombus or clot

Emboli may be released into the pulmonary or the systemic circulation.

Pulmonary embolism

The source of the thrombo-emboli is generally one of the leg veins. Small emboli block branches of the pulmonary arteries and produce either no effects or else infarction (p. 339). Large quantities of thrombus and propagated clot, however, produce the syndrome of massive pulmonary embolism. In this the main pulmonary artery and its branches are plugged

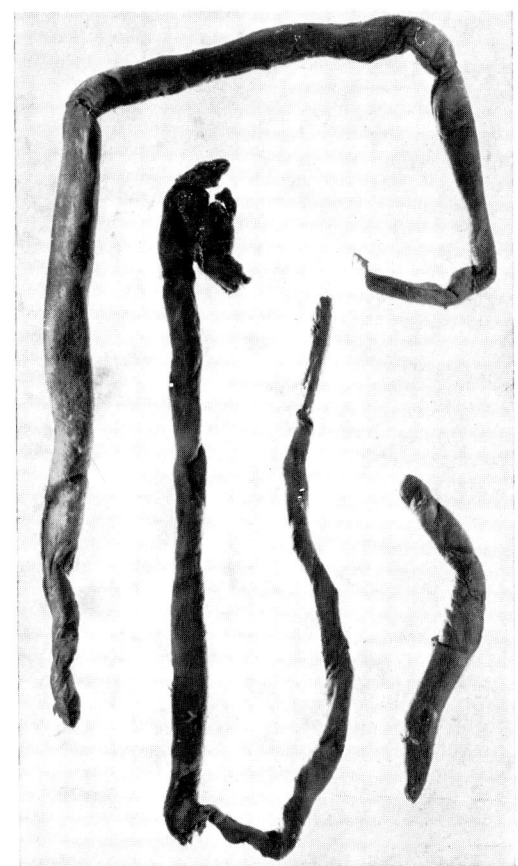

Fig. 27.5 Massive pulmonary embolism. These thrombi were removed from the pulmonary arteries of a man who died suddenly a week after an abdominal operation. There was extensive phlebothrombosis in both calves. Note that the calibre of the thrombi corresponds with the lumina of the leg veins. (C40.5. Reproduced by permission of the President and Council of the Royal College of Surgeons of England.)

by a mass of coiled thrombus (Fig. 27.5). The clinical effects are dramatic. The patient experiences sudden dyspnoea and chest pain. The obstruction of the right ventricular outflow results in a dramatic fall in left ventricular output; hypotension occurs and consciousness is lost. Death frequently follows. The prevention of massive pulmonary embolism is the prevention of deep-vein thrombosis (phlebothrombosis). Patients confined to bed must be given leg exercises to increase the venous circulation. Intramuscular injections of heparin, physiotherapy and early ambulation after surgery have done much to reduce the complication of deep vein thrombosis.

Systemic embolism

The emboli usually arise in the heart, commonly from the left atrium in mitral stenosis or heart failure. Other sources are the heart valves in infective endocarditis, a heart valve prosthesis, and the left ventricular wall overlying a myocardial infarct.

Gaseous emboli

Air

Air may inadvertently be introduced into a systemic vein, e.g. during a mismanaged blood transfusion or during operations on the head and neck. If in considerable quantity, it travels to the heart where it produces foaming in the right ventricle. The right ventricle compresses this foam but cannot expel it. Death therefore occurs rapidly.

During pleural aspirations air may inadvertently be introduced into the pulmonary venous circulation and reach the left side of the heart. From here it may block any systemic vessel. If a cerebral or coronary artery is blocked the result is serious and can be fatal.

Nitrogen: the decompression syndrome

Bubbles of nitrogen appear in the circulation in those who, having been exposed to a high atmospheric pressure, are suddenly decompressed. This occurs in divers, tunnellers, and pilots. Nitrogen, being soluble in lipids, also appears as bubbles in the central nervous system. This effect may result in considerable damage to the spinal cord. Severe pain is produced ('the bends'), and permanent damage or death may ensue.

Fat emboli

Globules of fatty marrow may enter the small veins after a fracture of a long bone; with multiple injuries this embolization may be quite extensive. Usually the emboli are trapped in the lungs and have no harmful effects because of the enormous capacity of the vascular bed. Occasionally, however, emboli pass through the pulmonary capillaries and enter the systemic circulation, where they produce the syndrome of systemic fat embolism. Multiple emboli lodge in the kidneys causing haematuria, the brain, where they lead to severe neurological changes, and the skin, where they cause small petechial haemorrhages.

Tumour emboli

It is probable that all malignant tumours invade the local blood vessels at an early stage of the disease, and that isolated malignant cells are of frequent occurrence in the circulation. The majority of these emboli are destroyed; only a small percentage develop into metastatic deposits. Occasionally a large mass of tumour invades a vein, becomes detached and forms a massive embolus.

Miscellaneous emboli

Foreign bodies. A large number of foreign bodies have been reported to undergo embolism, e.g. a polyethylene tube may become detached in a vein and travel to the right side of the heart. In therapeutic embolization foreign material (e.g. gelatin sponge or steel springs) is deliberately introduced into a vessel in order to reduce the vascularity of a part or to infarct a tumour.

Parasites. Various parasites and their ova are carried in the blood stream.

HYPOXIA

Hypoxia is a state of impaired oxygenation of the tissues. Four types are commonly described:

Hypoxic, due to a low oxygen tension (PO_2) in the arterial blood. This is a feature of central cyanosis (p. 352).

Anaemic, due to a low haemoglobin level.

Stagnant, or *ischaemic,* due to an inadequate supply of blood to the tissues. This, as will be seen, is due either to heart failure or some local vascular obstruction, and is a feature of peripheral cyanosis.

Histotoxic, due to cellular intoxication which prevents the uptake of oxygen, e.g. cyanide poisoning.

ISCHAEMIA

Ischaemia is defined as a condition of inadequate blood supply to an area of tissue. It produces harmful effects in three ways:

Hypoxia: oxygen deprivation is undoubtedly the most important factor producing damage in ischaemic tissue, especially in respect of very active cells, e.g. brain or muscle. On the other hand, it plays no part in the lesions produced by pulmonary arterial obstruction, because the alveolar walls derive their oxygen supply directly from the alveolar air.

Malnutrition: this is of little importance, because the blood contains much more glucose and amino acids than could be metabolized by its oxygen content.

Failure to remove waste products: the accumulation of metabolites is the most probable explanation of pain in ischaemic muscles. The presence of waste products or the failure to maintain important electrolyte or other balances is probably a factor in pulmonary infarction.

Causes of ischaemia

Ischaemia may be caused by an inadequate cardiac output; not all tissues are equally affected because of the redistribution of the available blood. The extremities (e.g. finger-tips) tend to be most severely affected, but the ischaemia is rarely sufficiently severe to cause structural damage. Not so, however, with the ischaemia that follows the sudden cessation of the heart's action. Sudden cardiac arrest may occur during the induction of anaesthesia or as a result of coronary thrombosis. The blood supply to the whole body is stopped, but manifestations are confined to the brain, which is particularly sensitive to hypoxia. If the arrest continues for 15 s, consciousness is lost, and if the condition lasts for more than 3 min, irreparable damage is done. The neurons degenerate and are replaced by glial tissue. If cardiac arrest lasts for more than about 8 min, death is inevitable. It follows that *all who deal with patients should be capable of diagnosing cardiac arrest (absent heart sounds) and dealing with it by the manoeuvre of external cardiac massage.*

Local causes

By far the most important cause of ischaemia is obstruction to the arterial flow. It should not, however, be forgotten that extensive venous and capillary damage can also produce ischaemia.

Arterial obstruction. The causes may be summarized:

Thrombosis.

Embolism. The effects of an embolus are potentiated by the reflex spasm of the arterial wall, and completed by the rapid development of thrombus over the embolus.

Spasm. See below.

Arterial disease. Atherosclerosis is the most important and produces partial obstruction of medium sized arteries, e.g. cerebral, coronary and renal arteries.

Occlusive pressure from without, e.g. tourniquets and ill-fitting plasters.

Venous obstruction. Extensive venous obstruction leads to engorgement of the areas drained by the affected veins. This may reach such an intensity that blood flow is impeded and ischaemia results. Mesenteric vein thrombosis is a good example of this; it leads to intestinal infarction.

Diseases of small vessels. See Chapter 28.

Vascular spasm. Although vascular occlusion is generally caused by an organic lesion, there are a number of conditions in which spasm of the vessel wall plays a most important part. Spasm may occur in either veins or arteries.

Venous spasm. Trauma applied directly to a vessel wall can cause marked spasm. This is sometimes a source of great difficulty during an inexpert venepuncture. Venous spasm has not been incriminated as a cause of tissue ischaemia.

Arterial spasm. Trauma to arteries frequently produces local spasm, a function which may be of life-saving importance. Cases of avulsion of a limb are on record in which, due to spasm of the main artery, the patient did not die of massive haemorrhage.

This ability of arteries to contract can be utilized by the surgeon who is faced with severe bleeding during the course of an operation. It is a wise policy to pack the wound and await the onset of spasm rather than make heroic though blind efforts with a pair of haemostats. Although this response of the arterial wall to trauma may be of benefit, its effects are sometimes detrimental. Trauma to an artery, e.g. by the close proximity of a bullet path, the pressure of a plaster, or the application of a tourniquet, may at times produce such persistent and widespread spasm that the area involved becomes ischaemic and infarcted. *Absence of the pulse of a limb beyond an area of trauma must be regarded seriously, and efforts should be made to relieve the spasm, lest permanent damage be caused.*

Spasm of small arteries is a feature of Raynaud's phenomenon. In this condition the digital arteries are unduly sensitive to the effects of cold and go into spasm. When cooled the hands or feet first become pale, then cyanosed and finally red with the onset of reactive hyperaemia. In many cases the phenomenon is a complication of systemic sclerosis or lupus erythematosus, while in other cases no cause or associated condition is evident. Widespread arteriolar spasm is a feature of shock (p. 295), and has also been incriminated in primary hypertension (p. 326).

Effects of ischaemia due to arterial obstruction

The effects depend largely upon the degree of ischaemia produced, and may range from sudden death to virtually no damage at all. The following are the possibilities:

No effects occur if the affected area is well supplied by blood vessels which form collateral anastomoses.

Functional disturbances: sufficient blood may reach the area to supply its needs under resting conditions but not under those of activity. This is the cause of the pain in the chest (*angina pectoris*) in patients with coronary artery disease, and the *intermittent claudication* in those with peripheral vascular disease (p. 345).

Cellular degeneration may affect the parenchyma of an organ and terminate in necrosis. This may be a patchy affair leading to atrophy; it is generally accompanied by replacement fibrosis or, in the central nervous system, gliosis. This type of lesion follows sudden complete arterial obstruction of short duration, or partial arterial obstruction of gradual onset.

Infarction, which is discussed below.

Sudden death occurs in massive pulmonary embolism and coronary occlusion.

Factors determining the extent of ischaemia in arterial obstruction. There are three crucial factors:

Speed of onset. If it is sudden the effects are more severe than if it is gradual, because there is less time for an effective collateral circulation to develop.

Degree of obstruction. A complete obstruction is obviously much more serious than a partial one.

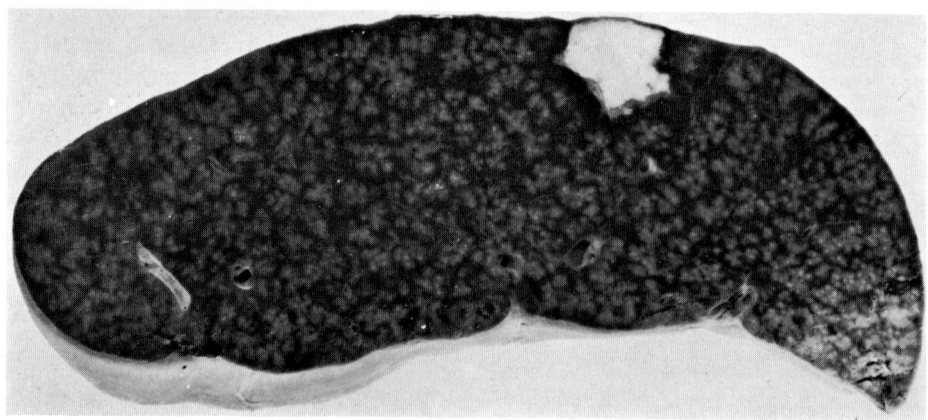

Fig. 27.6 Infarct of spleen. Note the pale, wedge-shaped infarct under the capsule. The lymphoid follicles are unduly prominent. The patient had *Strep. viridans* endocarditis. (H26.1. Reproduced by permission of the President and Council of the Royal College of Surgeons of England.)

Anatomy of the collateral circulation. Some arteries have no anastomotic channels; these are called *end arteries*, and if obstructed there is complete ischaemia of the area supplied. With most arteries there is sufficient anastomosis to ensure that the blood reaches the affected area even when a main branch is occluded. If the anastomotic vessels are well developed, ischaemia is an uncommon phenomenon. The stomach illustrates this well, for it is supplied by three separate arteries which anastomose freely.

Subsidiary factors. There are four subsidiary factors modifying the effects of arterial blockage:

1. *The pathology of the collateral circulation.* It stands to reason that if the collateral vessels are severely affected with spasm or atherosclerosis they are not likely to assist in maintaining a good alternative blood supply.

2. *The oxygenation of the arterial blood.*

3. *The efficiency of the heart.*

4. *The nature of the affected tissue.* Brain and heart are much more vulnerable to ischaemia than are any other organs. Connective tissue survives much better than does the parenchyma of an organ.

INFARCTION

Infarction may be defined as the circumscribed necrosis of tissue due to deprivation of blood supply. It usually leads to a circumscribed area of coagulative necrosis, which is subsequently organized into scar tissue. The process is as follows:

1. There is death of the cells in the area deprived of its blood supply. Blood, either from anastomotic vessels or by venous reflux, continues to seep into the devitalized area for a short time. Thus most infarcts contain a great deal of blood in the early stages, and are swollen and red in colour. The red cells entering the affected area escape from the damaged capillaries and lie free in the dead tissue. Infarcts of lax tissue, e.g. lung and intestine, are much more engorged than are those of compact organs, e.g. kidney and heart.

2. The dead tissue undergoes necrosis. In solid organs the associated swelling of the cells may squeeze the blood out of the infarct. In this

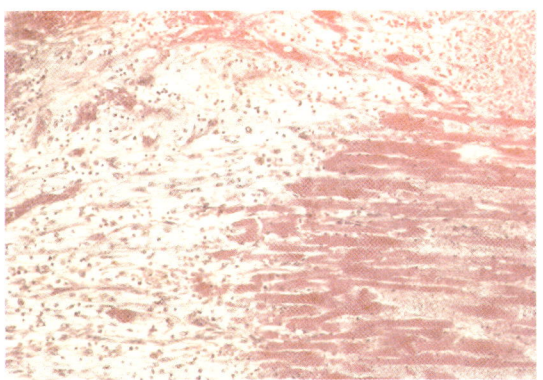

Fig. 27.7 Myocardial infarction. The muscle fibres on the right are necrotic and are being steadily replaced by vascular granulation tissue in which are inflammatory cells.

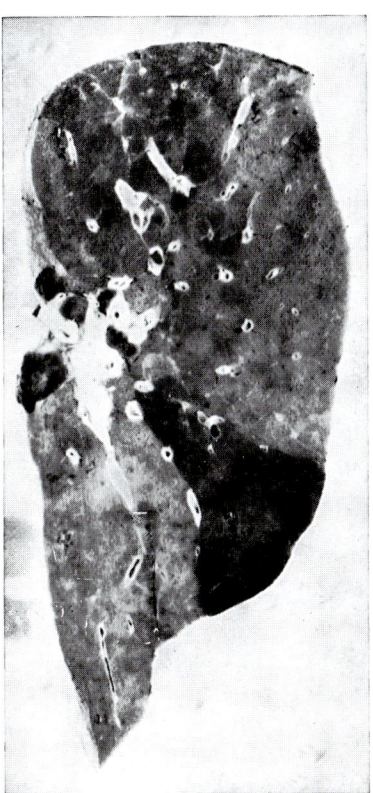

Fig. 27.8 Infarct of lung. Note the dark wedge-shaped infarct in this left upper lobe. It is stuffed with blood.(R27.3. Reproduced by permission of the President and Council of the Royal College of Surgeons of England.)

way it becomes paler. Infarcts of the spleen and kidneys are characteristically pale, and present a wedge-shaped area of coagulative necrosis, the apex of which is the blocked supplying artery, and the base the capsule of the organ (Fig. 27.6). Infarcts of the heart are also pale, but their shape is more irregular due to the arrangement of the vascular supply.

3. There is progressive autolysis of the necrotic tissue and haemolysis of the red cells. Microscopically an infarct shows a characteristic structured necrosis with the outlines of the cells being recognizable as ghosts without nuclei. This petrified-forest appearance may persist for many months. (Fig. 27.7).

4. At the same time the surrounding normal tissue undergoes an acute inflammatory reaction. The polymorph infiltration may be so intense as to simulate a pyogenic infection for a while. This is rapidly followed by macrophage activity.

5. The infarct gradually shrinks and becomes replaced by granulation tissue. Its central portion may, however, take many months to organize, and not infrequently shows dystrophic calcification.

Infarcts in particular organs present certain additional features. In the *lung* the infarct is so filled with blood that it remains red and generally organizes in this stage (Fig. 27.8). In the *intestine* the necrotic bowel wall is soon invaded by putrefactive organisms and becomes gangrenous. In the *limbs* sudden obstruction leads to infarction and wet gangrene, while slow obstruction produces the so-called dry gangrene (p. 47).

In the *central nervous system* the process is somewhat different, because the necrotic tissue undergoes rapid colliquative necrosis. The end-result is either a glial scar or else, if the infarct is large, a cyst surrounded by a layer of glial tissue.

Infarction of the lung does not occur in healthy people even if a major pulmonary artery is occluded. This is because the bronchial arteries supply well-oxygenated blood. If the bronchial arterial supply is itself impaired, as in heart failure, obstruction to a branch of the pulmonary artery may then lead to infarction. The usual cause of this is an embolus arising from one of the systemic veins. It will be recalled that phlebothrombosis is itself often associated with heart failure.

GENERAL READING

Gimbone M A 1986 Vascular endothelium in hemostasis and thrombosis. Churchill Livingstone, New York

Jaffe E A 1987 Cell biology of endothelial cells. Human Pathology 18:234,

Kaplan N K 1988 Systemic hypertension: mechanisms and diagnosis. In: Braunwald E (ed.). Heart disease 3rd edn. Saunders, Philadelphia

Leading Article 1988 What causes oedema? Lancet 1:1028

Mitchell J R A 1981 Prostaglandins in vascular disease: a seminal approach. British Medical Journal 282:590

Vanhoutte P M 1988 The endothelium-modulation of smooth-muscle tone. New England Journal of Medicine 319:512

Vane J R, Anggard E E, Botting R M 1990 Regulatory functions of the vascular endothelium. New England Journal of Medicine 323:27

Young A E 1981 Therapeutic embolism. British Medical Journal 2:1144

28. Diseases of arteries, veins and small vessels

DISEASES OF ARTERIES

Arterial disease and its complications are responsible for about 50% of all deaths in the Western World. Atherosclerosis is by far the most common contributor to this toll, but various inflammatory diseases and aneurysms play a significant role.

ARTERITIS

Infection is an occasional cause of arteritis but most examples are of unknown cause.

Infective arteritis

Arteritis may occur in pyogenic infections, and if the vessel wall undergoes necrosis, severe haemorrhage can result. A good example of this is the fatal haemorrhage from the lingual artery that sometimes ends the life of a patient with an ulcerating carcinoma of the tongue. Neoplastic invasion plays its part, but the major weakening effect is the result of infection. Similarly, destruction of an artery at the base of a gastric ulcer is a common cause of bleeding. Fortunately, in many chronic inflammatory lesions the artery responds by proliferation of its intimal lining so that the lumen becomes steadily occluded (*endarteritis obliterans*) and bleeding is restricted.

In pyaemia a localized suppurative arteritis may cause weakening of the arterial wall leading to the formation of a *mycotic aneurysm,* so named because of its mushroom shape. Syphilitic arteritis affecting particularly the thoracic aorta was common in the past but is now a rarity. A morphologically similar aortitis is associated with ankylosing spondylitis or may be of unknown aetiology.

Thromboangiitis obliterans

Otherwise called *Buerger's disease* this disease is seen predominantly in young men. It affects the veins and arteries of the legs, and causes ischaemia which leads to intermittent claudication (pain in the calf muscles on exercise) and ultimately gangrene commencing in the toes.

Giant cell arteritis

This is a disease of elderly people; the affected artery shows thrombosis and a chronic inflammatory granulomatous reaction with many giant cells formed around disrupted elastic fibres. The disease can affect any artery, but commonly it is the temporal one and pain in the temple is a marked feature. The ophthalmic artery is sometimes involved and blindness may result. Rarely the lingual artery is occluded, when ischaemia and pain can affect the oral structures, e.g. the tongue.

Polyarteritis nodosa

The classical type of this uncommon disease, first described in the last century, usually affects middle-aged males, and is characterized by an arteritis involving medium-sized muscular arteries of organs. The inflamed arterial walls become necrotic and infiltrated with both inflammatory cells and fibrin, which gives the appearance of *fibrinoid necrosis*. The weakened vessel walls bulge, and the aneurysms so formed are responsible for the designation 'nodosa'. The lumen of the affected vessels becomes obstructed by thrombus, and the disease is characterized by ischaemia and infarction affecting many organs, particularly nerves, spleen and kidney. Renal failure, often with hypertension, is a common end-result of this fatal disease.

Variants of polyarteritis nodosa

A number of clinical variants of polyarteritis nodosa have been described; often the involved vessels are small and the term *microscopic polyarteritis* has been applied. Sometimes the lesions of this group of conditions show an acute leucocytoclastic vasculitis and there is overlap with other conditions of small blood vessels termed acute vasculitis (see p. 349). Some of the recognized syndromes are as follows:

Progressive allergic granulomatosis. This variant usually commences with asthmatic attacks and pneumonia. Infarcted areas of lung excite a granulomatous reaction that closely resembles tuberculosis histologically.

Wegener's granulomatosis. This disease is defined as a microscopic polyarteritis affecting kidneys, lungs, and upper respiratory tract. In the last site, the lesions may resemble those described in lethal midline granuloma. Death is usually due to renal failure.

Lethal midline granuloma. This terrible disease usually affects young males and is characterized by extensive necrosis and gangrene affecting the nose and nasopharynx. It has been regarded in the past as a type of microscopic polyarteritis but it is now thought that most, if not all, cases are examples of a malignant lymphoma. Death from bleeding or bronchopneumonia was inevitable until the introduction of chemotherapy.

Hypersensitivity angiitis. The lesions of this group of conditions show an acute leucocytoclastic vasculitis that may affect several or many organs. Sometimes an immune complex mechanism appears to be important, and the disease may occur in SLE or complicate malignancy or an infection. If the skin, kidney and bowel are involved the condition is called Henoch–Schonlein purpura.

ARTERIOSCLEROSIS

This term embraces three conditions which are loosely called degenerative arterial disease. *Monckeberg's medial sclerosis* affects the tunica media of large muscular arteries, particularly of the legs. There is hyalinization and calcification of the tunica media. The lumen is not narrowed and the disease produces dramatic radiological changes but has little functional importance. *Arteriolosclerosis* causes thickening of the walls of small arteries and arterioles. It accompanies hypertension, causes nephrosclerosis and has been alluded to previously. *Atherosclerosis* is the third and most important component of the trio.

Atherosclerosis

Atherosclerosis is the commonest killing disease in all highly advanced civilized communities, and its lesions are present to some degree in almost every adult member. The disease characteristically affects the large elastic arteries like the aorta and its main branches. Of the medium-sized vessels the coronary and cerebral arteries are most commonly involved. This is extremely unfortunate in view of the vital nature of the organs they supply, and it accounts for the lethal effects of atheroma. Atherosclerosis may be considered as consisting of two types of conditions.

Basic lesions of atherosclerosis

Type I: Superficial yellow plaques in the intima. Lipid-containing cells (mostly macrophages but also muscle cells) accumulate in the subendothelial layer of the vessel and later break down to release their fatty content into the tunica intima. In this way are produced the yellow streaks that are a common necropsy finding in the aorta. When the fatty deposits occur in small arteries, they do not produce appreciable narrowing of the lumen. These early yellow plaques are sometimes referred to as *atheroma*.

Type II: Accumulation of fatty material in the intima with additional fibrosis. This is

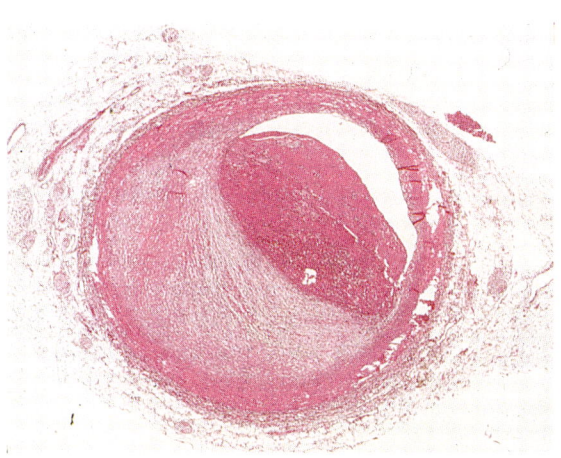

Fig. 28.2 Atherosclerosis of the coronary artery. The vessel has been cut transversely to show an atheromatous plaque causing intimal thickening and occlusion of the lumen by about 70%. As a terminal event an occluding thrombus has formed, and retracted enough to produce a demilune shaped lumen.

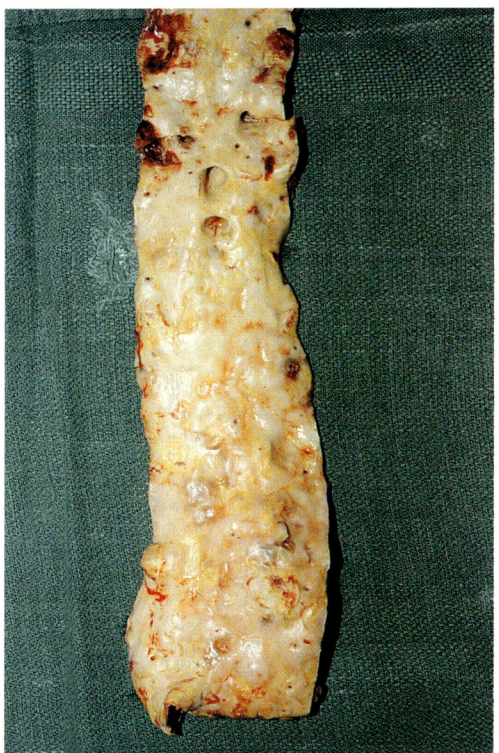

Fig. 28.1 Atherosclerosis of the aorta. The aorta has been opened from behind to show the intimal surface. The yellow areas are due to accumulation of atheromatous material; in places overlying fibrosis has produced white pearly plaques.

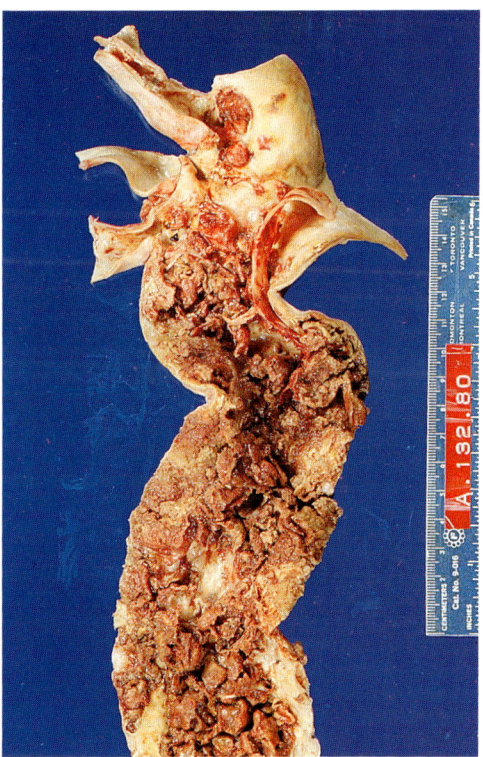

Fig. 28.3 Severe atherosclerosis of the aorta. The arch is relatively spared but the descending thoracic and abdominal aorta show severe atherosclerosis. The lining consists of ulcerated plaques and a covering of adherent thrombus.

the common type of lesion seen in middle age and old age (Fig. 28.1). The lesions consist of intimal plaques and contain a central mass of fatty, yellow, porridge-like material (from the Greek *athere* meaning porridge) consisting predominantly of cholesterol and its esters. This material is covered by dense fibrous tissue, which gives the plaque a white, pearly appearance. The intimal accumulation of atheromatous fatty material and the associated fibrous tissue encroach on the lumen of the vessel and reduce its lumen to a demilune (Fig. 28.2). This type of lesion is generally designated atherosclerosis.

Advanced and complicated lesions of atherosclerosis

Four further changes may be seen in the plaques as they progress:

Haemorrhage. Proliferation of vessels from the vasa vasorum produces increased vascularity in the connective tissue surrounding the atheromatous plaque. Rupture of one of these vessels leads to bleeding into the plaque. In a small vessel like the coronary artery this bleeding can produce acute obstruction.

Ulceration. The fibrous cap may rupture so that ulceration occurs. Atheromatous material may spill into the blood and lead to atheromatous embolism.

Thrombosis. Ulceration and turbulence around plaques can lead to superadded thrombosis (Fig. 28.3).

Calcification. The fatty material in the atheromatous plaque undergoes dystrophic calcification.

Effects of atherosclerosis

Gradual obstruction. Atherosclerosis of small vessels such as the coronary or cerebral arteries produces intimal thickening and progressive occlusion of the lumen. This leads to ischaemia of the area supplied.

Thrombosis. This leads to sudden complete obstruction and often to infarction.

Dilatation and aneurysm formation. The presence of an atherosclerotic plaque causes atrophy of the adjacent media. The wall consequently weakens, and the artery involved may show either a diffuse enlargement, called *ectasia*, or a localized dilatation, called an *aneurysm*. These effects are seen most often in the aorta, in which the atherosclerosis is most severe. The lesions of atherosclerosis tend to be more advanced toward the more distal regions of the aorta, and it is therefore in the abdominal portion that aneurysm formation is most common. The aneurysm is generally below the origin of the renal arteries, and rupture of such a lesion leads to exsanguination and death.

Embolism. It is not uncommon for atheromatous material, or overlying thrombus, to become detached and embolize distally. Usually such emboli are small and not apparent clinically. Nevertheless, the steady occlusion of many small vessels is probably a factor in the peripheral ischaemic disease of the lower leg as well as the progressive ischaemic renal disease that often accompanies atherosclerosis.

Risk factors

The cause of atherosclerosis is not known, but the disease is associated with a number of well-recognized risk factors. These may be listed: a family history of atherosclerotic related conditions, diabetes mellitus, cigarette smoking, and an abnormal plasma lipid profile (see below). The disease develops earlier in males, females being protected during their reproductive life but catching up after the menopause.

Plasma lipids in relation to atherosclerosis. The following are the main groups of lipoprotein present in the plasma:

Chylomicrons
Very low-density lipoproteins (VLDL)
Low-Density Lipoproteins (LDL)—this contains much cholesterol and is the form in which cholesterol is transported to cells for metabolism.
High-Density Lipoproteins (HDL).

Hyperlipoproteinaemia can occur as a result of diet, disease (e.g. alcoholism or diabetes mellitus) or be the effect of an inherited trait (e.g. familial hypercholesterolaemia). Those with a high level of LDL have a high incidence of atherosclerosis. A high level of HDL is protective.

Pathogenesis of atherosclerosis

The current hypothesis is that atherosclerosis is a *response to injury*. Damage to the arterial endothelium leads to an *influx of lipoproteins* into the intima, and also causes *adhesion of platelets*. The damage may be caused by an atherogenic pattern of hyperlipoproteinaemia, tobacco smoking, hypertension, abnormal shear stresses and probably other factors.

Endothelial cells normally secrete prostacyclin and play an important role in inhibiting platelet adhesion and aggregation. They promote the activation of protein C which inhibits coagulation, and secrete an activator of plasminogen, thereby helping to remove any fibrin that is formed. Damage to the endothelium therefore favours platelet deposition and fibrin formation.

The cells that accumulate in the intima in atherosclerosis are of two types:

Macrophages derived from blood monocytes which adhere readily to an intima damaged by hypercholesterolaemia.

Smooth muscle cells derived from the media. Platelets, macrophages, and endothelial cells release smooth muscle growth factors. Having been attracted into the intima, smooth muscle cells imbibe lipid to form foam cells. They also produce a variety of connective tissue components, namely glycosaminoglycans, elastin and collagen. In this way lipid, fibrous tissue and fibrin are formed in the lesions and the result is an atherosclerotic plaque.

Peripheral vascular disease

'Peripheral vascular disease' is an inclusive term that is used to describe all those conditions in which the blood supply to the limbs is impaired. Usually it is the legs that suffer. The following diseases all play their part:

Atherosclerosis. This tends to affect the large vessels such as the iliac and femoral arteries.

Buerger's disease. This is an occasional cause (p. 341).

Thrombosis. This may be secondary to atherosclerosis.

Embolism. Emboli may be large thromboemboli or small clumps of atheromatous material.

Small-vessel disease. Arteriolosclerosis associated with hypertension and diabetic microangiopathy are the most important.

Effects of peripheral vascular disease

The effects are serious and disabling. The ischaemia of the leg leads to atrophy of many structures, including the bones (osteoporosis) and the skin. Trivial injury can lead to chronic, persistent, extremely painful ulceration. Ischaemia of the muscle leads to pain on walking (intermittent claudication) and, ultimately, to pain at rest. Dry gangrene leading to a loss of the limb is an all-too-frequent end-result.

ANEURYSMS

An aneurysm is a local dilatation of an artery or a chamber of the heart due to a weakening of its walls. It may be localized and saccular or diffuse and fusiform.

Causes

The weakening of the wall may be due to:

1. Congenital deficiency, e.g. berry aneurysms of the circle of Willis (p. 423).
2. *Atherosclerosis.* This is by far the most common type of aortic aneurysm.
3. Inflammation, e.g. syphilitic aortitis and mycotic aneurysms.
4. Trauma. Sometimes an injury can damage not only an artery but also an adjacent vein, thereby establishing a connexion. This formation is called an *arteriovenous aneurysm*, or *fistula*. It is important, because so much blood can be diverted from the peripheral tissue that heart failure ensues.

Effects

Aneurysms produce harmful effects in a number of ways:

Pressure

An aneurysm of the thoracic aorta may press on the oesophagus and cause difficulty in swallowing, or on the recurrent laryngeal nerve and lead to changes in the voice.

Haemorrhage

Rupture of an aneurysm leads to bleeding; for a while this can be quite trivial because of the plugging effect of the thrombus lining the sac. Nevertheless, when an aneurysm, such as one of the abdominal aorta, has begun to bleed, it is not long before massive haemorrhage follows and the patient dies of exsanguination.

Thrombosis

The sac of an aneurysm soon becomes filled by laminated thrombus. This is due in part to the damage to the endothelial lining and in part to the local stasis. Parts of the thrombus may embolize.

Ischaemia

This is due to blockage of the branches of the artery at the site of the aneurysm, an effect produced either by local pressure or by thrombotic occlusion.

Dissecting aneurysm of the aorta

The basic defect is a change in the media of the aorta called *cystic medionecrosis* in which elastic fibres are lost and replaced by mucoid material. Bleeding occurs into the media either from rupture of one of the vasa vasorum, or through a tear in the intima. In either event a tear is invariably present in the ascending aorta. Blood is then forced in considerable quantity through this tear, and it produces an extensive stripping of the arterial wall, even down into the abdominal aorta (Fig. 28.4). The disease is quite common, and is usually heralded by the sudden onset of severe chest pain. The effects are serious because the dissection causes blockage of the ostia of important branches of the aorta. There is a vary-

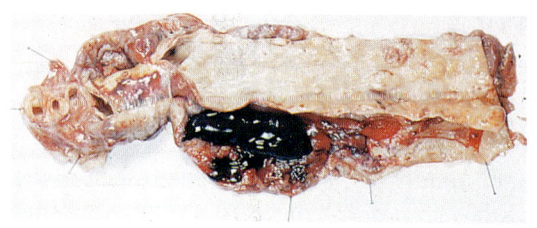

Fig. 28.4 Dissecting aneurysm of the aorta. The aorta has been opened from behind and a mass of blood clot and thrombus can be seen in the space created by the splitting of the media.

ing degree of obstruction to the arteries of the arms so that the pulses at the wrist are either unequal or weak. Furthermore, the signs change as the dissection proceeds. Blockage of the coronary ostia leads to myocardial infarction, while involvement of the renal arteries causes infarction and renal failure. In most cases, unless treated surgically, the outer coat of the aneurysmal sac ruptures into the pericardium, mediastinum or retroperitoneal space, and the patient dies of exsanguination.

DISEASES OF VEINS

Diseases affecting the walls of veins are uncommon, but thrombosis is common because stasis is particularly evident especially in the legs. Two distinct entities should be recognized: phlebothrombosis and thrombophlebitis.

PHLEBOTHROMBOSIS (DEEP VEIN THROMBOSIS)

In this important condition, commonly called deep vein thrombosis of the legs, there is extensive thrombosis and clot formation in the veins of the calf. It is due mainly to stasis, and is seen whenever the circulation in the legs is impaired. This occurs whenever the cardiac output is reduced, e.g. in heart failure, shock, and when the metabolic rate is reduced as when a patient is put to rest in bed. The venous return from the legs is greatly facilitated by the squeezing action of the surrounding muscles, and this important mechanism is in abeyance in the bedridden patient. The arms are much less likely to be affected, since they are in constant use in all conscious patients. Following trauma the increased platelet count, increased platelet adhesiveness, and decreased clotting time are further factors favouring thrombosis. Direct damage to the veins, e.g. by a fractured bone, or even the pressure of a pillow on the calf muscles, may be additional precipitating factors. It follows therefore that phlebothrombosis is common in the leg veins whenever a patient is put to bed, especially in the elderly, if the heart is failing, or if there is shock or severe trauma, such as after a major operation or a severe haemorrhage. Indeed, it occurs in about 35% of patients after major surgery, and is even more frequent in cases of recent myocardial infarction.

Pathogenesis

Five stages can be recognized (Fig. 28.5).

Primary platelet thrombus. Following some trivial intimal damage, platelets adhere to the vein walls and form a mass of pale thrombus.

This has been likened to the formation of a snow-drift during a snow-storm. Under normal circumstances this would produce no ill-effect, but if stasis is superadded, fibrin formation ensues and a large coralline thrombus is produced.

Coralline thrombus. As fibrin formation occurs and further platelets accumulate, the latter take the form of upstanding laminae growing across the stream. Between the laminae there is complete stasis, and fibrin is deposited; in it numerous red and white cells are trapped. This is an example of a mixed thrombus, and on section the alternating layers are seen (Fig. 28.6). The retraction of the fibrin layers lead to the characteristic ribbed or rippled appearance

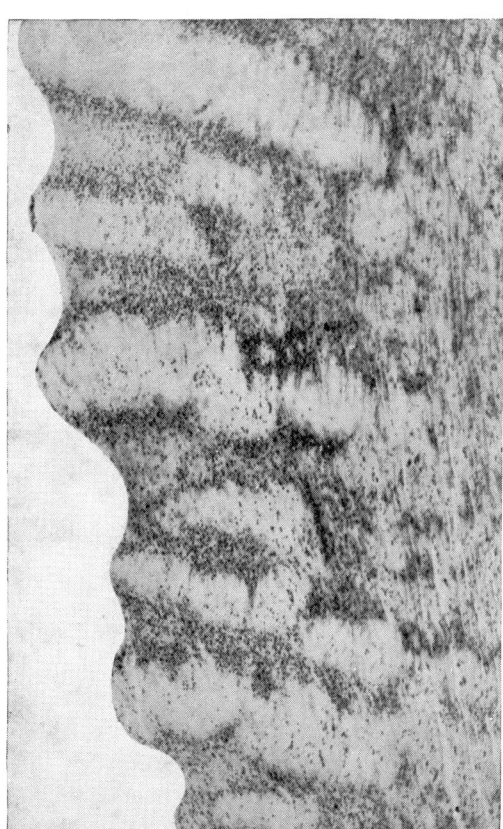

Fig. 28.6 Coralline thrombus. Photomicrograph of vertical section including free surface of a coralline thrombus adjacent to the wall of a large artery. Pale platelet laminae are seen projecting from the surface. Coagulated plasma containing leucocytes lies between them. Many leucocytes are adherent to the platelet laminae. (From Hadfield G 1950 Annals of the Royal College of Surgeons of England 6: 219.)

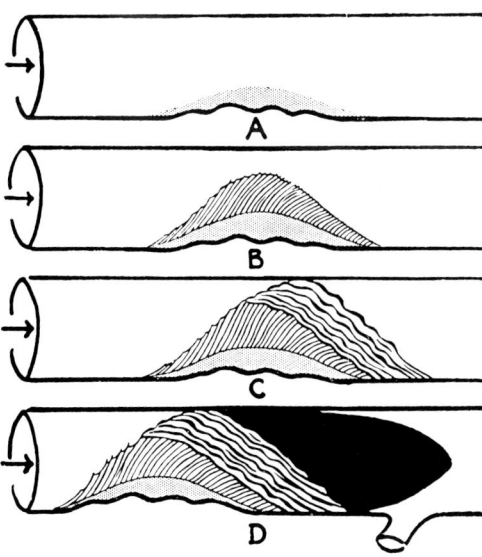

Fig. 28.5 The pathogenesis of phlebothrombosis. A, Primary platelet thrombus. B, Coralline thrombus. C, Occluding thrombus. D, Consecutive clot to the next venous tributary. (From Hadfield G 1950 Annals of the Royal College of Surgeons of England 6: 219.)

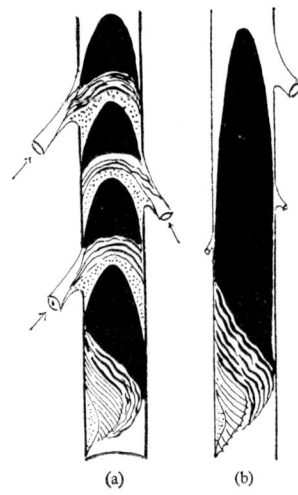

Fig. 28.7 Methods of propagation in phlebothrombosis.
(a) With thrombus formation at each entering tributary.
(b) Clotting en masse in an extensive length of vein.
(From Hadfield G 1950 Annals of the Royal College of
Surgeons of England 6: 219.)

seen when the surface of the thrombus is examined. The elevated platelet ridges are called the lines of Zahn, and are a characteristic feature of a thrombus formed in a fairly rapid stream of blood. Their presence is a useful indication that a structure found in a vessel is a thrombus formed during life and not a post-mortem clot (p. 334).

Occluding thrombus. The growth of the coralline thrombus progressively occludes the lumen of the vein, and the ensuing stasis rapidly leads to the formation of an occluding thrombus.

Consecutive clot. Once the vein is occluded, blood flow stops and with it stops the thrombosis. The stationary column of blood beyond the thrombus extending to the next entering tributary undergoes coagulation. This is called the consecutive clot (Fig. 28.7), and its free end, or tail, points like a dagger towards the heart.

Propagated clot. When stasis is marked, the clotting process extends up a considerable length of the vein past the entering tributaries to produce a long propagated clot (Fig. 28.7). As this retracts, it lies free in the lumen, and is attached only at the point of original thrombosis. This long, loose structure can easily become

detached and carried to the right side of the heart as an embolus.

Clinical features

Clinically phlebothrombosis is remarkably silent but the condition can be detected by special tests, e.g. phlebography and Doppler ultrasound. There is little pain in the limb, but direct squeezing pressure on the calf muscles may elicit tenderness. Careful measurement may detect slight oedema. Frequently the first indication of phlebothrombosis is the occurrence of pulmonary embolism.

The prevention of postoperative deep vein thrombosis involves leg exercises whilst the patient is in bed, early ambulation, avoidance of pressure on the calf and the administration of heparin.

Complications

Small emboli lodge in the lungs, and may produce infarction. A more serious complication is massive pulmonary embolism which can produce sudden death. This usually occurs from 7 to 10 days after injury or operation.

VARICOSE VEINS

In varicose veins or varicosities, the veins become elongated, irregularly dilated and tortuous. Sometimes the cause is increased intraluminal pressure as in the formation of oesophageal varicosities. This mechanism also plays a part in the formation of varicose veins of the legs, when the increase in pressure is related to the upright position, prolonged standing and the pressure of a gravid uterus. Sometimes there is a genetic basis for the disease and possibly some congenital defect in the valves of the veins is responsible. Certainly the veins are incompetent when the veins become dilated. The precise pathogenesis of this common condition is not known. Thrombosis is common because of the stagnant blood flow, but the vessels are so tortuous that embolism is very rare. Other effects are oedema of the ankles and congestion of the skin which, combined with a poor blood supply, result in the formation of *stasis ulcers*.

THROMBOPHLEBITIS

Inflammation of a vessel wall may follow the injection of irritant chemicals, e.g. anaesthetic agents, or be a complication of an adjacent area of infection, e.g. a staphylococcal abscess. In either event thrombosis occurs in the area of damage, but as stasis is not present, extensive propagation of the clot does not occur. The thrombosis is therefore relatively localized and firmly adherent. The condition is characterized by pain and swelling in the region of the vein, and is therefore clinically very obvious.

Embolism is most uncommon except in thrombophlebitis due to pyogenic infection, when the organisms invade the thrombus and cause its softening, so that small infected emboli are released into the circulation. The condition is called *pyaemia*, and the numerous infected emboli become impacted in distant organs, e.g. the lung, where they produce metastatic, or pyaemic, abscesses. If thrombophlebitis affects the portal vein, the *pyaemic abscesses* are found primarily in the liver. This is an occasional complication of suppurative appendicitis.

Thrombophlebitis migrans is a type of thrombophlebitis worthy of special note. It is characterized by thrombosis affecting many veins at different times. It is a well-recognized complication of malignant disease, especially carcinoma of the pancreas.

DISEASES OF SMALL VESSELS

In consideration of vascular disease the capillaries and arterioles are usually forgotten. There are, nevertheless, many conditions in which so many vessels in an area are occluded that ischaemia results. Because an additional effect is bleeding, petechial haemorrhages are a common feature of small-vessel disease even though the extent of the occlusion is insufficient to lead to ischaemia of the total area involved. Some causes of these diseases are briefly described below:

Frostbite. The harmful effects of cold on exposed parts are due in large measure to small vessel damage. In mild cases there is an inflammatory reaction causing large blisters to form; if the damage is severe, the vessels become completely occluded by thrombus and gangrene occurs.

Occlusion of capillaries by red cells. Patients with sickle-cell disease suffer from small vessel obstruction by deformed cells in areas of hypoxia, e.g. bone marrow, spleen and skin of the lower legs. Severe sludging as in shock is another example.

Occlusion by fibrin. This occurs in disseminated intravascular coagulation. The kidney is the organ most affected.

Occlusion by precipitated cryoglobulins. In cryoglobulinaemia exposure of the extremities to cold leads to vascular occlusion and petechial haemorrhages.

Fat embolism.

Decompression syndrome.

External pressure. The best example of this is a bedsore. Continual pressure on one area produces such ischaemia that necrosis of the skin and underlying tissues occurs. *It is a major duty of nurses to move non-ambulatory patients often enough that no pressure sores develop.*

Occlusion by antigen-antibody interaction. This is a feature of such immune complex phenomena as the Arthus reaction.

Vasculitis. This term is used to describe an inflammatory reaction in the walls of small vessels, and associated with necrosis of the vessel walls and fibrin deposition. Typical lesions occur in the Arthus reaction when immune complexes deposited in the vessel walls cause a type III reaction. The resultant damage is associated with a marked polymorph infiltration and thrombosis. The neutrophils break up into many nuclear fragments and the term *leucocytoclastic vasculitis* is used. This type of response is also seen in some drug eruptions and in septicaemia. Lesions occur in many organs but the kidney is most vulnerable. In the skin petechial haemorrhages occur and, as they can be felt, the condition is called *palpable purpura*. In some cases where no cause can be found there is overlap with the microscopic type of polyarteritis nodosa.

GENERAL READING

Gajdusek C, et al 1980 An endothelial cell-derived growth factor. Journal of Cell Biology 85:467

Roberts W C 1981 Aortic dissection: anatomy consequence and causes. American Heart Journal 101:195

Ross R, Glomset J, Harker L 1977 Response to injury and atherosclerosis.American Journal of Pathology 86:675

Ross R, et al 1980 The platelet derived growth factor. In: Gotto A M, Smith L D (eds) Atherosclerosis Five: Proceedings of the Fifth International Symposium. Springer-Verlag, New York

Ross R 1986 The pathogenesis of atherosclerosis—an update. New England Journal of Medicine 314:488

29. Diseases of the heart

Before commencing dental treatment it is particularly important to ascertain that the heart is normal, as dental treatment may precipitate serious disease in a patient with heart disease unless precautions are taken. Congenital lesions and valvular abnormalities predispose to infective endocarditis, and myocardial disease may lead to sudden death during anaesthesia.

The types and causes of heart disease are many and various; the effects, however, are few in number and stereotyped in nature. Since the heart is a pump, it follows that the diseased and failing heart often pumps inefficiently. The consequences of this are circulatory disturbances which together constitute the syndrome of heart failure. The main features of this will be described after individual diseases of the heart have been considered.

Two types of heart disease may be recognized: (1) the group of malformations which are present at birth and are due to faulty development (*congenital heart disease*); and (2) disorders occurring in a normal heart (acquired heart disease).

CONGENITAL HEART DISEASE

Congenital heart disease is a subject of importance to the dentist because the abnormality can predispose to infective endocarditis. Developmental anomalies range from those that are so severe as to be incompatible with continued fetal life (these lead to abortion), to others that are mild and symptomless. Between these two extremes there are those in which signs or symptoms become evident during infancy or childhood.

The incidence of congenital heart disease in newborn babies is at least 7 per 1000. Two-thirds of the affected infants die before their first birthday, so that only 2 or 3 of every 1000 school children have a cardiac malformation.

SIGNS AND SYMPTOMS

Factors that alert the clinician to the possibility of congenital heart disease include the following:

Murmurs

These are often loud and may be heard over the precordium. Indeed, they may be felt (*thrills*) by palm of the hand placed over the chest.

Evidence of heart failure

This may be either right or left heart failure.

Evidence of a right-to-left shunt, central cyanosis

This occurs whenever the cardiac defect allows deoxygenated blood to bypass the lungs and enter the systemic circulation, as in Fallot's tetralogy. It also occurs in severe lung disease as well as being a result of pulmonary arteriovenous shunts. Central cyanosis affects all the tissues. Peripheral cyanosis is due to stagnation and occurs in the skin when the temperature is reduced and there is vasoconstriction. Because the mucous membranes have a good supply, they are not affected in peripheral cyanosis. Cyanosis in 'blue babies' is usually due to Fallot's tetralogy.

Polycythaemia

This is due to the effects of hypoxia on the bone marrow.

Clubbing of the fingers and toes

This generally occurs when the cyanosis has been present for a long period. The pathogenesis is obscure. Clubbing is also found as an idiopathic congenital anomaly of little consequence; it is also a feature of chronic suppurative lung disease (e.g. bronchiectasis and lung abscess), lung cancer, and *S. viridans* endocarditis.

Squatting

Patients with cyanotic heart disease typically assume a squatting posture after exertion to obtain relief from their dyspnoea.

Hypoxic spells

The degree of hypoxia may suddenly progress to the extent that there is a loss of consciousness, seizures, and even death. Such alarming episodes are most common in young children.

Underdevelopment

Unless the congenital heart defect is corrected, the child tires easily and may show poor development. Respiratory infections are common; death may occur from them or from heart failure.

AETIOLOGY

Some types of congenital heart disease are familial and there is an evident genetic influence. The association with Down's syndrome is well established.

The heart develops during the third to eighth week of fetal life, and external agents acting during this period can cause damage to the heart. If the mother contracts rubella, heart malformations are likely to occur. Measles and mumps have also been suggested as likely aetiological agents in the developing fetus. Teratogenic drugs (e.g. thalidomide) are another important cause.

INDIVIDUAL LESIONS OF CONGENITAL HEART DISEASE

Patent ductus arteriosus (Fig. 29.1)

Before birth the pressure in the aorta is slightly below that of the pulmonary artery and the ductus transmits blood from the artery to the aorta. After birth the baby starts to breathe, and as the lungs inflate, so the pressure in the pulmonary artery falls and that in the aorta rises. Normally the ductus becomes obliterated. Should it fail to close, blood flows from the aorta to the pulmonary artery thereby increasing the volume of blood passing through the lungs and returning to the left atrium and ventricle. The heart can cope with this situation for a while, but pulmonary hypertension develops and eventually there is right-sided heart failure and a reversal of flow so that cyanosis ensues. If the shunt is large, it may cause cardiac failure in infancy, but more often the effects are less severe. Death generally occurs before the age of 40 due either to heart failure or the effects of infection (bacterial endarteritis). The treatment is division or ligation of the ductus, but it is essential that no other anomalies are present.

Ventricular septal defects (Fig. 29.2)

In ventricular septal defects the shunt of oxygenated blood from left to right through the defect causes the same changes in the heart and pulmonary blood flow as those of patent ductus arteriosus. Eventually pulmonary hypertension may lead to right-sided heart failure.

If the ventricular septal defect is large, early surgical intervention is required to save the child's life. With small defects there may be no symptoms and the condition may remain undiagnosed. In intermediate cases there is cardiac enlargement, diminished exercise tolerance, and a tendency to respiratory infections which ultimately lead to heart failure. Ventricular septal defects may close spontaneously during the first few years of life, and such children have a normal life expectancy. The treatment of ventricular septal defects is open-heart surgery and closure of the defect either by stitches or the insertion of a prosthetic patch.

Atrial septal defects (Fig. 29.3)

An atrial septal defect is the most common congenital anomaly found in adults. A left-to-right shunt results in overfilling of the right atrium and therefore an increased output of the right ventricle. Cardiac failure may develop between the ages of 20 and 40 years; if untreated, survival beyond the age of 45 years is rare.

Pulmonary stenosis (Fig. 29.4)

Pulmonary stenosis is relatively common and the obstruction may be supravalvular, valvular, or subvalvular. It usually occurs as a result of unequal division of the truncus arteriosus during development. Right ventricular hypertrophy results in all but the mildest cases; the limits of hypertrophy are eventually reached and cardiac failure occurs.

Aortic stenosis (Fig. 29.5)

Aortic stenosis is an uncommon form of congenital heart disease, but congenital bicuspid valves occur in about 2% of the population. It is generally symptomless, but prolapse of one leaflet may lead to regurgitation. This may be complicated by infection, or in later life cause calcification so that calcific aortic stenosis results.

Coarctation of the aorta (Fig. 29.6)

In this condition the aorta is narrowed either at the level of the entrance of the ductus arteriosus or immediately before or immediately after this. Blood then reaches the lower half of the body via collateral vessels. The importance of this condition is two-fold. Firstly the area of stenosis may become infected (infective endarteritis), and secondly there is systemic hypertension confined to the upper part of the body. This leads to left ventricular hypertrophy and failure, and an increased liability to cerebral haemorrhage. Unless treated, life is seldom prolonged over the age of 40 years. Coarctation is associated with Turner's syndrome.

Dextrocardia

The finding of an apex beat of the heart on the right side of the chest is an occasional surprise on examining a patient. The heart develops as a mirror image of the normal, and if all organs are similarly affected the patient lives a normal life. This is called *complete situs inversus*. However, if only the heart is affected other defects are present and the results are serious.

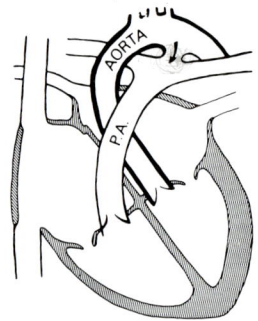

Fig. 29.1   Patent ductus arteriosus

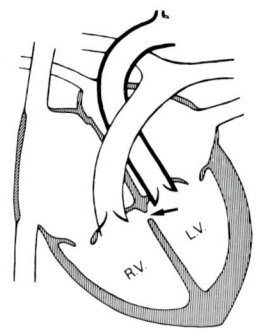

Fig. 29.2   Ventricular septal defect

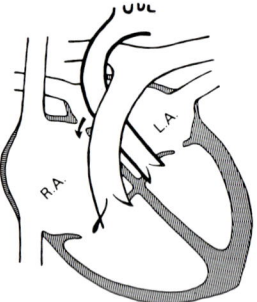

Fig. 29.3   Atrial septal defect

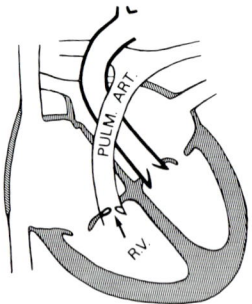

Fig. 29.4   Pulmonary stenosis

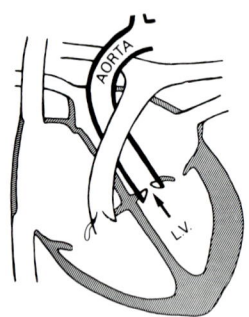

Fig. 29.5   Aortic stenosis

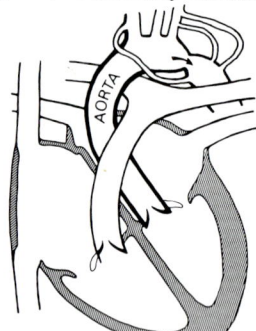

Fig. 29.6   Coarctation of aorta

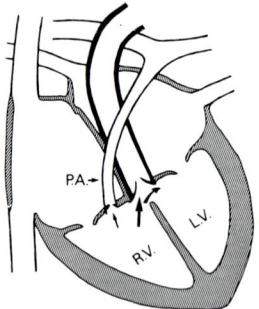

Fig. 29.7   Fallot's tetralogy

Figs 29.1 to 29.7 Congenital heart lesions. See the text for descriptions of the individual lesions. (Illustrations by the Photography Department, Birmingham Dental School).

Transposition of the great vessels

Transposition of the great vessels is a common fatal anomaly in children under 1 year of age. The aorta arises from the right ventricle and the pulmonary artery from the left ventricle as a result of a failure of rotation during development. A septal defect or some other anomaly is also present, otherwise life would be impossible.

Multiple defects

Developmental anomalies are often multiple. Not only may they be found in other organs, but several lesions may be present in the heart itself. A common combination is that found in the *tetralogy of Fallot* (Fig. 29.7). This comprises:

Pulmonary stenosis; ventricular septal defect; over-riding of the septum by the aorta, so that the blood from the right and left ventricles enters the aorta; hypertrophy of the right ventricle—this is compensatory.

In Fallot's tetralogy there is usually cyanosis at birth, but initially it may only be apparent during crying or feeding. Dyspnoea usually occurs early. The child exhibits the squatting phenomenon before the age of 3 years, and clubbing of fingers and toes is common. If untreated, survival past 21 years of age is uncommon.

ACQUIRED HEART DISEASE

The three important types of acquired heart disease are those associated with ischaemia, hypertension or rheumatic fever.

ISCHAEMIC HEART DISEASE

The myocardium is supplied by blood through the two coronary arteries. These vessels are commonly affected by atherosclerosis which steadily causes narrowing of the lumen. At any time the occlusion can become total, as a result of superadded thrombosis or haemorrhage into a plaque. The cause of atherosclerosis is considered in Chapter 28 but it should be noted at this stage that recognized risk factors predisposing to coronary atherosclerosis include a family history,

cigarette smoking, systemic hypertension, diabetes mellitus and hyperlipidaemia.

Myocardial ischaemia may be caused by other diseases affecting the coronary arteries. Compared with atherosclerosis they are uncommon; they include polyarteritis, embolism, dissecting aortic aneurysm. Sometimes ischaemia occurs in the presence of apparently normal coronary arteries. Spasm of the vessels appears to be the explanation in some cases. Severe hypotension, as in shock, can cause ischaemia as can marked tachycardia because the period of diastole is shortened (see later). Anaemia and thyrotoxicosis are other factors that cause hypoxia, so also can sudden violent exercise particularly in a subject with preexisting coronary disease. The presence of marked myocardial hypertrophy accentuates the hypoxia associated with other factors reducing coronary blood flow, because although the heart muscle fibres increase in size, there is no corresponding increase in supplying capillaries.

Effects of myocardial ischaemia

Sudden coronary occlusion tends to be associated with myocardial infarction and sudden death, whereas, gradual occlusion tends to cause angina pectoris or mild clinical symptoms. The association is by no means exact. In the account that follows, the main clinical syndromes will be described, and these will be related to the morphological and functional causes of ischaemia.

Acute functional derangements

An acute dysrhythmia such as ventricular fibrillation or complete heart block can cause sudden death. Immediate external cardiac massage or defibrillation can save the lives of some of these patients.

Angina pectoris

In some patients with myocardial ischaemia there are no symptoms at rest, but exercise causes pain which characteristically is felt in the precordium, spreads into the neck, sometimes up to the teeth, and down the inner side of the left arm. The pain may be precipitated by exercise, a heavy meal, or sudden exposure to a cold temperature. The pain is relieved by rest and by placing a tablet of nitroglycerine under the tongue. This drug is readily absorbed by the buccal mucosa, and acts by causing peripheral vasodilation, thereby lowering the systolic blood pressure and lessening the work load of the left ventricle. In addition, it causes coronary dilatation (see Chapter 27). In *variant angina* the pain occurs at rest and coronary artery spasm is the probable cause. In *unstable angina*, also called *acute coronary insufficiency*, the angina rapidly worsens and pain occurs with exercise and at rest. Severe coronary atherosclerosis with recent thrombosis is generally present and may be the forerunner of myocardial infarction or death.

Chronic ischaemic heart disease

Progressive myocardial ischaemia does not always cause angina. Sometimes there is patchy destruction of myocardium and replacement fibrosis. Clinically there is left ventricular failure.

Myocardial infarction

If the ischaemic muscle undergoes necrosis an infarct results (Fig. 29.8). Initially the area is pale, but within a few days the infarct appears as a firm, yellow area of coagulative necrosis with some surrounding haemorrhage and, later, inflammation. Microscopically no changes are evident until the lesion is 12–24 h old; the muscle fibres become eosinophilic, and early changes of acute inflammation are observed—interstitial oedema and an infiltration by neutrophils. By 3–7 days, the fibres are brightly eosinophilic, and their nuclei are either pyknotic, fragmented or completely absent. The inflammation is more intense and, in due course, macrophage activity removes the necrotic muscle and granulation tissue forms and evolves into scar tissue.

A localized infarct (*regional infarction*) is often associated with thrombosis of the corresponding branch of a coronary artery. Thus the anterior wall of the left ventricle and septum are involved when the anterior descending branch of the left coronary artery is thrombosed, while blockage of the right coronary artery is associated with infarction of the posteroinferior wall of the ventricle and adjacent septum. Regional infarcts may be transmural so that there is involvement of both the endocardium (with overlying *thrombosis*) and pericardium (with fibrinous *pericarditis*). A second pattern is *subendocardial infarction*, which involves a wide area of myocardium of the left ventricle. This is generally associated with widespread coronary disease without a localized thrombus.

Clinical features of myocardial infarction. A typical myocardial infarct is characterized by the acute onset of severe retrosternal pain, which is often described as having a crushing or squeezing character. Often it is severe enough to cause the patient to sweat. Unlike the pain of angina it is not influenced by exercise or the administration of nitroglycerine. Although severe pain is characteristic, many cases are encountered in which the pain is mild or indeed absent. It may be experienced in the epigastrium and mistaken for an attack of indigestion. As noted previously, there is an acute inflammatory reaction in the area of infarction and this is associated with fever, a raised ESR and a polymorphonuclear leucocytosis. Characteristic changes occur in the electrocardiogram, and their nature gives a good indication of the site of the infarct. The diagnosis is confirmed by finding an increase in the blood level of enzymes released from the necrotic muscle. The most specific is the MB fraction of creatinine pyrophosphate (CPK) the level of which rises within 6 h of the attack and peaks at 24 h. Other enzymes include the serum glutamicoxyloacetic acid transaminase (SGOT), and the lactic hehydrogenase (LDH). More recently, various nuclear imaging techniques have been introduced. Thus thallium scintigraphy shows areas of the heart that are perfused, while technetium-labelled pyrophosphate injected intravenously is concentrated in the area of infarction and is detected on scanning as a 'hot spot'. Positron emission tomography (PET) is another useful imaging technique.

Complications of acute myocardial infarction. A variety of dysrhythmias can result from involvement of the conducting system or the electrical excitation mechanism of the heart. The most serious is ventricular fibrillation, which is fatal unless reversed. Cardiopulmonary resuscitation with defibrillation can save the lives of these patients if it is immediately available.

Heart failure (pump failure) may be due directly to extensive myocardial necrosis or a severe dysrhythmia. A state of cardiac shock ensues and may be accompanied by pulmonary oedema and renal failure secondary to acute tubular necrosis. *Pericarditis* is another early complication, as is *endocardial thrombosis* with its danger of embolism to the systemic circulation. *Rupture of the myocardium* is a danger any time during the first 2 weeks. The rupture may be external into the pericardium leading to acute cardiac tamponade and rapid death. Rupture of the septum leads to right ventricular failure, while rupture of one of the papillary muscles of the mitral valve causes the sudden onset of mitral regurgitation and pulmonary oedema. An uncommon later complication is the *post-myocardial infarction syndrome*. It occurs within 3 months of infarction and is characterized by fever and pericarditis. It appears to be an autoimmune reaction to damaged heart muscle and is also encountered after cardiac surgery (*postcardiotomy syndrome*). Both conditions respond to glucocorticoid therapy. The end-result of a myocardial infarct is the formation of a scar. If large this may bulge to form an aneurysm of the left ventricle. This tends to bulge during systole so that some of the contractile force of the ventricular muscle is wasted. Heart failure may ensue and resection of the aneurysm is helpful.

The prognosis of acute myocardial infarction depends on the size of the infarct. On average over 70% of patients survive their first attack, but some are left with evidence of cardiac damage and further attacks may be expected.

HYPERTENSIVE HEART DISEASE

In systemic hypertension the left ventricle is subjected to a continuous strain. It responds by hypertrophy of its muscle fibres, and for a time bears the strain well, but eventually the enormously thick ventricular wall fails. Often there is associated coronary atherosclerosis. The chronic left ventricular failure is followed by congestive heart failure. In addition, some patients develop sudden nocturnal attacks of pulmonary oedema. The victim is seized by an ominous sense of suffocation; the condition is called paroxysmal (nocturnal) dyspnoea (p. 371).

RHEUMATIC HEART DISEASE

Rheumatic heart disease commences with an attack of acute rheumatic fever. The acute disease is now uncommon in the Western countries but is still rife in the Middle East, North Africa and in the Indian subcontinent. The first attack is generally in childhood, and follows 2–3 weeks after a streptococcal sore throat. The child develops fever, leucocytosis and a raised ESR. Pain and swelling affecting many joints is characteristic. Subcutaneous nodules develop over bony prominences and there is evidence of a pancarditis. Fibrinous pericarditis causes a friction rub audible clinically. Dilatation of the mitral and tricuspid valve rings cause regurgitation, and combined with myocarditis leads to heart failure. Microscopically the myocardium contains Aschoff's bodies. These have a central zone of fibrinoid necrosis surrounded by lymphocytes, macrophages and occasional neutrophils. Particularly characteristic are large mononuclear cells, termed Anitschkow's cells, and giant cells with up to four nuclei, termed *Aschoff's giant cells*. Fibroblasts are also present in the lesions and they ultimately form small scars.

The most important cardiac component of acute rheumatic fever is a valvulitis, involving particularly the mitral and aortic valves. In the acute phase the valves are swollen and small thrombi (called vegetations) form along the line of closure of the valve cusps (Fig. 29.9). These are well attached, do not embolize, and have little effect on valve function. However, rheumatic fever has a tendency to recur and with repeated attacks the valvulitis becomes chronic, with fibrosis being prominent. The valve cusps become thickened, rigid and adherent to each other. The result is stenosis of the valve orifice. If the mitral valve is affected the chordae tendinae are similarly affected, being thickened, rigid and shortened. The end-result is *mitral stenosis* combined with some degree of *regurgitation*. Similarly *aortic stenosis and regurgitation* can occur, but the valves of the right side of the heart are infrequently affected to any significant degree.

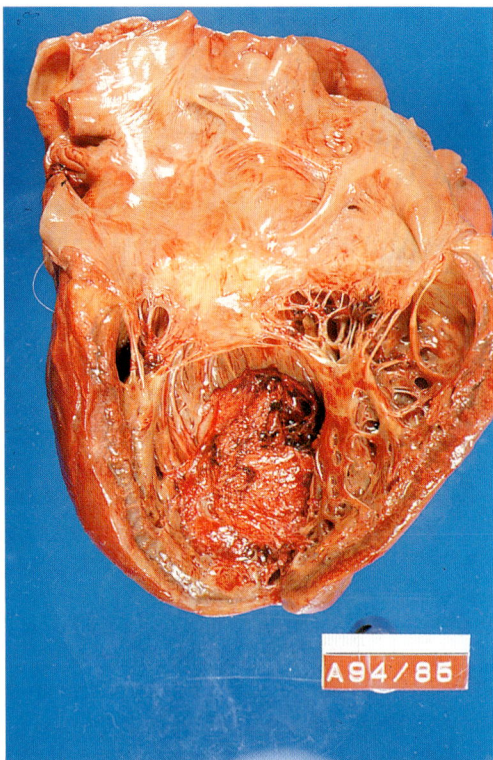

Fig. 29.8   Recent subendocardial myocardial infarct (7–10 days). The heart has been opened to show the left ventricle, mitral valve and left atrium. The cut surface of the left ventricular wall shows an extensive area of subendocardial infarction, which is yellow-grey in colour, replacing the deep red of normal muscle. The yellow mottling of the two papillary muscles is due to the underlying infarction. A recent thrombus covers the ventricular wall between the papillary muscles. (Photograph courtesy of Dr J Butany, University of Toronto.)

The precise pathogenesis of acute rheumatic fever is not known, but some immune mechanism is considered likely, either immune complex or T cell mediated. The relationship with streptococcal infection is well established, and long-term antibiotic therapy is employed to prevent recurrent infections with their attendant risk of continued heart damage.

ENDOCARDITIS

Non-bacterial thrombotic endocarditis

Small warty or friable vegetations along the line of closure of the mitral or aortic valves are not uncommon as a post-mortem finding. The veg-etations are sterile and may be formed on normal or deformed valves. They are of importance in two respects. Occasionally they become detached and embolize to the brain. About 10% of cerebral embolism has been attributed to this mechanism. Secondly the vegetations may form a nidus for the development of infective endocarditis. Usually however, the vegetations of non-bacterial thrombotic endocarditis are of no significance and are removed, probably by lysis.

Infective endocarditis

Colonization of the valves by organisms associated with inflammation and thrombus formation is a serious condition which without treatment is

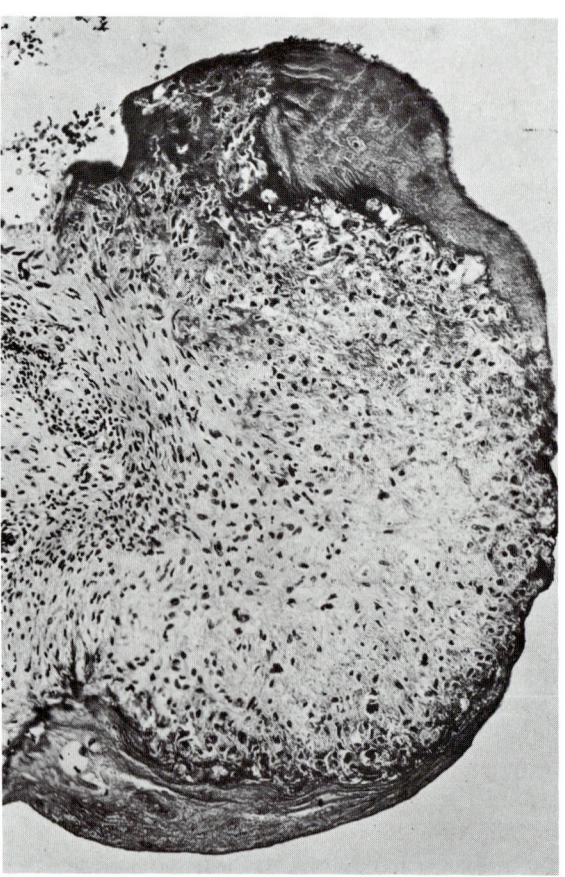

Fig. 29.9   Organizing rheumatic vegetation. The base of the thrombus has been invaded by granulation tissue, while a layer of fibrin (in which there are doubtless aggregations of platelets) still remains on the surface. × 110.

fatal. The severity of the illness and the clinical picture depends on the organism involved. In about 50% of cases infective endocarditis develops at the site of some pre-existing lesion, such a damaged valve (commonly rheumatic), a valve prosthesis, or a congenital malformation. Occasionally lesions develop in association with coarctation of the aorta or a patent ductus arteriosus. The disease is being encountered more frequently in the elderly than it was previously, and usually there is no preceding valvular disease to account for its localization. Perhaps minor degenerative lesions are present in the affected valve. The mitral and aortic valves are most commonly affected.

The presence of turbulence is believed to be important in the pathogenesis of endocarditis for it predisposes to thrombus formation. Should there be organisms present in the blood their incorporation in the thrombus initiates the endocarditis. If the organisms are highly virulent *acute infective endocarditis results*. Large friable vegetations are formed and the valve is rapidly destroyed: multiple infected emboli are released into the circulation and lead to the formation of multiple pyaemic abscesses or septic infarcts. Clinically the patient is gravely ill and there are signs of rapidly changing valvular lesions as well as multiple embolic phenomena. Common organisms are *Staph. aureus, Strep. pyogenes* and *N. gonorrhoea*. When the organisms are less virulent the vegetations are smaller, valve destruction is less marked and the disease is more protracted. The term *subacute infective endocarditis* is commonly used and in the classical disease, *Strep. viridans* was the most common organism involved. Since the introduction and wide use of antibiotics, at least half the cases are due to other organisms. The illness is protracted with fever, loss of weight and anaemia. Chronic bacteraemia is responsible for overgrowth of the MPS, as evidenced by splenomegaly. Multiple embolic phenomena are characteristic, and the lesions tend to remain sterile. Large emboli cause infarction in the brain, intestine, kidney or elsewhere. Immune complex vasculitis causes renal lesions with haematuria, palpable purpura and splinter haemorrhages under the nails.

A definite confirmation of a diagnosis of endocarditis hinges on obtaining a positive blood culture. However, the disease is so serious that if the clinical picture suggests endocarditis, it is justifiable to start treatment before pathological confirmation. Even with early treatment there may be so much valve damage with ultimate fibrosis and calcification that a replacement prosthesis is required.

Although it is traditional to describe endocarditis as subacute or acute, in practice intermediate types occur and it is more meaningful to describe the condition in relationship to the causative organism. With the current frequency of immunosuppressive therapy there are few organisms that have not been described as causing endocarditis! These include coliforms, bacteroides, fungi (particularly *Candida*), *Coxiella* and viruses. Open heart surgery and intravenous drug addiction have added to the predisposing causes of endocarditis.

Prophylaxis

Any patient known to have a valvular disease, a valvular prosthesis, or a congenital heart lesion should have adequate antibiotic cover before being subjected to invasive dental treatment affecting the soft tissues, or indeed any other treatment, such as catheterization, that is liable to cause bacteraemia. An antibiotic should be given an hour before surgery and repeated 8 h postoperatively. If given too early, there is a possibility of the development of a resistant organism.

VALVULAR DEFECTS

The heart-valve complex consists of the valve cusps, the valve ring, and the adjacent myocardium, including the papillary muscles in the case of the atrioventricular valves. Defects in any of these components causes dysfunction—stenosis, regurgitation, or a combination of the two. It is convenient at this stage to summarize these defects; details will be found elsewhere in this book.

Mitral valve disease

Mitral stenosis

Mitral stenosis is commonly rheumatic. The left

ventricle being under no strain is of normal size. The left atrium, however, is greatly dilated and there may be mural thrombus posteriorly above the valve. Embolism may result. The back pressure effect on the lungs causes chronic venous congestion and ultimately right sided heart failure. Atrial fibrillation is common.

Mitral regurgitation

Mitral regurgitation may also complicate rheumatic heart disease. A common cause is dilatation of the valve ring in heart failure from any cause. Fibrosed or ruptured papillary muscle, endocarditis and myxomatous degeneration of the mitral valve are other causes. The effects of mitral regurgitation are similar to those of mitral stenosis but in addition the left ventricle is enlarged.

Myxomatous degeneration of the valves. This condition is quite common, particularly in young women, but apart from a mid- or late-systolic click on auscultation it is clinically silent. The dense collagen of the valve cusps (usually of the mitral valve) becomes thinned and replaced by myxomatous tissue. The thin 'floppy valve' can prolapse and cause some degree of regurgitation. Infective endocarditis and rupture are two other complications.

Aortic valve disease

Aortic stenosis

Aortic stenosis may be congenital and supravalvular, valvular or subvalvular. The latter occurs in hypertrophic cardiomyopathy.

Calcific (calcareous) aortic stenosis. This condition, arising in a congenitally bicuspid valve, usually affects elderly men. The valve cusps become calcified, and fuse together producing a tight stenosis. The left ventricle is hypertrophied, but in spite of the overaction of this chamber an inadequate amount of blood is pumped into the aorta. In particular the blood supply to the coronary vessels is impaired, and these patients are in constant danger of sudden death. Surgical replacement of diseased valves by a graft or plastic prosthesis is therefore indicated.

Aortic regurgitation

Aortic regurgitation is generally due to dilatation of the aortic ring that may be idiopathic or accompany rheumatoid arthritis or syphilitic aortitis.

Tricuspid valve disease

Tricuspid regurgitation is common and accompanies right-sided heart failure as the valve ring dilates. Stenosis occasionally complicates rheumatic heart disease.

Pulmonary valve disease

Pulmonary valve involvement in rheumatic disease and endocarditis is rare. Congenital pulmonary stenosis is more common.

CARDIAC DYSRHYTHMIAS

In the normal heart the impulse that initiates cardiac contraction commences in the sinoatrial (S–A) node in the right atrium, spreads throughout the atria, reaches the atrioventricular (A–V) node, and then travels down the conducting bundle of His to reach the two ventricles. Any interruption in this process can cause irregularity in the heart beat. *Ectopic or premature beats* occur when the initiating site is not the S–A node. It may be in the atria, the A–V node or in the ventricles. Following the beat there is a compensatory pause before the next normal beat. This gives the patient the feeling of the heart 'turning over'. Ectopic atrial beats are common in normal people, but ventricular ones may be associated with myocardial ischaemia or digitalis overdose. In *paroxysmal tachycardia* repeated ectopic beats result in runs of rapid heart rate. Multiple ectopic foci discharging at varying rates lead to fibrillation. In *atrial fibrillation* only a few of the multiple impulses are passed to the ventricles, and the pulse is irregularly irregular, and each pulse varies in strength. Atrial fibrillation is a common complication of rheumatic heart disease, particularly mitral stenosis, but is also encountered in ischaemic heart disease and in thyrotoxicosis.

Ventricular fibrillation is a serious complication of ischaemic heart disease. There is no effective ventricular contraction and death is likely unless electrical defibrillation can be carried out.

In *heart block* there is depressed conduction between the atria and the ventricles. In the early stages the speed of conduction is merely delayed and the condition is diagnosed on the ECG. As the condition progresses, occasional impulses fail to reach the ventricles. Finally, in *complete heart block*, the ventricular beat is entirely initiated within the ventricles themselves. This intrinsic ventricular rate is slow—about 40 beats per minute. When complete heart block occurs suddenly there may be complete ventricular standstill for several seconds or minutes. The patient loses consciousness and seizures occur. These episodes are known as Stokes–Adams attacks.

HEART FAILURE

The most important chambers of the heart are the two ventricles. These fill during diastole from the low-pressured venous reservoirs, an effect aided by atrial contraction. Normally the heart is able to expel all the blood which flows into it. If the venous return is increased in volume, the increased filling of the heart stretches its muscle fibres and the force of the next contraction is increased. This is *Starling's Law of the Heart*. The cardiac output is thus gauged to the venous return, and the heart can satisfy the needs of the body under all normal circumstances.

Under resting conditions the ventricles do not empty completely with each systole, but with exercise their contraction results in more complete emptying. This is mediated by an increase in sympathetic tone,* and acting with the greater filling due to the increased venous return, it results in a larger volume (the stroke volume) of blood being ejected with each heart beat. In addition, the heart rate increases. Therefore the heart has a considerable *functional reserve*, and

can increase its output from the resting level of 5 litres per min to 25–30 litres per min.

Prolonged overwork of any chamber causes hypertrophy of the muscle of its walls. This is an additional cardiac reserve, but it should be remembered that the hypertrophied myocardium usually fails unless the strain on it is removed. A large heart is a diseased heart.

When, in the presence of an adequate venous return, the heart fails to supply blood to meet the needs of the body the condition is known as *heart failure*. At first the effects of this are to be seen on exercise, but as the failure increases so the effects are apparent even at rest. Either the left or the right ventricle may fail separately. More usually the heart fails as a whole, and the condition is called *congestive heart failure*.

Effects of right ventricular failure

Rise in central venous pressure†

A failure of the right ventricle to eject all the blood which it receives leads to distension of the right atrium by a back-pressure effect. The pressure in the great veins rises, and *the jugular veins are seen to be distended with blood* when the patient sits up in bed. To some extent this *aids* heart function, because the raised pressure causes increased filling of the heart. This by stretching the myocardium *increases* the force of contraction. However, a point can be reached beyond which increased stretching causes a *decrease* in cardiac contraction. Exercise, by increasing the venous return, further reduces the cardiac output; the patient is therefore bedridden. Once past this critical point, therapeutic bleeding increases the cardiac output by reducing the venous pressure. This is the basis for the time-honoured practice of bleeding as a treatment for heart failure. In right-sided heart failure all the organs of the body are congested. This is particularly well seen in the liver, where the centres of the lobules are deeply congested and red (see nutmeg liver, p. 362). Congestion is evident in the skin, especially of the face.

---

*A change in the force of contraction of the heart without a corresponding change in the initial length of the muscle is called an *inotropic effect*. The alkaloids of digitalis are used in heart failure because they have an inotropic effect.

†This is the pressure in the right atrium minus the negative intrathoracic pressure.

Cyanosis

The sluggish circulation allows a more complete deoxygenation of the blood as it passes through the tissues. In the skin this may be detected by the bluish colouration know as *cyanosis*. Cyanosis is evident when the capillary blood contains more than 5 g reduced haemoglobin per dl. It should be noted that cyanosis due to stasis (*peripheral cyanosis*) is not necessarily due to heart disease. It is seen whenever the circulation is sluggish, e.g. in polycythemia (where the blood is very viscous), in an area affected by venous obstruction, and in shock. Some people are so sensitive to cold that their ears, nose, and finger-tips become cyanosed even on exposure to a cool atmosphere.

Polycythaemia

An increased red-cell count occurs as a result of bone-marrow hypoxia.

Oedema

Oedema of the dependent parts is a prominent sign of heart failure. It accumulates around the legs and genitalia, and, during recumbency, the sacral region. The pathogenesis of the oedema is complex. In part it is due to the chronic passive venous congestion of the tissues, but a more important factor is the reduced cardiac output. The reduced output of the right ventricle leads to a corresponding fall in that of the left ventricle, for the quantity of blood entering this chamber is the same as the right ventricular output. This reduced cardiac output acts on the kidneys and causes salt and water retention (see congestive heart failure).

EFFECTS OF LEFT VENTRICULAR FAILURE

Rise in pulmonary venous pressure

The venous distension affects the lungs which become congested and tense. The effort of breathing is increased, and this causes distress (*dyspnoea*). *Pulmonary oedema* is an ever-present danger, and may come on with dramatic suddenness. Rupture of capillaries leads to *haemoptysis*,

and the blood which remains in the lungs is converted into haemosiderin. This produces a brown pigmentation of the lungs and stimulates fine fibrosis, a condition called *brown induration of the lung*. It is the result of longstanding chronic venous congestion.

It should be noted that in primary left ventricular failure the output of the two ventricles is the same, but the left is functioning with the aid of an increased venous filling pressure. The right ventricle, on the other hand, is working normally. This leads to a redistribution of blood, more being retained in the pulmonary circuit than is normal. In addition to producing pulmonary congestion and oedema, the rise in pulmonary pressure (*pulmonary hypertension*) ultimately causes the right ventricle to fail, and *congestive heart failure* ensues.

Effects of congestive heart failure

The inadequate cardiac output causes ischaemia of many organs. Selective vasoconstriction, e.g. of the skin vessels, causes sufficient redistribution of blood so that the important organs do not suffer damage in the initial stages. Cutaneous arteriolar constriction is an important factor in the pathogenesis of *peripheral cyanosis*. The two

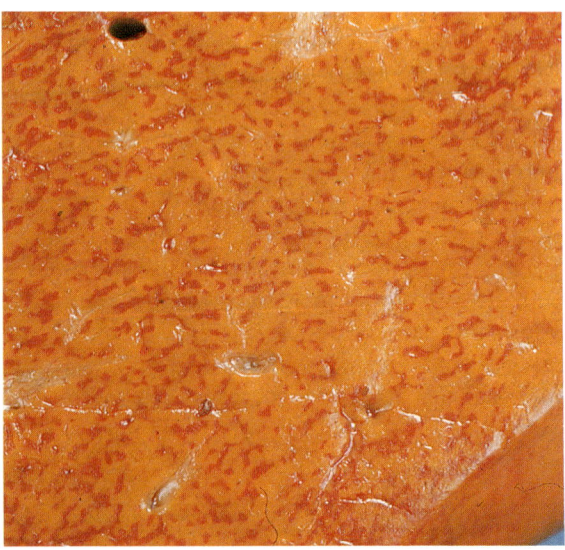

Fig. 29.10 Nutmeg liver. The pattern of alternating dark congestion and pale fatty change is apparent.

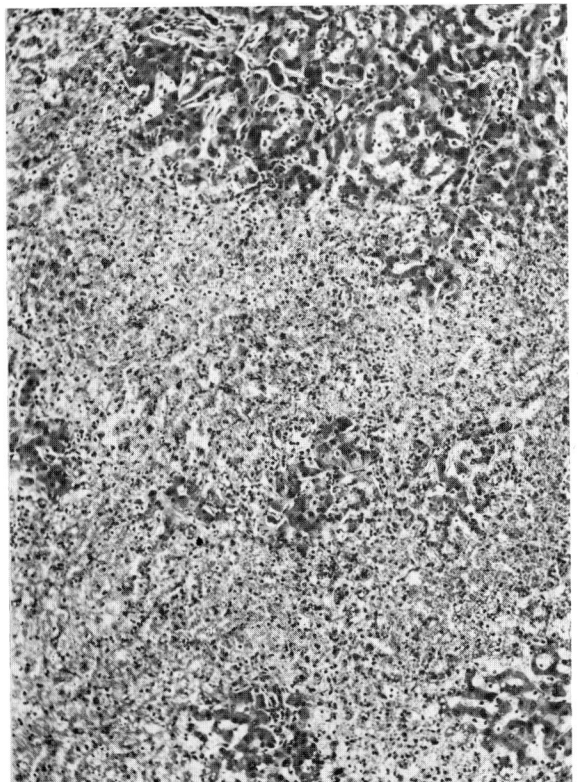

Fig. 29.11 Chronic venous congestion of the liver. There is virtual disappearance of the liver cells in the central zones of the lobules, and their replacement with engorged, dilated sinusoids. The peripheral cells show fatty change. × 90.

organs in which the effect of ischaemia is most marked are the liver and the kidneys.

In the liver the ischaemia leads to necrosis of the cells in the centres of the lobules, while the less severely affected peripheral cells show fatty change. The result is the characteristic *nutmeg liver* of congestive heart failure—the centres of the lobules are red and the peripheries yellow (Figs 29.10 and 29.11).

In the kidneys no morphological changes other than congestion are evident, but the impaired renal blood flow leads to *salt and water retention*. This is a very important factor in the causation of cardiac oedema. Venous distension plays its part in determining the location of the oedema rather than in causing its formation.

In the terminal stages of left-sided heart failure *the brain* receives an inadequate blood supply,

and this causes an impairment of consciousness and sometimes dementia.

THE CAUSES OF HEART FAILURE

As previously described, the heart can easily increase its output during exercise. It cannot, however, maintain the high output for long, nor can it continue to function in the face of a high-output pressure. Any condition which imposes a sustained burden on the heart will eventually lead to its failure. It may also fail because of myocardial damage. The causes of heart failure may be considered under three headings:

Overburdening due to a sustained increase in ventricular pressure

This occurs in systemic and pulmonary *hypertension* and also in *aortic and pulmonary valvular disease*. If the semilunar cusps fuse together to produce a narrowing, or *stenosis*, of the valve orifice, the chamber behind the diseased valve, the ventricle, has to generate a high pressure to force blood through the stenosed valve. Hypertrophy of the ventricle occurs, but in time failure ensues. It should be noted that when the mitral valve is diseased, the over-distension of the left atrium causes pulmonary hypertension such that *right ventricular failure soon follows*.

Myocardial disease

Myocardial disease is by far the most important cause of heart failure. It is generally due to ischaemia secondary to atherosclerosis of the coronary arteries (p. 344). Other causes of myocardial failure are *myocarditis* (e.g. rheumatic and viral), and a group of non-inflammatory myocardial diseases termed the *cardiomyopathies*. In the primary group the heart is the only organ involved. Some cases are believed to be associated with alcoholism, beriberi or viral infection. Others are familial. The secondary cardiomyopathies are a diverse group in which the cause is known or the heart condition is associated with some systemic disease. Examples include poisons (including alcohol and adriamycin, a drug used in cancer chemotherapy) amyloidosis, myxoedema and sarcoidosis.

Overburdening due to a sustained increase in cardiac output

Valvular defects.

With aortic regurgitation, blood flows back into the left ventricle during diastole. An increased volume of blood must therefore be ejected in systole. The actual output of the ventricle is increased, but the effective output is unaltered. A similar result is seen in mitral regurgitation, but here the wasted ventricular output is diverted to the left atrium. In both aortic regurgitation and mitral regurgitation left ventricular failure ensues. Pulmonary and tricuspid disease produce comparable effects on the right side.

High output failure

There are a number of conditions in which there is a sustained increase in the true cardiac output; for a while the heart copes with the load, but ultimately it fails. Even in failure the output may be above the normal, but is still inadequate to meet the demands of the body because these demands are themselves greater than normal.

This condition is called *high-output failure* in contrast to the more common type of heart failure, called *low-output* failure. The most easily understood example is thyrotoxicosis, where the increased metabolic rate demands an increased output from the heart. Anaemia and a large arteriovenous shunt have a similar effect. Paget's disease of bone, some types of chronic lung disease and cirrhosis of the liver are other causes, and the presence of small arteriovenous shunts in the affected organ is probably the explanation of the high output state.

Additional factors causing heart failure

Additional factors may contribute to heart failure although they are rarely the sole cause. Dysrhythmia, e.g. atrial fibrillation, contributes to failure by leading to inefficient ventricular contraction. Other examples are fever, which causes a rise in the metabolic rate, and pregnancy.

Anxiety raises the heart rate and blood pressure, thereby adding an additional burden on the left ventricle. Thus anxiety may precipitate an attack of paroxysmal nocturnal dyspnoea.

GENERAL READING

Braunwald E 1984 Pathophysiology of heart failure and clinical manifestation of heart failure: In Braunwald E (ed.) Heart disease. A textbook of cardiovascular medicine, 2nd edn. Saunders, Philadelphia

Conti C R 1983 Coronary-artery spasm and myocardial infarction. New England Journal of Medicine 309:238

Fuster Y, Chesebro J H 1986 Mechanisms of unstable angina. New England Journal of Medicine 315:1023

Hampton J R 1982 Falling mortality in coronary heart disease. British Medical Journal 284:1505

Leading Article 1985 Decline in Rheumatic fever Lancet 2:647

Olsen E G J 1979 The pathology of the cardiomyopathies. A critical review. American Heart Journal 98:385

Silver M D (ed.) 1991 Cardiovascular pathology, 2nd edn. Churchill Livingstone, Edinburgh

WHO 1980 Report of the WHO/ISFC Task Force on the Definition and Classification of Cardiomypathies 1980. British Heart Journal 44:672

Woodruff J F 1980 Viral myocarditis: a review. American Journal of Pathology 101:425

Zabriskie J B 1985 Rheumatic fever: the interplay between host genetics and microbe. Circulation 71:1077

30. Diseases of the respiratory system

Normal function

The function of the respiratory system is to enable gaseous exchange to take place between the blood and the atmosphere. Air is inhaled, and as it passes through the nose, nasopharynx, larynx, and trachea it is filtered and humidified. It eventually reaches the alveoli of the lung where it comes into close contact with blood in the capillaries. Conditions for gaseous exchange are ideal: oxygen is added to the blood and the carbon dioxide which is removed is exhaled. The gas in the alveoli is maintained at a fairly constant composition by the act of breathing. This has two components—ventilation and distribution.

Ventilation. This is the bellows-like action of the chest, by which fresh air is drawn in and stale air expired. The volume is approximately 7.5 litres per minute in the adult at rest.

Distribution. The inspired air is so distributed in relation to the volume of blood perfusing the lung that the composition of the alveolar gas is maintained at a constant level. Since the arterial blood, as it leaves the lung, is in equilibrium with the alveolar gas, it follows that the gaseous tensions of oxygen and carbon dioxide in the arterial blood are also maintained at this same constant level.

RESPIRATORY FAILURE

If through the dysfunction of the lungs there is oxygen lack or CO_2 retention, the condition is called *respiratory failure*. In the arterial blood under normal conditions the partial pressure of oxygen, usually written Po_2, is about 100 mmHg (or 13.3 kilopascals, abbreviated to kPa) and the partial pressure of carbon dioxide (Pco_2) about 40 mmHg (or 5.3 kPa). In respiratory failure the Po_2 is under 60 mmHg and the Pco_2 over 49 mmHg.

Hypoxaemia. The arterial blood is normally saturated with oxygen, but in respiratory failure both the tension and quantity of oxygen in the blood are reduced. As the blood passes through the tissues it becomes increasingly desaturated, and cyanosis of the exposed parts occurs. The hypoxia stimulates red-cell production in the bone marrow, and leads to polycythaemia. This increases the viscosity of the blood, and by causing stagnation in the tissues contributes to the cyanosis. In addition there is a further strain on the heart, and *heart failure* may occur. Usually the right ventricle is affected, because in most lung diseases causing respiratory failure there is considerable destruction of lung tissue and obliteration of pulmonary vasculature. This causes pulmonary hypertension and strain on the right ventricle.

Retention of carbon dioxide. An increased tension of CO_2 in the arterial blood (*hypercapnia*) produces vasodilatation of the vessels of the skin and brain. The skin is hot and flushed, and the brain becomes hyperaemic and oedematous. Clinically the latter is manifest as confusion, drowsiness, tremor, and finally coma and death.

DYSPNOEA

In a healthy person the rate and depth of respiration are so regulated that the individual is unaware of the movements involved in breathing. *Tachypnoea* is an increased rate of respiration, and is seen when pain restricts respiratory movement, as in pleurisy, or when the lungs become increasingly rigid, as in congestion or fibrosis. Tachypnoea is sometimes accompanied by an increase in depth of breathing, and the term *hyperpnoea* embraces both conditions. *Dyspnoea* is a condition in which the act of breathing causes distress. It occurs under two main circumstances: (1) *when tachypnoea or hyperpnoea are of marked degree;* (2) *when the ventilatory effect produced on inspiration is small in comparison with the muscular effort needed to produce it.* This occurs in any disease interfering with the respiratory excursions of the lungs, for instance, fibrosis or congestion. Obstruction to the major air passage, whether due to pulmonary disease like chronic bronchitis or to strangulation, has a similar effect, and produces intense dyspnoea.

BRONCHIAL OBSTRUCTION

The common causes of bronchial obstruction are:

Tenacious mucus which is not expelled from the respiratory passage, e.g. bronchial asthma and chronic bronchitis.

Inhaled foreign bodies, e.g. teeth and portions of food.

Tumours, commonly carcinoma.

The effects of obstruction depend on whether the obstruction is partial or complete. *Partial obstruction* of a bronchus impedes the ventilation of the lung distal to the obstruction. It follows therefore that the blood perfusing that part of the lung is inadequately oxygenated, and that in effect a quantity of venous blood is shunted directly into the pulmonary veins and thence to the left side of the heart. Since the blood leaving the lungs is normally fully saturated with oxygen, it follows that no amount of over-ventilation of the unaffected lung can compensate for this shunt effect. The arterial Po_2 is therefore lowered.

Infection commonly follows bronchial obstruction. Organisms that are inhaled into the affected lung segment becomes trapped in the mucus, their expulsion is impaired, and bronchopneumonia follows. The infection also involves the bronchial wall, and if long-continued will produce destruction of the muscle and cartilaginous component, so that the bronchus is weakened and tends to dilate (*bronchiectasis*). This is frequently seen distal to the obstruction caused by a carcinoma or a foreign body. Quite often bronchiectasis occurs in several parts of the lung as an idiopathic condition, and is thought to be the result of obstruction by mucus during some previous infection, such as measles or whooping-cough during childhood.

Where there is *complete obstruction* of a large bronchus, the lung distal shows a progressive absorption of its gas content until it becomes completely airless or *collapsed*.

PNEUMONIA

Pneumonia is defined as inflammation of the parenchyma of the lung and may be caused by physicochemical agents or infection. Two patterns of reaction are seen. In the first type, *pneumonia with alveolar exudation*, the inflammation is associated with exudation into the alveoli so that the lung becomes airless or consolidated; the unqualified term 'pneumonia' is generally applied to this type (Fig. 30.1). In the second type, the inflammatory exudate is largely confined to the interstitial tissues of the lung. This is *interstitial pneumonia*, also called alveolitis.

PNEUMONIA WITH ALVEOLAR EXUDATION

This type of pneumonia is invariably caused by bacterial infection. The pattern of reaction depends on the virulence of the organism and the immunity of the host. Classically two patterns are described but the advent of antibiotic therapy has modified the picture. The major difference between the two types is the extent of the lung involvement—either lobar or lobular.

Lobar pneumonia

Lobar pneumonia is caused by a highly virulent organism, most commonly one of the virulent types of *S. pneumonia*; it may affect healthy adults but some underlying condition such alcoholism predisposes to it. The onset is sudden with rigors, fever and pain in the chest. The inflammation affects the whole of one lobe of lung uniformly; occasionally, more than one lobe is involved. Initially there is a septicaemia, and the infection can also involve the meninges or elsewhere. Usually, however, the lung only is involved, and the lobe affected shows congestion followed by the formation of an acute inflammatory exudate containing numerous neutrophils within the alveoli. The whole lobe

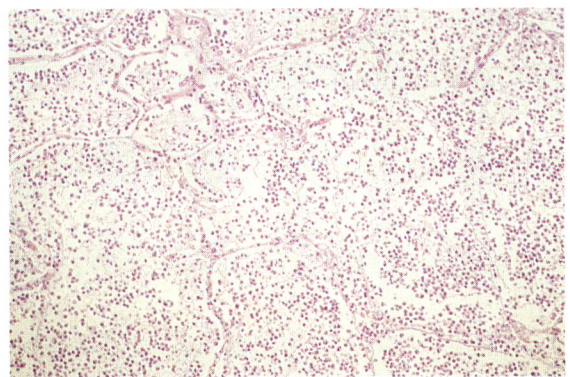

Fig. 30.1 Lobar pneumonia. The alveoli are uniformly filled with acute inflammatory exudate.

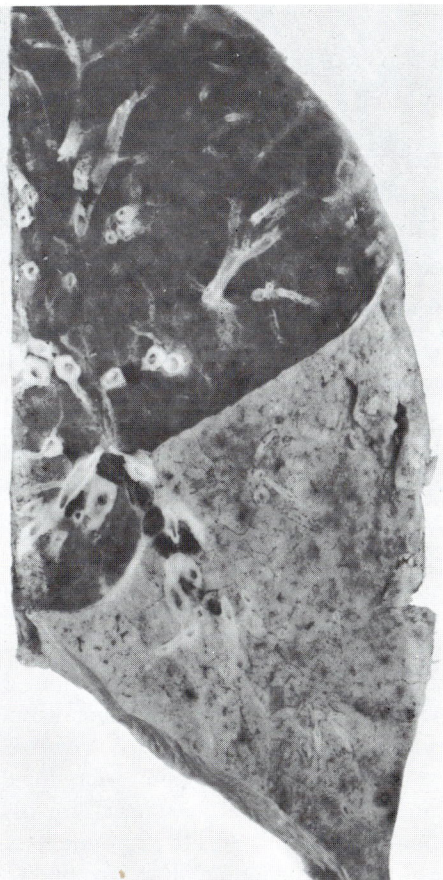

Fig. 30.2 Lobar pneumonia. The left lower lobe is consolidated in the stage of grey hepatization, while the upper lobe is unaffected. (R30.2. Reproduced by permission of the President and Council of the Royal College of Surgeons of England.)

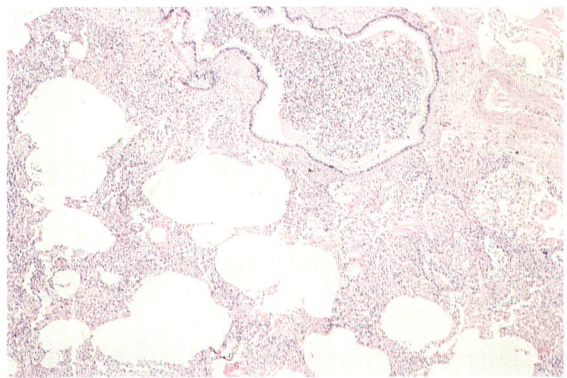

Fig. 30.3 Bronchopneumonia. Part of a terminal bronchiole is shown with its lining of ciliated columnar epithelium. The bronchiole is crowded with inflammatory cells, the majority of which are polymorphs. Some adjacent alveoli are either collapsed or contain inflammatory exudate. Others show compensatory dilatation.

becomes consolidated and the overlying pleura is involved (Figs 30.1 and 30.2). It is the fibrinous pleurisy that is responsible for the chest pain. The patient remains ill for 7–10 days and untreated may die during this phase. If the infection is overcome, the exudate is removed and the lung returns to normal. This is an excellent example of resolution. Clinically, if the patient survives, the disease terminates as suddenly as it started. Sweating leads to a return of the temperature to normal and a sense of well-being returns. This has been called termination by 'crisis'. In practice the clinical course is rarely seen because the disease responds promptly to antibiotic therapy.

Bronchopneumonia (lobular pneumonia)

This type of pneumonia is characterized by multiple discrete foci of bronchiolitis, with spread of the inflammation into the surrounding alveoli to produce small areas of consolidation (Fig. 30.3). The disease usually affects several lobes of the lung and is bilateral and basal in distribution (Fig. 30.4). The organisms causing the disease are either endogenous or exogenous.

Endogenous bronchopneumonia

The infecting organism is generally of low-grade virulence and is one of the commensal organisms of the upper respiratory tract—pneumococci, staphylococci, *Haemophilus influenzae* and various coliforms. These organisms cause infection under a variety of circumstances, which may be classified under the headings of general or local:

General causative factors. *Extremes of age.* Bronchopneumonia is commonest in infancy and old age.

General debilitating illness. The disease is a common terminal event in cancer, cerebrovascular accidents, and uraemia.

Impaired immune response. Any immunological deficient state, including glucocorticoid therapy, predisposes to bronchopneumonia.

Local causative factors. Local conditions interfering with ciliary action and the upward movement of mucus are liable to be followed by bronchopneumonia. The causes may be listed.

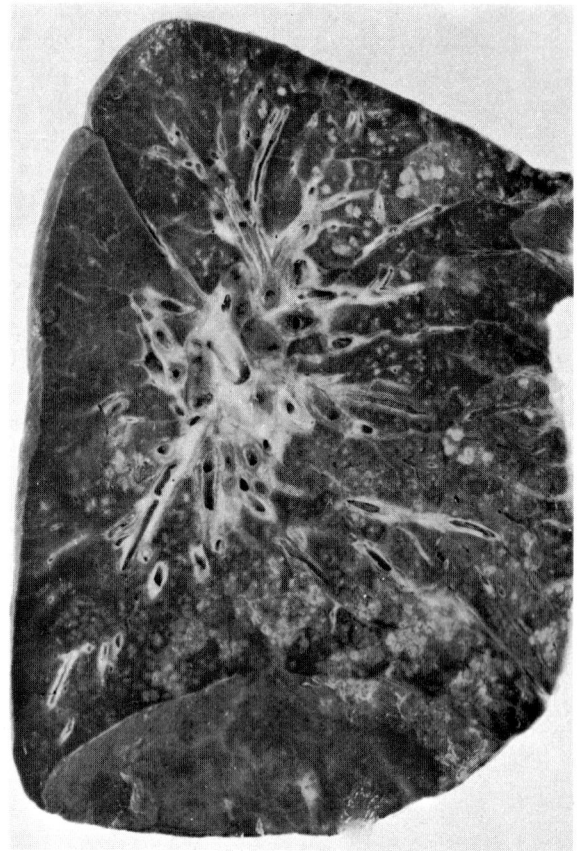

Fig. 30.4 Staphylococcal bronchopneumonia. There are discrete foci of consolidation scattered throughout the lung, and some have formed tiny abscesses. (R29.3. Reproduction by permission of the President and Council of the Royal College of Surgeons of England.)

Pre-existing acute respiratory disease. Bronchopneumonia often complicates influenza, measles, and whooping-cough. In these infections the ciliated bronchial epithelium is shed, and organisms which gain access to the lung cannot be removed.

Local obstruction. The trapped secretions form an admirable medium for bacterial growth, and bronchopneumonia is localized to the segment distal to the obstruction. Foreign bodies and tumours of the bronchi are well-known examples.

Chronic bronchitis and bronchiectasis. These are important predisposing causes of bronchopneumonia. Two factors are involved. In the first place the ciliated epithelium may be replaced by goblet cells or squamous cells; this impedes the upward flow of mucus. Secondly the mucus itself is often of viscid consistency, and cannot easily be removed. An excessive amount of mucus appears in the *chronic venous congestion* of heart failure due to the additional fluid contributed by transudation.

Pulmonary oedema. In oedematous lung tissue it seems likely that the macrophages are unable to perform their normal function. Infection is therefore quite a common sequel to oedema from whatever cause. The basal oedema which occurs in debilitated, bedridden patients, in those who are unconscious, and following operations often progresses to pneumonia, and is called *hypostatic pneumonia.*

Bronchopneumonia is of much longer duration than lobar pneumonia. If the primary condition is incurable, the pneumonia is merely a welcome terminal event, and there will obviously be little attempt at healing. Even in the childhood bronchopneumonias that follow measles and whooping-cough, a prolonged course is the rule, and is often punctuated by relapses and remissions depending upon whether the organism or the host is gaining the upper hand. Both the onset and the end of the disease are gradual.

Lesions. The disease is usually basal and posterior in distribution and is bilateral. If an area of bronchopneumonia is examined microscopically, it is found to consist of acutely inflamed bronchioles full of pus. Some of the surrounding alveoli contain oedema fluid in which there are macrophages and polymorphs, while others are filled with a dense fibrinous exudate in which there are innumerable polymorphs. Some are collapsed as the result of the absorption of air distal to the blocked bronchioles, whereas neighbouring alveoli are empty and distended due to compensatory dilatation. In contrast to lobar pneumonia, where all alveoli in a lobe are at about the same stage of the inflammatory process, in bronchopneumonia there is a very varied picture.

Clinical course. The onset of bronchopneumonia is insidious, the disease evolves slowly, and its course can become chronic even with antibiotic treatment. Complications such as fibrosis, abscess formation and empyema (pus in the pleural cavity) are more common than with lobar

pneumonia. Damage to the bronchial wall can lead to the development of bronchiectasis (Fig. 30.5).

Exogenous bronchopneumonia

A variety of virulent organisms when inhaled may lead to severe bronchopneumonia. The host may be a healthy adult, or else be enfeebled as a

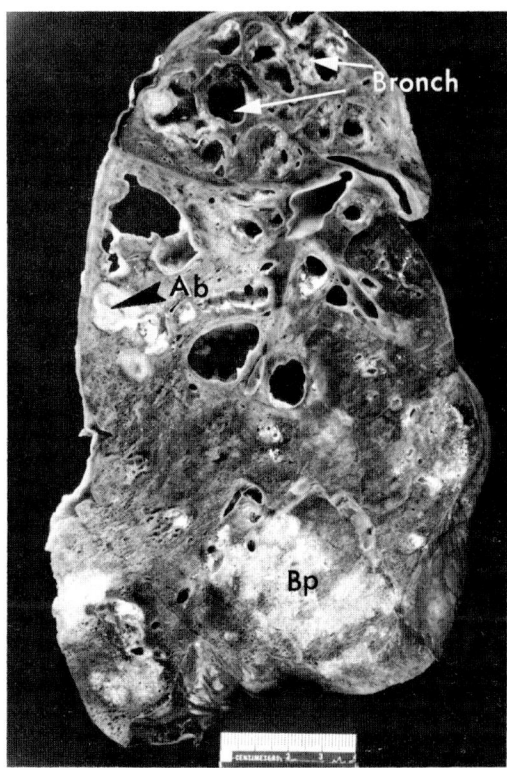

Fig. 30.5 Bronchiectasis with chronic lung infection. Since the age of 7 years this patient had had repeated attacks of pneumonia. When he was 24 years of age a diagnosis of cystic fibrosis was made (see p.212). He was treated with vitamins and pancreatic enzymes by mouth, but continued to be plagued by repeated lung infections. The terminal event was an overwhelming infection with *Pseudomonas aeruginosa*, and he died at the age of 32 years. This specimen shows the effects of repeated bronchopneumonia. Towards the base of the lung there are several areas of bronchopneumonia (Bp), and the discrete areas of consolidation have fused together to become confluent. Nevertheless, the appearances are not those of lobar pneumonia. In another area the pneumonia has progressed to abscess formation (Ab). Towards the upper part of the lung there is great dilatation of bronchi, and the upper lobe shows the typical appearances of advanced bronchiectasis (Bronch). Much of the intervening lung has been destroyed. From Walter J B (1992) An introduction to the principles of disease, 3rd edn., W B Saunders, Philadelphia.

result of a previous disease. Examples of virulent organisms causing exogenous bronchopneumonia are:

1. *S. aureus*, particularly as a result of hospital infection. Abscess formation is common.
2. *E. coli* and other gram-negative coliforms: *Pseudomonas aeruginosa* is common in patients with a tracheostomy and on mechanical ventilation.
3. *Legionella pneumophila*. This organism causes legionnaires' disease, a severe type of pneumonia that attained notoriety when it attacked delegates at the annual convention of the American Legion in Philadelphia in 1976. The organism is common in water supplies, and infection results when mist, created by showers and air conditioning units, is inhaled. The organism is difficult to stain and culture.
4. *Yersinia pestis*—pneumonic plague.
5. *Mycobacterium tuberculosis* and the deep-seated fungal diseases. This type of disease is quite distinct, as the lesions produced are characteristically chronic. They are described in Chapter 15.

INTERSTITIAL PNEUMONIA

This type of pneumonia is attaining greater importance now that the bacterial types of pneumonia can be controlled by antibiotics. In interstitial pneumonia the inflammatory process mainly affects the interstitial tissues, particularly the alveolar walls. The term *alveolitis* is therefore often used, and both acute and chronic forms are recognized. The causes of interstitial pneumonia are numerous and include infection (particularly viruses, mycoplasma, and *Pneumocystis carinii*), ionizing radiation, drugs (e.g. cyclophosphamide and antineoplastic agents), inhalation of noxious agents (e.g. smoke, metal fumes and high concentrations of oxygen), severe trauma, and collagen vascular diseases (particularly systemic sclerosis). In many cases, particularly in the chronic types the cause is unknown.

In *acute interstitial pneumonia* the initial damage is to the type I pneumocytes and the capillary endothelium. Inflammation in the alveolar walls is often followed by the formation of oedema within the alveoli. Since these are still ventilated, the fluid, with its plasma proteins and fibrin, is thrown onto the alveolar wall and condenses to form an eosinophilic hyaline membrane. Morphologically this is described as *alveolitis with hyaline membrane formation*. This is a feature of virus pneumonias and the alveolitis associated with drugs or inhaled agents. It is also encountered following severe trauma where the name *adult respiratory distress syndrome (ARDS)* is used. Acute interstitial pneumonia may resolve (e.g. a virus pneumonia) but all too frequently it evolves into chronic interstitial pneumonia.

Chronic interstitial pneumonia is a major medical problem and frequently its cause is unknown. Various morphological types are recognized, the commonest being *fibrosing alveolitis* also called *usual interstitial pneumonia (UIP)*. Progressive lung destruction and fibrosis lead to increasing disability and ultimately death.

OEDEMA OF THE LUNGS

The systolic pressure in the pulmonary artery is 15–25 mmHg, and being much lower than that in the systemic vessels, it follows that there is less tendency to oedema formation. The osmotic effect of the plasma proteins is relatively unopposed. Nevertheless, when oedema does occur, two factors tend to ensure that it persists and even spreads.

1. The loose nature of the lung prevents any appreciable rise in tissue tension, a factor which in other tissues limits the extent of oedema formation.
2. When once the lungs become oedematous, ventilation ceases, the vessels become hypoxic, and they tend to leak. It follows that in all examples of pulmonary oedema the fluid has a high protein content. It is not possible to distinguish between transudates and exudates as in other tissues.

Causes of pulmonary oedema

Acute inflammation. Oedema occurs in the early stages of bronchopneumonia and following the inhalation of certain gases, e.g. phosgene, chlorine, and nitrogen peroxide. Acute pulmonary oedema also follows the inhalation of gastric juice such as may occur if a patient vomits during the inexpert administration of a general anaesthetic.

Heart failure. Acute pulmonary oedema is a frequent complication of left ventricular failure and is also common in mitral stenosis. Although increased pulmonary venous pressure is the usual explanation offered for this complication, it is unlikely that this is the major cause. More important is the effect of a *redistribution of the blood volume*: attacks of acute pulmonary oedema occur quite suddenly, sometimes at night, and they are probably initiated by peripheral vasoconstriction. The amount of blood in the peripheral circulation is thus diminished, and the excess volume is displaced into the pulmonary circulation where it appears as oedema fluid. Support for this contention is the fact that acute pulmonary oedema is a well-known hazard of adrenaline administration. This drug causes peripheral vasoconstriction. It must never be given to patients with acute pulmonary oedema of cardiac origin. In bronchial asthma this drug is beneficial, but in cardiac asthma it can be lethal.

The terms *cardiac asthma* and *paroxysmal nocturnal dyspnoea* are often applied to these attacks of acute pulmonary oedema. The patient wakes up breathless with a sense of oppression in the chest and sits up, but the dyspnoea increases. Mounting restlessness drives the patient out of bed to seek the fresh air at the window. The sense of suffocation becomes intense, and with it there is profound distress. The skin has an ashen cyanosis, and there is profuse sweating. Blood stained sputum may be coughed up, and in severe cases a rapidly spreading pulmonary oedema results in death.

Overloading the circulation. If an excessive volume of fluid is administered intravenously, some of the excess is accommodated in the great veins, but the remainder is diverted to the pulmonary circulation and leads to oedema formation.

Cerebral damage. Acute pulmonary oedema is sometimes seen following damage to the brain, e.g. after trauma or cerebral haemorrhage. The most likely explanation is that there occurs considerable sympathetic activity, which by leading to peripheral vasoconstriction causes diversion of the circulating fluid to the lungs, as described above.

THE PNEUMOCONIOSES

This group of diseases, produced by the *inhalation of dust*, are mostly occupational in origin. The most important is *silicosis*, which is seen in miners and those who work with finely divided silica. Following the inhalation of this dust there results a chronic inflammatory condition which eventually leads to extensive nodular fibrosis. Silicosis predisposes to tuberculosis. Asbestosis produces a similar effect, but, unlike silicosis, the fibrosis is diffuse and the disease predisposes to cancer of the lung and mesothelioma of the pleura.

The commonest type of pneumoconiosis (*anthracosis*) follows the inhalation of soot particles and, to some extent, it occurs in every town dweller. It is particularly severe in coal miners due to the inhalation of coal particles; usually it causes little trouble but occasionally there is massive fibrosis—probably due to associated silicosis and tuberculosis.

CHRONIC OBSTRUCTIVE LUNG DISEASE

Chronic obstructive lung disease (COLD), also called chronic obstructive pulmonary disease (COPT), is a syndrome that is characterized by chronic or recurrent reduction of expiratory airflow within the lung. It includes chronic bronchitis, pulmonary emphysema, and small airways disease. These will be described separately, but they do in fact often occur together. They share a strong aetiological association with cigarette smoking. Bronchial asthma may be included but differs somewhat from the other three conditions and will be described separately.

CHRONIC BRONCHITIS

Definition and lesions. This is best defined as a condition in which there is a chronic or recurrent increase in the volume of bronchial mucus, sufficient to cause expectoration, and which is not due to localized bronchopulmonary disease. It is much commoner in tobacco-smokers than in non-smokers, and is very prevalent in England but less so in North America. The bronchial mucosa is thickened by hyperplasia of the mucous glands, and there is an increase in the number of goblet cells in the lining epithelium. True chronic inflammation is not a feature, and Laennec's 'bronchial catarrh' would be a better name.

Recurrent inflammation is a common complication, and may be due to infection or the effects of irritant chemicals—smog is particularly dangerous in this respect.

Effect. The effect of chronic bronchitis is impairment of ventilation due to bronchial narrowing. The mucosa is thickened and there is excess mucus in, and spasm of, the bronchi. Dyspnoea is a prominent symptom, and as the disease progresses respiratory failure develops. The arterial blood is unsaturated and cyanosis occurs. Hypercapnia and right ventricular failure are also common.

The administration of anaesthetics to chronic bronchitics and patients with bronchial asthma is particularly hazardous, since any further increase in mucous production or spasm of the bronchi is liable to precipitate respiratory failure.

PULMONARY EMPHYSEMA

Pulmonary emphysema is defined as a condition marked by an abnormal permanent increase in the size of airspaces distal to the terminal bronchioles, accompanied by destructive changes in the alveolar walls. The enzyme elastase, acting on the elastic content of the alveolar walls, is believed to be important in the pathogenesis of the disease. The effect of this lung destruction is to impair gaseous exchanges in the lung. Carbon dioxide can escape more easily than oxygen can be taken up. A common effect is therefore arterial desaturation and cyanosis. Dyspnoea is often marked.

Two conditions predispose to the development of emphysema. One is atmospheric pollution, particularly by tobacco smoke, and the other is α_1-antitrypsin deficiency. This has given rise to

the concept that there is an *elastase–anti-elastase imbalance* that leads to destruction of elastic fibres in the alveoli. Subjects with α_1-antitrypsin deficiency (an inherited error of metabolism) are prone to develop emphysema. α_1-Antitrypsin is the major anti-elastase in the lung. The part played by tobacco smoke is complex. It causes inflammation, and the polymorphs and macrophages that accumulate in the lung release lysosomal enzymes that contain elastase. Also it inhibits the action of α_1-antitrypsin. Regardless of the mechanism, tobacco smoking is a major cause of emphysema.

SMALL-AIRWAYS DISEASE

Goblet cell metaplasia and other changes in the bronchioles cause obstruction to these small airways and are an important contributor to COLD.

BRONCHIAL ASTHMA

Asthma may be defined as a condition of widespread narrowing of the bronchial airways, which *changes its severity over short periods of time* either spontaneously or under treatment, and is not due to cardiovascular disease. It is characterized by *paroxysms of wheezing dyspnoea*. The bronchial obstruction is caused partly by spasm of the bronchial muscle and partly by the presence of viscid mucus. The disease often has an hereditary basis, and is one of the manifestations of atopy (p. 138). Its pathogenesis is complex; attacks may be the result of hypersensitivity to some inhaled antigen, but psychological and other factors are undoubtedly involved.

TUMOURS OF THE LUNG

Benign tumours of the lung are rare, as is malignant lymphoma. Carcinoid tumours are occasionally encountered and form an infiltrating bronchial nodule that blocks the bronchus and is associated with haemoptysis and distal infection. By far the most important and common tumour is carcinoma.

Carcinoma of the lung

Cancer of the lung accounts for about 30% of all cancer deaths in the USA and is the commonest lethal cancer in males; until recently it was second to cancer of the breast in females, but in some societies this order has been reversed. Cigarette smoking is the major aetiological factor. Atmospheric pollution and industrial exposure to asbestos, uranium, nickel, chromium, arsenic and beryllium are contributory factors.

The peripheral type of tumour appears as a fairly discrete mass in the parenchyma of the lung. Symptoms are often absent until the pleura and chest wall are invaded, or distant metastases appear. The more common central type arises in one of the major bronchi. Ulceration leads to haemoptysis and bronchial obstruction results in collapse, bronchopneumonia, and bronchiectasis. Frequently the patient presents with fever, weight loss, cough, and episodes of bronchopneumonia.

Histological types. Although arising from a mucus-secreting epithelium, cancers of the lung are remarkable for their histological variation. *Squamous-cell carcinoma* is the commonest type. The tumour is usually poorly differentiated and arises from an area of epithelial atypia that progresses to carcinoma in situ before becoming invasive. *Adenocarcinoma* is usually a peripheral tumour; it is more common in women and is least associated with cigarette smoking. *Small-cell (or oat-cell) anaplastic carcinoma* is the third most common type. It is composed of elongated oat-shaped small cells with hyperchromatic nuclei and little cytoplasm (Fig. 30.6). It is thought to arise from cells of the diffuse endocrine system and is the malignant counterpart to the carcinoid tumour. It grows rapidly to produce a large fleshy mass, and early spread to lymph nodes leads to the formation of a large mediastinal mass that invades the pericardium and obstructs the great veins. The tumour is very radio-sensitive, and

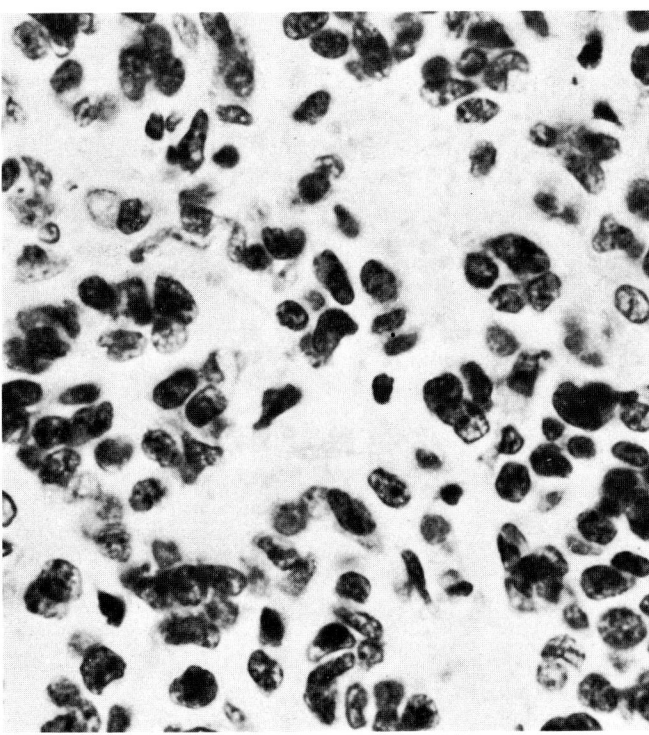

Fig. 30.6 Oat-cell carcinoma of the lung. The tumour is composed of sheets of uniform, small, darkly staining cells, nearly all the substance of which is nuclear. Many have a fusiform shape which gives rise to the descriptive term 'oat cell'. x 320.

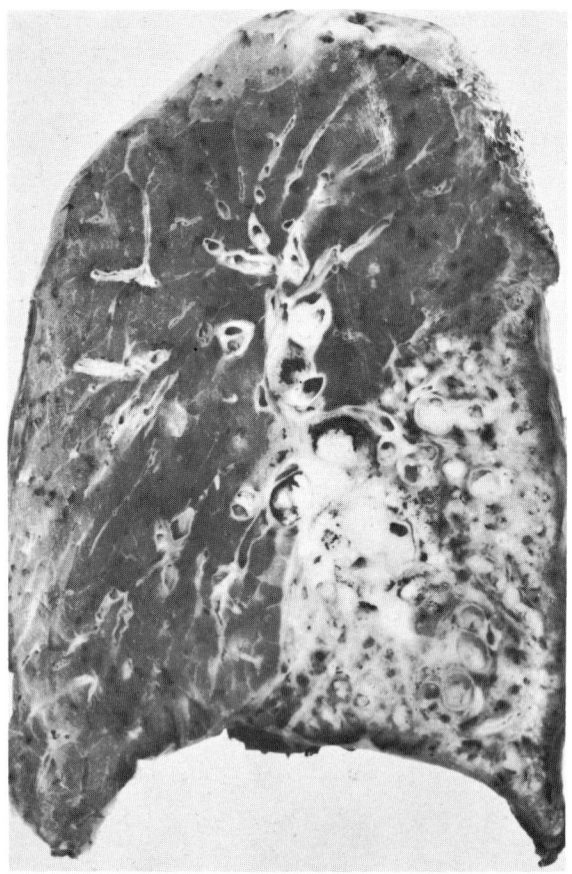

Fig. 30.7 Carcinoma of the lung. This has arisen from the left lower lobe main bronchus and has infiltrated into the lower lobe, which has also undergone fibrosis secondary to collapse, bronchiectasis, and bronchopneumonia. The local hilar lymph nodes are involved. The tumour proved to be a squamous-cell carcinoma. (R45.1. Reproduced by permission of the President and Council of the Royal College of Surgeons of England.)

radiotherapy with chemotherapy are commonly used rather than surgery. *Large-cell anaplastic carcinoma*, giant-cell carcinoma and other variants are the least common types.

Spread. Lung cancer spreads by all the classical routes:

Local spread to involve lung parenchyma, pleura, bronchi, arteries, and veins (Fig. 30.7).

Lymphatic spread to the hilar and mediastinal nodes. This usually occurs early, and is most marked with the oat-cell tumours.

Blood-borne metastases: secondary tumours are common in the *liver, bones, adrenals,* and *brain.* Even the spleen and bowel, organs not commonly the site of metastases from other tumours, may be involved. It is the frequency of distant spread which makes the prognosis so poor.

Diagnosis. Haemoptysis, recurrent or 'unresolved' pneumonia, or a persistent shadow on the radiograph should always lead to thorough investigation, particularly if the patient is a smoker. Sputum examination may reveal malignant cells. Bronchoscopy, mediastinoscopy or needle biopsy may provide tissue for diagnosis.

THE PLEURA

The pleural cavities are normally potential spaces situated between the visceral and parietal pleurae, each lined by flattened mesothelial cells. An accumulation of fluid in the pleural space is called a *hydrothorax,* or *pleural effusion.* There are two types:

A transudate. The fluid has a low protein content and few cells. The most common causes are congestive heart failure and the nephrotic syndrome.

An exudate. An exudate is formed as a result of inflammation or neoplasia involving the pleura. The protein content approximates that of the plasma; inflammatory or neoplastic cells are present in the fluid.

PLEURISY

Inflammation of the pleura (pleurisy or pleuritis) is usually secondary to underlying inflammatory or neoplastic lung disease. This may be apparent, as in lobar pneumonia or in a large area of infarction, or it may be inapparent, as in the pleurisy that accompanies a small tuberculous lesion. Occasionally the cause of the pleurisy is to be found below the diaphragm, e.g. a subphrenic abscess.

Fibrinous pleurisy. 'Dry pleurisy' is associated with an audible friction rub, and can be extremely painful, particularly on deep inspiration. Organization of the exudate leads to the formation of fibrous pleural adhesions.

Serous or serofibrinous pleurisy. 'Pleurisy with effusion' can lead to the accumulation of so much fluid that the affected lung is collapsed. Persistent pleural effusion should always be adequately investigated. Fluid can be withdrawn through a needle and sent for bacteriological and cytological examination. Tuberculosis and carcinoma (primary or metastatic) are two causes that must be considered.

EMPYEMA THORACIS

The presence of pus in the pleural cavity is called an 'empyema'. It is generally formed as an extension of infection from a contiguous structure, e.g. bronchopneumonia, a lung abscess, or a subphrenic abscess.

PNEUMOTHORAX

The presence of air in the pleural cavity is called a 'pneumothorax'. It may arise suddenly in an apparently healthy person (*spontaneous pneumothorax*), and it is usually due to the rupture of a small subpleural emphysematous bulla. The onset is sudden with severe pain in one side of the chest. Collapse of the lung causes dyspnoea and cyanosis; their severity depends on the amount of air that escapes into the pleural cavity. The condition tends to recur.

PLEURAL TUMOURS

The most common primary malignant tumour of the pleura is the mesothelioma. This tumour, which is related to asbestosis, forms an encasing mass around the lung. Metastatic tumours, particularly from carcinoma of the breast and lung, are frequent in the pleural cavity.

GENERAL READING

Becklake M R 1982 Exposure to asbestos and human disease. New England Journal of Medicine 306: 1480

Crystal R G et al 1985 Interstitial lung disease of unknown origin: disorders characterized by chronic inflammation of the lower respiratory tract. New England Journal of Medicine 310: 154, 235

Edelstein P H, et al 1984 Legionnaires' disease: a review. Chest 85: 114

Fletcher C M, Pride N B 1984 Definition of emphysema, chronic bronchitis, asthma and airflow obstruction: 25 years on from the Ciba Symposium. Thorax 39: 81

Leading Article 1986 Adult respiratory distress syndrome. Lancet 1: 301

Sobin L H 1983 Histological classification of lung tumours. Human Pathology 14: 1020

Spencer H 1985 Pathology of the Lung, 4th edn. Pergamon Press, New York

Wald N J, et al 1986 Does breathing other peoples tobacco smoke cause lung cancer. British Medical Journal 293: 1217

31. Diseases of the alimentary tract

Although the alimentary tract is usually regarded as being within the body, it is in fact a long tube exposed at each end to the exterior. Its contents, ranging from food in the mouth to faeces in the rectum, are never within the body proper. This is an ideal arrangement, for within the lumen the chemical changes necessary for digestion can occur under conditions which could not be tolerated inside the body itself. One effect of this arrangement is that many litres of digestive fluids are poured into the alimentary tract each day. Normally nearly all of this is reabsorbed, but it can readily be appreciated that if much escaped to the exterior the volume of fluid lost could reach alarming proportions. Vomiting and diarrhoea are potent causes of water and electrolyte depletion, and this is described in Chapter 27. In the present chapter the digestive aspects of the alimentary tract are considered as well as some of its common afflictions.

THE MOUTH, PHARYNX AND OESOPHAGUS

In the mouth food is masticated and mixed with saliva, which, by virtue of its mucus content, performs a lubricating action in addition to commencing carbohydrate digestion by the enzyme ptyalin.

Swallowing (*deglutition*) is triggered off by the voluntary contraction of the pharyngeal and buccal muscles. This, by raising the larynx and tongue, throws the bolus of food against the posterior pharyngeal wall. Thereafter a wave of peristalsis sweeps the bolus down the muscular oesophagus into the stomach.

Difficulty in swallowing (dysphagia). This is caused by a great variety of lesions, a few of which will be mentioned.

1. *Painful conditions* inhibit the voluntary initiation of the act of swallowing, e.g. aphthous ulceration and acute tonsillitis.

2. *Mechanical interference with deglutition* is seen when the pharynx or tongue is infiltrated with scirrhous carcinoma or amyloid.

3. *Mechanical obstruction.* This usually occurs in the oesophagus, and is caused by *carcinoma*, either squamous-cell, which is usually in the middle third of the oesophagus, or adenocarcinoma arising from the lower portion or the stomach. Less common are *benign strictures,* secondary either to chronic peptic ulcer at the lower end or to the destruction and scarring caused by swallowing corrosive acids and alkalis. The dysphagia of the *Plummer–Vinson syndrome* is associated with obstruction at the upper end of the oesophagus (p. 307); a web is often present in the anterior aspect of the cricopharyngeal area, but whether or not this causes a mechanical obstruction has been debated for years and is still undecided.

4. *Paralysis of the muscles of deglutition,* e.g. in poliomyelitis affecting the brain-stem and other lesions affecting the medulla.

5 *Neuromuscular incoordination.* In elderly people incoordination of the peristaltic waves and muscular spasm may produce a sensation of obstruction and severe pain. In *achalasia of the*

cardia there is a degeneration of the ganglion cells of the lower oesophagus, which results in disturbed peristalsis and a failure of relaxation of the cardiac sphincter. As a result the oesophagus becomes greatly dilated.

For clinical purposes dysphagia may be divided into two groups:

Oropharyngeal dysphagia, in which attempted swallowing may lead to the inhalation of food or its regurgitation through the nose.

Oesophageal dysphagia, in which the common symptom is a sense of obstruction in the chest during swallowing. Carcinoma is the lesion most to be feared, especially if the symptoms are progressive and difficulty in swallowing first affects solids and finally liquids.

Acute streptococcal sore throat. This is an acute infection of the tonsils and adjacent pharynx by *S. pyogenes.* The onset is sudden, and the sore throat is accompanied by fever, leucocytosis, and malaise. The tonsils and adjacent pharynx are swollen and red, and a white inflammatory exudate is seen on the surface. If the strain of streptococcus produces abundant erythrogenic exotoxin, and if the patient has no immunity to this toxin, the sore throat is shortly followed by an erythematous skin rash and is called *scarlet fever.*

Streptococcal sore throat is an important disease, because in a number of patients it is followed by acute glomerulonephritis or acute rheumatic fever—conditions that are considered elsewhere.

It should not be assumed that every sore throat is streptococcal. The gonococcus can cause a similar acute pharyngitis. Viral infections, for instance by the Epstein–Barr virus the causative agent of infectious mononucleosis (glandular fever), can have a very similar clinical appearance, although the onset is generally more insidious. In the past it was essential to consider diphtheria in the differential diagnosis; now, however, the disease is extremely uncommon in the Western world due to immunization. The diagnosis of diphtheria rests on obtaining a positive culture from a throat swab.

THE STOMACH

In the stomach the masticated food is softened, moistened, lubricated, and partly digested by the gastric juice. It is kneaded by strong muscular contraction into a semiliquid mass called *chyme,* which is passed steadily into the *duodenum.*

Wherever acid gastric juice comes into contact with a non-acid-secreting mucosa, peptic ulceration is liable to occur. It is therefore seen at the pylorus, along the lesser curve of the stomach, in the first part of the duodenum, at the lower end of the oesophagus, and at the site of anastomosis between the stomach and small intestine following gastro-enterostomy.

Acute ulceration

Acute erosions. Acute shallow ulcers, commonly called erosions, are often seen in the stomach. They are usually multiple, and appear to be caused by dietary indiscretions, alcohol, and the action of irritant drugs, e.g. aspirin. They are shallow and involve little more than the covering epithelium. Healing is rapid and complete. Slight bleeding is common, and may occasionally be severe.

Acute ulceration (also called *stress ulcers*) of the stomach or duodenum is also seen as a complication of burns and any severe injury, e.g. major surgery, and may be related to vagal overactivity. There are usually multiple ulcers and they usually heal rapidly with minimal scarring, but may occasionally erode a large vessel or perforate into the peritoneal cavity, giving rise to severe haemorrhage or peritonitis. Sometimes, after trauma, there is a generalized oozing of blood from the congested gastric mucosa. In this way much blood is lost without an obvious localized bleeding point.

Chronic peptic ulcer

Chronic ulcers are usually solitary, and present a characteristic appearance. The destructive process penetrates beneath the mucosa to the underlying muscle layers, and this produces a deep, round or oval, punched-out ulcer with straight edges (Fig. 31.1). The base of the ulcer consists of inflamed vascular granulation tissue covered by necrotic tissue which forms a slough. Bleeding is therefore common. Deeper in the base of the ulcer the

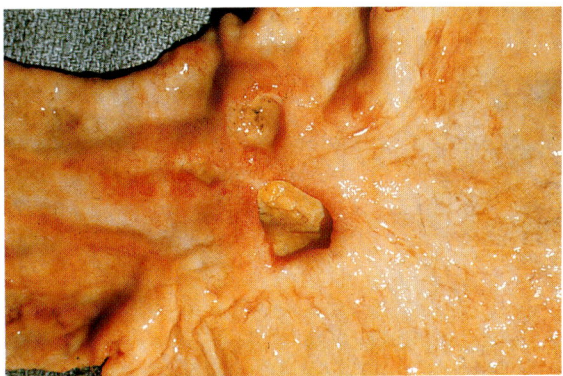

Fig. 31.1 Chronic peptic ulceration. The prepyloric region of the gastric mucosa shows two adjacent ulcers. Each ulcer is deep, having sharply defined rolled margins and slough covering its floor.

granulation tissue matures to form scar tissue.

Clinical features. Pain in the epigastrium is common and is related to the gastric acidity and spasm of the muscle. It is usually relieved by meals and especially by the administration of alkalis.

Complications. *Haemorrhage.* Repeated bleeding is a common cause of iron-deficiency anaemia. Sometimes the ulcer becomes attached to an adjacent structure, e.g. the pancreas, and a large artery is eroded. This leads to a massive haematemesis and melaena.

Perforation. When the ulcer penetrates to the peritoneal surface it produces a localized fibrinous inflammation which may cause adjacent structures to become adherent to it. If this does not occur the ulcer may perforate, and the gastric or dudodenal contents are poured into the peritoneal cavity. The patient immediately experiences excruciating pain, and generalized peritonitis soon develops.

Cicatrization. As an ulcer heals, the scar tissue is apt to contract and cause stenosis. Pyloric ulcers are particularly liable to this complication, and the resulting pyloric stenosis causes severe vomiting.

Cancer of the stomach

This tumour is not uncommon in Northern European communities, but its incidence is now lower than that of colonic cancer. It is very common in the Japanese. The tumour is either of the fungating, cauliflower type, or else it appears as a typical malignant ulceration. Occasionally the tumour cells invade the stomach wall so diffusely that no definite mass exists. Instead the whole wall is thickened by dense scirrhous tumour (*diffuse infiltrating carcinoma of the stomach* or *linitis plastica*). Histologically the cancer is usually a poorly-differentiated adenocarcinoma. Even with early excision the prognosis is extremely bad because there is usually early spread to the regional lymph nodes and the liver. In high-incidence areas, particularly Japan, the detection and treatment of early lesions has greatly improved the outlook.

THE SMALL INTESTINE

The function of the small intestine (duodenum, jejunum and ileum) is to receive the chyme from the stomach, complete the digestion of carbohydrates, fats and protein, and allow absorption of the products so formed. The succus entericus contains the enzyme *enterokinase* that converts trypsinogen in the pancreatic juice into the active enzyme trypsin, and this combined with pancreatic lipase completes the digestion of fats and protein. Bile salts assist in the absorption of fat. The final breakdown of disaccharides (e.g. lactose and sucrose) to monosaccharides is carried out by disaccharidases in the glycocalyx of intestinal cells. The complex villous structure of the small intestine and the microvilli of its cells appear well adapted for absorption. Of about 8 litres of fluid that enter the small intestine only 1.0–1.5 litres enter the colon daily. Any defect of absorption of fluid from the intestine can so overwhelm the colon with fluid that diarrhoea results and a large quantity of fluid and electrolytes is lost.

Diarrhoea is a common feature of intestinal disease and can be brought about in various ways. If there is impaired digestion of food, high-molecular-weight substances remain in the intestinal lumen and by an osmotic effect retain water. This is the mechanism of the *osmotic diarrhoea* in coeliac disease and lactase deficiency. Some bacterial toxins stimulate the formation of cyclic AMP such that there is an enormous outpouring of fluid into the small intestine. This *intestinal secretory diarrhoea* is typical of cholera. Finally, inflammation of the bowel wall, particularly the colon, leads to the outpouring of exudate, mixed with mucus and blood. This is described as *dysenteric diarrhoea*.

Acute inflammation of the small intestine is often accompanied by involvement of the stomach or colon so that gastritis, enteritis and colitis are frequently combined. The cause may be chemical (e.g. arsenic), or food may contain the preformed enterotoxins of *Staph. aureus* or *C. perfringens*. Usually there is an infective cause and organisms are present in the intestine. *Campylobacter, Yersinia, Salmonella, Shigella* and enteropathic strains of *E. coli* are common causes of an acute gastoenteritis. Rotaviruses and other viruses have been implicated in some cases, while in others no cause can be identified. The general term 'food poisoning' is used; traveller's diarrhoea is a variant of this. Some organisms, e.g. some strains of *E. coli*, produce a secretory type of diarrhoea like cholera. Others act by a different mechanism.

Typhoid fever

Typhoid fever is a specific type of enteritis and is described in Chapter 7.

Cholera

Cholera is acquired by ingesting water or food contaminated by *Vibrio cholerae* derived from human faeces. There is an acute onset of vomiting, and profuse diarrhoea with the passage of large quantities of 'rice water stools'. Loss of water and electrolytes leads to hypovolaemic shock and death within 2–3 days in about one-third of untreated cases. With efficient treatment by fluid and electrolyte replacement the mortality can be reduced to less than 1%.

Crohn's disease

This disease of unknown cause is a chronic recurrent inflammatory condition affecting the alimentary tract which causes major disability in young people. The terminal ileum is most commonly affected, but any part of the alimentary tract, including the colon, can be affected. The inflammation is transmural and characteristically there are small ulcers that penetrate the

bowel wall. Overlying peritonitis leads to adhesion between adjacent loops of bowel and other structures; with the formation of sinuses and fistulae, communication occurs between small bowel, colon, bladder and the skin surface. Thickening of the bowel wall leads to obstructions (Fig. 31.2). Diarrhoea, chronic abdominal pain and malabsorption are the salient clinical features. Oral lesions occur in around 6–20% of patients and include ulcers, labial and facial swelling, mucosal 'tags' or 'cobblestones' and proliferation of the oral mucosa.

The malabsorption syndrome

This is described in Chapter 18.

THE LARGE INTESTINE

The colon has two main functions: the absorption of water and electrolytes and the formation of a receptacle for faeces, so that they may be discharged when convenient. Acute inflammation of the colon results in a derangement of its functions, and the diarrhoea that results causes great inconvenience as well as a considerable loss of water and electrolytes. Two severe infections are recognized:

Bacillary dysentery

This is an acute infection of the colon caused by organisms of the genus *Shigella*. The incubation period is short (24–48 hours), and the disease is characterized by fever, abdominal pain, and diarrhoea which can lead to severe dehydration and death. The faeces are fluid and contain blood, mucus, and pus.

Amoebic dysentery

This is caused by a protozoon, *Entamoeba histolytica*, which invades the colonic mucosa and produces shallow ulceration. The disease may be acute with severe bloody diarrhoea, but more usually it is chronic, and the patient has several foul-smelling, sometimes blood-stained stools each day. Occasionally the amoebae invade the blood stream and cause *amoebic hepatitis*; a liver abscess may ensue.

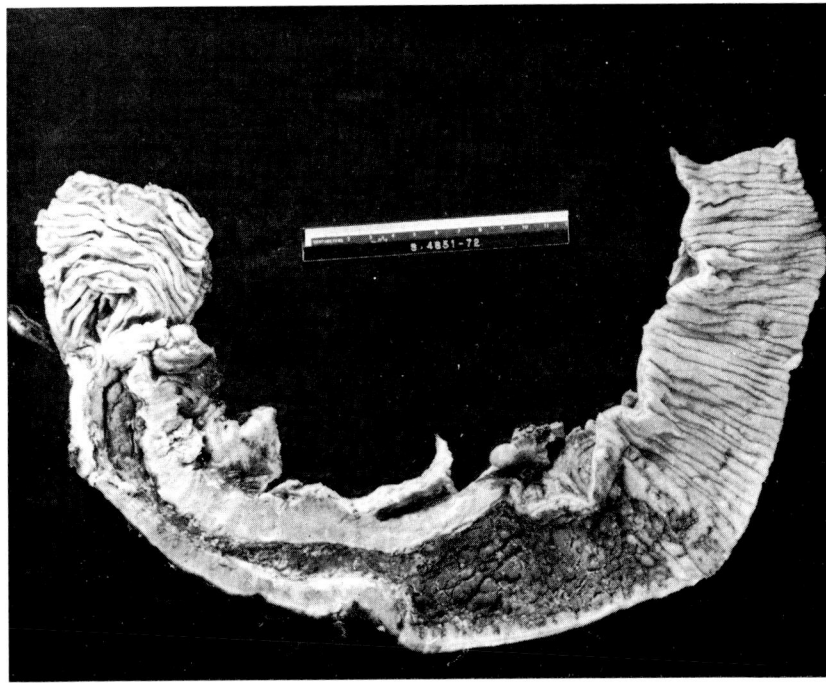

Fig. 31.2 Crohn's disease of ileum. Resected specimen of the terminal ileum, ileocaecal junction, caecum, and a small portion of the ascending colon from a man aged 22 years. The terminal ileum shows a great thickening and rigidity of its wall; the lumen is reduced in size and the mucosa has a characteristic cobblestone appearance. The disease stops sharply at the ileo-caecal valve. Microscopically, the affected bowel showed transmural oedema, fibrosis, and the presence of non-caseating tuberculoid granulomata. (Photograph by courtesy of Dr J B Cullen, University of Toronto.)

Both types of dysentery are most common in the tropics and in those who live under crowded, unhygienic conditions.

Idiopathic ulcerative colitis

Idiopathic ulcerative colitis shares many features in common with Crohn's disease. Both commonly affect young adults, both can affect the colon, and in both an autoimmune process has been proposed but remains unproven. Many possible causative infective agents have been proposed but none has been confirmed. In idiopathic ulcerative colitis there are recurrent attacks of colicky abdominal pain, diarrhoea and the passage of blood, pus and mucus in the faeces. Fever and malaise accompanies severe attacks.

The distal colon and rectum are generally first affected and in the acute phase the mucosa is deeply congested and bleeds at the slightest touch. Mucosal ulcers form but unlike Crohn's disease they do not penetrate the bowel wall, and fistulae are not a problem. The disease remains confined to the mucosa, but continued ulceration tends to undermine the adjacent mucosa so that tags or pseudopolyps are formed. Between 4 and 20% of patients with ulcerative colitis have recurrent apthous ulceration. These oral lesions respond when the colitis is treated medically or surgically.

A serious complication of idiopathic ulcerative colitis is the development of carcinoma. In patients who have had the disease for over 10 years the risk is 10–15% and for this reason, as well as to relieve the patient of the chronic symptoms of diarrhoea and blood loss, total colectomy is sometimes carried out.

Pseudomembranous colitis

This disease is described on p. 161.

Diverticular disease

Multiple diverticula of the colon (*diverticulosis*) are extremely common and form as outpouches of mucosa between the longitudinal muscle of the teniae coli. The muscle itself is greatly hypertrophied and the colon is shortened. It seems probable that diverticulosis results from chronic constipation secondary to the presence of small hard faeces that are the result of a diet low in cellulose roughage. Occasionally the orifice of a diverticulum becomes obstructed and inflammation ensues (*diverticulitis*). The condition therefore resembles appendicitis except that, since it is most common in the sigmoid colon, the lesion is on the left-hand side of the abdomen.

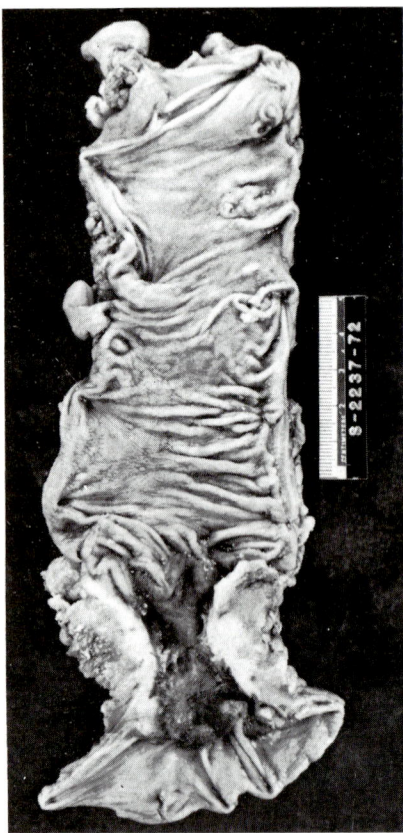

Fig. 31.3 Carcinoma of colon. This resection specimen from a man aged 66 years shows an adenocarcinoma at the recto-sigmoid junction. The tumour involves the whole circumference of the gut, and has produced stenosis. The pericolic fat has been invaded, and several regional lymph nodes contained metastatic carcinoma. (Photograph by courtesy of Dr J B Cullen, University of Toronto.)

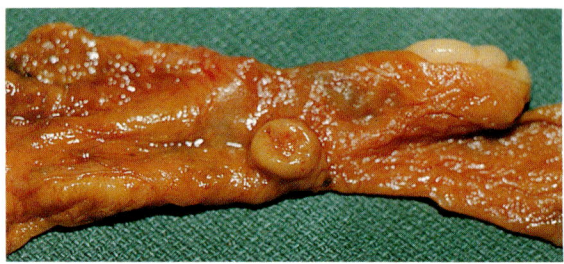

Fig. 31.4 Carcinoid tumour of small intestine. The tumour has a dull yellow colour and has produced a button-like elevation of the mucosa.

Colorectal cancer

The large bowel ranks with lung and breast as the most common site of fatal malignant disease in Europeans. The rectum and sigmoid colon are most frequently involved (Fig. 31.3). The tumour is usually a well-differentiated adenocarcinoma, and it breaks down to produce a typical carcinomatous ulcer. This tends to encircle the gut and produce obstruction. The passage of blood and mucus in the stools with constipation alternating with diarrhoea are the usual clinical features. The tumour invades locally, metastasizes to the regional lymph nodes, and finally invades the blood stream to give metastases in the liver and elsewhere. Growth is often relatively slow, so that the prognosis following resection is well correlated with the stage of the tumour.

Carcinoid tumours of the intestine

These are not common but are of great interest. They occur in the appendix, ileum, colon, and occasionally in the stomach and pancreas (Fig. 31.4). They are derived from cells of the diffuse endocrine system and are of intermediate malignancy. Tumours of the appendix tend to remain localized, but the ileal ones sometimes produce metastases in the liver. When extensive these lead to the *carcinoid syndrome*—diarrhoea, valvular lesions of the right side of the heart, asthmatic attacks, and periodic flushing of the face. The pathogenesis of this syndrome involves the release of 5-hydroxytryptamine by the tumour, the activation of the plasma kinins, and the deposition of platelets on the heart valves.

GENERAL READING

Almy T P, Howell D A 1980 Diverticular disease of the colon. New England Journal of Medicine 302: 324

Cohen S 1979 Motor disorders of the esophagus. New England Journal of Medicine 301: 184

Gorbach S L 1982 Traveller's Diarrhoea. New England Journal of Medicine 307: 881

Greenspan J S, et al 1985 Replication of Epstein–Barr virus within the epithelial cells of oral 'hairy' leukoplakia, an AIDS-associated lesion. New England Journal of Medicine 313: 1564

Kirsner J B, Shorter R G 1982 Recent developments in 'nonspecific' inflammatory bowel disease. New England Journal of Medicine 306: 775, 837

Leading Article 1982 Traveller's Diarrhoea. Lancet 1: 777

Lucas R B 1984 Pathology of Tumours of Oral Tissue, 4th edn. Churchill Livingstone, Edinburgh

Morson B C, Dowson I M P 1979 Gastrointestinal Pathology 2nd edn. Blackwell Scientific, London

Shklar G Oral leukoplakia 1986 New England Journal of Medicine 315: 1544

Thompson H 1982 Gastric Cancer. British Medical Journal 284: 684

Turnberg L A 1979 The pathophysiology of diarrhoea. Clinics in Gastroenterology 8(3): 551

32. Diseases of the liver

The liver is the largest organ in the body and its functions are manifold. Both anatomically and functionally it occupies a key position in relation to the digestive system, for nearly all the venous blood from the gastrointestinal tract reaches it via the portal vein. It is therefore not surprising that the liver performs many functions connected with fat, carbohydrate, and protein metabolism. The liver synthesizes many important proteins, e.g. all the clotting factors except factor VIII and many enzymes, e.g. alkaline phosphatase, and α_1-antitrypsin. It is a major site for the detoxicification of toxins and drugs. Related to this is the uptake, conjugation and secretion of bilirubin. The secretion of bile is an important factor in the digestion of food.

DEGENERATIVE CONDITIONS

The liver cells, or *hepatocytes*, are very susceptible to the effects of many poisons. Poisonous mushrooms (*Amanita phalloides*), carbon tetrachloride, chloroform, and many drugs (important among which is the anaesthetic agent halothane) can all cause severe liver damage, either by direct action or by an immune mechanism. Infections, in particular with the viruses of hepatitis, can also produce liver damage (see Ch. 16).

The effects of hepatotoxic agents can vary from mild cloudy swelling and fatty change to extensive necrosis.

Hepatic necrosis

Types. If the liver cells are severely affected, they die and undergo necrosis. This usually has a *zonal distribution*, which means that the cells of a particular zone in every lobule undergo necrosis—*centrilobular necrosis* is the most common (Fig. 32.1(b)). Sometimes the foci of necrosis are erratically distributed; this is termed *focal* or *spotty necrosis*, and is typical of viral hepatitis.

Occasionally the necrosis is more extensive and involves wide tracts of liver. Whole lobules are destroyed, and the name *massive necrosis* is applied.

Results. The outcome of necrosis depends upon the severity of the lesions:

Zonal and focal necrosis. The patient may have no symptoms, or suffer from an acute febrile illness with jaundice and gastrointestinal symptoms and then recover. The necrotic liver cells autolyse and are removed. The sinusoidal structure and reticulin framework of the liver lobules remain intact, and as the surviving liver cells divide, the destroyed ones are replaced, and there is complete restoration of the liver to normal (Fig. 32.1(a)).

Massive necrosis. The patient may die of liver failure in the acute phase—this is seen after acute poisoning and occasionally in viral hepatitis, but quite often no cause can be found. If the patient survives, the regenerating liver cells are held in correct anatomical position by the reticulin scaffold and the organ returns to normal. Rarely the scaffold collapses and regenerating liver cells form nodules that become surrounded by fibrous

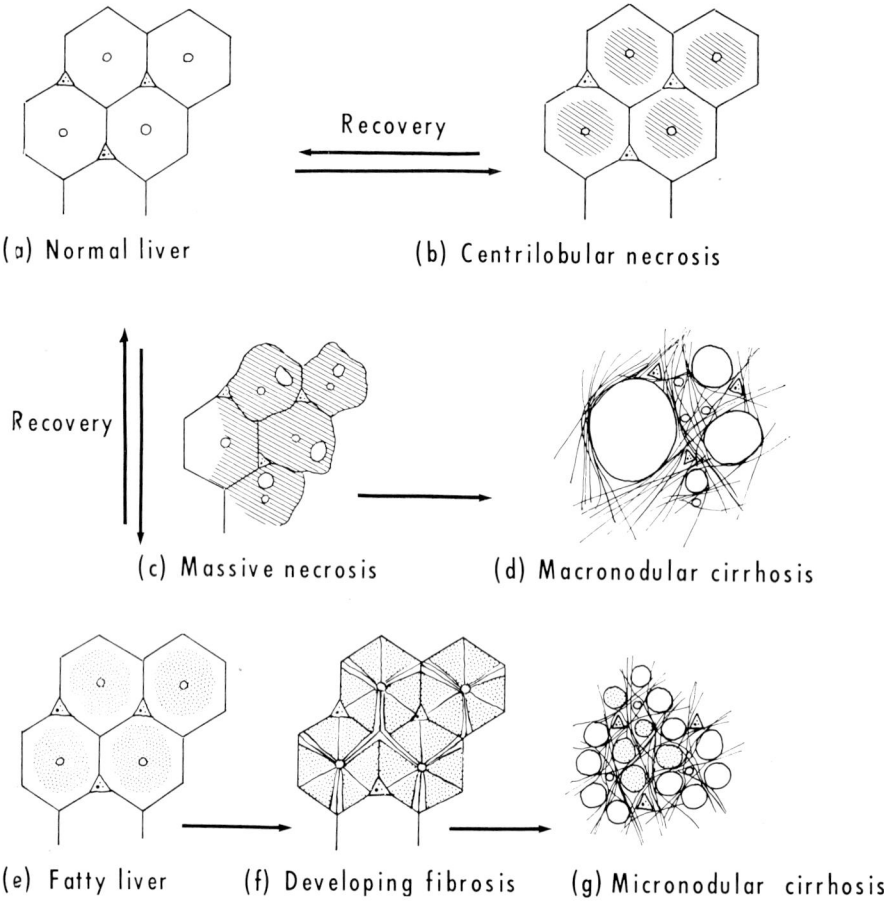

(a) Normal liver   (b) Centrilobular necrosis

Recovery

(c) Massive necrosis   (d) Macronodular cirrhosis

(e) Fatty liver   (f) Developing fibrosis   (g) Micronodular cirrhosis

Fig. 32.1 The pathogenesis of cirrhosis (a) Depicts four normal liver lobules as hexagonal structures each with a central hepatic vein. Between the lobules are the portal triads, each containing branches of the hepatic artery, bile duct, and portal vein. In (b) there is centrilobular necrosis, and when liver cell regeneration occurs there is complete return to normal. (c) Shows massive necrosis with collapse of the affected lobules. When regeneration occurs, a coarsely nodular cirrhotic liver is produced as depicted in (d); in some areas normal lobules will be found. A fatty liver (e) may return to normal. However, if it persists over a long period, fibrous septa form and these divide up the lobules (f). Some liver cells degenerate, and as regeneration occurs a finely nodular cirrhotic liver develops (g). No normal lobules remain. (Drawn by Margot Mackay, University of Toronto.)

tissue. A macronodular type of cirrhosis results. The final result is a form of *cirrhosis of the liver.* (Fig. 32.1(c,d)).

Hepatocellular degeneration and fatty change

The changes are described in detail in Chapter 4. Cloudy swelling, hydropic degeneration, and fatty change may all result from the effects of poisons, hypoxia, or infection. Fatty change is the most important lesion, and is often caused by an inadequate diet. It is also common in *chronic alcoholism.*

If the cause of the fatty liver is removed, complete recovery is usual—not so if the condition is due to chronic alcoholism. Gradually fibrous tissue forms, and hepatic cells become isolated as the lobules are split up (Fig. 32.1(f)). Some cells undergo necrosis, others regenerate, and micronodular cirrhosis results (Fig. 32.1(g)). The fatty liver of kwashiorkor does not predispose to cirrhosis.

Alcohol and the liver

There can be little doubt that alcohol abuse can adversely affect the liver; whether this is due to a direct toxic action of the alcohol on the liver cells or to an effect of the imbalanced diet of the addict has yet to be decided. The liver of the chronic alcoholic often shows fatty change, and in some subjects this progresses to cirrhosis. Acute episodes of alcohol intake results in patchy liver cell necrosis. The cells contain alcoholic hyaline, and foci of necrosis are accompanied by a polymorph infiltration. This condition, which is called *alcoholic hepatitis*, is a phase in the evolution of alcoholic cirrhosis.

HEPATITIS

Acute viral hepatitis

Two distinct types of acute viral hepatitis are known. Viral hepatitis A commonly occurs in institutions like schools and military camps. It is contracted by the ingestion of food and water contaminated with faeces. It has an incubation period of about 1 month. Viral hepatitis B is usually contracted by the use of contaminated syringes or needles and the injection of contaminated blood. The nature of hepatitis A virus, hepatitis B virus and other allied viruses is described in Chapter 16.

Symptoms. The onset is usually insidious with mild fatigue, lassitude, and sometimes fever. Nausea, vomiting, and diarrhoea are not uncommon, and an aversion to both food and cigarette smoking is a curious symptom. Such an influenza-like illness may be the only manifestation of hepatitis, but in other patients the disease progresses and jaundice appears, at first evident in the conjunctivae and later in the skin. Some tenderness over the liver may be noticed, and enlargement of the organ may be detected. Recovery is the usual end-result, but it may take 3 or 4 months, or even longer. The two forms of hepatitis have similar clinical features, although viral hepatitis B tends to be more severe, and in an appre-

ciable number of cases the disease progresses either to massive hepatic necrosis ending in death or to a chronic form of liver disease culminating in cirrhosis.

Chronic hepatitis

The term *chronic hepatitis* encompasses a number of different conditions that have three features in common:

1. Infiltration of portal triads by inflammatory cells, usually lymphocytes and plasma cells.
2. Necrosis of liver cells.
3. Fibrosis of the liver that may terminate in cirrhosis.

The diagnosis of chronic hepatitis is generally made on the liver biopsy. The following types can be recognized:

Chronic active hepatitis. This disease is characterized by recurrent attacks of hepatitis, ultimately developing into cirrhosis, usually of the macronodular type, which is fatal within 10 years. The disease was first described as affecting young people, 75% of the patients being women. Hypergammaglobulinaemia is a characteristic feature, and both antinuclear factor and rheumatoid factors are usually present. Although the disease was originally called *lupoid hepatitis*, there is no evidence that the condition is related to lupus erythematosus itself. Nevertheless, over half the patients

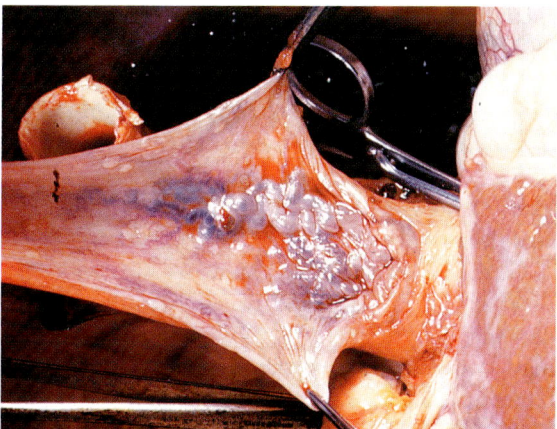

Fig. 32.2 Oesophageal varices. The lower part of the oesophagus has been opened to show tortous varices. The vessels are distended with thrombus.

also have arthritis. Antibodies that react with smooth muscle are present in most cases, and the disease therefore has a strong autoimmune component.

The syndrome of chronic active hepatitis has now been extended to include other groups of patients. Some are middle-aged women, and others are men who usually have HBsAg in their blood. Autoantibodies are usually present, but this autoimmune component is less striking than in the original lupoid hepatitis.

Other types of chronic hepatitis. There are other types of chronic hepatitis that do not fit into the entity designated chronic active hepatitis. Some are cases of patients who have recovered from an acute attack of viral hepatitis, and yet have evidence of continuing liver damage. Others are asymptomatic and yet are chronic carriers of the hepatitis antigen. Still others have neither HBsAg nor demonstrable autoantibodies in their plasma. Viral infection, resolving alcoholic hepatitis, and drug-induced liver damage are suggested as possible causes in the heterogeneous group of conditions labelled chronic hepatitis.

CIRRHOSIS OF THE LIVER

The term 'cirrhosis' (from Greek *kirrhos*, orange yellow, + *nosos*, disease) was introduced by Laennec, who was impressed by the tawny colour of the liver in this condition, but this is due merely to fatty change of the liver cells. The important structural features of cirrhosis are the *destruction of the liver parenchyma* and its *replacement by fibrous tissue*, thereby disrupting the normal lobular architecture. There is active regeneration of the liver cells occurring at the same time as this fibrous reparative process. The *formation of regenerative nodules* is the third essential component of cirrhosis.

Cirrhosis is best regarded as an *end-stage condition*, as it can be the end-result of liver damage due to many causes—poisons, alcohol, inadequate diet, infection, genetic error, etc. Classifications are very unsatisfactory since in many cases the cause is unknown (cryptogenic cirrhosis). A descriptive classification is the most useful and is based on the liver's nodularity. If the nodules are small and of uniform size the term *micronodular cirrhosis* is applied. This contrasts with *macronodular cirrhosis* (Fig. 32.1(d)), in which the nodules are of varying size and many of them are large. Micronodular cirrhosis may be idiopathic, but is often found in alcoholics with fatty liver; the macronodular type follows chronic hepatitis. It must be emphasized that there is no sharp line of division between these two types of cirrhosis.

Symptoms and complications. Cirrhosis is commonly asymptomatic until some complication makes the condition obvious. The appearance of jaundice, oedema of the ankles, or progressive abdominal enlargement may bring the disease to the attention of the patient. Increasing weakness, loss of weight, loss of body hair, and testicular atrophy are all features that may appear. Commonly the first symptom is massive haematemesis and the rapid development of hepatocellular failure with coma and death.

During the development of cirrhosis many branches of the portal and hepatic veins are obliterated. The pressure in the portal radicles rises (*portal hypertension*), and blood from the portal vein is shunted into the systemic veins following the development of anastomoses. This *portal-systemic shunting* of blood has serious effects:

Haemorrhage. An important group of anastomoses develops at the lower end of the oesophagus. The veins are thin-walled and tend to bleed (Fig. 32.2). Sudden, massive, and often fatal haemorrhage is the result. The blood is usually vomited up (*haematemesis*).

Intoxication. Products from the intestine bypass the liver and reach the remainder of the body. This leads to a *faecal odour* of the breath, and is thought to be the cause of the confused mental state and *coma* which patients dying of cirrhosis often develop.

Ascites. Fluid in the peritoneal cavity is common in cirrhosis, and is in part due to the portal hypertension. Hypoalbuminaemia and hyperaldosteronism are other factors in the pathogenesis of ascites and the generalized oedema which sometimes develops.

The main cause, however, appears to be obstruction of the flow of blood through the liver. This obstruction is postsinusoidal and results in an increased rate of formation of lymph in the liver. Normally the lymph is drained away by lymphatics into the thoracic duct, but in cirrhosis the vast excess of lymph produced oozes, or weeps, from the liver into the peritoneal cavity.

Hepatocellular failure. The other symptoms of terminal cirrhosis—including hepatic encephalopathy and haemorrhagic tendency—are described under hepatocellular failure (p. 390).

Biliary cirrhosis

Obstruction to the bile duct, particularly if combined with infection (cholangitis), can sometimes lead to such severe liver-cell damage that cirrhosis develops. There is, in addition, a *primary form of biliary cirrhosis.* This is most frequently encountered in middle-aged women. Itching is usually the first symptom, and this is followed by the development of obstructive jaundice. The disease has an autoimmune component, for the blood contains IgM antibodies active against bile-duct components as well as IgG antimitochondrial antibodies. The detection of the latter is a useful diagnostic feature of primary biliary cirrhosis.

BILE FORMATION AND JAUNDICE

Of all the symptoms of liver disease, *jaundice,* or *icterus,* is the most immediately apparent. Nearly all the tissues in the body are coloured a bright yellow. In addition to the skin, the conjunctivae and oral mucous membrane are discoloured, and in the early stages jaundice is sometimes most apparent in these sites, especially in dark-skinned individuals. Jaundice is due to an excessive amount of bilirubin in the plasma and tissues. Its development can be understood only in relation to bilirubin metabolism (Fig. 32.3).

Bilirubin metabolism

When red cells are broken down, the porphyrin moiety of the haemoglobin is converted into bilirubin in the cells of the mononuclear phagocyte system (MPS). Bilirubin is insoluble in water, and following its release from the MP cells it is carried in the blood stream attached to albu-

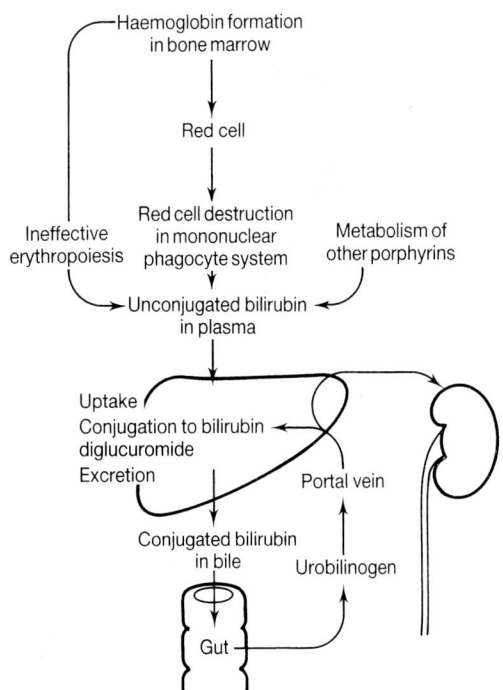

Fig. 32.3 Metabolic pathways in the formation and excretion of bilirubin. (From Walter J B (1992) An introduction to the principles of disease 3rd edn., W B Saunders, Philadelphia.)

min. The liver has three important functions in regard to bilirubin:

1. It *extracts* it from the blood.
2. It *conjugates* it with glucuronic acid to form bilirubin diglucuronide—this is water-soluble.
3. It *excretes* the conjugated bilirubin into the bile.

Under normal conditions 15–20% of the bilirubin excreted is derived from sources other than red-cell destruction. Some of this originates from the bone marrow during the formation of haemoglobin (*ineffective erythropoiesis*); the remainder is derived from the metabolism of porphyrins present in enzymes and elsewhere. The amount formed by ineffective erythropoiesis may be increased in disease, for example pernicious anaemia, and contribute to the jaundice.

Types of jaundice

Obstructive jaundice. Any obstruction of the flow of bile from the liver, through the bile ducts to the intestine causes bilirubin diglucuronide to be absorbed into the blood. Deep jaundice develops if the obstruction is complete. The conjugated bilirubin is water soluble and readily excreted in the urine which is therefore deeply coloured. This contrasts with the faeces, which are clay coloured due to the lack of bile pigment. Little urobilinogen is formed in the intestine, little is returned to the liver, and virtually none escapes into the urine. Two major types of obstructive jaundice may be recognized. In one (*extrahepatic cholestasis*) the bile duct is blocked, commonly by a gallstone in its lumen or by a carcinoma of the bile duct or of the head of the pancreas. In the second type the obstruction is in the liver itself (*intrahepatic cholestasis*). One important cause of this is the administration of certain drugs, for example chlorpromazine (Largactil) and other phenothiazine derivatives. Intrahepatic obstructive jaundice is sometimes present during early-stage acute viral hepatitis. It is also encountered in the acute fatty liver which sometimes follows an alcoholic binge; similar fatty liver with jaundice is an occasional complication of pregnancy.

Other characteristic features of obstructive jaundice include:

Malabsorption. Bile salts aid the absorption of fats and with chronic obstructive jaundice malabsorption with steatorrhoea may occur.

Pruritus. The severe itching that commonly complicates obstructive jaundice is attributed to the retention of bile salts.

Xanthoma formation. Obstructive jaundice causes the liver to synthesize an increased amount of cholesterol, and the resulting hypercholesterolaemia leads to the deposition of tumour-like masses of foam cells called xanthomata. These are most obvious in the skin and appear yellow due to the presence of carotene.

Haemolytic jaundice. This is the second type of jaundice to be considered. The excessive destruction of red cells causes an increased rate of bilirubin formation, and the liver is unable to deal with the increased load. The bilirubin in the blood is unconjugated, and is therefore insoluble in water and not excreted in the urine. This type of jaundice is said to be *acholuric*. The faeces contain an excess of stercobilin, and the amount of urobilinogen returned to the liver is increased. Haemolytic jaundice rarely reaches the intensity of the obstructive variety. An exception to this is that seen in haemolytic disease of the newborn. Because unconjugated bilirubin is relatively soluble in lipids, bile pigments pass into the brain tissue and can, if the jaundice is severe, cause severe damage to the developing central nervous system. This is called kernicterus.

Hepatocellular jaundice. This is considered below.

HEPATOCELLULAR FAILURE

It is convenient to complete this survey of liver disease by summarizing the important features of liver-cell failure. It is often called *cholaemia*, and may occur as a terminal event in many forms of liver disease. Thus it is seen in necrosis, cirrhosis, and occasionally when the organ is extensively involved by tumour.

Manifestations of liver-cell damage

Jaundice. This is due partly to a failure of the liver to take up bilirubin from the blood, conjugate it, or excrete conjugated bilirubin. This hepatocellular variety of jaundice is therefore of mixed type. Normally the liver converts most of the urobilinogen absorbed from the intestine into bilirubin, and excretes it in the bile. In liver-cell damage this function is impaired, and an excess of stercobilinogen reaches the kidney and is excreted as urobilinogen (Fig. 32.3).

Hepatic encephalopathy. Patients with chronic liver disease often exhibit forgetfulness, mental deterioration and other neurological signs. Ataxia and a characteristic 'flapping' tremor of the outstretched hands are noteworthy accompaniments. On the other hand, the syndrome may be acute and terminate in coma with convulsions.

The liver is the principal site of deamination of amino acids and is probably the only organ that can convert the ammonia so produced into urea. The other site of ammonia formation is the intestine, where it is formed by bacterial decomposition of protein. Shunting of this ammonia from the portal blood into the systemic circulation is a possible cause of cerebral dysfunction.

Acute encephalopathy is sometimes precipitated by bleeding oesophageal varices; the explanation is that the large quantity of protein-containing blood passes into the intestine and amounts to a heavy protein meal. Since bacterial action in the intestine appears to lead to the formation of damaging nitrogenous products, the administration of an insoluble antibiotic such as neomycin is useful.

Haemorrhagic tendency. The liver manufactures all the plasma clotting factors, with the exception of Factor VIII. In liver disease a haemorrhagic tendency is not uncommon. Surgery, even dental extraction, should be attempted with caution.

Hypoalbuminaemia. The liver also manufactures albumin, and it is not surprising that the plasma level falls in many chronic liver diseases. Hypoalbuminaemia contributes to the formation of ascites and generalized oedema.

Failure of detoxification. Many drugs, e.g. morphine and barbiturates, are detoxified or excreted by the liver. In patients with liver failure a normal dose of such a drug may precipitate coma and death.

A failure in the metabolism of oestrogen is the suggested cause of the testicular atrophy and gynaecomastia (enlargement of the male breast) that are associated with hepatic cirrhosis. Likewise, a failure to metabolize aldosterone may be the explanation of the hyperaldosteronism.

Fever. Pyrexia is not uncommon, but its cause is not known.

In the terminal stages severe electrolyte imbalance occurs. The patients sinks into a state of cholaemic coma with deepening jaundice, and the end is precipitated by renal, cardiac, or peripheral circulatory failure.

TUMOURS OF THE LIVER

Benign tumours are uncommon but a recent increase in the incidence of adenoma has been attributed to use of the birth control pill. Hepatocellular carcinoma is the most common primary malignant tumour. It sometimes complicates cirrhosis of the liver and where this is common so also is carcinoma. Indeed, hepatocellular carcinoma is the most common malignant tumour in some parts of the Orient. This has been linked to HBV carriage and the intake of aflatoxins.

Metastatic deposits of tumour are extremely common in the liver in cases of disseminated malignant disease. The common sites for the primary carcinoma are the breast, lung, and gastrointestinal tract.

A raised level of *alkaline phosphatase* in the plasma is characteristic of metastatic tumour and is a useful clinical test. Each nodule of tumour obstructs a number of small bile ducts, and the test is positive before there is significant retention of bilirubin. Jaundice is not common in tumours of the liver unless it is associated with cirrhosis or it occurs as a terminal event. This emphasizes the tremendous reserve capacity of the liver and its ability to regenerate (see also p. 95).

GENERAL READING

Leading Article 1986 Halothane-associated liver damage. Lancet 1: 1251
Leading Article 1984 Hepatic encephalopathy today. Lancet 1: 489

Sherlock S 1986 The spectrum of hepatotoxicity due to drugs. Lancet 2: 440
Sherlock S 1985 Diseases of the Liver and Biliary Tract, 7th edn. Blackwell Scientific, Oxford

33. Diseases of the kidney

THE FUNCTION OF THE KIDNEYS

The kidneys are essential for life because of the part they play in the excretion of the non-volatile waste products and in the regulation of the extracellular fluid. They control the concentration of its various electrolytes, contribute to acid–base balance, and are intimately concerned in the regulation of water balance. The kidney also has an endocrine function. Renin is involved in the regulation of blood pressure, erythropoietin plays a part in erythropoiesis, and vitamin D is hydroxylated to a more active compound that acts like a hormone. The major functions of the kidney depend on the secretion of urine and this entails two distinct processes:

1 The passive filtration of plasma through the glomeruli, so that the escaping fluid is similar to plasma except that it is virtually free of protein.

2 The passage of this filtrate through a complex system of tubules, where its content of solutes is altered and its pH is modified. The resulting fluid is urine.

The glomerulus and its tubule together constitute the *nephron*, and this opens into a large collecting tubule which empties into a calyx of the renal pelvis. From here the urine passes down the ureter to the bladder, where it is held until it can by voided by micturition.

Many alterations take place in the composition of the glomerular filtrate as it passes through the tubules:

There is reabsorption of all the glucose, about 80% of the water, and many electrolytes from the *proximal convoluted tubule*.

There is an active secretion of hydrogen and potassium ions by the *distal convoluted tubule*, and this is balanced by a reabsorption of sodium, chloride, and bicarbonate ions.

There is reabsoption of more water in the *distal convoluted tubules and the collecting tubules*—this function is under the control of the pituitary antidiuretic hormone, which makes the tubular cells more permeable to water exchange, while sodium reabsorption from the *distal tubule* is controlled by aldosterone.

RENAL FAILURE: URAEMIA

Renal failure is a state in which the body's metabolism is deranged as the result of dysfunction of the kidneys. Renal insufficiency usually first manifests itself in a disturbance of urine formation and this is followed by various systemic effects which culminate in a clinical syndrome described as *uraemia*. The most conspicuous biochemical feature of uraemia is the retention of nitrogenous substances in the blood. An indication of the extent of dysfunction may be obtained by measuring the plasma urea level—normally 2.5–6.0 mmol/L (15–35 mg/dl), or if expressed as blood area

393

nitrogen (BUN) it is 2.9–8.9 mmol/L (8–25 mg/dl). The plasma creatinine level rises similarly.

Clinical features of uraemia

Since the diagnosis of uraemia is largely clinical, it is convenient to describe its main features at this stage:

1 Cerebral symptoms, e.g. drowsiness, headache, convulsions, and coma. These are possibly due to disturbances of fluid balance and the retention of ill-defined waste products.

2 Deep, sighing respirations, which are due to metabolic acidosis.

3 Muscular twitchings, and occasionally muscular spasms, due probably to hypocalcaemia.

4 Nausea, vomiting, and diarrhoea. These are possibly due to the excretion of urea into the stomach and intestine, where it is converted into ammonia by the urease present in the gastric mucosa or secreted by colonic organisms.

5 Hiccup, gastrointestinal bleeding, pruritus (itching of the skin), purpura, and acute fibrinous pericarditis.

6 Infection, particularly bronchopneumonia, is common, and may be the terminal event.

Although many of the features of uraemia are unexplained at the present time, it seems certain that electrolyte imbalance and failure in acid–base regulation are more important than is the retention of nitrogenous substances.

Renal insufficiency may either appear acutely, or else develop gradually as a terminal feature of chronic destructive renal disease. These two types will be considered separately.

Acute renal failure. This manifests itself by a sudden diminution in the urinary output (*oliguria*), and this may be followed by complete cessation (*anuria*). This must not be confused with sudden failure to pass urine due to an obstruction, an event which commonly affects men with prostatic enlargement and is called *retention of urine*.

Acute renal failure is a common clinical emergency, and its causes may be classified as being *prerenal*, *renal* or *postrenal*. The most common prerenal cause is hypoperfusion of the kidney secondary to shock, for instance following severe injury in traffic accidents or following major surgery. The condition is often called *acute tubular necrosis* (ATN), but the term is not strictly accurate. Patients dying of ATN in shock may show focal tubular necrosis, but on the other hand the kidneys may appear remarkably normal at necropsy. The oliguria is mainly related to the functional defect—the underperfusion of the glomeruli.

If the patient survives, there follows a period when large quantities of urine are passed (*polyuria*), because the kidneys cannot conserve electrolytes and water. Life is then in jeopardy because of dehydration and electrolyte loss. Regeneration of tubular epithelium occurs quite rapidly, but a perfect functional recovery is unusual.

Renal causes of acute renal failure include acute renal diseases such as glomerulonephritis or pyelonephritis, malignant hypertension, acute vascular obstruction due to thrombosis, embolism, dissecting aneurysm of the aorta, or acute vasculitis. ATN may be included here when there is tubular necrosis due to the effects of poisons, e.g. carbon tetrachloride (used in fire extinguishers) or diethyl glycol (used in antifreeze).

Postrenal causes of acute renal failure include sudden obstruction to the urinary outflow, e.g. by stones, and rupture of the bladder.

The manifestations of acute renal failure are severe oliguria—complete anuria occurs in the worst cases—associated with the retention of nitrogenous substances, potassium, phosphate, and other anions in the blood. The pH of the blood falls due to the failure of tubular secretion of hydrogen ions (*metabolic acidosis*), and there is an increase in the volume of extracellular water. The patient may die of overhydration, potassium intoxication, infection, or the retention of unclassified toxic metabolic products.

Chronic renal failure. This too is common in clinical practice and is associated with the endstage of many chronic renal diseases—glomerulonephritis, chronic pyelonephritis, nephrosclerosis, diabetes mellitus, amyloidosis, hydronephrosis following chronic urinary obstruction (due to prostatic enlargement, urethral stricture, and malignancy in the pelvis), and polycystic disease of the kidneys.

The manifestations of chronic renal failure are complex and diverse. There is usually moderate dehydration, as the diseased kidneys cannot conserve water and sodium properly. Potassium is usually retained, and a metabolic acidosis develops. Phosphate retention is a prominent feature, and it may, if longstanding, lead to a reciprocal lowering of the plasma calcium level. Impaired metabolism of vitamin D can lead to impaired absorption of calcium from the gut due to hypovitaminosis D. Rickets or osteomalacia occur according to the age of the patient. Hypocalcaemia stimulates the parathyroid glands to activity and the bone lesions of hyperparathyroidism result. Often the bone changes are a complex combination, and the condition is termed *renal osteodystrophy*.

Many chronic renal diseases are complicated by *hypertension*. A fall in afferent arteriolar pressure stimulates renin formation (p. 326), but it is uncertain whether this is the means whereby hypertension occurs in renal disease.

Another feature of chronic renal failure is intractible anaemia, probably related to impaired erythropoietin production. Purpura is secondary to abnormal platelet functions.

Both acute and chronic renal failure, if unrelieved, culminate in uraemia, which is the harbinger of death.

THE PROTEIN-LOSING KIDNEY

Normally only a trace of protein escapes into the glomerular filtrate, and this is reabsorbed by the proximal tubule. There are a number of conditions in which the permeability of the glomerulus is increased, so that large amounts of protein escape into the filtrate and are voided with the urine. Albumin, the smallest of the plasma proteins, is affected the most severely, and hypoalbuminaemia results. The occurrence of proteinuria, hypoalbuminaemia, and oedema is called the *nephrotic syndrome*, and it may be a complication of chronic renal disease, e.g. certain types of glomerulonephritis (particularly the membranous and membranoproliferative types), diabetic nephropathy, and lupus nephritis. A common cause in children is minimal change disease (see later).

The main features of the nephrotic syndrome are:

1 Severe proteinuria

2 Hypoproteinaemia, especially affecting the albumin level of the plasma
3 Generalized oedema due in part to the hypoproteinaemia and perhaps also to hyperaldosteronism
4 Susceptibility to infection, due possibly to a loss of immunoglobulins in the urine
5 A raised level of lipids in the blood. The plasma cholesterol (normally 6.5 mmol/L or about 250 mg/dl.) may exceed 26 mmol/L or 1000 mg/dl. The cause of this is unknown.

In the early stages renal function is well maintained and the blood pressure is normal, but later renal failure and uraemia may occur.

GLOMERULONEPHRITIS

Glomerulonephritis is a term applied to a group of diseases that are not obviously of infective nature, and in which the glomeruli are primarily affected. Although many classifications have been proposed, none has been found to be satisfactory. The types at present recognized have been delineated on the basis of three parameters:

Clinical features. The onset may be acute with haematuria and oliguria (*acute glomerulonephritis*), or the onset may be insidious with signs of renal failure developing over a period of many months (*chronic glomerulonephritis*). Proteinuria is invariable, and if severe leads to the nephrotic syndrome. One important type of glomerulonephritis is associated with infection by *S. pyogenes*. This post-streptococcal glomerulonephritis may be either acute or chronic.

Immunological findings. Glomerulonephritis is a feature of immune complex disease, and is the result of the deposition of circulating immune complexes in the glomeruli. Immune complexes may form in the kidney when circulating antibody forms complexes with antigen in the kidney itself. The antigen may be exogenous and planted in the kidney, or it may be a renal antigen—commonly a component of the glomerular basement-membrane complex. The immune complexes can contain antigen derived from organisms (e.g. streptococci and malaria parasites), tumour antigen (the nephrotic syndrome can complicate malignancy), or endogenous antigen (e.g.

DNA-anti DNA complexes in lupus erythematosus).

The detection of antigens and immune complexes in kidney disease is performed by immunofluorescent techniques.

Histopathological findings. Light microscopy, aided by electron microscopy, reveals several types of changes. For example there may be proliferation of mesangial cells and deposits of material (mostly immunoglobulin) in the glomerular basement membrane zone (*proliferative glomerulonephritis*). Widening of the basement membrane zone may be sufficiently marked to be visible on light microscopy (*membranous glomerulonephritis*). Both these patterns may be combined (*membranoproliferative glomerulonephritis*). When the glomerular damage is severe, it often stimulates the parietal epithelial cells to proliferate and produce a *crescentic glomerulonephritis*.

A characteristic electron microscopic finding in glomerulonephritis is fusion of the foot processes of the epithelial cells (podocytes) of the glomeruli (see Fig. 33.1). This appears to be an effect of the increased permeability of glomerular vessels to protein and is therefore present whenever there is proteinuria.

The technique of needle biopsy, by which a core of kidney substance can be removed safely during life, has greatly aided the investigation of renal disease in patients. The material obtained is particularly suited for immunofluorescent studies and electron microscopy as well as for routine light-microscopic examination.

Types of glomerulonephritis

The diagnosis of glomerulonephritis is the task of the expert who has access to such sophisticated tools as electron microscopy and immunofluorescence: for a detailed account of the various types specialized texts should be consulted.

In one type of glomerulonephritis (*minimal-change* or *nil disease*) the glomeruli appear normal under light microscopy, but under electron microscopy fusion of the foot processes of the epithelial cells is revealed. Most patients with this type of disease are children with a nephrotic syndrome. In *post-streptococcal glomerulonephritis* the changes during the acute phase are those of a proliferative glomerulonephritis. The illness occurs from 1 to 6 weeks after a streptococcal infection, and is characterized by oliguria and haematuria with oedema, particularly of the face. Infection with certain strains of *S. pyogenes* (nephritogenic strains, e.g. type 12) are particularly liable to be followed by glomerulonephritis, and the organisms are thought to share an antigen with the human glomerulus. Cross-reacting antibodies are assumed to cause the renal damage. The majority of patients (about 80%) recover completely, and death rarely occurs from renal failure during the acute phase. A number of patients develop a rapidly progressive disease which terminates in uraemia. These patients show severe glomerular damage with crescent formation. The remainder develop a slowly progressive disease with the glomeruli ultimately being replaced by hyalinized collagenous tissue. The tubules undergo atrophy and there is fibrous replacement of the renal parenchyma (chronic glomerulonephritis). The disease may be silent for a long time apart from moderate proteinuria, but eventually the manifestations of chronic renal failure and uraemia develop. Hypertension and heart failure are common. Some cases develop a nephrotic syndrome.

At autopsy the kidneys are reduced in size and display a fine granular surface. At this stage it is frequently impossible to be certain of the nature of the original disease. Such *end-stage kidneys* can result from many types of glomerulonephritis, nephrosclerosis, chronic pyelonephritis, interstitial nephritis, diabetic nephropathy, etc.

DISEASES AFFECTING THE TUBULES

In this group of diseases the primary damage is to the tubules. It includes two distinct groups of conditions—acute tubular necrosis which has already been described, and tubulointerstitial disease in which there is tubular damage accompanied by interstitial inflammation.

Tubulointerstitial disease

Tubulointerstitial disease may be due to infection, and if accompanied by inflammation of the renal pelvis the term *pyelonephritis* is applied; it may be acute or chronic. This group is considered under the heading of urinary tract infection (p. 398). There is another group of tubulointerstitial diseases in which infection is not the cause and the renal pelvis is not involved. The term *interstitial nephritis* is applied to this group, and it too may be acute or chronic.

Acute interstitial nephritis is usually due to administration of a drug, the best known of which is methicillin. If the drug is not withdrawn the patient may die. *Chronic interstitial nephritis* has many causes including gout and the ingestion of poisons, particularly the heavy metals. Some cases occur after ingestion of large doses of analgesic drugs, particularly aspirin–phenacetin mixtures. The condition generally arises from self-medication and is called *analgesic nephropathy.*

OTHER TYPES OF RENAL DISEASE

Lupus nephritis. Glomerulonephritis of either a proliferative or a membranous type is common in systemic lupus erythematosus (Fig. 33.1). It often causes a nephrotic syndrome and ultimately leads to renal failure.

Nephrosclerosis. Nephrosclerosis is a term used to describe the renal lesions of systemic hypertension (see Ch. 27). In the *benign type*, the arteriolosclerosis causes patchy ischaemia. The affected nephrons become atrophic and are ultimately replaced by scar tissue. Hence, the kidneys in benign nephrosclerosis show thinning of the cortex and a granularity of the surface. In malignant hypertension the arteriolar necrosis causes extensive patchy foci of necrosis (*malignant nephrosclerosis*). Renal failure is a common cause of death.

Diabetic nephropathy. This condition is described in Chapter 17.

RENAL AND URINARY-TRACT INFECTIONS

Bacterial urinary-tract infection is a major medical problem and is particularly common in females.

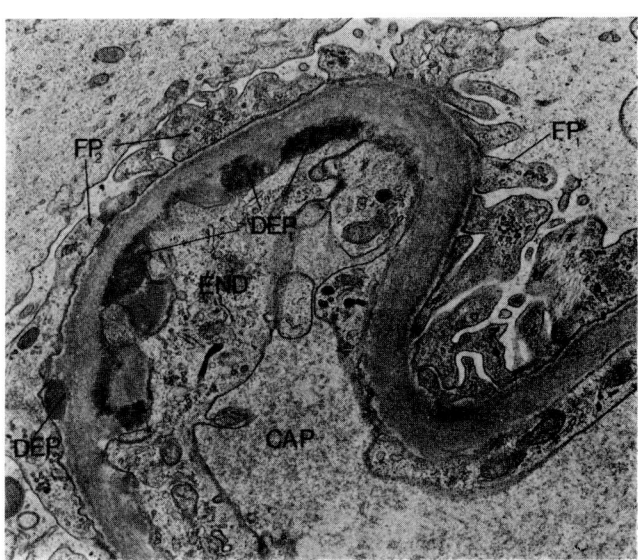

Fig. 33.1 Electron micrograph of glomerulus in systemic lupus erythematosus. In some areas the foot processes (FP$_1$) of the podocytes appear relatively normal, but elsewhere they are swollen and spread over the basement membrane (bm) of the capillary (FP$_2$). This change is commonly described as 'fusion of the foot processes'. Prominent subendothelial deposits are present (DEP$_1$). Subepithelial deposits are smaller and less obvious (DEP$_2$). In this patient the deposits were shown by immunofluorescence to contain IgG and components of complement. × 27 500. (Photograph by courtesy of Dr Y Bedard, Mount Sinai Hospital, Toronto. From Walter J B (1992) An introduction to the principles of disease, 3rd edn., W B Saunders, Philadelphia.)

The infecting organisms are usually derived from the patient's own faeces; *E. coli, P. aeruginosa, Proteus* species and *S. faecalis* are commonly implicated. The infection may be acute or chronic.

Acute infection. The common route of infection is an ascending infection from perineal organisms, and as might be expected this is a more common event in the female due to the short urethra. Catheterization with direct implantation of organisms into the bladder is a well-recognized cause. Haematogenous infection of the kidney is a less common cause. The initial effect of ascending infection may be inflammation of the bladder (cystitis), but in due course organisms reach the pelvis (to cause pyelitis) by retrograde ureteric peristalsis (*vesicoureteric reflux*). Inevitably the kidney is infected and *pyelonephritis* results. Certain individuals appear to be particularly susceptible to urinary-tract infection. A genetic factor has been suggested; their uroepithelium has receptors for certain organisms that then colonize the surface and cause infection. In children, vesicoureteric reflux is important. Obstruction to the urinary outflow is the most important factor predisposing toward infection. Thus unilateral pyelonephritis may follow the obstruction of one ureter. Pregnancy or, in the male, an enlarged prostate also predispose to infection.

Clinically acute pyelonephritis is characterized by rigors, fever and malaise. Pain on micturition and urgency are features of urethritis and cystitis, while pain in the loin occurs when the kidneys are involved. The kidneys show foci of acute inflammation and these may progress to suppuration.

Chronic pyelonephritis. Although chronic pyelonephritis may follow repeated attacks of acute infection and be associated with urinary-tract obstruction, this is uncommon. The disease usually has an insidious onset and becomes clinically evident when the patient develops signs of chronic renal failure or hypertension. Pathologically there is tubular destruction, interstitial fibrosis and an infiltration of the interstitial tissues by lymphocytes, macrophages and a varying number of neutrophils. The glomeruli are spared till late in the course of the disease. The picture is

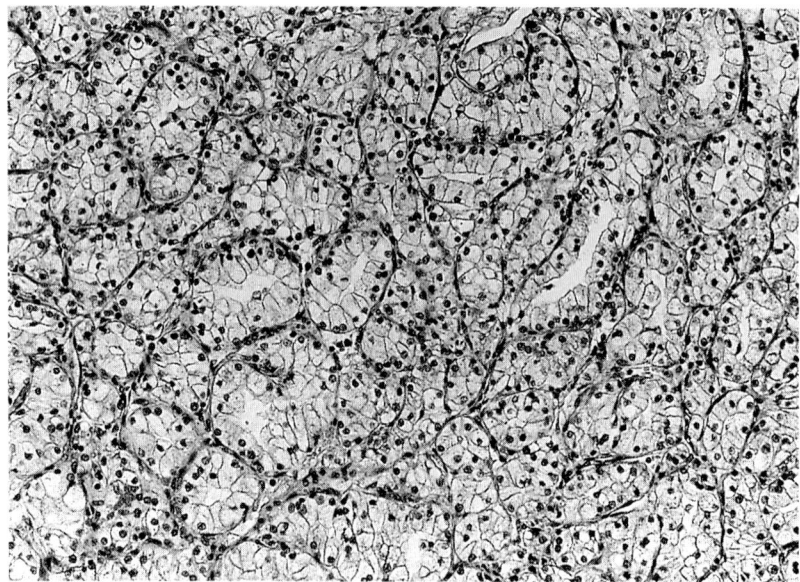

Fig. 33.2 Clear-cell carcinoma of the kidney. The tumour consists of masses of uniform cells with abundant clear cytoplasm. In places the cells are arranged to form tubular spaces. The clear cytoplasm is due to the high content of glycogen and lipid, both of which are removed during the preparation of the slide. (From Walter J B 1989 Pathology of Human Disease, Philadelphia: Lea and Febiger.)

very similar to that of chronic interstitial nephritis, and indeed in its later stages it resembles the end-stage kidney resulting from many other renal diseases. The pathogenesis of chronic pyelonephritis is not understood but chronic vesicoureteric and intrarenal reflux may be important even in the absence of infection.

The relationship between urinary-tract infection and urinary calculi (or stones) should be noted. Infection predisposes to the formation of *secondary stones* consisting of calcium salts. The presence of these stones predisposes to recurrent infection. Likewise primary calculi (these include stones composed of calcium oxalate, uric acid—sometimes associated with gout—and mixed calcium oxalate and phosphate—sometimes associated with hypercalcaemia and hypercalciuria as in hyperparathyroidism) may also cause urinary-tract obstruction and predispose to infection. Another noteworthy effect of calculi is the production of haematuria associated with severe pain (*renal colic*). This contrasts with the *painless haematuria* characteristic of carcinoma of the bladder or kidney.

TUMOURS OF THE KIDNEY

Renal-cell carcinoma and nephroblastoma are important tumours of the kidney.

Renal-cell carcinoma. This tumour presents at a pole of the kidney as a large encephaloid mass, which on section has a variegated appearance: areas of orange are interspersed amid white stroma and red foci of haemorrhage. Microscopically it consists of large cells with clear cytoplasm and sometimes arranged in tubular fashion (Fig. 33.2). The clear appearance of the cells is due to their high content of lipid and glycogen, both of which tend to be lost during histological processing. The carotenoids dissolved in the lipid give rise to the orange colour of the tumour. The tumour has also been called hypernephroma because of the mistaken belief that the tissue of origin was the adrenal cortex. The term is still in common use.

Clinically carcinoma of the kidney is often silent for a long time. Haematuria and an abdominal mass are two common presenting features. Distant lymphatic and blood-borne metastases are common, the liver, lungs, and bones being especially vulnerable. Indeed, a skeletal metastasis is sometimes the first indication of the tumour.

Another interesting feature is the phenomenon of dormancy (p. 253)—bony deposits may suddenly erupt many years after the successful removal of the affected kidney.

Nephroblastoma. The other important renal tumour is the *nephroblastoma*, or *Wilms's tumour*, an embryonic tumour of infancy discussed in Chapter 21.

GENERAL READING

Brenner B M, Rector F C Jr (eds) 1986 The kidney. 3rd edn. Saunders, Philadelphia
Bullock N, Sibley G, Whittaker 1989 Essential urology. Churchill Livingstone, Edinburgh
Heptinstall R H 1983 Pathology of the kidney. 3rd edn, Vols 1–3. Little Brown, Boston

Kaplan N K 1984 Systemic hypertension: mechanisms and diagnosis. In: Braunweld E (ed.) Heart disease, 2nd edn. Saunders, Philadelphia
Robinson R (ed.) 1984 Nephrology. Springer-Verlag, New York

34. The musculoskeletal system

INTRODUCTION

In early embryonic life condensations of mesenchyme are laid down at the sites of future bone formation, and by the end of the second month ossification commences. In the development of some bones, notably the cranium and the clavicle, there is a direct conversion of the membranous sheet of mesenchyme to bone. Bones formed in this way are called *membrane bones*. The base of the skull and the long bones develop in a different way: in these the mesenchyme differentiates into cartilage which is subsequently *replaced* by bone. The cartilage cells swell up and die, and the intervening matrix then calcifies. This *calcified cartilage* is eroded by osteoclasts, and at the same time osteoblasts lay down lamellar bone (see below); the process continues at the epiphyseal ends of long bones until adult stature is reached. This type of bone formation is called *endochondral ossification*. Some bones, for example the mandible, are formed by a mixture of the two processes of ossification.

Structure of bone

Bone is composed of calcified osteoid tissue; the latter consists of fibres of type 1 collagen embedded in a ground substance of glucosaminoglycans linked to the non-collagenous proteins osteocalcin and osteonectin. The calcium salts are generally considered to have a hydroxyapatite structure.

Depending upon the arrangement of the collagen fibres, two histological types of bone may be recognized.

Woven, immature, fibrillary, or non-lamellar bone. This shows irregularity in the arrangement of the collagen bundles and in the distribution of the osteocytes.

Formation. Woven bone is formed wherever ossification occurs primarily in loose connective tissue. This occurs in three situations:

1. During the formation of membrane bones
2. When bone forms in the midst of the differentiating granulation tissue of a healing fracture
3. In certain bone disorders and in osteogenic tumours.

Lamellar or mature bone. In this type of bone the collagen bundles are arranged in parallel sheets either in the form of concentric Haversian systems or flat plates.

In the outer dense *cortex* of a long bone Haversian systems predominate, while flat plates are seen under the periosteum and endosteum. This type of bone is called *compact bone.*

The central portion of long bones is hollowed out to form the medullary cavity, which contains marrow. Only a few spicules of bone remain. These are constructed of flat bundles of collagen, although in the wider trabeculae Haversian systems may be found. The central trabeculated part of the bone is called *cancellous,* and it should be noted that, like 'compact' bone, this is a term related to the gross appearance.

Formation. Lamellar bone is formed when bone is laid down on a previously calcified structure. This may be:

1. Calcified cartilage, as in normal endochondral ossification and in replacement of the cartilage which forms during the healing of a fracture
2. Woven bone, as during the early growth of membrane bones
3. Lamellar bone itself, as during the circumferential growth of all bones.

In the normal adult the entire skeleton is composed of lamellar bone.

Metabolic functions of bone

The relationship of bone to calcium metabolism and the functions of parathyroid hormone and calcitonin are described in Chapter 19. An important enzyme of osseous tissue is *alkaline phosphatase*; it is manufactured by osteoblasts, but its precise role in bone formation is not understood. Nevertheless, since some of the enzyme escapes into the blood, the plasma level is a good index of the overall osteoblastic activity within the body. The measurement of the alkaline phosphatase level in the plasma is therefore a useful aid in the diagnosis of generalized bone disorders.* The level is normally 30–110 units/litre, in adults and somewhat higher in children.*

Although bone appears rigid and inert, it is as susceptible as the soft tissues to adverse circumstances and deleterious agents; indeed, the effects on bone are often more severe and permanent.

There is a continuous process of remodelling throughout life with bone resorption by *osteoclasts* and bone deposition by *osteoblasts*, each keeping pace with the other. If either predominates osteoporosis or osteosclerosis results. *Osteoporosis* is a condition in which osteoid matrix, although reduced in amount, is normally mineralized. The bony trabeculae are greatly thinned, and the bone as a whole is weakened and liable to fracture.

Osteoporosis may be brought about by either excessive destruction of bone or defective formation, and may occur in a number of conditions in a localized or generalized form (see later).

In *osteosclerosis* there is excessive formation of osteoid, which being calcified, makes the bones appear dense on a radiograph.

Classification of generalized bone disorders

There is no very satisfactory classification of generalized bone disorders, but they may be considered under three headings:

1. *Developmental abnormalities,* of genetic or unknown cause
2. *Abnormalities due to metabolic disorders.* These include endocrine disturbances and vitamin deficiencies or excesses, and are described in Chapters 36 and 18, respectively
3. *Miscellaneous abnormalities* of bone.

Although this is a convenient classification, there is an overlap between the groups, and in some examples a localized form of the disease may occur.

---

*Very high plasma levels of alkaline phosphatase are found in obstructive jaundice. Liver disease must therefore be considered. The total plasma alkaline phosphatase activity consists of the summation of the effect of five isoenzymes. These can be measured seperately. Bone alkaline phosphatase is the most unstable and is the one referred to here. Another important alkaline phosphatase is derived from liver and its plasma level is raised in bile-duct obstruction. The level is not only raised in obvious jaundice due to main bile-duct obstruction, but also with multiple bile-ductule obstruction when jaundice is absent. A raised level is therefore a useful indication of the presence of multiple hepatic deposits of secondary carcinoma.

GENERALIZED BONE DISORDERS

Developmental abnormalities

There are a few rare conditions of bone which result in a failure during the developmental process.

Cleidocranial dysplasia. This condition is sometimes inherited as a dominant trait, and is characterized by the complete agenesis of a bone or part of a bone. The clavicle is most often affected, but defects have also been reported in the pelvic girdle and long bones. When the clavicles are absent, the subject is able to approximate the shoulders across the chest (Fig. 34.1).

There may also be retardation or failure of closure of the fontanelles, and the two halves of the frontal bone may not fuse. There is also asso-

ciated a general failure of eruption of the teeth and the presence of supernumerary teeth.

Osteogenesis imperfecta. Osteogenesis imperfecta is not a single entity but a group of inherited diseases in which the bones are abnormally thin and brittle. Six types have been described and they tend to fall into two groups. Those that are present at birth (*congenital type*) are usually inherited as autosomal recessive traits. Multiple fractures occur in utero or during birth, and the prognosis is poor. In the *tarda form*, usually inherited as a dominant trait, the condition is less severe.

The bones in osteogenesis imperfecta are generally thin and brittle. The cortex is thin, and there is a decrease in the amount of cancellous bone. The fragility results in the frequent occurrence of fractures which occur either spontaneously or as a result of trivial injuries. Although there is rapid healing of the fractures, the bone is of abnormal consistency. The multiplicity of fractures generally leads to severe deformities. Affected subjects are of short stature, and have lax ligaments which lead to hypermobility of the joints. In addition the sclera is sometimes thin and semi-translucent, so that it appears blue due to the pigmentation of the underlying choroid.

The pathogenesis of this group of diseases is not clear. In some forms an abnormal type of collagen is present in the bones. In others type 3 collagen is present in the bones and there is a diminished amount of type 1 collagen.

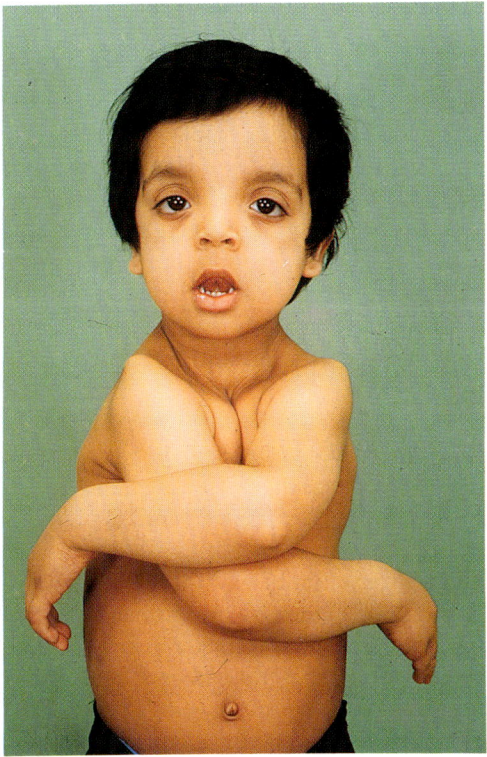

Fig. 34.1 Cleidocranial dysplasia. The shoulders can be approximated in this boy as a result of partial absence of the clavicles. There is evidence of bossing of the frontal and parietal bones. He had a number of supernumerary teeth and many teeth had failed to erupt. (Photograph courtesy of Dr L Shaw, University of Birmingham. Previously published in Rock W P, Grundy M C, Shaw L Diagnostic picture tests in paediatric dentistry. Wolfe Medical Publications, London.)

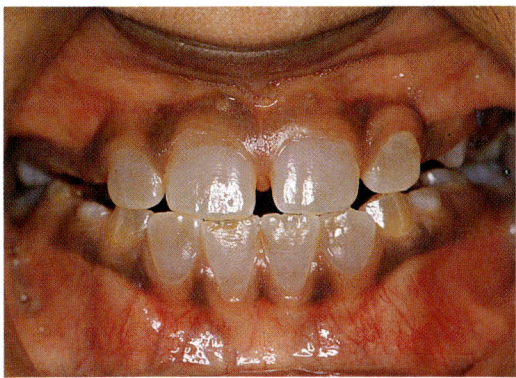

Fig. 34.2 Dentinogenesis imperfecta. The teeth have an opalescent hue due to the discoloured dentine showing through the translucent enamel.

Dentinogenesis imperfecta (hereditary opalescent dentine). This is a condition affecting that part of the tooth of mesenchymal origin (dentine), and may be seen in association with osteogenesis imperfecta or may occur without any bony involvement (Figs 34.2 and 34.3).

Fibrous dysplasia. The aetiology of this condition is unknown. It is characterized by the appearance of areas of bone resorption and replacement by fibrous tissue in which there are thin trabeculae of woven bone in the shape of Chinese characters. The marrow space is also obliterated in the affected areas. Any bone may be affected, either in its entirety or only focally. Fibrous dysplasia includes a wide variety of conditions which may well be excluded from this group as our knowledge increases. Two main types are described:

Polyostotic fibrous dysplasia. This manifests itself early in life. There is an insidious onset, and a pathological fracture may be the presenting symptom. The condition usually affects one side of the body only. When the skull and facial bones are involved there is much disfigurement. The disease process usually ceases when growth has ended.

Albright's syndrome, a more severe form of the condition, is accompanied by pigmentation of the skin (café-au-lait spots), endocrine dysfunction resulting in sexual precocity in young girls, and disturbances of growth and development. The reason for the pigmentation and endocrine disturbance is not known.

Monostotic fibrous dysplasia. Some authorities believe that this is a reparative reaction following trauma or infection. Despite the histological similarity to the polyostotic form it does not seem to progress to the latter. Monostotic fibrous dysplasia is much more common than the polyostotic form. It occurs in young people, and may affect any bone including the jaw in from 10 to 15% of cases.

Familial bilateral multilocular cysts ('cherubism'). This disease, first described by Jones in 1933, resembles monostotic fibrous dysplasia but is inherited as an autosomal dominant trait with incomplete penetrance. The bone is replaced by loose, oedematous fibrous tissue in which there are scattered giant cells. Bony trabeculae like those of fibrous dysplasia are not present.

Characteristically there is enlargement of the jaws and there may be submaxillary lymphadenopathy. Involvement of the orbital floor with upward displacement of the eyes combines with the large jaws to give a cherubic appearance.

Bony expansion of the jaws occurs particularly in the mandibular molar region—it commences in the first 2–3 years of life, and gradually ceases as growth terminates. There may be a premature loss of primary teeth and some disturbances of the permanent dentition with an absence of teeth and failure of eruption of those present.

Radiographs of the jaws show extensive symmetrical areas of radiolucency which have a multilocular appearance. Involvement of bones other than those of the skull and mandible can occur, but it is rare.

There is some doubt as to the exact nature of the condition. Jones, who coined the name cherubism, considered that it was an anomaly of dental development. Others regard it as a fibrous dysplasia or a bone dysplasia. Others do not commit themselves, and consider the condition a familial osseous dysplasia or fibrous swelling of the jaws.

Achondroplasia (chondrodystrophy fetalis). This disease is transmitted as an autosomal dominant trait. The essential feature is defective endochondral bone formation, and the long bones of the limbs are therefore short. The trunk and head are of normal size, but the middle third

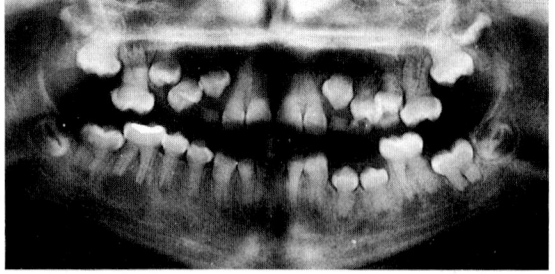

Fig. 34.3 This panoramic radiograph shows the classic appearance of the dentinogenesis imperfecta. Note the bulbous crowns, short roots and almost complete lack of pulp chambers in this 8-year-old. There is also radiolucency in the apical region of the first permanent molars as a result of non-vital pulpal tissue which has become infected.

of the face is depressed due to the early closure of cartilaginous growth centre, the spheno-occipital synchondrosis, resulting in maxillary hypoplasia and relative mandibular protrusion. This type of dwarf, who has normal intelligence, is very muscular and agile, and is frequently seen in the circus ring.

Osteopetrosis (Albers–Schönberg disease, marble-bone disease). This disease occurs in various forms and with varying severity. The infantile form is inherited as a Mendelian recessive trait and is severe. Cases with dominant inheritance tend to be more benign and be manifest in adult life. There is increased deposition of bone in this condition so that the bones are thickened, hard, heavy, and inelastic. This renders them liable to fracture easily. The cortex is greatly thickened, and the marrow cavity is much reduced in size. Leuco-erythroblastic anaemia may result. Later on blindness, deafness, and facial paralysis develop, due to constriction of the cranial nerves as they pass through the bony foramina of the skull.

Miscellaneous abnormalities of bone

Generalized osteoporosis. Osteoporosis is a condition of bone atrophy, and has been aptly defined as a lesion in which the volume of bone tissue per unit volume of anatomical bone is reduced. There is a reduction in the amount of osteoid tissue, which, however, remains normally mineralized. It must be distinguished from *osteomalacia*, in which osteoid is present in abundance but is poorly calcified. The radiological appearance of osteoporosis is a reduction of bone density; it must, however, be remembered that this can be detected in routine films with certainty only when the content of calcium is reduced by at least a half. Refined techniques may be more sensitive.

Causes. Disuse osteoporosis. Prolonged recumbency produces considerable osteoporosis in most bones. It would seem that stress and strain are a necessary stimulus for the maintenance of bone structure. Immobilization leads initially to osteoclastic resorption of bone and the mobilization of excessive amounts of calcium, which results in hypercalciuria and sometimes renal-stone formation. This is then followed by a phase of quiescence in which the bone shows little

osteoclastic or osteoblastic activity. If movement is resumed, the bones gradually return to normal. The blood levels of calcium, phosphate, and phosphatase are normal in disuse osteoporosis.

Idiopathic osteoporosis. Osteoporosis, especially of the pelvis, spine, and ribs, is not uncommon in old age (*senile osteoporosis*), and compression of the vertebral bodies causes backache as well as a considerable loss of height. The condition is also seen in women who have passed the menopause (*post-menopausal osteoporosis*), and this has been attributed to hormonal imbalance (Fig. 34.4). Occasionally osteoporosis occurs in a younger age-group for no very obvious reason.

Other types of osteoporosis. Osteoporosis is also seen when collagen formation is impaired as in:

1. Scurvy
2. Excessive glucocorticoid levels, e.g. Cushing's disease and with prolonged administration of adrenocortical hormones
3. Impaired supply of protein, e.g. starvation and the malabsorption syndrome.

Effects. Symptoms are generally referable to the spine and pelvis, which are the parts of the skeleton most severely affected in generalized osteoporosis. Chronic backache and kyphosis are common, and collapse of the vertebrae may produce episodes of acute pain. Diminution in height is characteristic, and may be as much as 8 inches before being noticed by the patient. Fractures may complicate osteoporosis; thus minimal trauma may cause the fracture of a limb bone, particularly the lower forearm bones and the femur.

Paget's disease of bone (osteitis deformans). Described first by James Paget in 1876, this condition is considered by some to be an inflammatory disease. However, despite much study its aetiology and nature are unknown. It occurs in people over the age of 40 years, predominantly in the male sex. It is perhaps more common than was originally thought, as routine radiographs sometimes reveal solitary lesions in the spine and pelvis without clinical manifestations. The involved bones show much thickening of the cortex due to the dominance of osteoblastic activity.

Initially the bone is softened due to osteoclastic resorption, and the affected area shows increased

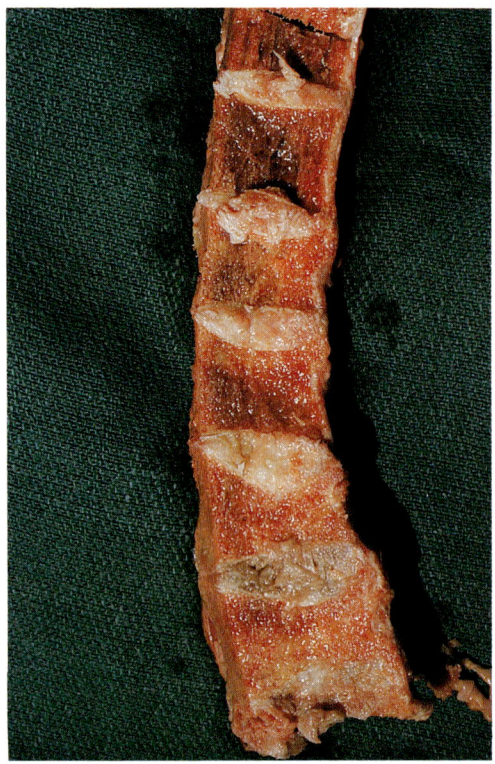

Fig. 34.4 Osteoporosis of the spine. The large lumbar vertebral bodies show severe compression. The intervertebral discs have bulged into the vertebrae further reducing the vertical height of each vertebra.

vascularity. The bending of softened, weight-bearing bones results in deformities, and is adequate reason for the alternative name of osteitis deformans. Later there is irregular subperiosteal deposition, and the bones become hard and thickened (Fig. 34.5). Microscopically the irregular new-bone formation results in a characteristic mosaic appearance (Fig. 34.6). The plasma calcium and phosphate levels are within normal limits, but the alkaline phosphatase may be raised as much as fifty times above normal.

The skull is frequently affected, and later it may become obviously enlarged. When the jaws are affected the teeth show marked hyper-cementosis. Bone pain may be an early feature. Blindness, deafness, headaches, and facial paralysis are complications that may occur as a result of compression of the nerves due to the increased bone formation. Sarcoma of bone

complicates the condition in about 1 per cent of patients. The reasons for this is not known; it appears that the excessive proliferative activity of the bone leads eventually to neoplastic growth.

BONE DISORDERS CAUSED BY PHYSICAL DISTURBANCES

Localized osteoporosis

Due to immobilization. The local disuse of a bone causes osteoporosis in the same way as does total recumbency, and the immobilization of a joint leads to marked osteoporosis of the adjacent bones. This occurs after fractures and also in diseases of the joints themselves, e.g. tuberculous and rheumatoid arthritis. It is very pronounced in paralysed limbs; indeed, if paralysis occurs in childhood, as after poliomyelitis, the whole limb including the bones fails to attain adult size.

Sudeck's acute bone atrophy is probably an example of disuse atrophy. It follows quite trivial trauma to the hands, and more rarely the feet. Examples of this condition have also been noted in the mandible. This condition is associated with marked pain and swelling, and there is radiological evidence of rapidly progressing osteoporosis. The pain is usually out of all proportions to the extent of the injury, and the most likely explanation of both the osteoporosis and the oedema is disuse consequent on the pain.

Pressure atrophy. Expanding lesions which exert pressure on the surrounding bone cause local ischaemia due to compression of the blood vessels, and atrophy results. Thus a benign tumour or cyst may produce a sharply-defined area of rarefaction. In an attempt to offset the weakness that ensues more bone is produced by the periosteum opposite the lesion, so that the mass appears to cause expansion of the bone. This is well seen in the giant-cell tumour and in the ameloblastoma. It should be noted that cartilage, being avascular, does not undergo pressure atrophy. Therefore an aneurysm of the descending aorta pressing on the vertebral column causes atrophy of the vertebrae but spares the intervertebral discs. For the same

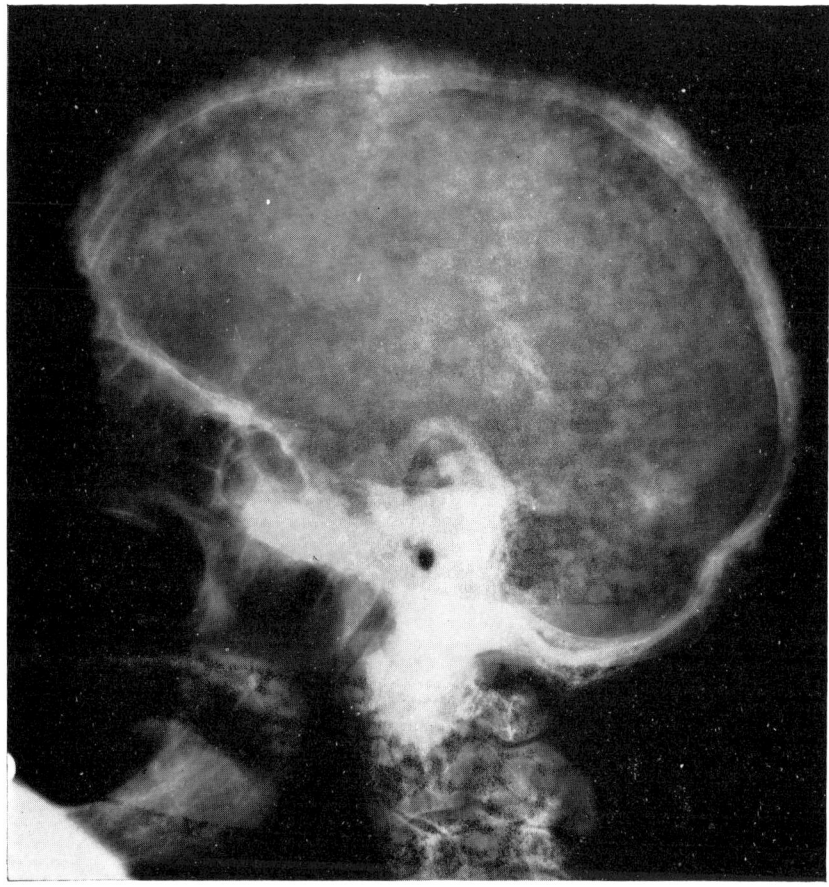

Fig. 34.5 Paget's disease affecting the skull. Note the uneven thickening of the outer table and the blurring of the demarcation between the inner and outer tables. (Radiograph by courtesy of the late Professor H C Killey.)

reason benign tumours and cysts do not destroy the epiphyseal cartilage of a long bone.

Fractures

Causes

Excessive mechanical force.

Direct violence, e.g. depressed fracture of the skull.

Indirect violence, e.g. fractures of the condyles of the mandible following a blow on the chin.

Muscular action. Sudden unexpected strains during violent exercise may cause fractures in normal bones (*spontaneous fractures*). Likewise the violent convulsive movements of tetanus and strychnine poisoning may result in the collapse of a vertebral body, causing wedging.

Abnormal bone. A fracture may occur in a diseased bone subjected to a normal strain (*pathological fracture*). Any lesion which causes weakness may be responsible, e.g. osteitis fibrosa cystica, osteogenesis imperfecta, simple bone cyst, and tumour. Secondary carcinoma must always be borne in mind, and indeed a pathological fracture may be the first indication of a malignant lesion, e.g. carcinoma of lung or breast.

Stages in fracture healing (bone regeneration)

The stages in healing of a fracture are illustrated diagrammatically in Fig. 34.7. It must be remembered that the entire area is not all at the same stage of healing; while the centre may be at an

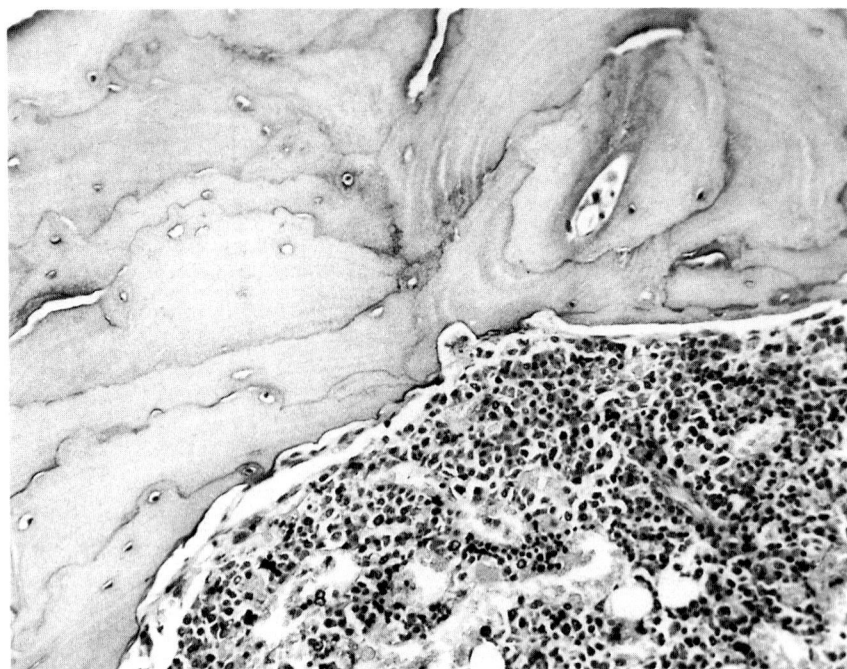

Fig. 34.6 Paget's disease of bone. There are massive, irregular trabeculae of bone that have been deposited haphazardly on one another during the process of new-bone formation that follows the initial osteoclastic resorption of bone. The disorientated blocks of bone are joined together by irregular cement lines which produce the mosaic pattern that is virtually specific to Paget's disease, and characteristic of its final, burnt-out phase. The bone marrow is hypercellular, being packed with neoplastic plasma cells. The patient also had multiple myeloma.

early stage, the changes adjacent to the bone ends are much more advanced. However, for descriptive purposes it is convenient to divide the healing process into separate stages.

Stage 1: haematoma formation. Immediately following the injury there is a variable amount of bleeding from torn vessels, and a haematoma is formed.

Stage 2: inflammation. The tissue damage excites an acute inflammatory response, with vasodilatation and a polymorphonuclear leucocytic infiltration. The hyperaemia has been held responsible for the decreased density of the adjacent bone ends often noted radiologically. This 'decalcification' is presumably a form of osteoporosis due to osteoclastic activity, but the pathogenesis is not clear. The connective-tissue changes that accompany the inflammatory reaction cause a loosening of the attachment of the periosteum to the bone. The haematoma therefore attains a fusiform shape.

Stage 3: demolition. Macrophages invade the clot and remove the fibrin, red cells, inflammatory exudate, and debris. Any fragments of bone which have become detached from their blood supply undergo necrosis, and are attacked by macrophages and osteoclasts.

Stage 4: formation of granulation tissue. Following the demolition there is an ingrowth of capillary loops and mesenchymal cells derived from the periosteum and endosteum. The importance of the periosteum in fracture union has been much disputed in the past. The cells of its deeper layer certainly have osteogenic potentiality, and together with its blood vessels contribute to the granulation tissue.

In fractures of the neck of the femur the head is dependent upon the periosteum for its blood supply. If this is damaged, there is ischaemic necrosis of the head. Hence in this situation the integrity of the periosteum is of great practical importance. In a rib following subperiosteal

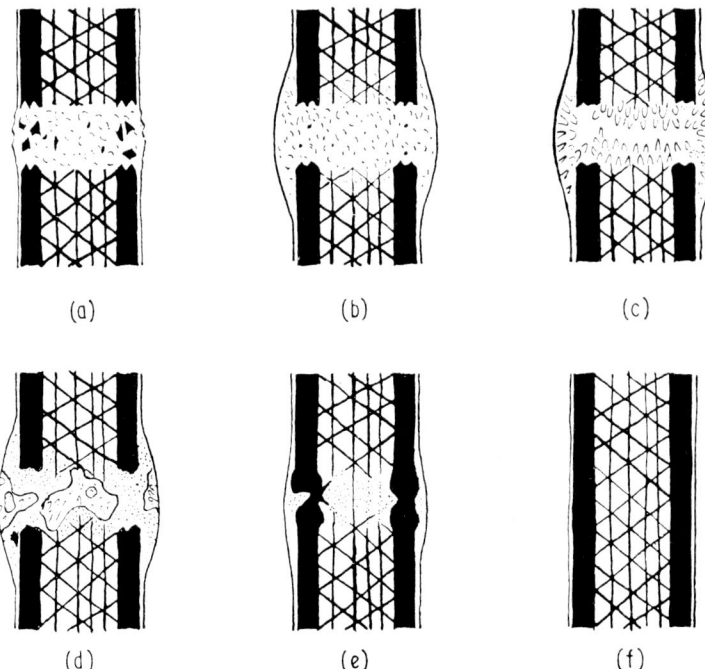

(a) (b) (c)

(d) (e) (f)

Fig. 34.7 Stages in the healing of a fracture. (a) Haematoma formation. (b) Stages 2 and 3. Acute inflammation followed by demolition. Loose fragments of bone are removed, and the bone ends show osteoporosis. (c) Stage 4. Granulation tissue formation. (d) Stage 5. The bone ends are now united by woven bone, cartilage, or a mixture of the two. The hard material is often called callus, and can be divided into three parts—internal, intermediate, and external. The intermediate callus is that part which lies in line with the cortex of the bone, while the external callus produces the fusiform swelling visible on the outside of the bone. (e) Stage 6. Lamellar bone is laid down, and calcified cartilage and woven bone are progressively removed. (f) Stage 7. Final remodelling.

resection the periosteum alone is capable of effecting complete regeneration. Here it probably acts partly by forming a limiting membrane around the haematoma, and partly by providing cells and blood vessels for the granulation tissue.

In fractures of the long bones, however, it must not be forgotten that a very extensive area of cancellous bone is exposed. From this the endosteal osteoblasts and the medullary blood vessels grow out to form the granulation tissue. Under these circumstances the periosteum is of much less importance.

During these early phases the pH is low, and this is spoken of as the *acid tide.*

Stage 5: woven bone and cartilage formation. The mesenchymal 'osteoblasts' next differentiate to form either woven bone or car-

tilage. The term '*callus*', derived from the Latin and meaning hard, is often used to describe the material uniting the fracture ends regardless of its consistency. When this is granulation tissue the 'callus' is soft, but as bone or cartilage formation occurs it becomes hard. The word is used loosely by surgeons, radiologists, and pathologists, but exact definition of its various stages is difficult and serves no useful function. If the term is used, it is probably best to apply it to the calcified hard tissue uniting the bone ends.

Formation of woven bone. The osteoblasts form both the collagen fibres and the ground substance, in which they are embedded. The osteoid is in this way formed by the maturation of granulation tissue, and as in the repair of ordinary connective tissue progressive devascularization occurs. The collagen bundles are irregularly arranged with no attempt at lamellar structure.

After about 10 days the pH of the uniting fracture increases. During this *alkaline tide* the osteoid undergoes calcification, and thereby becomes woven bone. Osteoblasts produce an alkaline phosphatase which may play a part in the calcification, in that it may lead to a local supersaturation of phosphate due to its effect on hexose phosphates. Resorption of bony spicules may at the same time produce a local super-saturation of calcium ions.

The bone ends thus become united by woven bone. It forms a fusiform mass which is arbitrarily divided into internal, intermediate, and external callus (Fig. 34.7).

Woven-bone formation is found whenever the bone ends are adequately immobilized (Fig. 34.8). It normally occurs in human fracture healing, and is a predominant feature in healing of tooth sockets. In experimentally produced fractures in animals adequate immobilization is difficult to attain, and then the granulation tissue matures not to woven bone, but to hyaline cartilage as described below.

Formation of cartilage. The mesenchymal cells ('osteoblasts') behave as chondroblasts and form cartilage, i.e. the cells actively lead to the formation of a specialized ground substance in which the collagen fibres are embedded (Fig. 34.9). These cartilage cells swell and die, and the intervening matrix undergoes calcification. Cartilage formation is seen in fractures in which movement occurs, not only in experimental fractures in animals, but also fractures in the human where complete immobilization is impractical, e.g. ribs.

In many fractures both cartilage and woven bone are formed. Both are capable of forming a calcified scaffold on which the final adult-type, lamellar bone can later be built. The two embryological methods of bone formation, endochondral and intramembranous ossification, are faithfully repeated in later life during the regeneration of bone.

Stage 6: formation of lamellar bone. The dead calcified cartilage or woven bone is next invaded by capillaries headed by osteoclasts. As the initial scaffolding ('provisional callus') is

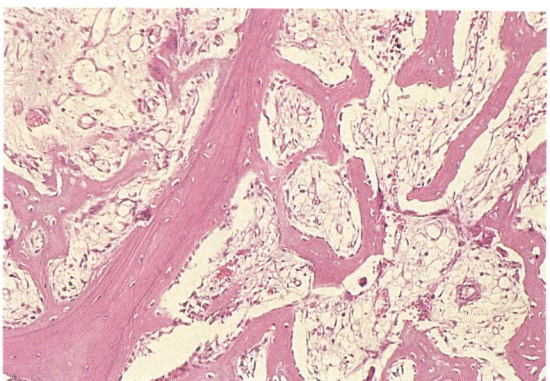

Fig. 34.8 Fracture healing. The callus consist of vascular granulation tissue in which irregular shaped areas of woven bone are forming. The large strut of bone to the left is lamellar bone.

removed, osteoblasts lay down osteoid which calcifies to form bone. This time its collagen bundles are arranged in orderly lamellar fashion. For the most part they are disposed concentrically around the blood vessels, where they form Haversian systems. Adjacent to the periosteum and endosteum the lamellae are parallel to the surface as in the normal bone. This phase of deposition of definitive lamellar bone merges with the last stage.

Stage 7: remodelling. The final remodelling process, involving the continued osteoclastic removal and osteoblastic formation of bone, results in the formation of a bone which differs remarkably little from its previous state. The

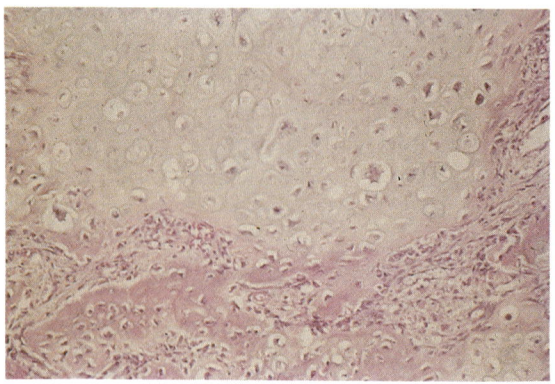

Fig. 34.9 Fracture healing. The callus consist of hyaline cartilage, adjacent to which is granulation tissue and early woven bone.

external callus is slowly removed, the *intermediate callus* becomes converted into compact bone containing Haversian systems, while the *internal callus* is hollowed out into a marrow cavity in which only a few spicules of cancellous bone remain.

The healing of a socket following the extraction of a tooth is similar to that of a fracture. After an extraction the socket fills with blood which forms a clot, which within a few days is replaced by granulation tissue. Woven bone is laid down in the socket and this is later replaced by lamellar bone. There is a covering of compact bone. As the alveolar bone is no longer required to support the tooth, remodelling takes place and results in a reduced ridge in that area. The extraction of a tooth produces an open wound, and the healing process also includes epithelization over the granulation tissue.

A complication that sometimes occurs is the condition known as a 'dry socket'; this is a focal osteomyelitis and may occur if the blood clot disintegrates or is lost. The exposed bone becomes necrotic, and sequestration follows. The condition is extremly painful and healing is slow.

It is interesting to note that the healing of a fracture has some features in common with the process of axial regeneration in amphibia. Thus there is dedifferentiation of cells and the formation of a blastema in which the cells subsequently differentiate along several lines.

Abnormalities of fracture healing

Fibrous union. Although the cells of the granulation tissue are called osteoblasts, they are capable of differentiation along several lines. They can form bone, but if immobilization is not complete, cartilage may develop. When movement is even more free, the cells behave as fibroblasts, and the bone ends become united by ordinary scar tissue. Whether this can ever undergo ossification is debatable. It is claimed by some authorities that fibrous tissue can become replaced by bone, but that it is a very slow process. From a practical point of view fibrous union is an unsatisfactory end-result of healing, because in many cases it is permanent.

Occasionally with excessive movement the cells differentiate into synovial cells, and a false joint,

or *pseudarthrosis*, results. This is a well-recognized sequel of fractures of the tibia.

Non-union. Complete lack of union between the fracture ends results from the interposition of soft parts. Muscle or fascia separating the bone ends may prevent the formation of a uniting haematoma. Under these conditions union of any sort is impossible. This phenomenon is utilized in the treatment of some disorders of the temporomandibular joint in order to create a new joint.

Delayed union. In the presence of a continuous haematoma any of the causes of delayed healing (p. 92) retard bone regeneration.

Causes of impaired healing. If the adverse conditions are severe, fibrous union may be the end result. In practice the following are the most important:

Movement. Movement of any sort is harmful, because it causes damage to the delicate granulation tissue, and thereby excites an inflammatory reaction. In surgical practice every attempt is made to reduce movement to a minimum. In the case of impacted fractures this is usually easy, but in other instances where the bone ends are mobile, recourse may have to be made to pins, plates, or other forms of internal splinting. The bone ends must not be over-distracted, for this leads to slow healing. Indeed, if on the contrary the bone ends are brought together under high compression, there is rigid immobilization and healing is accelerated.

Infection. By prolonging the acute inflammatory phase, infection is an important cause of slow union or non-union. Since the tension engendered by the formation of exudate in a bone is liable to lead to extensive ischaemic necrosis with sequestrum formation, it is particularly important to avoid contaminating previously closed fractures during open reduction. Rigorous asepsis must be maintained by employing a no-touch technique.

Poor blood supply. While complete loss of blood supply results in necrosis of bone, poor blood supply leads to slow granulation tissue formation and therefore slow union. Certain sites are notorious for this complication, e.g. fractures of neck of femur, shaft of tibia, and the carpal scaphoid. In these situations the avoidance of other possible causes of delayed healing, e.g. movement, is particularly important. The slow healing of fractures in old age is probably due to ischaemia.

Traumatic myositis ossificans. If there is an extravasation of the fracture haematoma into the surrounding muscles, its subsequent organization and ossification results in the condition of *traumatic myositis ossificans*.

DISORDERS OF THE BONE MARROW

Disorders of the haematopoietic tissue of the marrow produce obvious effects in the circulating blood, and are considered in Chapter 26. There remain a number of disorders of uncertain nature which affect the mononuclear phagocyte system as a whole, and are considered elsewhere.

TUMOURS OF BONE

The tumours of bone form a complex group of neoplasms, for in spite of the apparent simplicity of bone structure, the histogenesis of some of the tumours which arise from it is quite obscure. The occurrence of tumours in the adjacent marrow and the frequency of skeletal metastases add further to the confusion.

Pain and swelling are the common early features of a bone tumour, but quite often the initial diagnosis is made on radiological grounds. Histological confirmation by biopsy is essential before treatment is attempted. The 'characteristic' appearances of certain tumours, e.g. osteosarcoma, are often absent, and furthermore may be mimicked by other lesions.

On the basis of the World Health Organization's classification, the following six groups of bone tumours are recognized: bone-forming tumours, cartilage-forming tumours, connective-tissue tumours, giant-cell tumour of bone, marrow tumours and finally a group of other tumours. The common types in each group will be described.

Bone-forming tumours

Osteoma and osteosarcoma are important examples.

Osteoma. The osteoma is a benign tumour composed of compact bone (ivory osteoma) or cancellous bone, or a mixture of the two. The skull is the common site and the tumour may grow into the orbit or into one of the nasal sinuses. Pressure effects or cosmetic disfigurement may necessitate removal.

Osteosarcoma. Osteosarcoma is the most common and the most malignant of this rare group of primary bone tumours. It usually occurs in children and young adults, but is found in older persons as a complication of Paget's disease or as a result of the deposition of radioactive substances in the bone. The tumour is composed of malignant osteoblasts which are usually very pleomorphic; giant cells are often abundant. Well-differentiated tumours produce variable amounts of cartilage together with osteoid, which may or may not calcify to form bone (Fig. 34.10). The surrounding normal bone is destroyed, and radiologically a poorly-differentiated tumour appears *osteolytic*, as there is an irregular bony defect. The tumour lifts up the periosteum, and if neoplastic bone is formed, it tends to be laid down around the periosteal vessels as they penetrate the tumour mass. This leads to the characteristic sun-ray appearance of the *osteosclerotic* type of tumour (Fig. 34.11). The outlook for a patient with osteosarcoma is extremely poor, for blood-borne metastases to the lungs appear early.

Cartilage-forming tumours

Two examples will be described.

Chondroma. Various types of chondroma are recognized. *Osteochondrama* is present at the metaphysis of a long bone. It is probably a malformation consisting of a cartilage capped spur of bone that has become separated from the epiphysis. When growth stops at puberty the cartilage disappears and the lesion becomes an exostosis.

Chondrosarcoma. This malignant tumour is composed of atypical cartilage cells and most commonly involves the axial skeleton—spine, pelvis and scapula. It is about half as common as osteosarcoma. The tumour is often very large; local invasion and later distant metastases are other features.

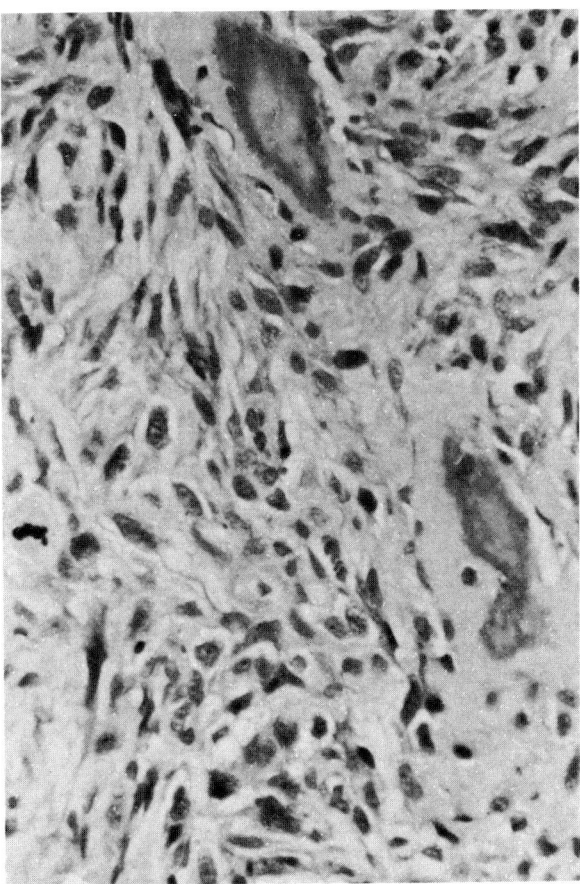

Fig. 34.10 Osteosarcoma. The tumour consists of sheets of spindle-shaped cells intimately connected with the intervening stroma. Two spicules of osteoid are included. Note the mitotic figure at the left edge of the section. × 350 (Photograph by courtesy of Dr A D Thomson.)

Connective tissue tumours

These tumours are uncommon and may be either benign (fibroma, angioma, etc.) or malignant (e.g. fibrosarcoma or angiosarcoma).

Giant-cell tumour of bone

This tumour of uncertain histogenesis is usually found in patients between 20 and 40 years of age. It is composed of a mixture of spindle cells and giant cells resembling osteoclasts (Fig. 34.12). The tumour destroys bone locally by pressure atrophy and in some cases by actual invasion. This produces the characteristic soap-bubble appearance seen radiologically. About 15% of giant-cell tumours metastasize to the lungs.

The tumour is usually seen in the long bones, and is very rare in the jaws. In the past it was commonly reported in the jaws, but this was probably due to the misdiagnosis of other non-neoplastic conditions. Some of these should be noted:

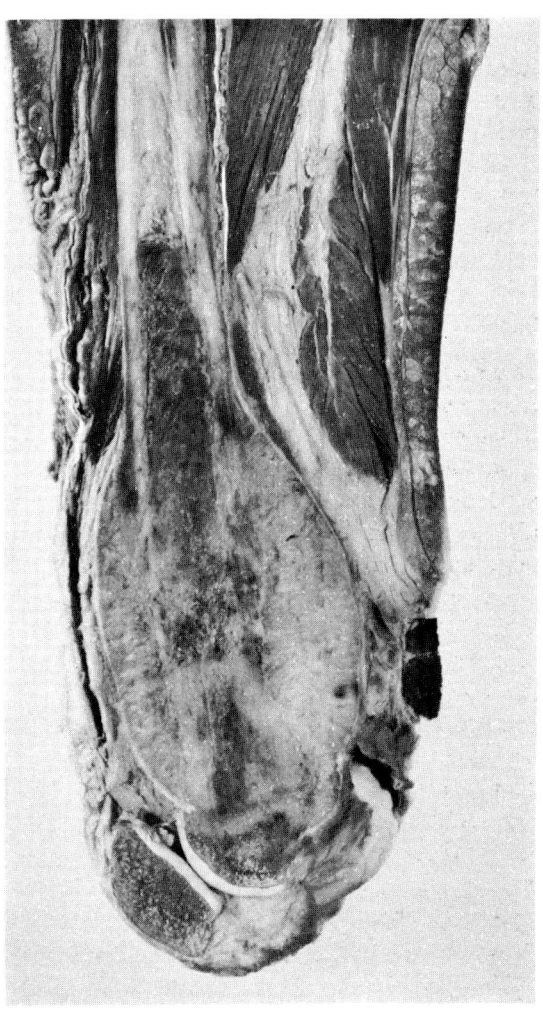

Fig. 34.11 Osteosarcoma. This has arisen from the lower end of the femur and has spread almost to the knee joint. The tumour has lifted up the periosteum, and has assumed a fusiform shape. There is a radiating ('sun-ray') disposition of newly-formed bony spicules in this spindle-shaped mass. (S72.5. Reproduced by permission of the President and Council of the Royal College of Surgeons of England.)

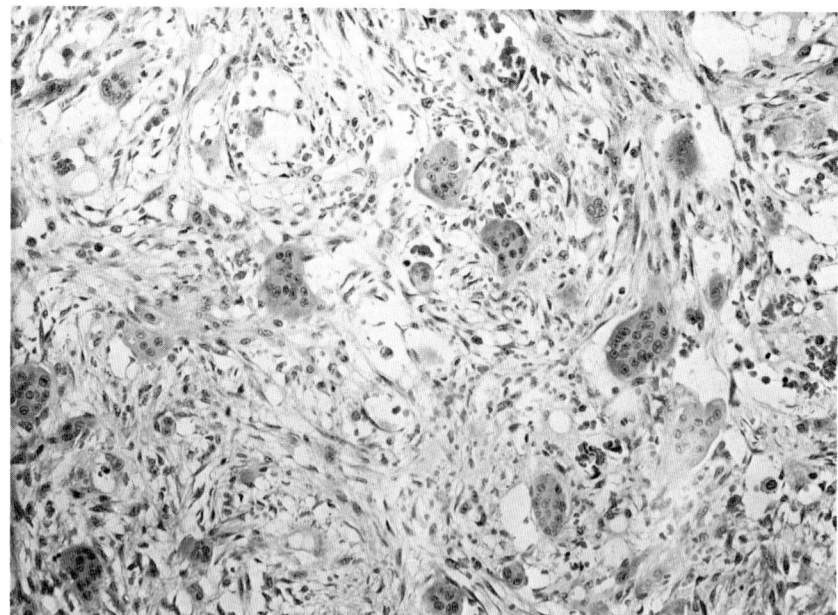

Fig. 34.12 Giant-cell tumour of bone. The tumour is composed of very large giant cells resembling osteoclasts and also a smaller spindle-shaped fibroblastic element. × 200.

Central giant-cell reparative granuloma. This appears as a central, expanding lesion in the tooth-bearing portion of the jaw, usually the mandible. It occurs between the ages of 10 and 25 years, and closely resembles a giant-cell tumour histologically. Nevertheless, it is thought to be non-neoplastic; it never metastasizes, and is perhaps a reaction to haemorrhage.

Brown tumour. See p. 219

Peripheral giant-cell reparative granuloma (giant-cell epulis). This should not be confused with a giant-cell tumour. It arises from the gingivae or periosteum as a result of chronic infection or irritation (see Fig. 20.11, p. 235).

Aneurysmal bone cyst. This lesion also consists of spindle cells and giant cells but these are associated with cavernous blood spaces. The lesion is probably not neoplastic and is easily cured by surgery. It is most common in the vertebrae or the metaphysis of a long bone.

Marrow tumours

This group includes Ewing's tumour, lymphoma and myeloma.

Ewing's tumour. This tumour occurs in young children, and most often affects the shaft of a long bone. It is composed of sheets of small round cells, and is osteolytic. The raised periosteum may produce layers of new bone around the tumour, leading to an onion-like appearance radiologically. The nature of Ewing's tumour is obscure. It appears to be a distinct entity, but can be closely mimicked by lymphoma and metastatic neuroblastoma. The tumour has a bad prognosis because it usually metastasizes to other bones and viscera. Nevertheless, with modern treatment, some cases are curable.

Lymphoma. This tumour occurs in an older age-group. It is osteolytic, and nearly always appears as an isolated tumour. It is radiosensitive, and the prognosis is better than that of Ewing's tumour.

Myeloma. A B-cell tumour composed of monoclonal neoplastic plasma cell precursors is occasionally encountered as a *solitary myeloma* in the tonsil or nasopharynx. More commonly the tumours are multiple and are found in the bones, especially the vertebrae, ribs, sternum, and skull, bones that normally contain red marrow (*multiple myeloma*). The disease occurs in patients over the age of 40, and the osteolytic tumours produce characteristic punched-out areas on a radiograph (Fig. 34.13). The results of these tumours are serious. Not only do they lead to the destruction of the surrounding cortex and cause spontaneous fractures and collapse of the vertebral column, but they may also produce so much demineralization of the skeleton that hypercalcaemia and renal failure may follow. Pain is an early and often severe symptom.

The monoclonal tumour cells form large amounts of a homogeneous immunoglobulin called *myeloma protein*. Some tumours produce an excess of its component light chain, which has a molecular weight of about 22 000 daltons. (*Bence–Jones protein*), and is small enough to escape from the glomeruli and pass into the renal tubules where it precipitates and may obstruct them; combined with the effects of nephro-calcinosis, pyelonephritis and amyloidosis this renal damage (producing the myeloma kidney) leads to death from renal failure.

Other tumours of bone.

This group includes ameloblastoma, chordoma, and a variety of unclassified tumours. Amelo-blastoma is described in Chapter 21. The *chor-*

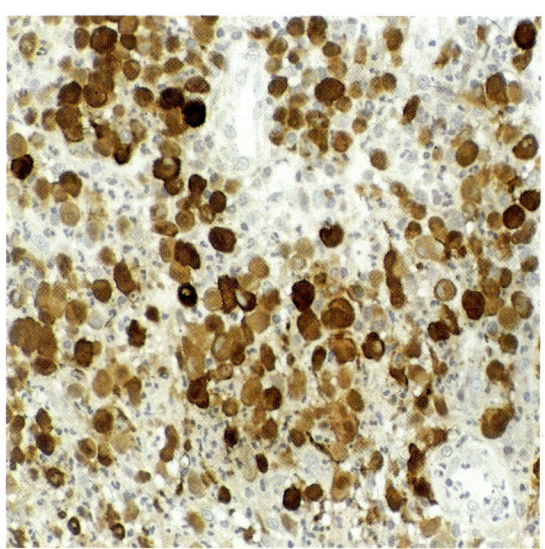

Fig. 34.14   Immunoperoxidase method. This section of skin in histiocytosis X has been stained to show the presence of S 100 protein. The large cells stained brown are malignant Langerhans' cells. (The same figure appears in colour on p. 4.)

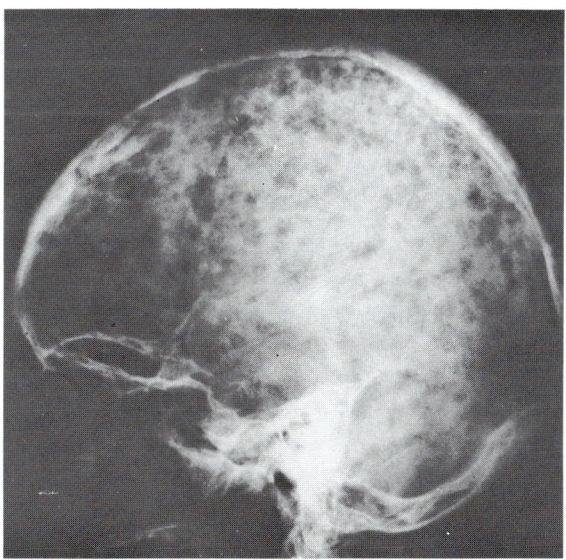

Fig. 34.13   Multiple myeloma. This radiograph of the skull shows numerous osteolytic tumour deposits that produce a typical moth-eaten appearance resulting from the punched-out areas where bone has been destroyed. An appearance similar to this can be produced by secondary carcinoma. (Photograph by courtesy of Dr D E Sanders, Toronto General Hospital, Toronto.)

doma is derived from notocordal remnants, either in the sacrococcygeal region or in the base of the skull. It forms a gelatinous mass and is of low malignancy. Nevertheless, because of its location, removal is often impossible.

Histiocytosis X. This disease is considered here because it commonly involves bone, although it is not primarily a tumour of bone. Its cell of origin is believed to be the Langerhans' cell of the skin, a cell of bone-marrow origin and a member of the MPS. They are S100 positive (Fig. 34.14). The alternative name of Langerhans'-cell histiocytosis has been proposed. The disease covers a spectrum of conditions but traditionally they have been divided into three categories.

Letterer–Siwe disease. This is the most severe form of the disease and generally affects children under the age of 3 years. It can occasionally affect adults, particularly elderly men. There is widespread infiltration of the skin, spleen, liver, bone marrow and other sites by large histiocytic type cells that contain the characteristic Birbeck granules or Langerhans' bodies. The cells show atypical mitotic activity and invade tissues, and the picture is that of a malignant disease. This is in keeping with the rapid, fatal course of the disease.

Multifocal eosinophilic granuloma. The lesions are widespread, involving skin, lungs, bones, spleen and other organs. In distribution it resembles Letterer–Siwe disease, but the course is more protracted and lesions often resolve under treatment. Some cases, labelled Hand-Schüller-Christian disease, exhibit the triad of involvement of the bones of the skull, diabetes insipidus, and exophthalmos.

Solitary eosinophilic granuloma. This variant usually affects a bone (calvarium, ribs and femur) but the lungs are also a common site. The lesion is made up of histiocytes, lymphocytes, lipid-containing macrophages and eosinophils. The latter are often present in striking numbers, as the name implies. Local treatment effects a cure and the picture is that of a benign lesion.

Metastatic tumours

Secondary tumours of bone are much more common than the primary ones. They develop from blood-borne metastases of carcinoma commonly of the prostate, breast, bronchus, kidney, stomach, or thyroid. They are characteristically osteolytic, with the exception of carcinoma of the prostate which is osteoplastic. Pathological fractures and pain are the usual presenting symptoms.

The jaws are rarely affected, but when secondary deposits do occur it is usually in the mandibular molar area. A deposit in the jaws has been known to give rise to symptoms before the primary growth manifested itself.

DISEASES OF JOINTS

A joint consists of two or more opposing *cartilage-covered bone ends* united by a sleeve of connective tissue called the *capsule*, the innermost layer of which is modified into a secreting membrane called the *synovium*. This consists of one or more layers of flattened or cuboidal cells that secrete a clear, pale, viscid fluid (*synovial fluid*) which contains small quantities of albumin and globulin and also a significant amount of mucin. Not only does the synovial fluid lubricate the joint, but it is also the main, if not the only, source of nourishment of the hyaline cartilage covering the bone ends. The amount of synovial fluid in the joint is very small—there is only about 0.5 ml in the knee joint.

Arthritis

This is an inflammation of a joint. There is usually an increased amount of synovial fluid present due to a concomitant inflammation of the synovial membrane (*synovitis*). Arthritis may be traumatic, as after the twisting or the forcible hyperextension or hyperflexion of a joint. This may lead to a minor tear of the capsule, called a sprain, but if more severe the rupture of the capsule may cause a partial or complete displacement of the bone ends. A partial displacement is called a subluxation, and a complete one a dislocation. Simple sprains heal spontaneously, but the weakness of a ruptured capsule may predispose to a recurrent dislocation.

Another type of arthritis is *infective* in aetiology. This may follow a penetrating joint injury, when the infection is introduced from outside, or it may be blood-borne during the course of a systemic illness. The most important type of haematogenous arthritis is the suppurative arthritis that occasionally occurs in the course of such pyogenic diseases an gonorrhoea, lobar pneumonia, and staphylococcal septicaemia. Sometimes the infection may be of a more chronic type, e.g. tuberculosis and syphilis. Suppurative arthritis, unless energetically treated in the early stages with antibiotics, leads to the rapid destruction of the articular cartilages, and the whole cavity is filled with exudate which organizes and obliterates the space. In this way the joint is destroyed, and the bone ends are united by fibrous tissue. This is called an *ankylosis*, and it may undergo ossification later. A bony ankylosis is characteristic of a burnt-out suppurative process, whereas tuberculous arthritis usually terminates in a fibrous ankylosis.

By far the most important types of chronic arthritis are *rheumatoid arthritis* and *osteoarthritis*.

Rheumatoid arthritis

This common disease occurs most frequently in young adults, especially women. It is characteristically polyarticular (affecting many joints) and symmetrical. The small joints of the hands and feet are usually worst affected, but the knees also suffer badly. It is a systemic disease, and in the active phases there is mild pyrexia, weight loss, and sweating bouts. A moderate anaemia often develops.

The affected joints are swollen, tender, and painful. In the early stages the synovial membrane is acutely inflamed; it proliferates into villous folds in which there is a heavy infiltration of lymphocytes and plasma cells. Later on the lymphocytic infiltration becomes more copious and lymphoid follicles may also develop. There is a steady encroachment of granulation tissue from the articular margin on to the cartilage. This inflammatory tissue forms a *pannus* over the cartilage and destroys it. The joint space is gradually obliterated by fibrous adhesions, and eventually ankylosis occurs. In this late stage there is severe atrophy of the adjacent bones and muscles, and the overlying skin is smooth and shiny. The results of advanced rheumatoid arthritis are tragic to see. Progressive contractures lead to flexion deformities seen especially in the distorted hands with the characteristic ulnar deviation of the fingers, and the flexed, ankylosed larger joints which render the patient immobile (Fig. 34.15). There may be limited movement in the temporomandibular joints, and occasionally ankylosis occurs.

The nature of rheumatoid arthritis is unknown, but the basic lesion seems to be a fibrinoid necrosis of collagen. It is therefore classed among the collagen disease (Ch. 13). The disease is not confined to the joints but affects many other organs and is best regarded as a systemic disease—*rheumatoid disease. Subcutaneous nodules* develop over pressure points. The nodules have a central area of necrotic tissue surrounded by a palisade of histiocytic cells around which are lymphocytes and plasma cells (Fig. 34.16). Involvement of the heart is commonly manifest as pericarditis, and lung involvement leads to pleurisy and a type of fibrosing alveolitis. Regional lymphadenitis may occur and if associated with lymphoid hyperplasia in liver and spleen constitutes Still's disease. Involvement of the eye (keratoconjunctivitis sicca) may occur in rheumatoid arthritis alone or be combined with a dry mouth (xerostomia).

The triad constitutes *Sjögren's syndrome*. If the eye and mouth lesions occur alone the term *Sicca syndrome* is used; it occurs in other diseases with an autoimmune component.

Amyloidosis is an important complication. Indeed, it is the only significant fatal lesion in rheumatoid arthritis, which may otherwise smoulder on for many years and produce complete crippling.

The sera of about 80% of patients with rheumatoid arthritis contains an antibody directed against a site in the third domain of the heavy chain of IgG. Possibly antigen–antibody complex are formed in the joints and neutrophils accumulate following the activation of complement. However, autoantibodies are not present in all patients, and rheumatoid factor can be found in patients without rheumatoid arthritis.

Ankylosing spondylitis.

This condition resembles rheumatoid arthritis and has been regarded as a variant which attacks the spinal column and sacroiliac joints. Nevertheless it is probably a distinct disease and differs from rheumatoid arthritis in several important ways, primarily: (1) young men are usually affected, (2) the vertebral joints and the large peripheral joints are affected, whereas the small distal joints are seldom involved, and (3) there is bony ankylosis of the spinal and peripheral joints, and the spinal ligaments and the margins of the intervertebral discs undergo ossification. In due course the spinal column is converted into a composite bony mass, the so-called bamboo spine. Subcutaneous nodules are not present, nor is the rheumatoid factor. (4) Uveitis and aortitis are recognized associations. There is a strong association between ankylosing spondylitis and histocompatibility type HLA-B27.

Osteoarthritis

Osteoarthritis, despite its name, is not an inflammatory disease of joints but rather a degenerative one; for this reason it is often called degenerative joint disease, or osteoarthrosis. It is one of humanity's commonest afflictions, for it is essentially an accentuation of the normal

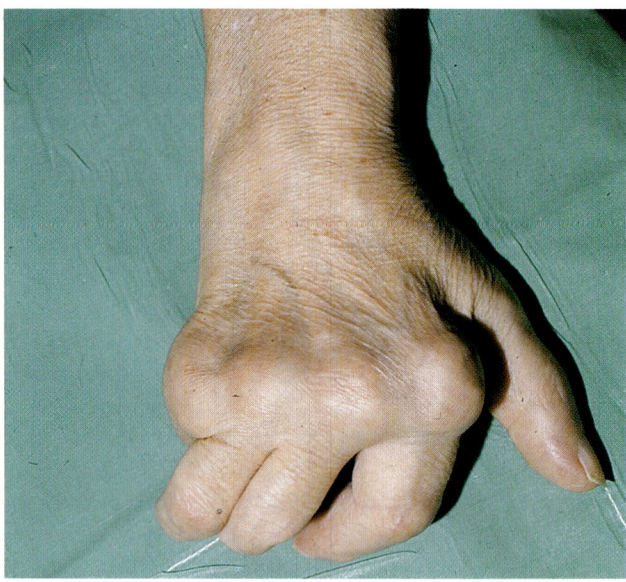

Fig. 34.15 Rheumatoid arthritis. The enlarged joints and ulnar deviation of the fingers are characteristic. Note how the extensor tendons stand out because of the atrophy of the small muscles of the hand.

ageing process of articular cartilage. The nourishment of the hyaline cartilage is normally rather precarious, depending on the synovial fluid. The constant wear and tear on the joints after many years' activity leads to a gradual deterioration of the central parts of the articular cartilage; for this reason obesity predisposes to osteoarthritis of the weight-bearing joints. This process is greatly aggravated by concomitant trauma to a joint, for example that sustained during athletics. Osteoarthritis is a disease of later life, but it can affect a traumatized joint in a younger person. The spine and the large weight-bearing joints, especially the hips, are most severely affected, but the smaller joints do not escape. Osteoarthritis, unlike the rheumatoid variety, is not a systemic disease. The general health is not affected.

The condition commences with a softening and fraying of the articular cartilage. It becomes progressively thinner, and ultimately the underlying bone is exposed. This increases in density, and its surface becomes hard, worn, and polished, a change called *eburnation*. Meanwhile there is a proliferation of cartilage cells at the margin of the articular area. The new cartilage that is formed soon ossifies. The result is that the periphery of the articular cartilage is raised and bossed; this is called *lipping*, and is an important radiological finding. The peripheral new bone may become elongated into irregular *marginal osteophytes*. Not only do these interfere with the range of the joint's movement, but they may also become nipped off to form *loose bodies*

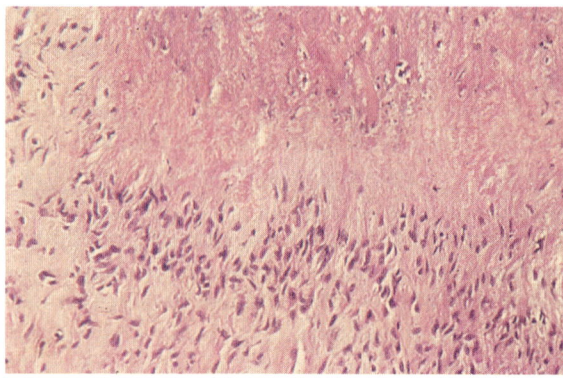

Fig. 34.16 Rheumatoid nodule. The centre of the nodule consists of amorphous, eosinophilic, degenerate collagen; it is bordered by a palisade of histiocytes.

(also called 'joint-mice'). These are a constant nuisance because they tend to be caught between the opposing bone ends during movement; the result is 'locking' of the joint, which may be excruciatingly painful if a fringe of synovium is included. A prominent site for osteophytes is the terminal interphalangeal joint of the fingers of elderly people. These produce the painless bony swellings called *Heberden's nodes*.

There is no primary synovial change, but later the membrane is thrown up into vascular villous folds. There is no inflammatory change except after locking, which produces a traumatic synovitis. These joints do not become ankylosed, but the destruction of articular cartilage and the osteophyte formation seriously limit movement, which may be very painful. Fortunately the operation of arthroplasty is now so successful that many people crippled with osteoarthritic hips have been restored to activity with artificial metallic or silastic joints.

Tumours of the synovium

Synoviosarcoma is an uncommon tumour that characteristically has an epithelial and connective tissue element, thereby somewhat resembling the malignant mesothelioma.

GENERAL READING

Gardner D L 1983 The nature and causes of osteoarthritis. British Medical Journal 286:418
Hamerman D 1989 The biology of osteoarthritis. New England Journal of Medicine 320:1322
Hosking D J 1981 Paget's disease of bone. British Medical Journal 283:686
Krane S M, Simon L S 1986 Rheumatoid arthritis: clinical features and pathogenetic mechanisms. Medical Clinics of North America 70:263

Lichtenstein L 1975 Diseases of Bone and Joint Disease. 2nd ed. Mosby, St Louis
Raisz L G, Kream B E 1983 Regulation of bone formation. New England Journal of Medicine 309:29 & 83
Revell P A 1986 Pathology of bone. Springer-Verlag, Berlin
Teitelbaum S L, Bullough P G 1979 The pathophysiology of bone and joint disease, a teaching monograph. American Journal of Pathology. 96:283

35. Diseases of the central nervous system

COMPONENTS OF THE CENTRAL NERVOUS SYSTEM

The brain and spinal cord are of such complexity that only those features of neuropathology which are relevant to dental surgery will be described in this chapter.

Cellular components

The important component of the central nervous system is the nerve cell, or *neuron*. The highly specialized neurons with their long axonal processes are held in position and insulated from each other by a specialized connective tissue called *neuroglia*. This has three components:

The *astrocytes* are closely associated with the bodies of the nerve cells and the blood vessels.

The *oligodendroglia* enclose the axons and forms their myelin sheaths, an insulating function which is essential for the conduction of nerve impulses.

The *microglia*, as the name implies, is composed of small cells. They are mesodermal, and members of the mononuclear phagocyte system (MPS).

The extreme susceptibility of the neurons to hypoxia has been noted previously (p. 336). Permanent brain damage can easily occur if the brain is rendered ischaemic; this may occur during periods of hypotension in the course of a surgical operation. Inadequate ventilation of the lungs with oxygen is not uncommon during the inexpert administration of nitrous oxide as an anaesthetic, and is another important cause of cerebral hypoxia.

Meninges

The coverings, or *meninges*, of the central nervous system are three:

The *pia mater* closely envelops the brain and spinal cord.

The *dura mater* is closely adherent to the bony-ligamentous protective housing provided by the skull, vertebral column, and the connecting ligaments.

The thin, translucent *arachnoid* covering lies between the pia and the dura.

The space between the arachnoid and the pia is called the *subarachnoid space* and contains *cerebrospinal fluid (CSF)*. This fluid originates in the choroid plexuses, perfuses the ventricles, and finally escapes through the foramina in the roof of the fourth ventricle to reach the subarachnoid space.

EFFECTS OF INCREASED INTRACRANIAL PRESSURE

Although the rigid bony enclosure of the brain is a necessary protective shield, its presence has some attendant disadvantages. Any lesion which takes up space within the skull (*space occupying lesion*) tends to cause a rise in intracranial pressure, and this increases the pressure in the veins. Initially some CSF and venous blood are displaced, but soon, as venous obstruction is produced, there is a marked rise in CSF pressure, which has very serious effects. If of sudden onset, the blood supply to the brain is so reduced that the cerebral hypoxia causes rapid *loss of consciousness*. When the lesion develops gradually, severe *headaches* are common, and there is also progressive *mental impairment*. Pressure around the optic nerve impedes the venous return and leads to oedema of the nerve. The result is swelling of the optic disc (*papilloedema*). Eventually *blindness* follows. *Haematoma*, *abscess* with inflammatory oedema, and *tumour* are examples of space occupying lesions.

Brain herniations

The brain can be forced into abnormal positions if there is an expanding lesion in one area. The results are serious and often fatal. Thus if the lesion is in one cerebral hemisphere it can force part of that hemisphere to pass under the falx cerebri to the other hemisphere. If there is expansion of the hemispheres, part of the brain (the uncus) is forced through the gap in the tentorium cerebri and surrounds the brain stem. This is called *uncal herniation,* and the resulting pressure on the midbrain causes unconsciousness while pressure on the third cranial nerve leads to changes in the pupil; ultimately it becomes fixed and dilated. For this reason the pupils are carefully observed in patients with intracranial lesions such as bleeding following head injury. Increased pressure can also be transmitted to the cerebellum so that the cerebellar tonsils are forced out of the cranial cavity into the spinal canal. This tonsillar herniation is commonly termed 'coning' and is an extremely serious condition because the cone of cerebellar tissue presses on the medullary centres causing death from respiratory or circulatory failure.

TRAUMATIC LESIONS OF THE CENTRAL NERVOUS SYSTEM

An injury involving the jaws is sometimes accompanied by a much more important injury to the brain. Blows on the head produce damage to the region underlying the injury and to the brain at the opposite pole—this is the *contre-coup injury*. Minor injuries cause petechial haemorrhages and traumatic inflammatory oedema, while more severe ones may actually tear the brain (*laceration*), and haemorrhage may be of sufficient magnitude to cause death. Some degree of haemorrhage into the subarachnoid space is common in all head injuries, and can be detected by examining the cerebrospinal fluid obtained by lumbar puncture.

Subdural haemorrhage. It sometimes happens that a bridging vein is torn, and blood escapes into the loose subdural space to produce a subdural haematoma. If small, this is of little importance. If large, it organizes at the periphery and its centre remains fluid. The cyst which is formed imbibes fluid, and enlarges to form a *chronic subdural haematoma* which acts as a space occupying lesion. The injury which causes this type of lesion is often relatively mild, and in an elderly or alcoholic patient may be completely overlooked. Headaches and other signs and symptoms of raised intracranial pressure develop several weeks later.

Extradural haemorrhage. This occurs when the *middle meningeal artery* is torn, usually in association with a fracture of the skull involving the temporal region. Unconsciousness may occur immediately after the injury, but the patient often recovers and feels well for a few hours. This *lucid interval* is deceptive, for presently, as the bleeding proceeds, increasing signs of raised intracranial pressure appear, and are followed by coma and death. It is evident that *all cases of head injury, except the most trivial, should be observed carefully for 24 hours*. This word of caution applies particularly to persons suspected of being drunk —a state which may be mimicked by the combination of medicinal brandy given by a wellwisher and an extradural haemorrhage.

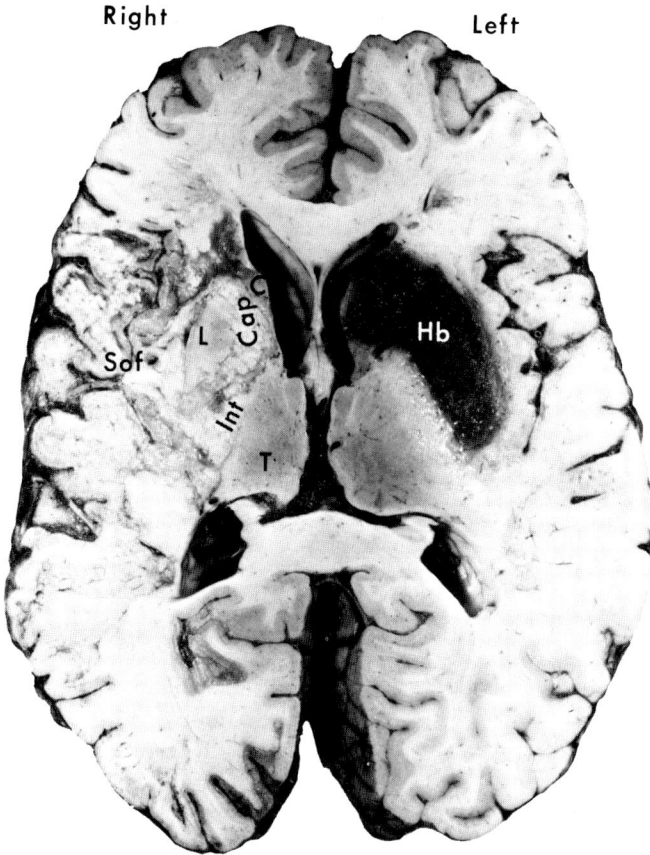

Right   **Left**

Fig. 35.1 Cerebral softening and haemorrhage. The brain has been sectioned horizontally, and is viewed here from below. There is severe damage. On the right-hand side there is extensive softening (Soft). Note the shrunken appearance of the affected area, which extends outwards to involve the grey matter of the cerebral cortex. The internal capsule (Int Cap) is severely affected. It lies between the lentiform nucleus and thalamus (T) posteriorly. Loss of the corticospinal fibres leads to an upper motor neuron lesion of the opposite side of the body. The patient had had a stroke three months before death. The attack, which had been attributed to a cerebral thrombosis, left the patient with left-sided hemiplegia. She subsequently had another stroke involving the opposite side. Note the extensive haemorrhage (Hb) that has occurred into the area of softening on the left side. (Photography by courtesy of Dr N B Rewcastle. From Walter J B (1992) An introduction to the principles of disease, 3rd edn., W B Saunders, Philadelphia.)

NON-TRAUMATIC VASCULAR LESIONS

Subarachnoid haemorrhage. This is not uncommon in the 20–50 year age-group. The haemorrhage stems from a ruptured aneurysm of one of the major cerebral arteries in the neighbourhood of the circle of Willis. The aneurysms lie in the subarachnoid space and are from 0.5 to 1.0 cm in diameter—because of this size they are often called *berry aneurysms*. They are thought to arise at the site of congenital defects in the elastic coat of the arteries. Sometimes they are multiple.

Cerebral haemorrhage and infarction. Atherosclerosis and hypertension both predispose to cerebral haemorrhage (sometimes called cerebral apoplexy). The common site is from the lenticulostriate artery, well named the artery of cerebral haemorrhage, and the region of the brain

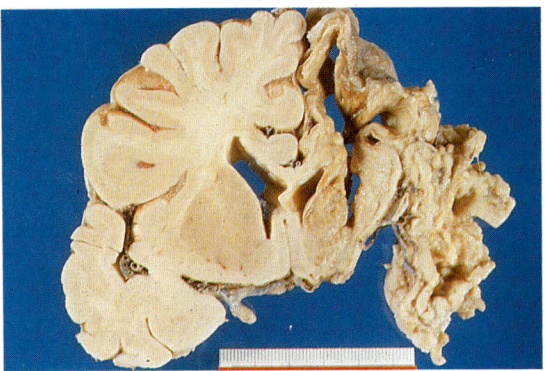

Fig. 35.2 Infarction of brain. This coronal section through the brain shows that much of one hemisphere has been destroyed by an infarct. It has been replaced by a cyst with a glial wall.

affected is therefore the basal ganglia. The immediate effects of haemorrhage tend to be more severe than those produced by thrombosis. In both there is the clinical picture commonly called a 'stroke' (Fig. 35.1).

With *haemorrhage* there is usually sudden loss of consciousness, and as blood disrupts the substance of the brain, coma deepens and death ensues. This is not, however, inevitable, and the bleeding may stop.

Thrombosis often occurs during sleep, and although consciousness may be lost this is not invariable. Thrombosis causes *infarction*, which can itself lead to later haemorrhage in the damaged area.

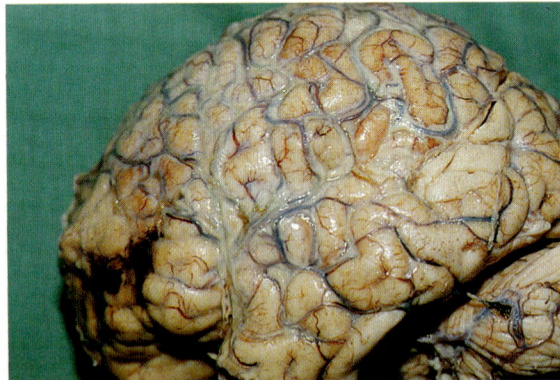

Fig. 35.3 Acute meningitis. The surface of the hemisphere is covered by acute inflammatory exudate which is most obvious in the sulci where it is obscuring the meningeal vessels.

The infarct is usually pale, and in those patients who survive the area softens (colliquative necrosis). The microglial cells enlarge, become phagocytic, and appear as large foamy macrophages. The damaged nerve fibres are not replaced to any extent, and the area heals by proliferation of astrocytes to produce a *glial scar.* The area of brain thus collapses, and sometimes a central cyst remains where once were the long tracts from the motor cortex to the spinal cord. It should be noted that any nerve cells destroyed are not replaced (Fig. 35.2).

Cerebral embolism is another common cause of a stroke. The embolus generally originates from the heart, and the onset of the stroke is sudden.

In cerebral infarction the neurological picture is commonly that of *hemiplegia*—loss of voluntary movement on the side of the body opposite to that of the lesion.

In addition to acute episodes of thrombosis or embolism, cerebral athersclerosis can lead to multiple, bilateral, ischaemic lesions in the brain. The characteristic mental deterioration of old age is one effect, but if the lesions are extensive there may be severe bilateral damage to the corticospinal tracts. Pseudobulbar palsy results if bilaterrally innervated muscles such as those of the tongue and pharynx are affected.

INFECTIONS OF THE CENTRAL NERVOUS SYSTEM

Baterial infections

Pyogenic bacteria may produce a diffuse infection of the subarachnoid space, which is called *meningitis*, or a localized suppuration in the brain substance (*cerebral abscess*).

Meningitis

Mode of infection. Two routes of infection are common:

Blood-borne. S. *pneumoniae*, H. *influenzae* and N. *meningitidis* (meningococcus) gain entry to the blood, presumably from an infection in the upper respiratory tract. The meninges are probably infected via the chroroid plexuses, where the organisms are filtered out of the blood. The infection spreads through the ventricular system and reaches the subarachnoid space in the region of the basal cisterns. It is here that the most severe effects are encountered. The pia and arachnoid are acutely inflamed, and there is a massive polymorph and fibrinous exudate into the subarachnoid space (Fig. 35.3). With modern chemotherapy the patients often survive, but even then the exudate may undergo organization, and the foramina in the roof of the fourth ventricle become blocked. Cerebrospinal fluid accumulates in the ventricular system which expands accordingly—this is one mechanism whereby *hydrocephalus* develops. In the young child the pressure exerted on the developing bones leads to a tremendous enlargement of the vault of the skull.

Tuberculous meningitis is mentioned on p.166.

Local spread. Meningitis may follow the spread of infection from the middle ear or mastoid air cells—sites of infection that were once quite common in childhood. It is also a complication of a fractured skull when the wound is exposed to the exterior or the nasal cavity. Fracture of the cribriform plate of the ethmoid is followed by an escape of cerebrospinal fluid into the nose (*cerebrospinal rhinorrhoea*). Meningitis may follow.

Cerebral abscess

As with meningitis there are two modes of infection:

Blood-borne. Patients with chronic chest infections (empyema, lung abscess, and bronchiectasis) sometimes develop a cerebral abscess. The infection is presumably blood-borne; an alternative explanation is that spread occurs from an infected nasal air sinus—a common accompaniment of chronic chest suppuration.

Local spread. As with meningitis this occurs from an infected middle ear or nasal air sinus.

Viral infections

A large number of virus types cause infection of the central nervous system, e.g. the viruses of mumps, rabies, and the various forms of arbovirus encephalitis. Poliomyelitis is described on p. 190.

Other infections

Fungal infections are now a common complication in patients who are immunologically suppressed, particularly AIDS. Candidiasis is the most common, followed by aspergillosis, mucormycosis, histoplasmosis and cryptococcosis.

Amoebic meningoencephalitis is also encountered in the immunosuppressed, as is toxoplasmosis.

DEMYELINATING DISEASES

The myelin sheath of nerve fibres degenerates following the degeneration of the enclosed axon, for example as when the nerve cell dies. In addition there are a number of diseases in which the sheath undergoes degeneration due to some immune mechanism or the effects of a toxin. The most important disease in this group is multiple sclerosis.

Multiple sclerosis

This disease generally starts in patients between the ages of 20 and 40 years. The lesions consist of foci of demyelination in the white matter of the brain or spinal cord; the axons tend to be preserved so that some recovery of function can occur. The disease pursues a fluctuating course, with repeated attacks during which some part of the brain or spinal cord is affected; the effects depend on the exact location of the lesions. Sudden impairment of vision or speech, paralysis due to pyramidal tract damage, and ataxia associated with impaired cerebellar function are common. Remissions occur and there is some degree of recovery, but with each episode further damage is inflicted so that ultimately the effects are permanent, widespread and severe. Paralysis due to pyramidal tract damage, cerebellar ataxia, emotional lability and bladder dysfunction are common.

The cause of multiple sclerosis is not known, and both hereditary and environmental factors have been incriminated.

Other demyelinating diseases

Acute post-infectious encephalomyelitis is an

uncommon acute disease following a virus infection or vaccination against rabies. It is characterized by demyelination and is probably due to an autoimmune reaction triggered by the antigenic stimulus of the infection or the vaccine.

TOXIC, DEFICIENCY AND METABOLIC DISORDERS OF THE BRAIN

Many exogenous toxic substances adversely affect the central nervous system. *Alcohol* is a familiar example and the effects on the brain differ widely. Sometimes the effects are functional, e.g. tremor, hallucinations and seizures. Cerebral atrophy and particularly cerebellar atrophy are common neurological abnormalities and are a feature of the fetal alcohol syndrome. Other exogenous poisons are arsenic, lead, mercury and carbon monoxide.

Thiamine deficiency is responsible for a variety of effects that include confusion, loss of memory, ataxia and paralysis of external eye muscles. Vitamin-B12 deficiency leads to degeneration of the posterior and lateral columns of the spinal cord.

Metabolic disorders include a great array of conditions. There are numerous inborn errors of metabolism in which the nervous system is involved and their diagnosis is the task of the specialist. Tay–Sachs disease may be cited as one of the most common. Of the acquired conditions, *hepatic encephalopathy* is the best defined. Patients exhibit a decrease in the level of consciousness and a characteristic flapping tremor of the extremities called asterixis. Astrocytes undergo a characteristic change with loss of cytoplasm and enlargement of the nuclei. The effects of *hypoxia* may be included under the heading of metabolic disorders. The brain has a high metabolic rate and is so sensitive to lack of oxygen that permanent damage can be inflicted by a short period of hypoxia.

DEGENERATIVE NEUROLOGICAL DISEASE

Degeneration of neurones is the salient feature of a number of neurological diseases, mostly of unknown cause, that for convenience are grouped under this heading. Alzheimer's disease is the most important.

Alzheimer's disease. This is a disease of middle-aged and older people and is characterized by steady loss of the higher mental functions. Loss of short-term memory, confusion and disorientation are the chief early symptoms. Patients often wander off and become lost. This provides a great problem for those who must tend them, particularly because the disease has no treatment and invariably progresses to dementia and death. Characteristically there is loss of neurones and the formation of neuritic plaques that contain amyloid.

Multi-infarct dementia. Numerous small infarcts can cause a type of dementia. The disease is diagnosed less frequently now, and in the past cases of Alzheimer's disease were almost certainly included.

Huntington's disease. This disease is inherited as a Mendelian dominant trait and symptoms generally commence before the age of 30 years. Bizarre involuntary movements and progressive dementia are the clinical manifestations of nerve-cell loss that affects the basal ganglia and the cerebral cortex.

Parkinson's disease. This common disease commences in middle life and is characterized by increased skeletal muscle-tone combined with a fine tremor affecting particularly the hands. The face has a characteristic immobile mask-like appearance; dementia develops in about one-quarter of patients. Pathologically there is degeneration of the pigmented cells in the brainstem.

Motor neurone disease. In this disease there is degeneration of the upper motor neurones in the cerebral cortex and the lower motor neurones of the brain stem and spinal cord.

EPILEPSY

The term epilepsy comes from the Greek and means a seizure. It should be regarded as a syndrome rather than a disease entity because epilepsy is a symptom of an underlying brain disorder. It occurs in about 1% of the population, and only about 5% of the sufferers are mentally subnormal.

Epilepsy consists of a sudden, uncoordinated burst of impulses from a group of nerve cells. The seizure that results may be limited to a particular part of the brain and this constitutes *partial*, or *focal*, *epilepsy*. On the other hand, the seizure may cause loss of consciousness and may be accompanied by widespread brain dysfunction. This is *generalized epilepsy*.

Focal epilepsy

There are many areas of the brain in which epileptic discharges may originate and there are therefore many clinical variations of local seizures. If the temporal lobe is affected, the patient experiences hallucinations which may be of smell, taste, hearing, or sight. Sometimes there is a feeling of great familiarity of the surroundings—this constitutes the 'déjà vu phenomenon'. In *Jacksonian epilepsy* the motor areas of the brain are affected, and the patient experiences muscular twitching confined to a particular area (e.g. a hand), and the twitching slowly extends to involve the whole limb or even the whole body. Sometimes after recovery from a Jacksonian fit the affected part remains paralysed—this is called Todd's paralysis. In any type of partial epilepsy the focal discharging area may steadily extend its effect so that the initial local disturbances progress to involve a wide area and the condition then becomes an example of generalized epilepsy.

Generalized epilepsy

In generalized seizures there is loss of consciousness; two major types are described.

Grand mal seizures. There may be a *prodomal phase* lasting several hours or even days when the patient becomes aware that an attack is imminent. Often a change of mood is the forerunner of the attack itself. Grand mal seizures may commence with some sensory manifestation (a strange taste or feeling, or seeing flashes of light) or some motor activity (movement of one part of the body) which is described as the *aura*. This precedes loss of consciousness by a few seconds. Then follows the generalized convulsion. At first the muscles exhibit *tonic contraction*, and as the chest muscles contract the patient may emit a characteristic cry as air is forced past the glottis. The tonic phase is followed by a *clonic phase*, in

which the muscles exhibit powerful jerking movements. Movement of the jaw and tongue causes saliva to froth at the mouth, and at this stage, which lasts about half a minute, the tongue may be bitten and the patient may sustain damage. The final phase is one of relaxation, and the patient passes from a comatose state into normal sleep. During the tonic and clonic phases the patient is often incontinent of urine and less frequently of faeces also.

Petit mal seizures. In petit mal seizures, sometimes described by the patient as 'dizzy spells' or 'fainting turns', there is a transient loss of consciousness. The patient develops a staring expression and there may be an upward rolling of the eyes. If a child is doing something, he will discontinue the activity for a few seconds, and then when the seizure is ended resume the action as though nothing had happened. The condition is most common in children, and attacks may cease at puberty.

Causes of seizures

Seizures can be induced in anyone provided a powerful enough stimulus (e.g. an electric current) is applied. There is indeed a *threshold level* for each individual, and any stimulus above this will result in an epileptic fit. In subjects with a 'normal' threshold there are many conditions (e.g. hypoglycaemia) which will induce seizures. Sometimes a local brain lesion will lower the threshold, and this results in epilepsy. When such lesions can be recognized the disease is labelled symptomatic epilepsy. When no cause can be identified resort must be made to the term idiopathic epilepsy.

Symptomatic epilepsy. Amongst the numerous organic causes of epilepsy the following should be noted:

Cerebral tumours. This is the commonest type of symptomatic epilepsy, and in 10 per cent of the cases a seizure is the initial sign of the tumour. Glioma or metastatic carcinoma should always be considered as a likely cause of seizures commencing in patients over the age of 40 years.

Cerebral trauma. Trauma may cause seizures immediately or after a period of time, in which event it is presumed that scarring of the brain is the cause.

Cerebrovascular disease. Seizures may occur in cerebral haemorrhage and infarction.

Cerebral infections. Brain abscess and encephalitis may precipitate a seizure.

Metabolic diseases. Hypoglycaemia (insulin overdose), hypocalcaemia (tetany), uraemia, and hypoxia provide examples.

Sunstroke. See p. 283.

Drug intoxication. Certain drugs such as strychnine cause convulsions, but seizures may also follow the withdrawal of a drug (e.g. alcohol or barbiturates) in addicts.

Miscellaneous brain diseases. There are many diseases associated with seizures, for example, tuberous sclerosis and cerebral palsy.*

Convulsions are more common in infants due presumably to the fact that the nervous system is immature and more unstable. Many children have convulsions during the eruption of teeth, or with a sudden onset of fever. Hence, convulsions are encountered with pneumonia, otitis media, and in the common viral infections. Such convulsions may be an isolated incident due presumably to some metabolic defect, or they may be the forerunner of more persistent seizures in later life. Seizures may occur following general anaesthesia, and patients prone to epilepsy require supervision for several hours postoperatively. Seizures may occur in the dental chair, and it is important to protect the patient from injury on equipment or biting the tongue.

Idiopathic epilepsy. When no morphological or biochemical cause of the seizures can be found the disease must be labelled idiopathic. Often when seizures begin in childhood no cause can be found, and it is possible that there is some specific genetic defect in cerebral metabolism. Patients with epilepsy may have their seizures precipitated by a variety of circumstances. Thus hyperventilation can cause a fit, as also may a flickering light or emotional disturbance. If such triggers can be recognized, then both idiopathic and symptomatic seizures may be averted.

In the treatment of epilepsy a variety of drugs are in use. One of the commonest is phenytoin (dilantin), and an important complication of the administration of this drug is gingival hyperplasia. Indeed this occurs in about 50% of patients taking this medication. Good oral hygiene reduces the effect; if marked hyperplasia occurs, the advisability of using some other drug should be raised with the attending physician. Gingivectomy may be necessary if the hyperplasia is severe.

TUMOURS OF THE CENTRAL NERVOUS SYSTEM

Primary tumours

The majority of primary tumours of the brain originate in the glial cells and are called *gliomata*. The tumours are locally invasive and the most malignant ones may also metastasize via the cerebrospinal fluid to other parts of the brain. Metastasis outside the central nervous system is rare but is occasionally encountered following surgery, particularly if a shunt is created between the ventricles and the peritoneum. The commonest glioma is the *astrocytoma*, which may be well-differentiated and grow slowly or be poorly differentiated and have a poor prognosis; the latter type is also called a *glioblastoma multiforme*. Less common are tumours derived from oligo-dendroglia and ependyma.

In children the commonest tumour is the *medulloblastoma*, a tumour thought to arise from primitive neuroectodermal cells. It occurs in the posterior cranial fossa and although fast-growing and highly malignant, is very sensitive to radiation so that, with combined radiation and surgery, a 50% cure rate may be obtained.

The *meningioma* is a tumour derived from cells of the arachnoid mater. It is about as common as the gliomata, and usually affects middle-aged

---

Cerebral palsy is a popular term for a condition in which there is a major disturbance of motor function that is generally non-progressive and has been present since infancy. Upper-motor-neuron damage with spasticity is the dominant feature. Cerebral palsy is not a distinct entity, but is the end result of many processes—inherited defect, infection, birth trauma, etc. The term has been adopted by fund-raising societies (e.g. the Spastic Society), and is unlikely to disappear readily from medical terminology.

adults. The majority of meningiomata are benign but can produce atrophy of adjacent brain tissue by pressure. Simple removal effects a cure but sometimes this is impossible because of the tumour's position, e.g. adjacent to the medulla. Occasionally the tumour is locally malignant and invades the adjacent skull.

Secondary tumours

These are as common as primary growths. Carcinoma of the lung in males and carcinoma of the breast in females are the common primary tumours in these cases.

GENERAL READING

Adams J H, Corsellis J A N, Duchen L W (eds) 1984 Greenfield's Neuropathology, 4th edn. Edward Arnold, London

Leech R W, Shuman R M 1982 Neuropathology: a summary for students. Harper & Row, Hagerstown
Okazaki H 1983 Fundamentals of neuropathology. Igaku-Shoin, Tokyo

36. Diseases of the endocrine glands

While the nervous system exerts major control of the activity of higher animals, there is an additional mechanism whereby one group of cells can influence another. This is by their secretion into the blood stream of potent chemicals (hormones), which, being carried by the circulation, can exert influence on some distant part. Secreting cells which perform this endocrine function are being recognized in increasing numbers, for not only are they situated in the well-known endocrine glands, but are also found scattered in other tissues. For instance, when food enters the pylorus, the hormone called *gastrin* is secreted, and this stimulates the fundus of the stomach to produce hydrochloric acid. When acid enters the duodenum, *secretin* is formed, and this causes the pancreas to pour out its alkaline juice. Some cells produce substances that act locally on adjacent cells. This is called paracrine secretion.

This chapter deals only with the common disorders of the major endocrine glands and the more recently recognized diffuse endocrine system.

MODE OF ACTION OF HORMONES

Hormones have an extremely potent and highly specific action on their target cells. This selective action is due to the binding of the hormone to specific cell receptors. The water-soluble hormones, such as adrenaline and glucagon, act on receptors situated in the cell membrane; cyclic AMP is formed, acting as a second messenger to stimulate or depress a characteristic biochemical activity (see Fig. 2.2, p. 9). The lipid-soluble steroid hormones act on receptors in the cytoplasm, and the hormone-receptor complex, after modification, enters the nucleus and then acts by influencing the expression of the cell's genetic material.

THE HYPOTHALAMUS

The hypothalamus consists of a complex collection of nerve cells and fibre tracts that help regulate, many functions of the body (Fig.36.1). It controls the circadian rhythms such as the rhythmic daily variations of many bodily functions, e.g. temperature regulation and hormone secretion; a specific cycling centre is responsible for regulating the menstrual cycle.

In addition the hypothalamus contains cells that have an endocrine function. Two groups of hormones are recognized:

1. *Oxytocin* and *antidiuretic hormone (ADH)*, also called *vasopressin*. These are considered in the section on the neurohypophysis (p. 433).
2. *Releasing and inhibiting hormones or factors.* These hormones are secreted into capillaries

that form portal vessels, reach the adenohypophysis and either stimulate or inhibit it.

HYPOTHALAMUS

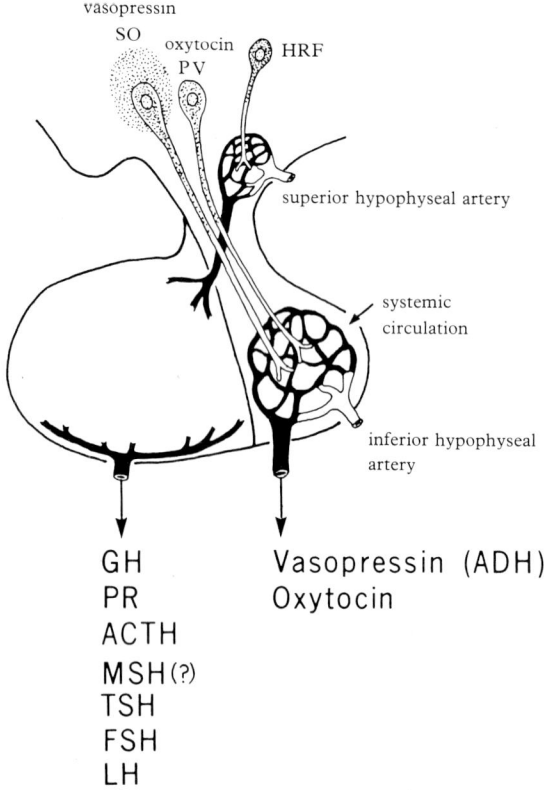

GH
PR
ACTH
MSH(?)
TSH
FSH
LH

Vasopressin (ADH)
Oxytocin

Fig. 36.1. The relationship between the hypothalmus and the pituitary gland. Vasopressin (antidiuretic hormone, or ADH) and oxytocin are manufactured in nerve cells in the supraoptic (SO) and paraventricular (PV) nuclei of the hypothalamus. These hormones are not released into the circulation until they have reached the neurohypophysis. The shaded area surrounding the SO cell body represents the 'osmoreceptor' that is responsive to changes in osmolality of the fluid perfusing it. HRF represents an ill-defined group of cells that secrete a series of releasing factors into the primary capillary network of a portal vein. This vein passes in the pituitary stalk to the adenohypophysis, where cells manufacture the 7 hormones of this lobe of the pituitary: growth hormone (GH); prolactin (PR); adrenocorticotrophic hormone (ACTH); melanocyte-stimulating hormone (MSH), which is present in some species; thyroid-stimulating hormone (TSH); follicle-stimulating hormone (FSH); and luteinizing hormone (LH). (Drawn by Margot Mackay, University of Toronto. After a drawing by Blackstock E. In: Ezrin C, Godden J O, Volpe R, Wilson R (eds) 1973 *Systematic endocrinology.* Harper & Row, New York.)

Releasing hormones

Growth hormone-releasing hormone (GHRH).
Corticotropin-releasing hormone (CRH).
Thyrotropin-releasing hormone (TRH). This also acts as a prolactin-releasing factor.
Gonadotrophin-releasing hormone (GnRH). This causes the release of both follicle-stimulating hormone and luteinizing hormone.
Prolactin-releasing factor. This is distinct from TRH.

These hormones or factors act on their target cells in the adenohypophysis and cause secretion of the appropriate hormone. Thus, CRH stimulates the pituitary corticotropes to secrete ACTH. This in turn stimulates the cells of the adrenal cortex to secrete cortisol. Each cell type is regulated by a negative feedback mechanism; for instance a rise in ACTH blood level inhibits CRH secretion, while a rise in cortisol level inhibits both ACTH and CRH secretion.

Inhibiting factors. The hypothalamus also secretes inhibiting factors that inhibit the release of thyroid-stimulating hormone (TSH), prolactin, growth hormone (GH) and others. The inhibitor of growth hormone is called *somatotropin release-inhibiting factor* or *somatostatin*. In addition to inhibiting the release of GH it also inhibits the release of other hormones, e.g. thyrotropin (from the adenohypophysis) and insulin (from the pancreas). *Prolactin-inhibiting factor* is the main regulator of prolactin secretion.

DISEASES OF THE HYPOTHALAMUS

The hypothalamus is a complex part of the brain and can be affected by events in other parts of the brain. Psychological and physical stress can lead to altered function; for example psychological events and severe physical exertion, as in athletics, can cause amenorrhoea in young women. In the *maternal deprivation syndrome*, emotional stress can delay a child's growth.

Many pathological processes can cause hypothalamic dysfunction. These include infections such as meningitis, encephalitis and tuberculosis; sarcoidosis, histiocytosis X, head injury, hamartoma, and tumours both primary and secondary. The effects can be complex and differ widely; they include *obesity*, due to overeating, *somnolence* or *restless overactivity*, and *failure to maintain body temperature*. These are attributable to direct damage to the hypothalamus. *Visual disturbances* are caused by pressure effects on the optic chiasma. Other syndromes associated with hypothalamic disease are related to hormonal effects:

Diabetes insipidus. This results from lack of vasopressin.

Hypothalamic hypogonadism. This results from lack of GnRH. When the delayed puberty is combined with obesity the term *Fröhlich's syndrome* is applied.

Dwarfism. This results from lack of GHRH.

Hyperprolactinaemia. This causes amenorrhoea, galactorrhoea and decreased libido. It results from impaired production of prolactin-inhibiting factor. Syndromes associated with hypersecretion of other pituitary hormones (causing precocious puberty, acromegaly or hypercortisolism) are rare.

Hypothyroidism and *hypocorticoidism* are rare.

THE PITUITARY GLAND (HYPOPHYSIS)

The pituitary gland or hypophysis is situated in the sella tursica and is flanked by the optic chiasma. It consists of two parts—the neurohypophysis that develops from a diverticulum of the developing brain, and the adenohypophysis that develops from a diverticulum of the foregut.

THE NEUROHYPOPHYSIS

The neurohypophysis consists of the posterior lobe of the pituitary gland, the pituitary stalk and part of the adjacent hypothalamus. It releases two peptide hormones—vasopressin or ADH, and oxytocin. These are synthesized in neurones of the hypothalamus and stored in the neurohypophysis until their release is stimulated. *Oxytocin* causes contraction of the uterine muscle during labour. It also plays a minor role in breast-feeding when the act of suckling stimulates its release and causes ejection of milk from the nipple. Antidiuretic hormone acts on the distal tubule of the kidney and causes water to be retained. Its release is determined by hypothalamic osmo-

receptors and other receptors in the left atrium and the great vessels that respond to volume depletion. If the secretion of ADH is reduced or absent large quantities of very dilute urine are passed (*polyuria*), and in turn thirst leads to a large intake of water (*polydypsia*). The condition is called *diabetes insipidus*. It may occur as an idiopathic condition or result from any local destructive disease.

THE ADENOHYPOPHYSIS

In spite of its small size the anterior lobe of the pituitary is remarkably complex. Electron microscopy and immunochemistry have delineated five types of cells;

Somatotropes. These cells are the most numerous and secrete bursts of GH during the day. This hormone stimulates the formation of *somatomedins* in the liver and probably elsewhere. They are a family of insulin-like growth factors that stimulate the growth of many tissues especially bone and cartilage. They antagonize the actions of insulin and inhibit lypolysis.

Lactotropes (prolactin cells). These cells secrete prolactin (PL) which is important in initiating and maintaining lactation.

Corticotropes. These cells release ACTH (corticotropin) that stimulates the adrenal cortex and also has a melanocyte stimulating action similar to *melanocyte stimulating hormone (MSH)*. The cells also form *β-lipotropin* a large molecule that can be split to form *MSH* and *endorphins*. MSH is of importance in amphibians, but little is formed in humans. Endorphins have a morphine-like action and resemble the encephalins that are neurotransmitters in the central nervous system.

Thyrotropes. These cells secrete thyrotropin (TSH).

Gonadotropes. This type of cell secretes follicle-stimulating hormone (FSH) and luteinizing hormone (LH) that play a vital role in the functions of the ovary and testis.

Disorders of the adenohypophysis

The effects of diseases of the pituitary may be considered under three headings: local pressure effects, hyperpituitarism and hypopituitarism.

Local pressure effects. Enlargement of the pituitary, generally by tumour, causes three important pressure effects. Pressure on the optic chiasma causes loss of the temporal fields of vision (*bitemporal hemianopia*). Pressure on adjacent bone causes *enlargement of the sella tursica*. Pressure on other components of the pituitary gland leads to diminished hormone secretion (*hypopituitarism*).

Hyperpituitarism. Excess formation of pituitary hormones is generally due to a tumour, commonly an adenoma. Three syndromes are common:

Excessive prolactin. This causes amenorrhoea, infertility and inappropriate secretion of milk (galactorrhoea) in females. In males the symptoms are less obvious—impotence and sometimes galactorrhoea.

Excessive growth hormone. Gigantism results if the condition arises during childhood. In addition to excessive skeletal growth there is also an increase in the size of the viscera. If hypersecretion of GH occurs after closure of the epiphyses, the distal or acral parts of the body are affected, and acromegaly results. The typical acromegalic appearance is one of overgrowth of the mandible (*prognathism*), prominence of the supraorbital ridges and malar bones, and enlarged hands and feet. The prognathism is the result of stimulation of the condylar growth centre of the mandible; this normally ceases activity in the teens but persists throughout life, and can be reactivated. Diabetes mellitus is present in 10–15% of cases.

Excessive ACTH. The effect is *Cushing's disease* due to excess secretion of cortisol (hypercorticism) by the adrenal cortex. Excess MSH is also produced and its effects become striking, causing darkening of the skin, if adrenalectomy is performed in a case of Cushing's disease, because the negative-feedback effect of ACTH is removed and the pituitary gland secretes excessive amounts of ACTH and MSH.

Hypopituitarism. If hypopituitarism occurs in children, the effects are due to lack of growth hormone and gonadotropins. The result is dwarfism and failure of puberty to occur. The pituitary dwarf is quite different from the achondroplastic dwarf, for the head, body and limbs are all well-proportioned though diminutive. General growth processes are slow, and become arrested at an early stage. There is also a delay in the eruption of the teeth. In hypopituitarism with predominant gonadotrophin deficiency there is impaired gonadal maturation. Puberty does not occur and if growth hormone secretion is normal, bone growth continues for a while since sex-hormone secretion is low. These eunachoid patients have long arms, their arm span exceeding their height (normally the two are equal). Gonadotrophin deficiency in adults leads to amenorrhoea* and loss of the secondary sex characteristics in females and testicular atrophy and impotence in males. Another type of hypopituitrism in adults is associated with lack of TSH and hypothyroidism results.

Hypopituitarism associated with extreme wasting is called Simmond's disease and is due to total destruction of the adenohypophysis. Apathy is characteristic and death is usually due to adrenal insufficiency. It must be distinguished from anorexia nervosa, in which the patients are restless and aggressive rather than apathetic (see Chapter 18).

THE THYROID GLAND

The thyroid gland has the unique property of being able to trap iodine from the blood and incorporate it as thyroglobulin in the colloid of its vesicles. By the action of a proteolytic enzyme, the iodine-containing thyroid hormones thyroxine and triiodothyronine are released. This occurs when the gland is stimulated by TSH from the anterior pituitary. TSH secretion is itself stimulated by a low blood level of thyroid hormone.

The inconspicuous C-cells of the thyroid secrete calcitonin, but so far no syndrome has been described in relation to an excess or deficiency of this hormone.

Amenorrhoea is the absence of the menses or the menstrual periods. In *primary amenorrhoea* the periods have never commenced, whereas in *secondary amenorrhoea* the menses were at one time normal and have then stopped.

Action of the thyroid hormones

In spite of much research the precise mode of action of the thyroid hormones is not known. However, much has been learned by comparing the normal individual (*euthyroid*) with those who suffer from excessive or diminished secretion (*hyperthyroid* and *hypothyroid)*.

Excessive secretion increases the metabolic rate. The effects are described under hyperthyroidism (see later).

A deficiency causes:

A reduction in metabolic rate.
Impaired mental and physical growth. This is
    most marked in childhood.
Anaemia—this is less constant.

Goitre

Any enlargement of the thyroid is called a goitre, and to a minor extent this occurs at times of stress, e.g. puberty and pregnancy. Indeed, in ancient Egypt the rupture of a thread tied round the neck of a bride was used as an indication of pregnancy. A more potent cause is a diet deficient in iodine, because the thyroid, being unable to manufacture its hormone, cannot check the secretion of TSH which stimulates it to activity. Before iodine was added to table salt, goitres were common in many parts of the world for this reason—in the Great Lakes area of North America, the Andes, the Himalayas, and Derbyshire, England. Repeated phases of hyperplasia followed by involution led to the formation of large nodular goitres containing many colloid-filled areas, some of which showed necrosis and dystrophic calcification (*nodular colloid goitre*).

The goitres associated with hyperthyroidism, Hashimoto's disease, and neoplasia are described later.

Hypothyroidism

Hypothyroidism used to be frequent in areas of endemic goitre, but it may also be due to causes other than iodine lack—for instance, a congenital absence of the thyroid gland or a defect in one of the enzymes involved in thyroxin synthesis. Hypothyroidism is also a feature of some thyroid diseases, e.g. Hashimoto's disease, and follows surgical removal. The effects in the child differ from those in the adult.

Cretinism. An insufficiency of thyroid hormone in the infant leads to cretinism. The child has a bloated face, protruding tongue, and vacant expression, and becomes mentally defective. There is a retardation of growth with delayed ossification and delayed epiphyseal union. There is also delay in dental development.

Myxoedema. This is the manifestation of hypothyroidism in the adult. There is a reduction in mental and physical activity, and the patient exhibits a characteristic bloated appearance due to a curious oedema of the skin. The patients are intolerant of cold, and hypothermia may develop in cold climates. There may be an increase in bone density due to a diminution in excretion of calcium and phosphorus.

Hyperthyroidism

This is also known as *thyrotoxicosis*, and occurs in two forms.

Primary hyperthyroidism (Graves' disease). This disease is characterized by a diffuse enlargement of the thyroid gland (goitre) due to a marked hyperplasia of its epithelial elements (Fig. 36.2). There is a raised metabolic rate which manifests itself by a persistent increase of the heart rate, and the individual is typically jumpy

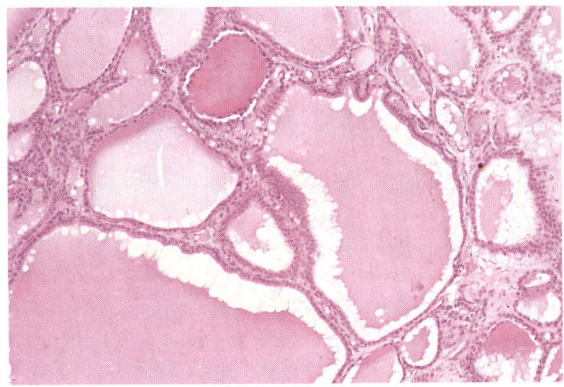

Fig. 36.2 Graves' disease. The acini are lined by tall columnar epithelium; there are vacuoles where colloid abuts the epithelium, and in the large acini these vacuoles have fused to form a wide zone of colloid loss.

and nervous. The hands are warm and sweating; they are seldom at rest, and exhibit a fine tremor when the fingers are stretched out.

Muscular weakness is a common symptom, and can be severe (*thyrotoxic myopathy*). The eyes have a characteristic appearance: the eyelids are retracted, giving the patient a staring expression (Fig. 36.3), while in severe cases the globe is actually pushed forward. If these changes are very severe, the eye muscles can become paralysed and sight can be lost. This is called *malignant exophthalmos*. The skin overlying the tibia may show a focal accumulation of proteoglycans, a condition called *pretibial myxoedema*.

If left untreated, thyrotoxicosis often terminates in heart failure. In long-standing cases osteoporosis may occur. This is due to an increased osteoclastic activity which leads to the excessive excretion of calcium and phosphorus in the urine.

The stimulus to thyroid hyperplasia is an IgG autoantibody, termed *thyroid-stimulating immunoglobulin*, directed against TSH receptor sites on the thyroid cells. Its formation may be related to depressed T-cell function, but the cause for this is not known. A genetic factor is probably involved, and there is an increased incidence of the disease in subjects who have HLA-DR3. Another

antibody, termed long-acting thyroid stimulator (LATS), may be involved in the production of the exophthalmos and pretibial myxoedema.

Secondary hyperthyroidism (toxic nodular goitre or focal primary hyperplasia). This occurs as a secondary phenomenon in a patient who is already suffering from goitre from some other cause, e.g. iodine deficiency. One or more focal nodules of hyperplastic thyroid are present and are evident as 'hot spots' on ^{131}I-scintiscanning. This is in contrast to most tumours which are 'cold'. The disease is less severe than Graves' disease, and exophthalmos does not occur.

Hashimoto's disease

Like most thyroid disease this is more common in women than men. The gland is diffusely enlarged, showing atrophy of its epithelial elements and a massive infiltration with lymphocytes and plasma cells. Hypothyroidism is common, especially in the later stages of the disease. Hashimoto's disease has a strong autoimmune basis; many autoantibodies are present in the blood, including ones reacting with thyroglobulin and various thyroid cell components including microsomes, TSH receptors, and DNA. Antibody-dependent cytotoxicity by T or K cells may be involved in the pathogenesis of the disease. There is also an association with HLA-B5 and HLA-DR5. The pathogenesis has features in common with Graves' disease but instead of stimulating the gland to activity, the antibodies are destructive.

Tumours

Benign encapsulated nodules in the thyroid gland are common, but the majority are probably focal areas of hyperplasia. These are usually multiple (nodular colloid goitre).

Carcinoma was apparently not uncommon in goitrous districts, but is nowadays distinctly rare.

THE ADRENAL GLANDS
THE ADRENAL MEDULLA

The phaeochromocytes of the adrenal medulla are derived from the neural crest. They liberate

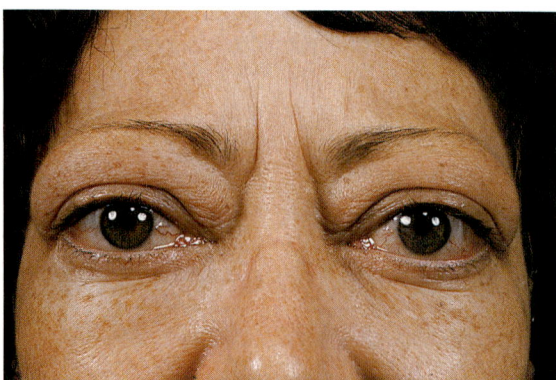

Fig. 36.3 Ocular manifestation of Graves' disease. The patient noted that her eyes had become prominent at the same time as other symptoms of Graves' disease had developed. The eyelids and periorbital tissues are swollen and the conjunctiva is congested and moist as a result of excessive lacrimation. The globe is pushed forward (*proptosis* or *exophthalmos*) by an accumulation of mucoprotein in the orbital tissues. (Photograph courtesy of Dr N Pairaudeau, New York General Hospital, Willowdale, Toronto.)

adrenaline (epinephrine) and noradrenaline (nor-epinephrine) in response to sympathetic stimulation. These hormones cause a redistribution of blood such that the individual is better adapted to fight or flight. The *phaeochromocytoma*, an uncommon tumour derived from phaeochromocytes in the medulla, secretes these agents in excess and causes systemic hypertension which is classically paroxysmal.

The medulla also contains ganglion cells and from their precursor neuroblasts the *neuroblastoma* arises. This is one of the most common malignant tumours of childhood. It is a remarkable tumour in that it occasionally undergoes spontaneous regression, or its cells differentiate into neurones and a benign ganglioneuroma results.

THE ADRENAL CORTEX

Three major groups of hormones (corticosteroids) are secreted:

Glucocorticoids, e.g. cortisol (hydrocortisone). In physiological concentrations cortisol accelerates the synthesis of glucose from non-carbohydrate precursors, and inhibits the actions of insulin.

Mineralocorticoids, e.g. aldosterone. This primarily affects electrolyte metabolism. It causes sodium retention and increases potassium loss in the urine.

Sex hormones. These are predominantly androgens.

Adrenal insufficiency—Addison's disease

Idiopathic atrophy, perhaps by an autoimmune process, or destruction, usually by tuberculosis, is the cause of Addison's disease. A low blood pressure, loss of appetite, loss of weight, weakness, and eventual death are the main features. As would be expected there is hypoglycaemia, a fall in plasma sodium (*hyponatraemia*), and a rise in plasma potassium (*hyperkalaemia*). The skin and mucous membranes, including the oral mucosa, show increased melanin pigmentation. This is because the low plasma cortisol level stimulates the excessive production of pituitary ACTH and MSH. Both these hormones, especially MSH, cause a darkening of the skin by an effect on the melanocytes.

Acute adrenal insufficiency. This is generally encountered when patients who are unable to increase their corticosteroid production are exposed to sudden stress, such as trauma, haemorrhage, or severe infection. This is seen most often in patients with Addison's disease or panhypopituitarism who are on a maintenance dose of glucocorticoids. Acute adrenal insufficiency is characterized by shock, hypotension, collapse, and sometimes fever.

Adrenal hypersecretion

Three patterns of disease occur depending on which adrenal steroid is produced in excess. Mixed cases also occur.

Adrenogenital syndrome. This syndrome is characterized by masculinization. In boys, puberty may occur prematurely, even as early as 4 years ('infantile Hercules'). In girls, male characteristics may develop. In adult women this maculinization is called *virilism*, e.g. atrophy of breasts, cessation of menstruation, enlargement of the clitoris, growth of beard, deepening of the voice, etc.

Conn's syndrome. Excess aldosterone secretion produces systemic hypertension accompanied by low potassium, with sodium and water retention.

Cushing's syndrome. The major features are obesity, hyperglycaemia, osteoporosis, hypertension, and increased body hair growth in women. Rounding and swelling of the face is particularly characteristic (moon faces). Cushing's syndrome is caused by glucocorticoid therapy, adrenal hyperplasia or neoplasia, or ectopic ACTH production, e.g. by carcinoma of the lung. When the adrenal hyperplasia is secondary to an ACTH-secreting tumour of the pituitary the condition is termed *Cushing's disease*.

Glucocorticoid therapy

Replacement glucocorticoid therapy is logical and useful in patients with adrenal insufficiency. However, when used in massive (pharmacological) amounts, the glucocorticoids have two additional actions that can be useful.

Anti-inflammatory action. This action of the glucocorticoids is used to inhibit unwanted inflammatory reactions. Topically they are used on the skin in dermatitis and other skin diseases. Systemically they are useful in many diseases, e.g. interstitial pneumonia, cerebral oedema, etc.

Suppression of the immune response. This action may be used to advantage in treating graft rejection, pemphigus vulgaris, rheumatoid arthritis, lupus erythematosus and bronchial asthma.

Complications of glucocorticoid therapy. Prolonged administration of large doses of glucocorticoids can have serious and sometimes fatal consequences. Important complications are:

Cushing's syndrome.

Opportunistic infections. Overwhelming fungal or viral infections may prove fatal in some patients. A quiescent tuberculous focus can be reactivated and lead to miliary tuberculosis.

Osteoporosis. Severe disabling widespread osteoporosis can be complicated by fractures after trivial injury. Collapse of vertebral bodies is common.

Avascular necrosis of the head of the femur. The cause of this is not known.

Peptic ulcer. Peptic ulcer and its complications, especially bleeding, are common.

Eye changes. Cataracts may form. Topical treatment can precipitate glaucoma.

Diabetes mellitus. See Chapter 17.

Inhibition of wound healing. Wound contraction, granulation tissue formation and collagen synthesis are inhibited.

Mental effects. An acute mental breakdown (psychosis) may be precipitated. Suicide is an important cause of death.

Systemic hypertension. The development of hypertension or the accentuation of existing disease appears to be due to the salt-retaining activity of most glucocorticoids.

Acute adrenal insufficiency. This emergency, characterized by hypotension, shock and sudden death, occurs if steroid therapy is suddenly withdrawn. It may also occur if a patient who is taking a steroid develops a severe infection or is subjected to severe injury such as major surgery and does not have his dose increased. It is vital that all patients on glucocorticoid therapy as well as their medical attendants be aware of this possibility.

THE DIFFUSE ENDOCRINE SYSTEM

The diffuse endocrine system* includes a widely distributed group of cells that are arranged either singly or in small groups. Their special feature is that they secrete regulatory peptides that act either locally (paracrine secretion) or are liberated into the blood stream and act as hormones. They are inconspicuous in routinely stained sections but can be demonstrated by special staining techniques. On electron microscopy the cells are seen to contain characteristic secretory granules which contain the stored peptide. More recently immunohistochemical techniques have been used to detect their hormonal product.

The following groups of cells are included in the diffuse endocrine system:

The chromaffin cell system. These cells are found prodominantly in the adrenal medulla and in relationship to the paravertebral sympathetic plexuses. They contain granules that have an affinity for chromium salts due to their content of catecholamines. Somewhat similar are the cells found in the non-chromaffin paraganglia, notably the carotid body, aortic body, glomus jugulare, and similar structures.

The diffuse gastroenteropancreatic cell system. There are about 30 cell types distributed in the gastrointestinal tract, pancreas (islets of Langerhans), and other areas derived from the primitive endodermal tube—e.g. salivary glands and bronchial mucosa. In some areas the cells are termed argentaffin because they can be demonstrated with silver stains. The cells of this system are responsible for secreting 5-hydroxytryptamine, or polypeptide hormones including gastrin, cholecystokinin, secretin, glucagon, somatostatin, and many others. Insulin is produced by the B cells of the islets of

---

APUD is an acronym for a group of monoamine-metabolizing and polypeptide-containing cells derived from their capacity for Amine Precursor Uptake, and Decarboxylation. The APUD cells have been regarded as being derived from the neural crest during embryogenesis, but while this is certainly the origin of some of its members, it is difficult to prove with others, e.g. the parathyroid glands. The boundaries of the APUD system are vague, and term 'diffuse endocrine system' has replaced it. Likewise the term *apudoma* for a tumour of this system is now rarely used.

Langerhans. Immunohistochemical methods are now used to identify each cell type.

Other members of this ill-defined group of diffuse endocrine cells include the melanocytes, parathyroid C cells (secreting calcitonin) hypothalamic neuroendocrine cells, autonomic neurones and cells of the adenohypophysis and parathyroid glands.

Neoplasms of the diffuse endocrine system

Tumours of this system may be described as adenomata or carcinomata but many are of intermediate malignancy and have been called carcinoid tumours. This term is commonly used, but tumours so described vary greatly in behaviour. In the appendix they infiltrate but almost never metastasise. In the remainder of the intestine and lung their behaviour is more malignant. Some tumours derived from the diffuse endocrine system, e.g. the oat-cell carcinoma, are highly malignant. The present trend is to name the tumours according to their secretion or exact cell type of origin, e.g. G-cell tumour or gastrinoma.

GENERAL READING

Bloodworth J M B (ed.) 1982 Endocrine pathology: general and surgical, 2nd edn. Williams and Wilkins, Baltimore

De Lellis R A, et al 1984 Carcinoid tumors. Changing concepts and new perspectives. American Journal of Surgical Pathology 8:295

Ezrin C, et al (eds) 1980 Pituitary disease. CRC Press, Boco Raton

Freisen, S.R 1982 Tumors of the endocrine pancreas. New England Journal of Medicine 306:508,

Kovacs K, Howath E 1986 The pituitary gland: atlas of tumor pathology, Fascicle 21, Series 2. Armed Forces Institute of Pathology, Washington

Leading Article 1981 Thyroid autoimmune disease: a broad spectrum. Lancet 1:874

Moore-Ede M C, Czeisler C A, Richardson G S 1983 Circadian timekeeping in health and disease. New England Journal of Medicine 309:469

Orth D N 1984 The old and the new in Cushing's syndrome. New England Journal of Medicine 310: 649

Pearse A G E 1974 The APUD concept and its implications in pathology. Pathology Annual 9: 27

Phillips L S, Vassiloupou-Sellin R 1980 Somatomedins. New England Journal of Medicine 302: 371, 438

Reichlin, S 1983 Somatostatin. New England Journal of Medicine 309: 1495, 1556

Rosai J, Carcangiu M L 1984 Pathology of thyroid tumors: some recent and old questions. Human Pathology 15: 1008

Strakosk C R, et al 1982 Immunology of autoimmune thyroid diseases. New England Journal of Medicine 307: 1499

37. Diseases of the skin

The number of diseases of the skin which have been described in the literature far exceeds that of any other individual organ. There are many reasons for this: the skin is exposed to the external environment and is a complex, composite organ. It contains hair follicles with associated sebaceous glands, eccrine and apocrine sweat glands, a surface epithelium, and a connective tissue element with a loose papillary dermis between the epithelial elements and the reticular dermis, itself composed of dense collagenous bundles and coarse elastic fibres. The ease with which the skin can be examined and biopsied and the importance that mankind has given to its appearance have further added to the complexity of dermatology. This chapter describes some common skin reactions, particularly those that affect the face or the oral mucosa. Some diseases, e.g. pemphigus vulgaris and lichen planus, can affect the mouth either initially or to a major extent. Biopsy of these mucosal lesions is sometimes difficult, and histological interpretation can be unsatisfactory. The finding of more typical lesions on the skin is therefore rewarding, since skin biopsy is easy and pathological interpretation clear-cut.

TERMINOLOGY

An area of altered skin, usually red (erythematous), whether pigmented or non-pigmented is, if flat and not palpable, called a *macule* if less than 1.0 cm in diameter and a *patch* if larger. Similar areas which are palpable (usually they are raised and indurated, but in atrophic conditions may be depressed) are called *papules* if small and *plaques* if over 1.0 cm in diameter. A lesion containing a visible accumulation of clear fluid is a *vesicle* if small and a *bulla* if large (over 0.5 cm or 1.0 cm according to definition). *Pustules* contain pus. If flakes of keratin are seen obviously adherent to the lesion it is called *squamous*. Since most such lesions can be felt, they are therefore called *papulosquamous*. The presence of visible abnormally dilated vessels is called *telangiectasia*. Shallow ulcers or erosions are called *excoriations* if they are produced by scratching.

In attempting to arrive at a diagnosis of a skin disease, several aspects must be considered. The morphology of the primary lesions of the rash should be assessed because certain types are characteristic of certain diseases. For example vesiculation is characteristic of many forms of dermatitis but is never found in psoriasis or syphilis (in the adult). The next most important observation is the distribution of the rash. Thus, psoriasis characteristically affects the extensor surfaces, while seborrhoeic dermatitis affects the flexures. Both occur in the scalp. A dermatitis on one wrist suggests sensitivity to the wrist-band or watch-strap. If affecting both ear lobes, sensitivity to costume jewelry is a strong possibility. A localized rash suggests a localized cause. Pruritus denotes itching and its presence is characteristic of scabies, lichen simplex chronicus, certain drug eruptions and atopic dermatitis. It may occur in psoriasis but is rarely marked. In syphilis it is very uncommon.

DERMATITIS AND ECZEMA

Dermatitis and eczema are commonly used as synonymous terms to describe a particular skin reaction in which there is inflammation and obvious epidermal involvement. Three histological types are recognized: acute, subacute, and chronic.

Histopathological types of dermatitis

Acute dermatitis. The epidermis shows intercellular oedema (*spongiosis*) that terminates in the separation of epidermal cells with the formation of vesicles or bullae (Fig. 37.1). There is an acute inflammatory reaction in the dermis with oedema and, surprisingly enough, a lymphocytic infiltrate. The sparcity of polymorphs is noteworthy but the explanation is not understood. The spongiotic vesicles formed in the epidermis rupture, and clinically this produces a 'weeping' or crusted surface.

Subacute dermatitis. Spongiosis and vesicle formation are evident, but in addition the epidermis reacts by increasing mitotic activity so that it becomes thicker (*acanthosis*). Keratinization is disturbed, with the result that in places the keratin layer retains cellular nuclei. This condition is called *parakeratosis*. The term spongiotic dermatitis is used by some authorities to denote acute and subacute dermatitis.

Chronic dermatitis. Spongiosis is scanty, and vesicles are not formed. Chronic dermatitis is characterized by acanthosis, together with the formation of excessive keratin (*hyperkeratosis*) and, in places, parakeratosis (Fig. 37.2). Clinically, chronic dermatitis appears as indurated, scaly papules or plaques, and the skin markings tend to be accentuated. This latter feature is known as *lichenification* and is particularly marked in lesions that are rubbed frequently.

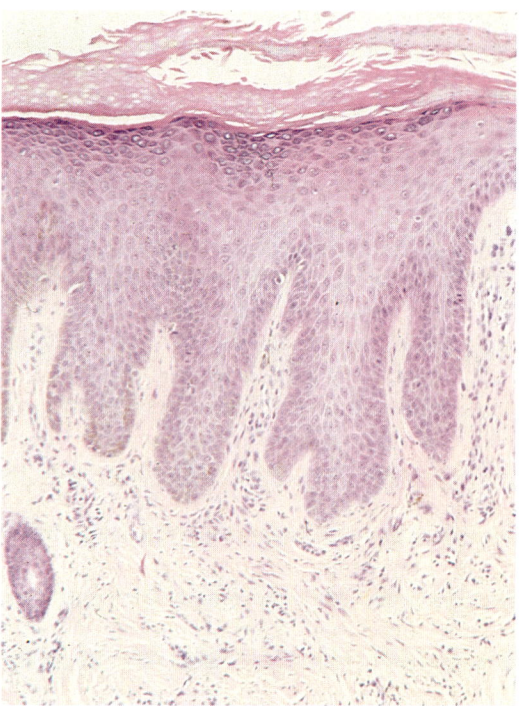

Fig. 37.2 Chronic dermatitis. The epidermis shows marked hyperkeratosis and acanthosis with irregular elongation of the rete ridges. There is a focus of parakeratosis, and the dermis shows a sparse infiltration by lymphocytes. The changes should be compared with normal skin present on the left-hand side of Fig. 37.1. × 120.

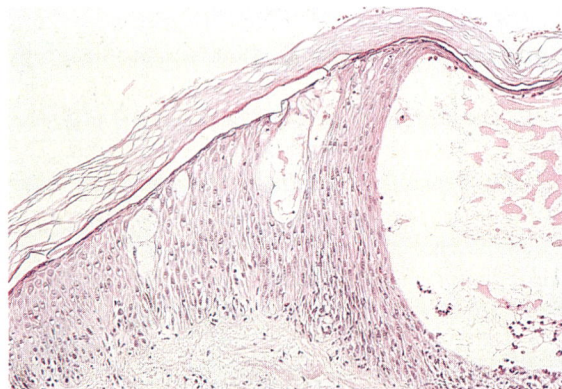

Fig. 37.1 Acute dermatitis. This is an example of acute allergic contact dermatitis due to poison ivy. The epidermis shows spongiosis, and in many places the cells have torn apart to produce intra-epidermal vesicles. The largest of these is on the right-hand side, and contains coagulated exudate and a number of inflammatory cells, mainly lymphocytes. The dermis shows a mild inflammatory reaction, again with a lymphocytic infiltrate. × 120

Clinical types of dermatitis

The clinical types of dermatitis are many and various. They cannot be distinguished from each other histologically but differ in their causes and clinical presentation.

Primary irritant dermatitis. Externally applied chemical irritants are a frequent cause of dermatitis (*contact dermatitis*): a common example is the chronic lichenified hand eczema seen in housewives whose hands are brought repeatedly into contact with water, detergents, and other household agents. Alkalis, acids, and many industrial chemicals can act as primary irritants, and if applied over a long period they lead to a refractory chronic dermatitis. Elderly individuals with dry skin may develop a dermatitis that is due to exposure to agents such as water, soap, and detergents that would be harmless in a younger person. Dentists and surgeons who have to wash their hands repeatedly with detergents and antiseptics are also liable to develop contact dermatitis of this type. Sensitization to components of talc and rubber gloves is another hazard of these professions.

Allergic contact dermatitis. The development of type-4 hypersensitivity toward chemicals results in the production of *allergic contact dermatitis*. Iodine, formaldehyde, dyes, plants (e.g. poison ivy), and nickel (used in costume jewellery) are among the many agents that can cause this type of allergic dermatitis (Fig. 37.3). It is noteworthy that certain parts of the skin are more sensitive to irritants than others. Thus, allergic contact dermatitis is more common on the backs of the hands than it is on the palms. Likewise, the face is particularly sensitive and may react to agents that elsewhere cause little trouble. Dermatitis around the eyes can be due to nail polish, which causes little trouble when applied to the hands or feet.

Photodermatitis. This diagnosis is suggested if the rash is confined to the sun-exposed skin. Ultraviolet light can act on chemicals (either applied topically or taken systematically) present in the sun-exposed skin and so alter them that direct irritant effects (*phototoxic dermatitis*) or new antigen formation and subsequent sensitization (*photoallergic dermatitis*) results. Agents that are well known to cause this sensitizing effect when applied topically

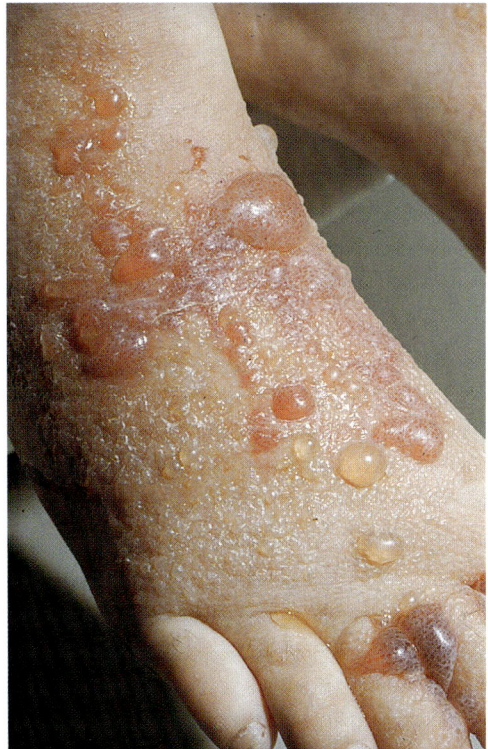

Fig. 37.3 Acute dermatitis. This acute vesiculo-bullous rash appeared a few days after contact with poison ivy.

are perfumes, coal-tar derivatives, and halogenated salicylanilides (used in deodorant soap).

Some drugs taken internally can have a similar effect. Common examples are chemotherapeutic agents such as sulphonamides and tetracyclines, diuretics (e.g. chlorothiazide), and tranquillizers (e.g. chlorpromazine), to name a few. It is of great importance to enquire of any patient with a skin disease if drugs have been applied locally or used systemically.

Infantile eczema and atopic dermatitis. These two conditions occur in atopic (allergic) individuals, but the pathogenesis is obscure, for although the associated respiratory diseases such as hay-fever and bronchial asthma appear to be mediated by IgE, the skin lesions are more complex and the damage is probably a type-4 response.

Nummular dermatitis. This descriptive term is applied to localized, well-demarcated plaques of subacute or chronic dermatitis. Itching is usually marked. The cause is unknown but the disease is more common in atopic individuals.

Seborrhoeic dermatitis. Seborrhoeic dermatitis or dandruff most often affects the scalp and results in the formation of greasy scales. Although it is extremely common, its precise nature is not understood. The dermatitis can extend beyond the scalp and affect the face (Fig. 37.4). Occasionally there is involvement of the trunk, particularly the front of the chest, and the flexural regions such as the axilla or under the breasts. This type of dermatitis can be encountered in all age groups, ranging from infants (cradle cap) to old people. Patients with AIDS are particularly susceptible.

Lichen simplex chronicus. Any itchy rash (e.g. atopic dermatitis) tends to cause scratching, which in turn accentuates the itch. A vicious circle is established, so that the lesions persist even after the initial cause has been removed. Localized plaques of chronic dermatitis are formed at any site that can be easily scratched, e.g. back of the neck and front of the ankles. If the lesions are widespread the term *neurodermatitis* is sometimes used.

PAPULOSQUAMOUS ERUPTIONS

The description of this wide group of dissimilar diseases, which includes secondary syphilis and ringworm, will be restricted to two common examples, both of unknown aetiology.

Psoriasis

This is a chronic disease that fluctuates in intensity both spontaneously and under the influence of treatment. It occurs as well-demarcated erythematous plaques with a dry, silvery scale. Common sites are the elbows, knees, and other extensor surfaces (Fig. 37.5). The palms, soles, and scalp are also frequently affected. Psoriasis is not usually itchy, and vesicles are never formed. This distinguishes it both clinically and histologically from dermatitis.

Histologically, it resembles chronic dermatitis, but acanthosis involves a regular elongation of the rete ridges, and the intervening papillary dermis is vascular and often oedematous (Fig. 37.6). Inflammatory cells including neutrophils are present in the papillae. The neutrophils migrate through the epidermis to form small collections called *Munro microabscesses*. The microscopic changes are very

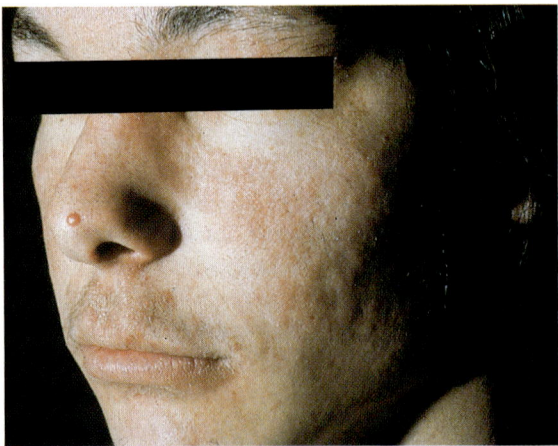

Fig. 37.4 Seborrhoeic dermatitis. There is an erythematous papulosquamous eruption involving the nose, cheeks, moustache area, and chin. The papule on the nose is likely to be either an angiofibroma or a melanocytic naevus.

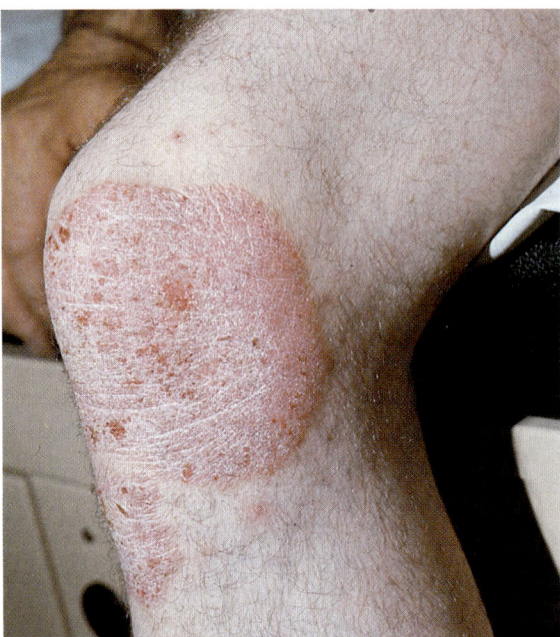

Fig. 37.5 Psoriasis. The psoriatic plaque on the extensor surface of the leg overlying the knee is sharply delineated, erythematous and covered by a silvery scale.

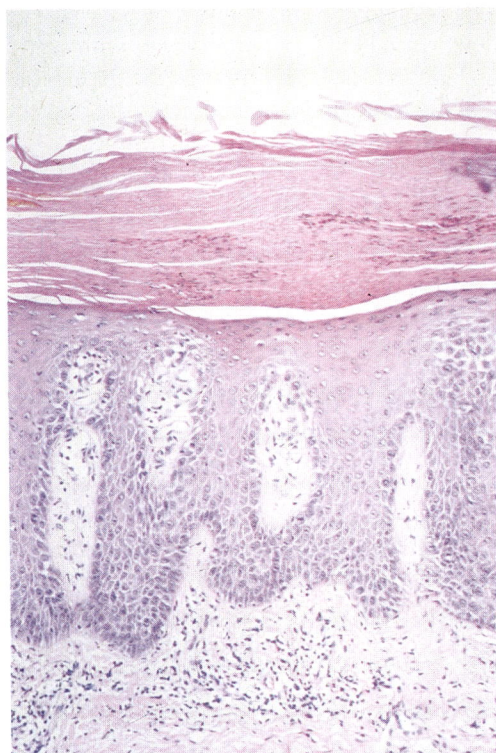

Fig. 37.6 Psoriasis of the skin. The epidermis shows marked hyperkerotosis, parakerotosis, and acanthosis. The elongation of the rete ridges is particularly well shown, and the broad club-shaped processes are seen to anastomose on the right side of the picture. The papillae between the rete ridges exhibit the highly characteristic vasodilatation and oedema.There is a sparse inflammatory infiltrate in this part of the dermis, and cells are seen to be migrating through the epidermis.

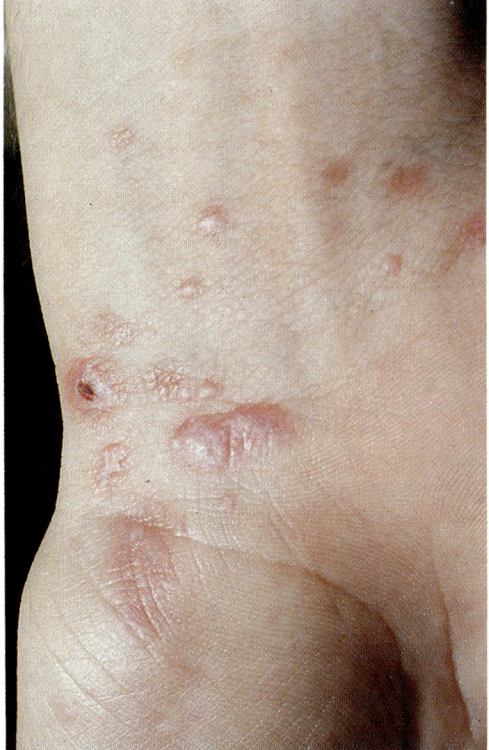

Fig. 37.7 Lichen planus on the anterior aspect of the wrist. The lesions are flat-topped papules and show the diagnostic white lines called Wickham's striae. In this case they are well shown around the periphery of the larger papules. The faint dark circle near the edge of the large central papule indicates the area which is biopsied. It showed the typical appearance of lichen planus, and the changes, particularly the prominent granular layer, were most pronounced in the region of the striae.

similar to those of superficial migratory glossitis (geographic tongue) but there appears to be no connection between the two diseases.

Lichen planus

Lichen planus occurs as pruritic, often violaceous, plat-topped papules (Fig. 37.7). Any site may be involved but common areas are around the wrists and ankles. The mucous membranes are affected, and in about 15% of cases these are the only areas involved. In the oral mucosa the lesions are white and form a lace-like network on the buccal mucosa (Fig. 37.8). Superficial erosions may occur. The glans penis is another common situation. Lichen planus of the oral mucosa is sometimes followed by malignancy, but less frequently so than in dysplastic leukoplakia.

Lichen planus of the skin has a very characteristic histological appearance (Fig. 37.9). There is acanthosis, hyperkeratosis and focal accentuation of the granular cell layer (hypergranulosis). Three features distinguish typical lesions from chronic dermatitis or psoriasis:

1. Parakeratosis is absent.
2. There is liquifactive (also called hydropic or vacuolar) degeneration of the basal cell layer of the epidermis. Degenerate cells form eosinophilic structures termed Civatte bodies.

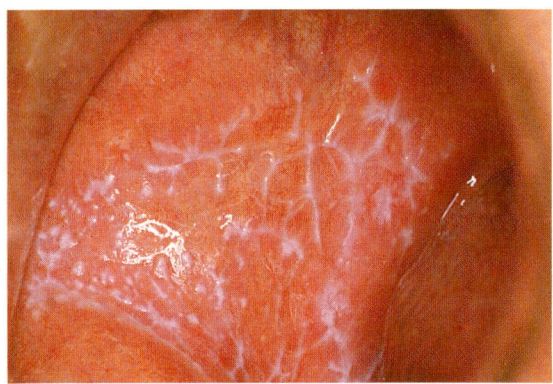

Fig. 37.8 Lichen planus. There are small white punctate lesions connected by white lace-like striae in the buccal mucosa. (Courtesy of Mr J Hamburger, University of Birmingham.)

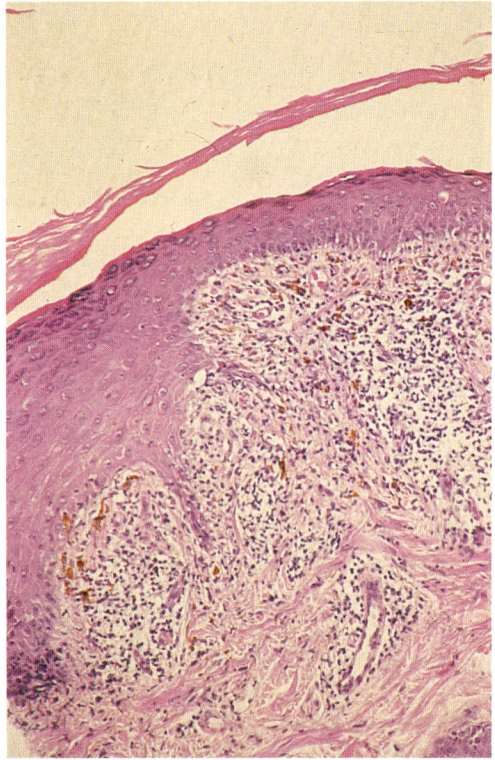

Fig. 37.9 Lichen planus of the skin. The epidermis shows marked hyperkeratosis, but there is a complete absence of parakeratotic nuclei. The granular layer is increased in prominence, and the epidermis shows acanthosis with elongation of some rete ridges. The basal layer of the epidermis has been replaced by flattened cells, and the epidermis has a saw-toothed appearance. The characteristic band of lymphocytic infiltrate in the papillary dermis is well shown. × 120.

3. The papillary dermis shows a dense well-demarcated band of lymphocytes with scattered melanophages. This obscures the dermoepidermal junction, and is so characteristic that such an infiltrate is described as 'lichenoid'.

The oral lesions are similar in appearance except that parakeratosis may be present.

Although plasma cells form a conspicuous feature of the inflammatory infiltrate in many oral lesions, they are inconspicuous in lichen planus.

DISEASES CHARACTERIZED BY A DERMAL INFLAMMATORY REACTION

An inflammatory reaction in the dermis is present in many skin diseases including those which appear primarily to affect the epidermis, e.g. dermatitis and psoriasis. A localized area of dermal inflammation is a feature of many infections, e.g. tuberculosis and erysipelas, but there is a group of conditions in which a widespread vascular reaction occurs. The most mild example in this group is urticaria.

Urticaria

In acute urticaria ('hives'), there is an acute inflammatory reaction in the dermis with vasodilatation, mild polymorph accumulation, and marked oedema. Clinically the area appears red, but central pallor appears as oedema produces a weal. The lesions resemble changes seen in a mosquito bite or the triple response of Lewis (p. 60). Acute uticaria may be a type I hypersensitivity reaction mediated by IgE, but is also seen in immune-complex disease. It follows the ingestion of a particular food or drug, and as with other hypersensitivity reactions, small quantities of the agent can be sufficient to induce an attack. Thus, the menthol in a cigarette or toothpaste can precipitate acute urticaria in a sensitized person. Repeated attacks of urticaria may occur over many years (chronic urticaria), and in these patients the cause is rarely found.

Urticaria affects the dermis. When the subcutaneous tissues are also involved, the condition is termed *angio-oedema*. In both urticaria and angio-oedema the mucous membranes, including that of the tongue, can be involved. In one type of hereditary angio-oedema, there is a deficiency of C1-esterase inhibitor. This is a serious condition, for lesions occur in the intestine causing colic, and in the larynx causing death from asphyxiation.

Toxic erythema

This general term is applied to many conditions in which the epidermis is normal, at least in the early stages, but in which there is a dermal inflammatory reaction showing vasodilatation and a perivascular collection of cells, chiefly lymphocytes. As an acute condition toxic erythema accompanies many viral infections (e.g. measles, German measles, and infectious mononucleosis) and is a common component of a drug eruption (Fig. 37.10). Itching is generally marked. Damage to blood vessels by immune complexes is the probable pathogenesis.

VESICULO-BULLOUS DISEASES

The formation of vesicles or bullae is the outstanding feature of this group of diseases, and for

accurate diagnosis a biopsy of an *early* lesion is often necessary, because the situation of the vesicle is of vital importance in differential diagnosis. Some vesicles are intra-epidermal, while others are subepidermal. It should be noted that a late subepidermal vesicle becomes intra-epidermal as tongues of regenerative epidermis cover the base. This is one of the reasons for biopsying an early lesion.

Subepidermal vesicles

Erythema multiforme. This is an acute generalized disease of unknown cause that in about 50% of cases is precipitated by some event such as the intake of a drug or an infection, commonly herpes simplex. The disease tends to recur, particularly if the precipitating cause such as a cold sore recurs. The onset of the disease is sudden and the patient rapidly develops symmetrical lesions of varying types—urticarial, erythematous macules and papules, and sometimes vesicles. Target shaped or iris lesions are characteristic (Fig. 37.11). Microscopically there is a dermal lymphocytic inflammatory reaction with marked papillary oedema which, if severe, culminates in the formation of a subepidermal vesicle. The dermal reaction causes secondary degenerative changes in the epidermis. The severity of the

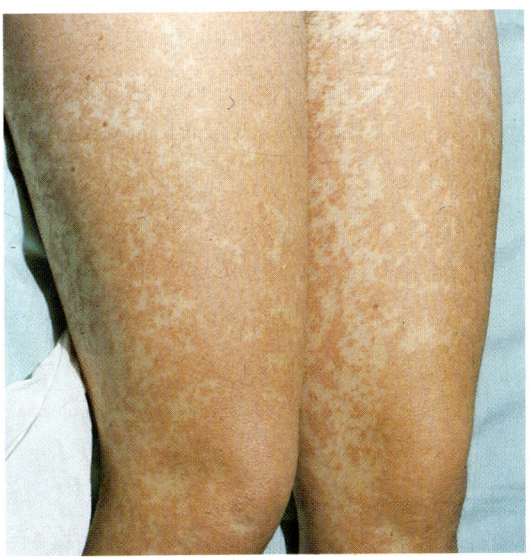

Fig. 37.10 Drug eruption. There is a widespread erythematous maculopapular eruption that in many areas has become confluent. Itching was severe. The rash appeared about 1 week after commencing penicillin treatment.

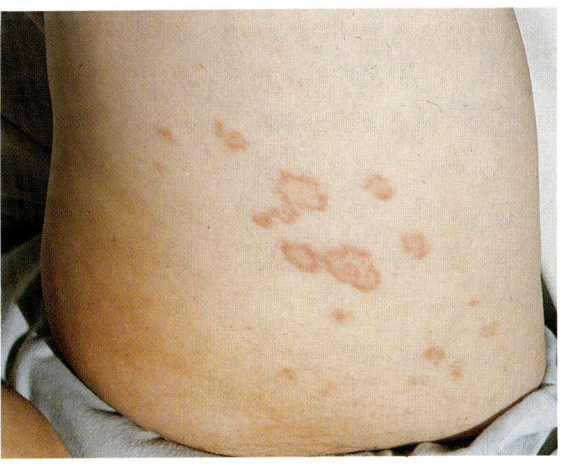

Fig. 37.11 Erythema multiforme. One of the lesions show the characteristic target-like configuration.

dermal inflammatory reaction, the absence of eosinophils and the degenerate appearance of the epidermal roof of the vesicle serve to distinguish lesions of erythema multiforme from those of bullous pemphigoid. The severity of erythema multiforme varies from case to case. With very severe disease the epidermis can undergo extensive necrosis and a condition resembling a severe, widespread burn can result (toxic epidermal necrolysis); involvement of the mucous membranes (Fig. 37.12), oral and genital, leads to the *Stevens–Johnson* syndrome, which can be fatal.

Bullous pemphigoid. A dermal inflammatory reaction is followed by the formation of a subepidermal vesicle. The disease is not uncommon, and is characterized by the occurrence of crops of tense vesicles and bullae (Fig. 37.13) appearing on the trunk and sometimes on the mucous membranes. The disease is chronic and tends to occur in elderly people. A disease with similar histology, *benign cicatrizing mucosal pemphigoid*, affects the oral mucosa and the conjunctiva (Fig. 37.14). Numerous eosinophils are a feature of the dermal inflammatory infiltrate.

Porphyria cutanea tarda. In the porphyrias there is an upset in porphyrin metabolism such that an excess of certain porphyrins is formed; some of these are photosensitizers. Porphyria cutanea tarda is the commonest example of this group of disease.

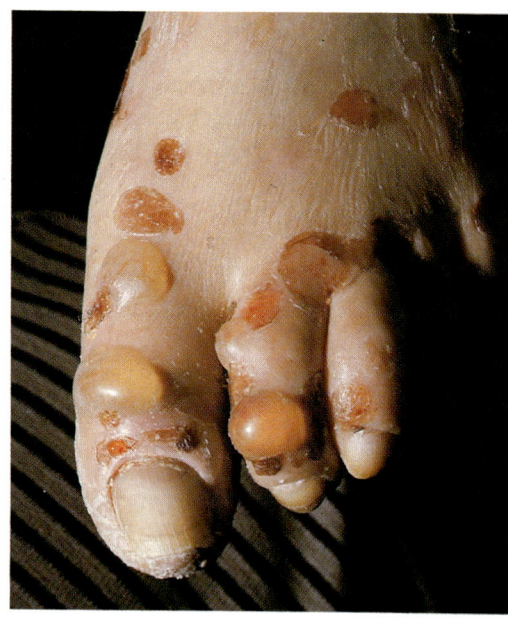

Fig. 37.13 Bullous pemphigoid. Numerous tense vesicles and bullae are present. Some of the lesions have ruptured.

It is associated with alcoholic liver disease and leads to fragility of the skin and great sensitivity to light. Exposure to light results in bulla formation, best seen on the backs of the hands.

Epidermolysis bullosa. This is a complex group of at least six diseases in which the skin is abnormally fragile so that minor trauma can cause the formation of bullae (Fig. 37.15). The

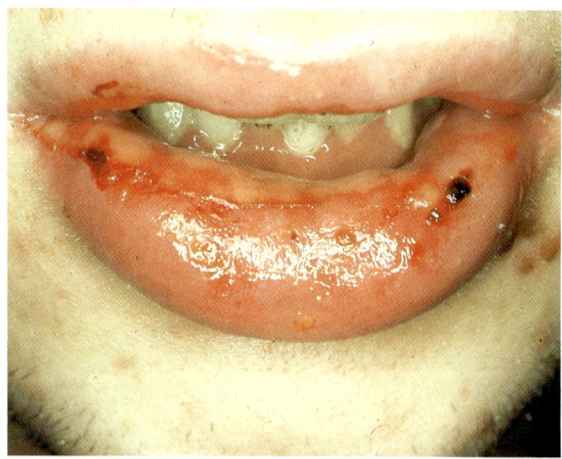

Fig. 37.12 Erythema multiforme. Shallow erosions in the lower lip with haemorrhagic areas and small areas of crusting. (Courtesy of Professor J W Frame, University of Birmingham.)

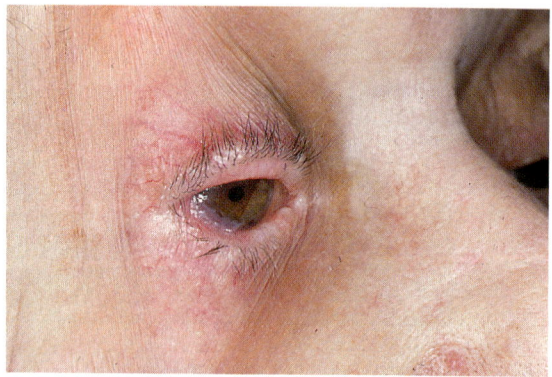

Fig. 37.14 Benign mucosal pemphigoid. The eyelids are firmly bound to the globe of the eye as a result of previous vesicular lesions involving adjacent surfaces.

epidermis becomes detached from the dermis such that on routine microscopy a subepidermal vesicle is formed; subsequently there is an erosion. Electron microscopy is required to delineate the exact site of separation—whether in the basal layer of the epidermis itself, the basement membrane zone or in the upper dermis. The oral mucosa may also be involved.

Intra-epidermal vesicles

The superficial subcorneal vesicles and pustules of candidiasis and impetigo can generally be diagnosed clinically without the aid of biopsy. So also can the spongiotic vesicles of acute and subacute dermatitis. The fluid in these vesicles contains inflammatory exudate. This contrasts with an important group of blistering diseases in which the vesicles are formed as a result of a loss of adherence between adjacent epidermal cells. The detached epidermal cells become rounded off and lie free in the fluid. This process is called *acantholysis*, and is a dominant feature of two groups of diseases.

The pemphigus group. In pemphigus vulgaris the acantholytic process commences immediately above the basal layer of the epidermis, so that a suprabasal acantholytic cleft is formed

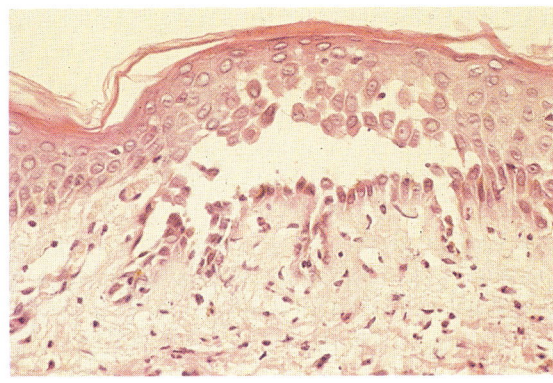

Fig. 37.16 Pemphigus vulgaris. Suprabasal acantholysis has lead to the formation of an intraepidermal cleft or vesicle in which free acantholytic cells are present. The cells in the roof of the vesicle are well preserved.

(Fig. 37.16). The papillae of the dermis are covered by a layer of relatively unaffected basal cells that have been likened to a row of tomb-stones. Clinically, the patient develops *flaccid* vesicles and bullae which rupture leaving extensive raw areas. The distinction from bullous pemphigoid is important, because pemphigus vulgaris is often fatal and can be kept under control only by heavy immunosuppression. Bullous pemphigoid is chronic and tiresome but rarely fatal. Pemphigus vulgaris often affects the oral mucosa; in about 50% of cases this is the predominant and presenting symptom (Fig. 37.17).

The vesicular viral group. In zoster, varicella, smallpox, vaccina, and herpes simplex,

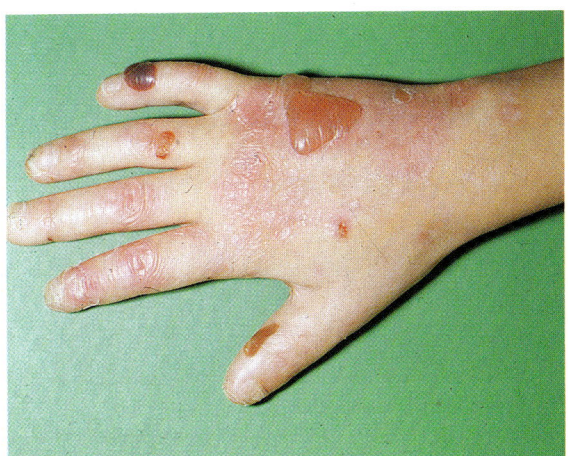

Fig. 37.15 Epidermolysis bullosa dystrophica. There are bullous lesions and extensive scarring on the hand of this young boy. (Previously published in Rock W P, Grundy M C, Shaw L Diagnostic picture tests in paediatric dentistry Wolfe Medical Publications, London.)

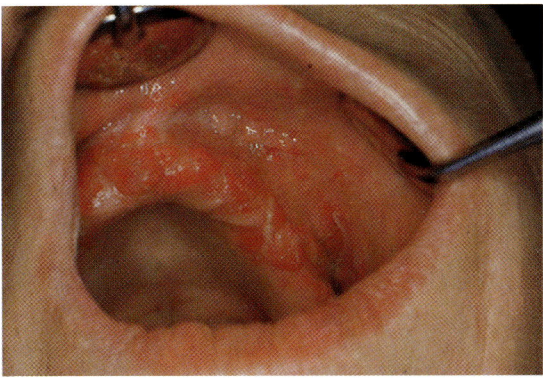

Fig. 37.17 Pemphigus vulgaris. There are extensive shallow erosions affecting the labial aspect of the upper edentulous alveolus.

acantholytic intra-epidermal vesicles are formed. Fusion of epidermal cells may produce multi-nucleate giant cells; some of these are acantholytic and floating free within the vesicle. There is a marked dermal inflammatory reaction present in most examples. The distinction between the individual members of this group is difficult to make histologically, but electron microscopy of the vesicle fluid and other virological techniques can be used to identify the cause.

Immunopathology of the vesiculo-bullous diseases

Patients with pemphigus vulgaris commonly have an IgG auto-antibody in their plasma, and its titre reflects the activity of their disease. The antibody is directed against intercellular substance of squamous epithelium. Hence a patient's skin or mouth biopsy treated with fluorescein-labelled anti-human IgG shows brilliant fluorescence around each epidermal cell when examined under ultraviolet light (Fig. 37.18). This is a *direct test*. The plasma antibody is detected *indirectly* by incubating normal human skin (or monkey oesophagus) with patient's serum; the skin is then washed, and labelled anti-IgG serum is applied.

In bullous pemphigoid an antibody directed against skin basement membrane is often found. The direct test shows a linear band of fluorescence in the basement membrane zone (Fig. 37.19). The indirect test shows antibody to be present in the serum of about 70% of patients. In the cicatricial form of the disease serum antibodies are found less frequently.

ACNE

Inflammatory disease of the pilosebaceous unit is termed acne. In the common type (*acne vulgaris*) commonly affects teenagers. The primary lesion is keratin plugging of the pilosebaceous follicles to form the familiar comedo or blackhead. Proliferating *Propionibacterium acnes*, a common

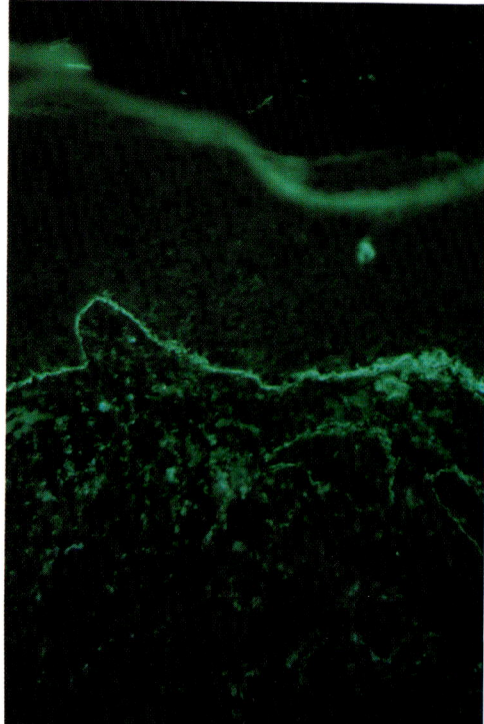

Fig. 37.19 Deposition of IgG antibody in the basement membrane of skin in bullous pemphigoid. A frozen section of skin taken adjacent to a recent vesicle was stained with fluorescein-labelled anti-IgG and examined microscopically under ultraviolet light. The linear staining of the basement membrane is characteristic of this disease. The ill-defined fluorescence on the surface of the skin is non-specific staining of the stratum corneum.

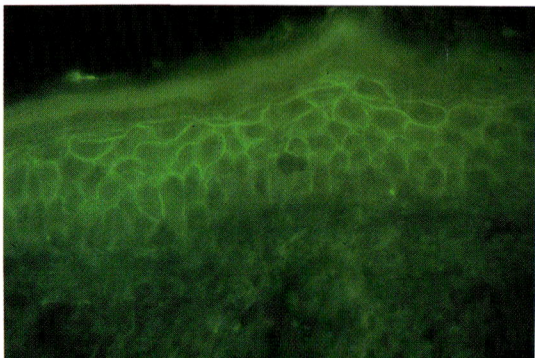

Fig. 37.18 The immunofluorescence pattern of pemphigus vulgaris. A frozen section of a skin biopsy taken from a patient with active pemphigus vulgaris was stained with fluorescein-labelled anti-IgG and examined under ultraviolet light. The staining of the intercellular material of the epidermis is well shown. (Photography by courtesy of Dr Susan Ritchie, University of Toronto.)

commensal of the skin, splits the lipids of retained sebum to form irritating fatty acids that cause a chemical inflammation. Pustules and abscesses (often termed acne cysts) result. Rosacea (acne rosacea) has many features in common with acne vulgaris but tends to affect an older group—generally over 30 years of age. In addition to papules, pustules and cysts, there are two other features—persistent erythema with telangiectasia, and sebaceous gland hyperplasia. The disease affects the central area of the face and can therefore resemble lupus erythematosus.

HAMARTOMATA OF SKIN

Hamartomata of the skin or birthmarks are termed naevi. Vascular naevi ('haemangiomata') are described in Chapter 20. Epithelial naevi and the most common type of naevus—the melanocytic naevus—are described below.

Melanocytic naevi

The common mole, also called a pigmented or naevocellular naevus, arises from melanocytes, cells which are believed to originate from the neural crest and migrate with the peripheral nerves to the skin where they become incorporated in the basal layer of the epidermis. During childhood abnormal focal proliferation of these cells forms a naevus which may be regarded as a type of hamartoma. The naevus is at first junctional with the naevus cells lying at the dermoepidermal junction. This is a junctional naevus (Fig. 37.20(b)). The naevus cells are shed into the dermis during childhood to form a compound naevus (Fig. 37.20(c)), and by about the age of 30 years, most naevi have lost their junctional component to become intradermal naevi (Fig. 37.20(d)). As the naevus cells mature in the dermis they tend to loose the ability to make melanin. Hence while junctional and compound naevi are pigmented, intradermal naevi appear as flesh coloured papules.

Certain types of naevi deserve special attention:

Spindle cell-naevus of Spitz. This is a type of naevus, usually compound, which occurs in young people, and because of its rapid growth imitates a malignant melanoma. Histologically the predominant cell type is spindle-shaped or epithelioid, and the presence of mitoses can easily lead to a diagnosis of malignant melanoma. The lesion is usually not pigmented, but is vascular. The spindle-cell naevus is entirely benign, and its old name 'juvenile melanoma' is misleading.

Dysplastic naevus. The dysplastic naevus was first described in subjects with a personal or family history of melanoma. This constitutes the dyplastic naevus syndrome and the naevi are generally multiple, on the trunk, and over 0.6 mm in diameter. They have an irregular flat border and microscopically show a wide junctional element with some degree of atypia of the cells. It has become apparent that 'dysplastic naevi' may occur as isolated lesions and are very common, affecting perhaps 5% of the population. It is not known whether these naevi in the absence of a family history predispose to melanoma. They probably do not, in which event the term 'dysplastic' is unfortunate. The term Clark's naevus has been suggested in recognition of the work done on this subject by the Philadelphia dermatopathologist of that name.

Blue naevus

This type of naevus shows focal accumulation of dendritic melanocytes in the dermis, and has a different mode of formation to that of the common naevocellular naevus. The blue naevus is generally present at birth, and appears blue because the pigment is situated entirely in the dermis. A localized nodular form of the lesion is called a *common blue naevus*. Sometimes the naevus is diffuse and produces a wide area of hyperpigmentation that somewhat resembles a tattoo. When the eye and surrounding skin are involved, this is called the *naevus of Ota*. It is quite common to find a similar type of lesion at birth over the sacral region in the Oriental races. This *Mongolian spot* differs from the blue naevus described above in that it invariably fades as the baby grows up.

TUMOURS OF THE SKIN

Squamous-cell papilloma

This is generally used as a descriptive term which covers a number of separate entities. One variety

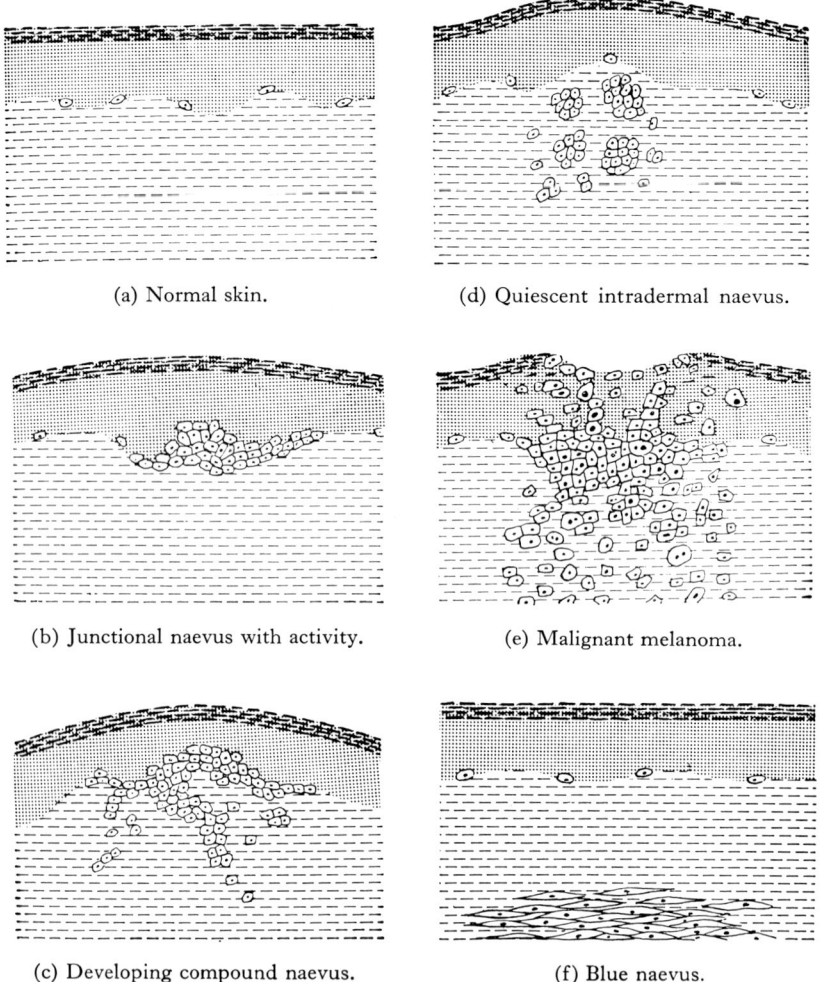

(a) Normal skin.

(d) Quiescent intradermal naevus.

(b) Junctional naevus with activity.

(e) Malignant melanoma.

(c) Developing compound naevus.

(f) Blue naevus.

Fig. 37.20 Sketches to show the various types of melanotic naevi: the only cells drawn are melanocytes and naevus cells. In the normal skin melanocytes are present only in the basal layer of the epidermis. A focal proliferation of these cells produces a junctional naevus (b) which may be regarded as a stage in the development of a compound and intradermal naevus. (c) the formation of a compound naevus by the invasion of the dermis by melanocytes. When the junctional activity regresses, the naevus cells remain in the dermis as an intradermal naevus (d). (e) A malignant melanoma which shows invasion of the epidermis as well as the dermis and deeper structures. Atypicality of the cells and the epidermal invasion help to distinguish it from the compound naevus, which an early malignant melanoma may resemble. (f) The strap-like naevus cells situated deep in the dermis impart the colour to the blue naevus.

is present at birth and is a type of hamartoma termed an *epithelial naevus*. Frequently the lesions are linear. The common wart (*verruca vulgaris*) is a type of papilloma due to an infection by one of the papovaviruses. In elderly people it is very common to find multiple *seborrhoeic keratoses* on

the backs of the hands, trunk, and face. They are papillomata often with considerable acanthosis and melanin pigmentation. Clinically they appear to be 'stuck on' the surface of the skin either as elevated warty papillomata or as flat, roughened, pigmented plaques (Fig.

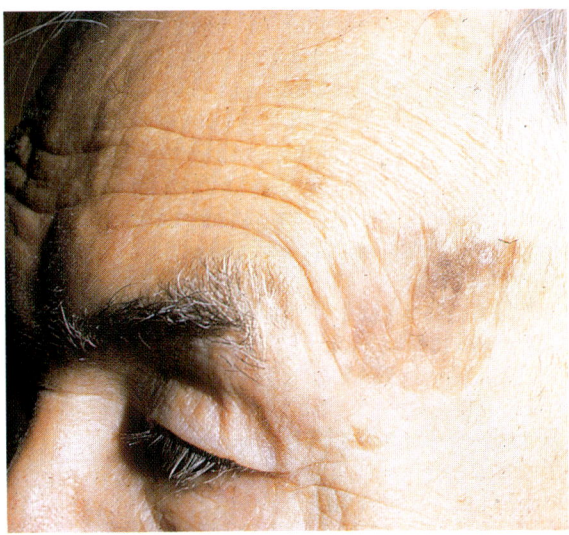

Fig. 37.21 Seborrhoeic keratosis. The lesion has a rough surface and its pigmentation can lead to misdiagnosis.

37.21). Curettage effects an easy cure. They are not premalignant, but when heavily pigmented are liable to be confused with other pigmented lesions— melanocytic naevi, pigmented basal-cell carcinoma, Hutchinson's freckle, or malignant melanoma.

Other benign tumours are not uncommon: dermatofibroma, lipoma, neurofibroma, etc. These will not be further considered.

MALIGNANT TUMOURS

The most common malignant tumour of the skin in white races is the basal-cell carcinoma. See Fig. 37.22.

Basal-cell carcinoma

The common type of basal-cell carcinoma is found on the skin of the face of fair-skinned people exposed to the sun. It appears as an indurated nodule or ulcer with a firm rolled pearly border (Fig. 37.22). Microscopically the dermis is invaded by small basophilic round or fusiform cells with prominent darkly staining nuclei. The layer of cells at the edge of each clump is usually arranged in the form of a palisade, and resembles the germinative layer of the epidermis from which it arises (Fig. 37.23).

Basal-cell carcinoma shows progressive local invasion and destruction of tissue. Growth is usually very slow, and it is common to find small tumours in patients who have had the lesion for years. On rare occasions the tumour exhibits a relentless course of invasion so that the nose, orbit or meninges are involved. Very rarely indeed are there metastases.

Squamous-cell carcinoma

This tumour commonly arises on the sun-exposed skin in a pre-existing *actinic keratosis*. Actinic keratoses are areas of epidermal dysplasia caused by prolonged, repeated exposure to sunlight. They appear as scaly erythematous areas on the face or hands, and in contradistinction to seborrhoeic keratoses, they must be regarded as precancerous. Squamous-cell

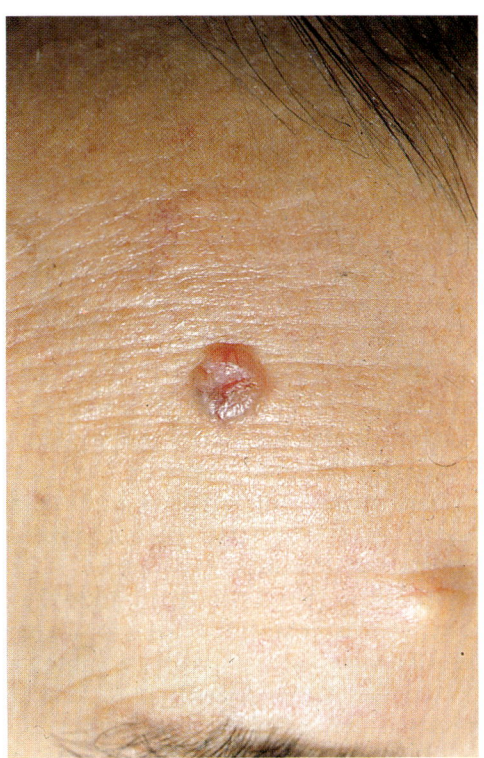

Fig. 37.22 Basal cell carcinoma on the forehead of a 56-year-old man. The picture shows the typical appearance with a depressed centre and raised and rolled edge. The dome-shaped swelling on the right of the picture is an epidermoid cyst or sebaceous cyst.

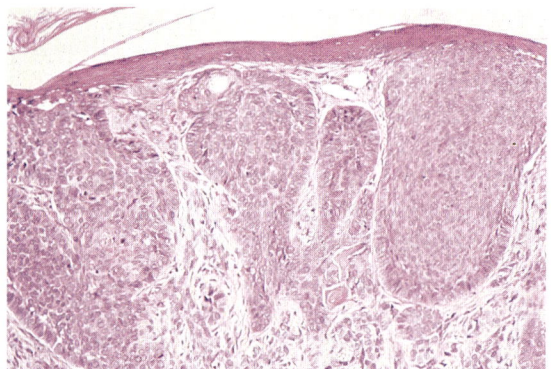

Fig. 37.23 Basal-cell carcinoma. Groups of cells with basophilic cytoplasm are seen to be arising from the undersurface of the epidermis. The outer layer of the tumour masses tends to show palisading.

carcinoma arising in an actinic keratosis is invasive, but metastasis is late and the prognosis is good. Squamous-cell carcinoma may also arise in normal skin or in a chronic erythematous lesion called *Bowen's disease*. This is a type of *carcinoma-in-situ*, and can occur on any part of the body. This type of squamous-cell carcinoma is more malignant than that arising in an actinic keratosis. Squamous-cell carcinoma must be differentiated both clinically and pathologically from a keratoacanthoma, which it closely resembles and which also occurs on a sun-exposed area (see p. 235).

Malignant melanoma

The incidence of malignant melanoma in the population is increasing rapidly and this has been attributed to increased exposure to sunlight. Occasional severe burns are thought to be more damaging than continued chronic exposure. Melanoma may arise in several ways:

In normal skin. Some tumours invade the dermis early so that their vertical growth produces a nodule. This *nodular type* has a poor prognosis. Other tumours spread laterally both in the epidermis itself and in the papillary dermis. Radial growth exceeds vertical growth. This *superficial spreading type of melanoma* has a much better prognosis.

In a pre-existing melanocytic naevus. The incidence of malignancy in naevi is unknown, but

considering the number of naevi in the average person, it must be very uncommon. The chances of developing a melanoma appears to be related to the number of naevi that a person has. Another risk factor is a family history of melanoma. Possibly about one-third of melanomata arise in naevi. Danger signals suggesting malignancy are a recent increase in size, a change in colour, an irregular shape, ulceration and bleeding. The possible relationship to dysplastic naevi has been described in the section of naevi.

As in-situ melanoma. The best known example of in-situ melanoma is *lentigo maligna* or *Hutchinson's freckle.* This is apparent as a pigmented patch or plaque on the sun-exposed part of the face. It slowly increases in size, has irregular pigmentation and an irregular border. Microscopically there is proliferation of atypical melanocytes in the basal layer of the epidermis. At some stage, often after many years, the melanocytic cells invade the dermis and invasive malignant melanoma develops. *Acral lentiginous melanoma in situ* occurs on the palms, soles or around the nails. Rapid evolution to an aggressive melanoma is common.

Microscopically malignant melanoma shows proliferation of atypical melanocytes at the dermoepidermal junction (Fig 23.24). Irregularity in size, shape and staining of the cells helps to distinguish them from benign naevus cells. The melanoma cells invade the epidermis itself either

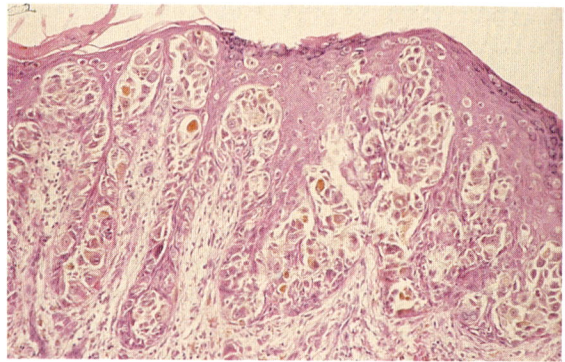

Fig. 37.24 Malignant melanoma of skin. The tumour consists of plump atypical melanocytes, some of which have invaded the acanthotic epidermis to produce a pagetoid appearance. Dermal invasion is also present, but only one small group of cells is seen in this photograph.

as small groups of cells or as individual cells; the appearance is well termed pagetoid, because the picture resembles Paget's disease itself. With vertical growth, tumour cells invade the dermis.

The prognosis of melanoma is related to many factors, including the site of occurrence and the histological type. In the skin, the thickness of the tumour as measured with a micrometer on the histological slide is important. Metastases occur to the regional lymph nodes and later involve many organs by blood spread.

Other malignant skin tumours

Many other types of malignant skin tumours are known but they are uncommon. *Mycosis fungoides* is a malignant T-cell lymphoma that affects the skin primarily, although terminally can involve lymph nodes and other organs. By infiltrating the skin it can produce disfiguring plaques and tumours.

Kaposi's sarcoma

This tumour has recently become more common because of its association with AIDS. It is a tumour of endothelial cells and appears to arise multicentrically. It occurs in two forms. In Europe, particularly around the Mediterranean coast, it is an indolent disease first appearing as a purple discolouration of the skin of one ankle and slowly spreading to the other leg and later the arms. The formation of tumour nodules and further spread to other organs occurs after many years. In Black Africans a different type of tumour is encountered. It appears as erythematous or purple nodules on the skin. As further nodules erupt on the skin, spread to internal organs is rapid. It is this type of the disease that afflicts patients with AIDS.

The management of skin tumours is beyond the scope of the book, but it should be emphasized that before radical treatment is undertaken a positive biopsy must be obtained. The hypothetical possibility of disseminating tumour by biopsy, even in the case of malignant melanoma, is more than offset by the tragedy of treating a benign lesion by radical means. The study of skin tumours has highlighted several curious pseudomalignant lesions. Thus, keratoacanthoma closely mimics carcinoma and nodular fasciitis resembles sarcoma. Before diagnosing malignant lymphoma of the skin it is necessary to exclude certain pseudolymphomatous lesions which may arise spontaneously (pseudolymphoma of Spiegler-Fendt) or as a result of trauma such as an arthropod bite.

GENERAL READING

Greene M H, et al 1985 Acquired precursors of cutaneous melanoma. The familial dysplastic nevus syndrome. New England Journal of Medicine 312: 91
Maize J, Ackerman A B 1987 Pigmented lesions of the skin: clinicopathologic correlations. Lea & Febiger, Philadelphia
Lever W F, Schaumburg-Lever G 1990 Histopathology of the skin, 7th edn. Lippincott, Philadelphia

Index